Production Dynamics for Life Quality
in the Incipient 21st Century

Chau-kiu Cheung

Production Dynamics for Life Quality in the Incipient 21st Century

Springer

Chau-kiu Cheung
Department of Social and Behavioural
Sciences
City University of Hong Kong
Hong Kong, China

ISBN 978-981-19-3826-9 ISBN 978-981-19-3827-6 (eBook)
https://doi.org/10.1007/978-981-19-3827-6

This Springer imprint is published by the registered company Springer Nature Singapore Pte Ltd.
The registered company address is: 152 Beach Road, #21-01/04 Gateway East, Singapore 189721, Singapore

Contents

Chapter 1
Introduction

Statics and dynamics for producing life quality in the general person in the world during 2004–2012 connect to the tracking and predicting life quality. In this work, quality refers to a person's life quality in living and comprises the maintenance of health, satisfaction, avoidance of worry, and delight, including happiness, autonomy, and financial adequacy. This quality depends on production, which uses resources acquired or experienced (Lindenberg 2001; van Bruggen 2000). Specifically, life quality is a current or recent feeling or state resulting from experiences, practices, and personal and environmental background characteristics that existed or formed in the past. The processes thus proceed successively from background characteristics to experiences and practices and finally to life quality. These production processes unfold the statics or structural mechanisms of influence, which are changeable over time to reflect influence dynamics. Statics represent general influences regardless of time, whereas dynamics reveal changes in the influences across time.

To show the statics and dynamics of life quality production, this study employed Waves 5 and 6 of the World Values Survey conducted from 2005 to 2012. In addition, the study incorporated national data from the World Bank and the Quality of Government Basic Dataset (Dahlberg et al. 2018) and the Standardized World Income Inequality Database (Solt 2016) to reveal life quality production at the personal level. The national data of 2004 and 2009 preceded Wave 5 and Wave 6 personal data, respectively. To represent any person in the world generally, the study applied weighting to the data to make them representative of the world population. The statics of the production concern successive effects from personal and national background characteristics to personal life experiences, personal life practices, and personal life quality appraisals. Personal background characteristics include age, gender, marriage, education, and social class. National indicators include population size, economic development per capita, technology export per capita, income inequality, globalization, democracy, liberty, human development, and carbon dioxide (CO_2) emission. Personal life experiences include economic hardship, victimization, security, and neighborhood nuisance. Personal practices comprise private and public ones. Private practices include e-activity, learning, risk aversion, spiritual activity, and

C. Cheung, *Production Dynamics for Life Quality in the Incipient 21st Century*,
https://doi.org/10.1007/978-981-19-3827-6_1

weapon carrying. Public practices include appealing, civic organizational participation, strike participation, political voting, and green activism. Life quality appraisals include health, life satisfaction, happiness, autonomy, and worry. Meanwhile, the dynamics of the production concern the main and interaction effects of time (Wave 6 vs. Wave 5) on personal life experiences, practices, and quality appraisals. The interaction effects mean the time effects on the influences of personal and national characteristics and personal experiences and practices. Essentially, the dynamics concern the strengthening or weakening of the statics.

Concern about the dynamics of production processes leading to life quality stems from a broader concern about the dynamics of social and environmental changes, such as modernization, postmodernization, individualization, globalization, and denaturalization or humanization. The most notable among these concerns is the conservation or volatility of the static, structural mechanism over time (Fein 2015). The conservative view emphasizes the stasis of the mechanism because of the crystallization of norms, stratification, decentralization, and other structures in society. Notably, decentralization or differentiation suggests the erosion of a central institution to enforce concerted and pervasive changes. By contrast, the liberal and populist views expect changes or even revolutions in the structural mechanism over time (Fein 2015). These views posit the importance of individuals in shaping changes collectively according to a centralized or bureaucratic institution to counter the stasis imposed by established norms or structures. That is, people are capable of mustering collective power to overthrow structures through democratic or populist means. This notion is compatible with a broader, generalist view that people and their creations and structures are flexible (Fein 2015). These differing views expose the need to clarify dynamics in the production of life quality during the inception of the twenty-first century.

The twenty-first century is clearly of imminent concern for research and clarification. The inception of the century has been noteworthy for spawning many changes in life, technology, work, politics, and the world (Hicks et al. 2008; Jang 2016; Lou et al. 2011). For instance, it has generated new skills in information communication technology, interpersonal relationships, and applications in science, technology, engineering, and mathematics (Jang 2016; Mainemelis et al. 2002; Markauskaite 2007). As such, the skills trigger changes in communication, information processing, socializing, cooperation, management, and problem-solving. These changes are germane to education and other ways to prepare for future life (Lou et al. 2011). Such education notably emphasizes innovation to cater to changes toward decentralization, transparency, interoperability or orchestration with multiple devices, and so on (Flogie et al. 2018). Innovation has also been prominent in robotics, satellite applications, networking, leisure activity, and income generation (Lou et al. 2011; Nugent et al. 2010; Suzuki and Best 2003). The spate of innovation necessarily demands attention and research to harness it to benefit life quality.

This innovation exemplifies social and environmental changes that are the focus of dynamics. These changes include modernization, postmodernization, individualization, globalization, and denaturalization or humanization to leave the required human footprint in the natural environment. Modernization has its primal characteristic in industrialization and Westernization, which means a change to resemble Western, industrialized, or advanced society (Harper and Leicht 2011). The other basic characteristics of modernization include diversifying occupation and social life to increase social complexity and heightening productivity by using inanimate energy to raise income. As a further advanced, and probably revolutionary form of modernization, postmodernization features the multiplication of ideas, voices, and forms in society (Adams 2007). Nevertheless, the "post" condition in postmodernization raises questions about the significance of modernization elements, such as industrialization. Meanwhile, individualization and globalization connect to both modernization and postmodernization. On the one hand, individualization principally means progress toward disintegration from or downplaying of classes, roles, and other conventional statuses that group people (Beck and Beck-Gernsheim 2002). On the other hand, globalization means the increasing flow of people, materials, and information worldwide (Harper and Leicht 2011). Accordingly, globalization implies denationalization to reduce the legitimacy of the national state. Moreover, denaturalization or humanization registers the environmental change due to the increasing presence of people and their deeds. This change can be detrimental to the environment and/or people, such as increasing environmental degradation, destruction, and deforestation (Black et al. 2011; Hengeveld 2012; Jorgenson et al. 2009). Nevertheless, the change can happen by improving the environment or at least making it more suitable for people. Given these changes, the critical question concerns their impacts on life quality and its formation. The latter is especially crucial because of its uncertainty. This uncertainty is the topic of dynamics that this research needs to address.

Research on the statics and dynamics of life quality builds on the grand theoretical framework of analytical functionalism (Lackey 1987; Munch 1987, 1988; Parsons 1968; Savage 1981; Schwinn 1998; Turner 2013). Within this framework, the orienting idea is the need to elaborate the functions required to sustain the whole system. These functions are analytically the products of just two dimensions: internal versus external and instrumental versus consummatory functioning. Internal functioning deals with concerns inside, whereas external functioning deals with interaction with the outside. Meanwhile, instrumental functioning is about the means to achieve goals, whereas consummatory functioning is about the satisfaction of goals. Four functions evolve from the combination of the two dimensions: goal attainment of the fulfilling function of external and consummatory functioning, adaptation function of external and instrumental functioning, integration function of internal and consummatory functioning, and latency function of internal and instrumental functioning. These four functions further buttress four mechanisms: those concerning power realization for the fulfilling function, utility optimization for the adaptation function, norm conformity for the integration function, and idea consistency for the latency function (Munch 1987). Specifically, the realization mechanism emphasizes the driving force of power, the optimization mechanism emphasizes the attractive force of gain, the conformity mechanism emphasizes the assimilating force of the norm, and the consistency mechanism emphasizes the exhibiting or rationalizing force of ideology. The realization mechanism encompasses conflict or power theory and psychoanalytic theory; the optimization mechanism encompasses rational choice and exchange theories; the conformity mechanism encompasses social learning, norm, and cultural theories; and the consistency mechanism encompasses symbolic-interactionist and cognitive consistency theories. The mechanisms of the analytical-functionalist framework already cover materialist theory, structuration theory, and idealist theory. The analytical-functionalist framework likewise differentiates between voluntaristic and deterministic levels in applying the mechanisms. Whereas the voluntaristic level focuses on the mechanisms of internal forces, the deterministic level focuses on the mechanisms of external forces. In applying to the person, voluntaristic mechanisms emphasize the forces of personal power, gain (expected), norm exposure, and idea. By contrast, deterministic mechanisms emphasize forces external to the person, including those from the polity or authority, economy or market, community or social network, and culture or religion. These forces arise from society when it functions well. Apart from being influential through their impacts on voluntaristic forces, deterministic forces are influential directly on the person through coercing, shaping, channeling, and even providing and substituting, which means acting for the person.

Voluntaristic and deterministic forces are engaged in personal and national factors, respectively, when the framework elaborates statics in the production process, including experiences, practices, and life quality. Reflecting the power realization mechanism, voluntaristic forces include personal resources, ability, education, income, marriage, access to resources from family and other sources, and resource deficiency in terms of age, divorce, widowhood, and immigration. Representing the utility optimization mechanism, voluntaristic forces include personal gains expected from employment, work quality, security, and saving, and losses expected from unemployment, hardship, nuisance, and victimization. Registering the norm conformity mechanism, voluntaristic forces include personal exposure to norms from employing organizations and the media. Revealing the idea consistency mechanism, voluntaristic forces include personal ideas or religious beliefs and their manifestations in actions and habits. In addition, deterministic forces include the basic national conditions of PISTOL (i.e., population, information, space, technology, organization, and life standards) (Bailey 1994). These forces also include the modernization factors of economic development, globalization, government effectiveness, democracy, liberty, human development, and human capital (Dahlberg et al. 2018). Modernization factors include the side effect factors of income inequality and CO2 emission. These national factors provide external forces, including resources and conflicts, to determine the production process.

The dynamics of the production process involving experiences, practices, and life quality center on time impacts. Concerning the World Values Survey, the impacts refer to changes from 2004 to 2012 or from Waves 5 and 6 of the survey. Theoretically, the passage of time indicates social and environmental changes in modernization, postmodernization, individualization, globalization, and denaturalization. The World Values Survey indicated tremendous and statistically significant increases in the national indicators of population (*partial* $r = 0.798$, controlling for countries), bank credit to the private sector (*partial* $r = 0.757$), gross domestic product

(GDP, *partial* $r = 0.790$), globalization (*partial* $r = 0.784$), government effectiveness (*partial* $r = 0.575$), human development (*partial* $r = 0.932$), and human capital (*partial* $r = 0.920$). Meanwhile, land per capita greatly decreased (*partial* $r = -528$). At the personal level, increases were substantial and significant in independent work (*partial* $r = 0.315$), public employment (*partial* $r = 0.255$), and e-activity (*partial* $r = 0.224$). Meanwhile, full-time employment evidenced a substantial and significant decrease (*partial* $r = -0.345$), demonstrating modernization, postmodernization, globalization, individualization, and denaturalization. Specifically, increases in bank credit, prosperity (i.e., GDP), globalization, government effectiveness, human development, and human capital indicate modernization. Globalization and e-activity reflect both postmodernization and modernization. The increase in independent work and the decrease in full-time employment illustrate individualization. Meanwhile, the increase in population and the decrease in land per capita manifest denaturalization or humanization.

Precisely, the dynamics of the production processes depict the effects of time on the production of life experiences, practices, and quality. Such dynamics reasonably reflect modernization, postmodernization (including globalization), and individualization. In brief, the dynamics of modernization highlight the increasing influence of rationality, thus strengthening the effects of personal adaptation (or utility optimization) and latency (or idea consistency), which entail instrumental and substantive rationality, respectively. Conversely, the dynamics of modernization suggest the diminishing influences of resources and social factors, including personal power realization, norm conformity, and external determination. By contrast, the dynamics of postmodernization emphasize the increasing unpredictability of personal experiences, practices, and quality. These dynamics thus champion blanket declines in the effects of any factor. Alternatively, the dynamics of individualization stress the increasing influences of personal factors and the declining influences of non-personal factors.

The dynamics of modernization that indicate rationality factors increase their influences with time, whereas non-rationality factors reduce their influences with time register rationalization in modernization. Accordingly, rationalization is a characterizing component of modernization (Brand 1999; Gibbins and Reimer 1999; Heaphy 2007; Venkatesh 1999) and refers to the elevation of instrumental reasoning and purposive reasoning (Heaphy 2007; Venkatesh 1999). Reasoning involves personal calculation and expectation of optimizing utility, gain, or the achievement of valued goals and the consistency maintained among ideas, values, beliefs, and attitudes. Consequently, reasoning means upholding instrumental and substantive rationality. Conversely, rationalization means disenchantment and the dispelling of tradition or external demand or norms (Heaphy 2007). For instance, religious affiliation would reduce its influence in the face of modernization. This condition indicates the impact of secularization, which is a feature of modernization (Gibbins and Reimer 1999; Inglehart 1999; Inglehart and Baker 2000; Martinelli 2005). A source of secularization in modernization is expanding education or enlightenment, which would demystify and downplay superstitious and religious influences (Best and Kellner 2001; Martinelli 2005). This process relates to the increasing favor for humanism in modernization (Best and Kellner 2001). Such an increase underlies the increasing reliance on science and technology in modernization (Best and Kellner 2001; Martinelli 2005; Zhen and Wu 1996) and facilitates industrialization as another critical feature of modernization (Heaphy 2007; Martinelli 2005). Industrialization, in turn, expedites socioeconomic development, notably prosperity or progress visible in the economy (Gibbins and Reimer 1999; Inglehart and Welzel 2005; Martinelli 2005; Mouzelis 1999). This development enables rationalization, notably the increase in self-reflection or reflexivity (Beck et al. 1994; Han and Shim 2010). Reflexivity builds on the personal awareness about information, which is increasingly available in modernization (Beck et al. 1994; Diolae and Seda 2001). In all, rationalization hinges on secularization, educational expansion, scientific and technological development, socioeconomic development, and popularization of information, all of which characterize modernization.

The dynamics of postmodernization emphasize the unpredictability of personal experience, practice, quality, and other aspects. Unpredictability is a defining characteristic of postmodernization and the central proposition of postmodern theory or postmodernism (Gibbins and Reimer 1999). Moreover, unpredictability connects to indeterminacy, ambiguity, contingency, and chaos arising in postmodernization (Boje 1995; Heaphy 2007; Tester 2004). Essentially, postmodern theory rejects determinism (Heaphy 2007). These features stem from change, volatility, fluidity, and liquidity, as emphasized in postmodernization (Blackshaw 2005; Gibbens and Reimer 1999; Heaphy 2007; Martinelli 2005). The emphasis champions constant search and reconstruction (Gibbins and Reimer 1999; Goulding 2000). Postmodern fads and catchwords are short-lived, instant, unstable, and insecure (Blackshaw 2005; Gibbins and Reimer 1999; Martinelli 2005; Pilisuk et al. 1996) because of the liberal, permissive, and tolerant orientation treasured in postmodernization (Martinelli 2005; Peritore and Karina 2000). Postmodern fads are intricate, bricolaged, ambivalent, and variegated (Blackshaw 2005; Heaphy 2007; Jacques 1998). Adding to unpredictability are the arational and anti-scientific features of postmodernization, such that it is unintelligible, illogical, and independent of rationality and knowledge (Crook et al. 1992; Gibbins 1998; Ritzer 1997). Postmodern incidents, such as buying and playing, are whimsical, impromptu, situational, and ephemeral (Martinelli 2005), all of which characterize the transient self in postmodernization (Jacques 1998). Moreover, arationality happens in incoherence or inconsistency among ideas, values, orientations, and other mental concepts (Geser 1999). Alternatively, it represents perversity to obstruct predictability (Gibbins and Reimer 1999). Unpredictability also arises from diversification, decenteredness, discontinuation, and mixing or dedifferentiation in postmodernization (Brand 1999; Gartman 1998; Gibbins and Reimer 1999; Rojek 1995; Scambler 2002). Specifically, the gist of the postmodern object is unidentifiable. This idea connects to fragmentation or the loss of an identifiable whole in postmodernization (Gibbins and Reimer 1999; Martinelli 2005; Venkatesh 1999). For example, the postmodern self can play many conflicting roles simultaneously, just like in a drama (Blackshaw 2005). This ability stems from nihilism prevailing in postmodernization to deny anything central or essential (Gibbins and Reimer 1999; Scambler 2002). It also results from the multiplicity, multidimensionality, plurality, or perspectivism or acceptance of multiple perspectives emphasized in postmodernization (Boje 1995; Gibbins and Reimer 1999; Heaphy 2007; Peritore and Karina 2000). This emphasis underlies the debate and negotiation to defy common understandings in postmodernization (Alvarado 1996), resulting in noisiness which impedes understanding and predictability (Blackshaw 2005). Another source of unpredictability is experimentation and risking or the lack of intention, planning, and solid knowledge in postmodernization (Blackshaw 2005; Heaphy 2007). Furthermore, the emphasis on particularism, idiosyncrasies, and uniqueness impedes predictability in postmodernization (Gibbins and Reimer 1999; Inglehart 2000; Leonard 1997; Venkakesh 1999). This outcome means upholding personal images instead of objective reality in postmodernization, thus dampening predictability (Gibbins and Reimer 1999; Heaphy 2007; Sampson 1999).

The dynamics of individualization hold the increasing influences of individual-based or internal factors and dwindling social or external influences over time because of the growing importance of personal agency (Beck et al. 1994; Beck and Beck-Gernsheim 2002). Such agency transpires in personal awareness, choice, autonomy, self-culture, self-orientation, self-determination, self-reference, self-reflection, and self-influence (Bauman 2001; Beck and Beck-Gernsheim 2002; Beck et al. 1994; Burgess 2018; Heinz 2002; Sorensen and Christiansen 2013). Remarkably, the agency tends to engage in applying science or technology (Elliott 2003). The application also stems from liberation, disembeddedness, disengagement, separation, and disintegration from groups such as classes (Bauman 2001; Beck et al. 1994; Beck and Beck-Gernsheim 2002). Institutional influence also declines with individualization (Burgess 2018). Consequently, habit, attachment, commitment, and obligation to tradition and other social establishments lose their influences with individualization (Bauman 2001; Burgess 2018; Gibbins and Reimer 1999).

Study Needs

Statics and dynamics in sustaining or producing life quality in the average person in the contemporary world of the incipient twenty-first century require theoretical and empirical elucidation. Such production involves inputs from national and personal backgrounds through the throughputs of life experiences and practices to engender the output of life quality appraisal. All these factors are prominent and essential. Life quality, well-being, or the good life is of crucial concern, associated with civilization, morality, and policy (Diener et al. 2009; Ng et al. 2003; Veenhoven 1984). Pursuing personal life quality is the lifelong goal of ethics and politics (Helliwell and Putnam 2005; Lane 2000; Marks and Shah 2005). This personal aspect necessarily respects the person rather than the collective. As each person counts, personal life quality is noteworthy rather than collective national life quality, though collective life quality is also valuable. Importantly, life quality, experiences, practices, and the production processes apply to the average adult in the world, not to the American, Chinese, Brazilian, Nigerian, or other specific nationality. As in most other studies, the current study needs to understand the average person rather than the Westerner. National boundaries are unnecessary for general understanding, especially in the globalized world (Smith 2004; Sorensen and Christiansen 2013). Hence, national identity is a factor rather than a delimitation or filter for this study to avoid Eurocentrism or Sinocentrism.

In the average contemporary adult, both the statics and dynamics of life quality production, comprising their influential input and throughput factors, are obscure. Most available knowledge about the statics and dynamics comes from national or Western studies of individuals or cross-national studies of nations. This knowledge tends to be Eurocentric (i.e., centered on the West, including Europe, North America, and their descents). Moreover, the knowledge is commonly devoid of a comprehensive theoretical framework for understanding. Hence, it can be atheoretical, short-term, and even whimsical (Ryff 1989; Veenhoven 2008). Knowing the universal truth is crucial and required, particularly regarding life quality production (Nevarez 2011; Veenhoven 2000). This knowledge appeals to human nature or interest in curiosity, authenticity, and truth-seeking (D'Raven and Pasha-Zaidi 2016; Huta 2017; MacLeod 2015; Maslow 1999; Seligman 2002; Veenhoven 2014; Waterman 2008). People also have a strong desire to tackle their problems concerning life quality (Cummins et al. 2009). This desire tends to hold because of the prevalence of personal and collective melancholy, dysfunction, and crisis in the contemporary world (Cummins et al. 2009; Lane 2000). Life quality in the new millennium is under challenge (Lyubomirsky 2001). Meanwhile, people are long-lived and perfectionistic, thus desiring more knowledge about life quality production (Phillips 2006; Veenhoven 2008).

The comprehensive theoretical framework underlying the statics and dynamics of life quality production has not engaged enough theorizing and empirical work. On the one hand, a promising theorizing work builds on analytical functionalism to incorporate both voluntaristic and deterministic mechanisms that thoroughly cover personal and impersonal or collective factors. Theorizing the mechanisms and factors of life quality production has not been pervasive and systematic. Therefore, theorizing is necessary to enhance people's understanding and meet their need for a complete explanation or cognitive closure (Kruglanski et al. 2002). It also needs to address atheoretical work on life quality production (Ryff 1989; Veehoven 2008). On the other hand, demonstrating empirical findings about the effects of the theoretically plausible factors is necessary to meet people's need for truth (Maslow 1999; Salagame 2014). These findings are always necessary for understanding life quality production (Megone 1990). They need to indicate general knowledge about the average adult globally based on statistical analysis (Sachs 2003). Hence, the knowledge is objective and representative. Crucially, such knowledge highlights statistically and practically significant static and dynamic factors in life quality production.

Especially for the voluntaristic mechanism of power realization, statistical analysis reveals significant resources, strengths, and drives that power the production, such as education, income, and marriage. Regarding the voluntaristic mechanism of utility optimization, the analysis is to probe significant gains that attract life quality production, such as from security, self-employment, and independent work.

Regarding the voluntaristic mechanism of norm conformity, the analysis is to screen norms and social experiences that assimilate with the production. For the voluntaristic mechanism of idea consistency, the analysis is to identify beliefs, roles, and behaviors that rationalize the production. Moreover, to clarify the deterministic mechanism, the analysis identifies national factors that enable personal life quality production, including population size, economic development or living standards, and democracy. These deterministic factors, which incorporate social and material resources, will push, coerce, empower, channel, put, and/or even replace one in the production. Replacing means that a person obtains life quality or related experiences because other people act for the person's life quality production. An example is an adult behaving just like a child to receive feeding from other people.

In addition to improving the understanding of the functionalist mechanisms and their factors, this study needs to clarify the dynamics of social and natural changes, including modernization, postmodernization, globalization, individualization, and denaturalization, diminishing natural properties due to human intervention. The clarification appeals to human interest in understanding and predicting changes and the future (Hassenzahl et al. 2015; Prenda and Lachman 2001). That is, understanding the dynamics enables the prediction of the future. Of vital concern for the understanding and prediction is change, improvement, or deterioration in life quality production (Brockmann et al. 2009; Phillips 2006). This concern is necessary for planning, preparing, and/or coping with the change in the production (Baylis 2005; Gattino et al. 2015; Navarez 2011; Prenda and Lachman 2001). Nevertheless, understanding and planning are presently uncertain in the face of diverse views about social and natural changes and their dynamics. These views include the changes as challenging, colonizing, conflicting, unequalizing, fragmenting, evolutionary, revolutionary, and teleological or planned (Adams 2007; Cole 2003; Fararo 2001; Fein 2015; Harper and Leicht 2011; Schmidt 2010; Turner 2003). Specifically, controversy is raging over the dynamics of modernization, postmodernization, globalization, individualization, and denaturalization concerning life quality (Munck 2018; Nederveen Pieterse 2010; Rabbani 2011), raising issues about progress, risk, crisis, limitation, sustainability, indeterminacy, and nihilism (Johnson 2009; Schroeder 2013). The diverse views entail different responses in adaptation, conformity, competition, migration, social movements, and anxiety (Adams 2007; Fein 2915; Harper and Leicht 2011; Turner 2003). Thus, clarification of the diverse views is necessary.

Specifically, the dynamics of modernization, postmodernization, globalization, individualization, and denaturalization for life quality production require clarification because, while the dynamics tend to be real and prevailing, their impacts on life quality production are obscure. Accordingly, modernization, characterized by rationalization and industrialization, has engendered peace, autonomy, and stress (Delhey 2010; Dioake and Seda 2001). Postmodernization, which maintains discontinuity, volatility, uncertainty, and unpredictability in society, has raised consumption and fear (Haller 2002; Tester 2004). Globalization, which underlies postmodernization, has enlarged revenue, stress, and resistance (Arnett 2002; Brady et al. 2007; Tsai 2006). Individualization, which springs from both modernization and postmodernization, has sustained liberation and peace and risks, anomie, insecurity, and anxiety

(Bauman 2001; Beck et al. 1994; Burgess 2018; Castells 2000; Frank and Meyer 2002; Turner 2010). The effects of dynamics on static influences on life quality production have likewise remained uncharted. Specifically, how the influences of personal and national determinants of life quality production transform over the incipient twenty-first century remain unclear. These influences can reflect increasing rationality in modernization, increasing unpredictability in postmodernization, and personal influence in individualization. All these possible changes require empirical scrutiny.

Study Plan

Following the above introduction, the study unfolds its theory and findings in seven subsequent chapters before arriving at conclusions. Individually, the chapters concern identification of life quality appraisals, experiences, and practices (Chap. 2); theory about life quality production (Chap. 3); findings on life quality production (Chap. 4); theory about life experience production (Chap. 5); findings on life experience production (Chap. 6); theory about life practice production (Chap. 7); findings on life experience production (Chap. 8); and conclusions (Chap. 9).

Chapter 2 is about identifying life quality appraisals, experiences, and practices. It displays findings from the statistical analysis of World Values Survey data in the twenty-first century concerning the factor structure and reliability of the appraisals, experiences, and practices. All the analyses involved person-level data weighted to represent the average adult in the world. For current life quality appraisal, factor analysis identified two factors to represent worry and delight: happiness, autonomy, and financial satisfaction. Concerning recent life quality, factor analysis showed that health and life satisfaction were separate factors. Regarding experiences, factor analysis identified four factors pertaining to economic hardship, neighborhood nuisance, victimization, and security. In addition, the analysis found family saving to be a stand-alone experience (i.e., not falling into any factor). For private practice or activity, factor analysis identified five factors about e-activity, learning, spiritual activity, risk aversion, and television watching. Factor analysis also found weapon carrying to be a stand-alone private practice. For public practice or activity, factor analysis identified four factors about civic organizational participation, appealing, strike, and voting. In addition, factor analysis showed that participation in green demonstrations and green donation were stand-alone public practices. The identified factors were all reliable. Partial correlation analysis then showed relationships among personal factors, national factors, and time while controlling for indicators of the nation (i.e., Brazil, China, Egypt, and so on). The analysis indicated significant and relatively large increases in e-activity, public employment, and independent work over time in the early twenty-first century. By contrast, the analysis revealed significant and relatively large decreases in learning, civic organizational participation, spiritual activity, full-time employment, and private business employment with time. Moreover, the analysis displayed very strong increases in population, bank credit, economic development, globalization, human development, and human capital with time. These changes demonstrate modernization, globalization, and individualization in the world.

Chapter 3 is about the theory of life quality production and details the conceptualization and explanation of life quality. Life quality in terms of health, happiness, life satisfaction, financial satisfaction, and no worry primarily identify the hedonist good life, whereas life quality in terms of autonomy reflects the eudemonic or humanist good life. In any form, life quality is explicable with the voluntaristic mechanisms of power realization, utility optimization, norm conformity, and idea consistency and the deterministic mechanism of external force within the analytical-functionalist framework. This framework incorporates explanations predicated on resources, exchange, comparison, temperament, and others. Life quality appraisal involving health maintenance, satisfaction, feeling happy, independence, and worry-free is both a voluntaristic action and a deterministic response. At the personal level, sociodemographic characteristics, experiences, and practices produce life quality according to the voluntaristic mechanism. Recent life quality likewise produces current life quality considering the voluntaristic mechanism of consistency. Furthermore, national factors such as population and economic development produce life quality initially and directly through the deterministic mechanism and indirectly through the voluntaristic mechanism. The deterministic mechanism holds that a person's life quality results from other people's production efforts. For instance, national human development in terms of education, life expectancy, and income provides people with increased capability to help one another sustain life quality. Due to modernization, postmodernization, globalization, individualization, and denaturalization, life quality can also change with time. Additionally, the effects of personal and national factors on life quality can change with time. The dynamics of effects or time or zeitgeist are explicable with the deterministic mechanism.

Chapter 4 is about findings concerning life quality production and primarily exhibits the main and interaction effects of personal and national factors on the life quality of health, life satisfaction, delight, and worry. Among the significant main effects, the most pervasive was the positive effects of education and family saving and the negative effects of economic hardship and neighborhood nuisance. In addition, independent work and national human development displayed positive effects, while national land per capita exhibited negative effects. The effects are explicable with the voluntaristic and deterministic mechanisms of the functionalist framework. Among voluntaristic mechanisms, power realization and utility optimization are particularly applicable. The significant interaction effects with time manifest the modernization, postmodernization, and individualization dynamics. That is, non-rational factors decreased their influences in line with modernization dynamics. Similarly, influences became weaker, or life quality became more unpredictable, thus supporting postmodernization dynamics. In addition, social factors decreased their influences, and individual-based factors increased their influences in support of individualization dynamics. Notably, modernization, postmodernization, individualization, and their dynamics prevail simultaneously and are not mutually exclusive.

Chapter 5 is about the theory regarding the production of life experiences as precursors to life quality appraisals. These experiences consist of the adversities of economic hardship, neighborhood nuisance, victimization, and the benefits of security and family saving. They also represent the objective or experiential indicators of life quality. Their production reflects the voluntaristic and deterministic mechanisms of the functionalist framework. On the one hand, life experiences, including economic hardship and neighborhood nuisance, can be voluntaristic in that they involve personal selection, awareness, perception, and interpretation. Thus, these talents enable one to encounter favorable experiences according to the voluntaristic mechanism of power realization. Alternatively, favorable expectations, norms, and beliefs can induce favorable perceptions and experiences according to the voluntaristic mechanisms of optimization, conformity, and consistency. On the other hand, life experiences can be involuntary responses to deterministic factors external to the person. Static national and dynamic factors conveyed through modernization, postmodernization, and others can determine personal life experiences.

Chapter 6 exhibits findings on the production of life experiences. The findings primarily show the main and interaction effects of personal sociodemographic and national factors on the experiences. The main effects indicate the statics about the production, whereas the interaction effects gauge the dynamics or change due to the time about the production. The interaction effects particularly manifested individualization dynamics such that individual-based factors became more influential on life experiences with time. The individual is increasingly responsible for his or her life experiences.

Chapter 7 discusses the theory concerning the production of life practices, which produce life quality. These practices consist of the private activities of e-activity, learning, risk aversion, and weapon carrying and the public activities of civic organizational participation, appealing, strike, voting, green demonstrations, green donation, and spiritual activity. They also count as the objective or behavioral indicators of life quality. Their production reflects the voluntaristic and deterministic mechanisms of the functionalist framework. The voluntaristic mechanisms involve personal, sociodemographic factors, whereas the deterministic mechanisms hinge on national factors. National factors such as national technology and organization would shape or require the person to do something, such as e-activity, when the deterministic mechanisms operate. These mechanisms also identify the statics and dynamics in producing life practices. The dynamics, which underlie changes over time, reflect modernization, postmodernization, individualization, and others.

Chapter 8 concerns findings on the production of life practices. The findings primarily show the main and interaction effects of personal sociodemographic and national factors on the practices. The main effects illustrate the statics about the production, whereas the interaction effects unfold the dynamics of the production. The interaction effects showed that the practices were increasingly predictable with time, thus refuting postmodernization dynamics.

Chapter 9 concludes the findings on statics and dynamics in producing life quality, including its subjective dimensions of appraisal and objective indicators of life experiences and practices. Both statics and dynamics rest principally on the analytical-functionalist framework, encompassing voluntaristic and deterministic mechanisms engaging personal and national factors. The statics highlight the importance of the voluntaristic mechanism of power realization, which hinges on resources or various kinds of capital. At the same time, the statics reveal the deterministic mechanism, which builds on national factors. This mechanism suggests that national factors can directly influence life quality production through external provision, coercion, and/or channeling. The dynamics reflect the deterministic mechanisms of time or social change in terms of modernization, postmodernization, globalization, individualization, and denaturalization. Such dynamics consist of the main effect of time and its interaction with personal and national factors. The interaction effects particularly illustrate that modernization, postmodernization, and individualization underlie the dynamics in producing life quality.

Chapter 2
Life Quality, Experiences, and Practices: Identification

Life quality or its appraisals or feelings generally is the end for predication by such predictors as experiences and practices. The feelings include current worry and delight and existing health and life satisfaction. Delight includes satisfaction, happiness, and a sense of autonomy. The experiences include those of economic hardship, neighborhood nuisance, victimization, security, and family saving. Meanwhile, practices include such private activities as e-activity, learning, spiritual activity, risk aversion, weapon carrying, and public activities such as active organizational participation, appealing, joining strikes, voting, and environmentalist involvement.

Life feelings, experiences, and practices are crucial because they are functional or dysfunctional to bolster and materialize the social system. On the one hand, the bolstering rests on practices and their underlying dispositions and attitudes, typically prosocial. Such bolstering emanates from the voluntaristic functions of goal attainment, adaptation, integration, and latency, or their respective mechanisms of power realization, utility optimization, norm conformity, and idea consistency. Accordingly, personal feelings, experiences, and practices engender personal practices relevant, functional or dysfunctional, to the social system. Those functional ones would be sustainable, famous, or prominent, whereas those dysfunctional ones would be unsustainable, unpopular, and marginal. On the other hand, the materialization happens when personal feelings, experiences, and practices exemplify discourses, such as conservatism, liberalism, and socialism prevailing in the social system. The materialization or exemplification engages the latency function of idea consistency or rationalization. Those materializing discourses in the social system would be functional and sustainable, whereas those contradicting discourses in the social system would be dysfunctional and unsustainable. Herein, such discourses are functional to the social system with the latency function of rationalization. In other words, discourses are the superstructure or spiritual pillars of the system.

C. Cheung, *Production Dynamics for Life Quality in the Incipient 21st Century*,
https://doi.org/10.1007/978-981-19-3827-6_2

Life Quality Feelings

Life quality resides in one's appraisal or feeling about life (Huta 2017). Feeling means a conscious, subjective psychological state (Reber 2016). It is crucial for acting, such as problem-solving, maintaining homeostasis, and retaining and rejecting memories (Heller 2009; Reber 2016). That is, feeling good retains memories of something good. The contributions of feeling to action and homeostasis reflect the functions of adaptation and goal attainment in the analytical-functionalist framework. Accordingly, feeling provides the guide for action in achieving adaptation and sets the goal for homeostatic attainment. In addition, feeling is justifiable or of concern through some discourses. Empiricist discourse posits that feeling is factual, real, and experienceable (Ratcliffe 2008). By contrast, phenomenological discourse maintains that feeling is a reflection as opposed to a display of dogmatism (Ratcliffe 2008). Hence, feeling is active or lively. Feeling is also vital as a kind of romance, which is treasurable in romanticism (Heller 2009; Reber 2016). Moreover, feeling is a basis for virtue, guiding virtuous action (Reber 2016). For instance, feeling bad drives virtuous action to redress something terrible. Feeling is crucial in Confucian and stoic ethics or virtues (Reber 2016). Whereas Confucian ethics emphasizes associating feeling with music, ritual, and reading moral maxims, stoic ethics advocates the deprivation of longing from feeling.

Life quality feeling is noteworthy in positive psychology (Cowen and Kilmer 2002; D'raven and Pasha-Zaidi 2016). This approach casts doubt on the objective treatment of life quality in medicine, neglecting the positive aspect of life. The positivist approach thus emphasizes personal strengths, including appreciation, gratitude, hope, humor, love, spirituality, and vitality, which also characterize life quality or well-being. In the approach, feeling well broadens and builds one's repertoire and its enactment, which are constructive and productive (Diener et al. 2009; Fredrickson 2008). They can contribute to one's employment, health, income, relatedness, resources, solidarity, trust, and upward social mobility (Diener et al. 2009; Fredrickson 2008; Oishi and Koo 2008; Veenhoven 2008). In a broader view, feeling well induces longevity as opposed to pathology and dysfunction (Cummins et al. 2009; Veenhoven 2008). Such individual achievement follows and accords with individualization (McKenzie 2016). Individualization is a social trend to connect individual well-being to societal functioning (Cummins 2016). Feeling well is the ultimate motivator for personal and societal development action (Lai et al. 2007). Considering the analytical-functionalist framework, such motivation illustrates the goal-attainment function of feeling well as energy or resource.

Life quality feeling is justifiable or essential in humanist, individualist, neoliberal, utilitarian, and other discourses. Humanist discourse maintains that the feeling is necessary to fulfill needs, such as for fairness, parity, and worth in life (Burnett 2012). Individualist, egocentric, person-oriented, or Western discourse posits that feeling well is necessary for agency, autonomy, self-actualization, self-development, and self-fulfillment (Barrow 2019; Burnett 2012; Ganesh and McAllum 2010). Utilitarian discourse asserts that feeling well is essential for capitalism, characterized by competitiveness and productivity, freedom, individualism, and market operation (Burnett 2012; Duncan 2014). The good feeling evolves from and contributes to leisure and work. This contribution is helpful to generate maximum utility in a maximum number of people. Essentially, feeling well is the core of utility. Standing on individualism and utilitarianism, neoliberal discourse similarly treasures the role of feeling well in capitalism, consumerism, economic growth, and rationality (Cabanas 2016; Daraei and Mohajery 2013). That is, feeling well plays a vital role in consumption, economic activity, and thus capitalism. Rationality is relevant for the person to optimize the good feeling. Hence, feeling well is adaptive, representing a requisite function in the analytical-functionalist framework. According to World Values Survey data, the feeling or appraisal can take the forms of happiness, satisfaction with life and finance, particularly autonomy, health, and having no worry.

Worry, as a negative form of good or life quality feeling, is a dysfunction in need of minimization (Bouton et al. 2001; McNally 1990). Such a dysfunction is indicative of danger and threat, which are stable and intrusive (Flinkfeldt 2020; Zeidner and Matthews 2011). Moreover, worry is an irrational, problematic arousal reflecting feeling about uncertainty in need of vigilance (Frink et al. 2004; Zeidner and Matthews 2011). Worry tends to be a feminine characteristic associated with emotionality, inferiority, and vulnerability as opposed to choosing, control, and reasoning (Nelson 2015). Nevertheless, worry is prevalent because of its susceptible to social construction, including that in the media and social atmosphere (Hubbard 2003). The prevalence is visible in worry about terrorist attack, unemployment, war and civil war particularly, and wiretapping or the lack of privacy.

Terrorism or terrorist attack is violence against civilians or non-combatants in clandestine ways to arouse worry (Orr 2012; Taylor 2018). The attack thus inflicts damage, insecurity, intimidation, and even war (Morin 2016; Orr 2012; Taylor 2018). Moreover, terrorism aims to provoke publicity because of its exceptional adversity (Morin 2016; Orr 2012). Terrorism can transpire in extortion, extremism, killing, and paralysis, as well as an attack (Bjorgo 2016; Dugan and Chenoweth 2012; Neumayer and Plumper 2009; Onursal and Kirkpatrick 2021). Based on the clash of civilization and media circulation and amplification, terrorism becomes prevalent (KhosraviNik and Amer 2022; Morin 2016). The clash registers unresolvable entrenched cultural or ideological conflict fueling terrorism. Terrorism is blameworthy according to discourses about care, consequentialism or utilitarianism, contractualism, and deontology. Care discourse wrongs terrorism for its harm, violence, and worrying (Held 2008). Instead, the discourse embraces empathy, equality, fraternity, mutuality, and relatedness. This discourse rests on the premise of interrelated conditions in society. Consequentialist or utilitarian discourse faults terrorism for undermining peace and utility (Held 2008; Taylor 2018). Contractualist discourse criticizes terrorism for violating the law, liberty, and rationality or reasoning (Taylor 2018). Deontological discourse condemns terrorism for its violation of rights (Held 2008). In addition, terrorism is objectionable because of its barbarism, evilness, extremism, fanaticism, scapegoating, tyranny, victimization, and provocation of war (Bhatia 2009; Blain 2015; Fragnon 2019; Jackson and Hall 2016).

Unemployment is a worrisome problem concomitant to such social changes as labor deregulation and technologization (Francesconi and Golsch 2005; Schellenberg 1996). Such deregulation originates from globalization or global employment and an associated decline in unionism. Globalization also capitalizes on technologization to replace labor with technology. Consequently, unemployment signifies disqualification and stigmatization imposed on unemployed people (Gallie and Paugam 2000; Paugam and Russell 2000). Unemployment is also blameworthy for income inequality and poverty (Francesconi and Golsch 2005). All these register the risk society characterized by insecurity and vulnerability (Tam and Ip 2017). Furthermore, unemployment is problematic, considering discourse on agency, which treasures personal control, growth, and independence (Dooley and Prause 2004). The lack of agency introduces stress to the person (Dooley and Prause 2004). In addition, unemployment is symptomatic of skill mismatch, reflecting problems in education to suit the job market (Adely et al. 2021). Unemployment is worrisome because it provokes economic hardship, homelessness, hospitalization, and victimization (Lelli 2008; Kaukinen 2004; Muhlau 2014). That is, unemployment jeopardizes one's health and wealth (Lelli 2008; Reeskens and Vandecasteele 2017). Conversely, unemployment has eroded one's social capital (Manturuk et al. 2010; Webber and Huxley 2007). As such, unemployment indicates dysfunction in goal attainment or fulfillment in the analytical-functionalist perspective.

War is worrying, as is politically institutionalized lethal violence (Olsson and Maleevi 2018). It operates collectively and solidly through fighters of either side (Malesevic 2010). Its worry is understandable with the discourses of consequentialism, feminism, pacificism, and virtue. Consequentialist discourse problematizes war that results in disadvantage and misrule (Gorman 2010; Graham 2008). Feminist discourse condemns war for its origin in patriarchy, particularly unfair to women (Owens 2010). Based on consequentialist, deontological, and teleological ethics, pacificism castigates war for harm to pleasure, happiness, welfare, dutifulness, and virtues such as charity, faith, hope, justice, love, and moderation (Orend 2006; Owens 2010). Furthermore, virtue discourse accuses war for undermining such additional virtues as charity, dignity, fortitude, freedom, prudence, and temperance (Gorman 2010). War is unjust when it is arbitrary, clandestine, invasive, illegal, irresponsible, sudden, unreasonable, and violating human rights (Orend 2006).

Civil war, as a kind of war involving opposing parties within a country, is worrying because of its domestic havoc (Bentrovato and Nissanka 2018). Such war commonly comes with rebellion, revolution, resistance, and subversive struggles for power (Meis 2017). Civil war is disharmonizing and upsetting peace (Bentrovato and Nissanka 2018). Often, civic war involves different ethnic parties in a country, thus registering ethnic conflict or struggle (Corstange and York 2018). Civil war can arise from democracy, which appeals to the pursuit of freedom and rights, which becomes a cause of civic war (Bentrovato and Nissanka 2018). Such war is worrying or unjustifiable with collectivist, counter-terrorist, evil or irrationality, and security discourses (Bentrovato and Nissanka 2018; Seoighe 2016; Sorial 2012; Whiting 2012). Accordingly, civil war undermines national collectivity, solidarity, and security, especially when it foments terrorism which is evil and irrational. Civil war is justifiable, pardonable, or common according to discourses on defense, history, humanitarianism, liberation, loyalty, pragmatism, self-determination, separatism, terrorism, traitors, and victimization (Nackers 2015; Seoighe 2016). Accordingly, civil war is a necessary defense for certain parties, including separatists, to uphold their liberty and rights practically or effectively, rather than being victims of misrule. Hence, destruction through terrorism or civic war is acceptable. In addition, civil war just follows some historical tradition to declare loyalty to a specific party in a country. Moreover, when a party betrays the country with treason, civil war erupts to safeguard national interests.

Wiretapping is worrying as an intrusion into personal privacy (Hampton 2016). Privacy emphasizes autonomy and opposes being in public (Connor and Doan 2021). In justifying privacy, privatism encompasses self-interest and familialism or family orientation as opposed to being civic or public and privileging helpfulness, social order, and the state (Cook 2001; Dowling et al. 2010; Hampton 2016; Pospech 2020). Privacy or privatism arises from depoliticization, desire, marketing, and technology, notably concerning information and communication (Cook 2001; Hampton 2016). These factors register the basis for self-interest and self-sufficiency, hence privacy or privatism. Notably, depoliticization means that one does not need to care about politics, as the emphasis is on the market, which rests on self-interest. Privacy or privatism, in turn, stands on liberal, neoliberal, and right discourses. Liberal discourse favors the market (Huber 2012; Tapper and Kobayashi 2018). In addition to favoring the market, neoliberal discourse treasures commerce, competition, deregulation, and the privatization of public services, as opposed to state planning and welfare (Dowling et al. 2010; Huber 2012; Tapper and Kobayashi 2018). In addition, rights discourse privileges personal rights (Lokot 2020). By contrast, privacy or privatism is questionable according to formal or rationalist, order, and theological discourses. Formalist or rationalist discourse, stemming from enlightenment, advocates transcendence or going beyond the person (Dell'Oro 2002). Discourse order favors order and its conformity (Fritz et al. 2022). In addition, theological discourse upholds sharing and commonality and demeans privacy or privatism, and it regards people as the common subjects of God (Dell'Oro 2002).

Education as a kind of human capital and a way of learning is noteworthy for worrying (Dolton et al. 2004; Nordin 2011). Thus, education embodies the functions of human capital, rationalization, and social control that are common everywhere (Munk 2003; Nordin 2011; Papastephanon 2015). Education has nurtured such ideologies as capitalism, communitarianism, conservatism, environmentalism, expressivism, humanism, individualism, liberalism, meritocratism, moralism, multiculturalism, neoliberalism, postmaterialism, postmodernism, populism, progressivism, relativism, socialism, and traditionalism (Derks 2004; Engels and Jacobson 2007; Evans et al. 2010; Gilberbloom and Markham 1995; Hood and Deopere 2002; Hraba et al. 2001; McCright and Dunlop 2008; Norris and Inglehart 2009; Pichler 2009; Sotirovic 2000; Sharp and Josyla 2008; Tranter and Western 2009; Wernet et al. 2005; Yuchtman-Yaar 2002; Welzel 2013). Meanwhile, education has eroded such ideologies as authoritarianism, Buddhism, egalitarianism, familism, humanitarianism, leftism, nationalism, patriotism, pronatalism, and racism (Achterberg and

Houtman 2009; Barker and Tinnick 2006; Billiet et al. 2003; Jones and Brayfield 1997; Norris and Inglehart 2009; Rossi 2001; Tang 2001; Vernby and Finseraas 2010; Wodtke 2012), Moreover, education has raised the values of autonomy, childrearing, conformity, imagination, independence, need, reasoning, voting, and work (Armon and Dawson 2003; Gelissen 2002; Fjellvang 2011; James and Luo 1999; Ulbig 2002; Weimann and Brosius 1994; Wu and Macneill 2003; Xiao 2000). Conversely, education has discounted the values of ascription, conservation, evaluation, obedience, and survival (Datler et al. 2013; Fjellvang 2011; Forgas et al. 1995). All these effects reflect the integration or norm conforming function of education through its variegated contents. Alternatively, education has enhanced civic skill, conscientiousness, intelligence, knowledge, memory, morality, openness, physical functioning, susceptibility, and verbal ability (Norris and Inglehart 2009; Opp 1989; Pratt et al. 1996; Rossi 2001; Shin 2012; Stevens et al. 2001; Straughn and Andriot 2011; Verba et al. 1995). These contributions indicate the functions of goal attainment and integration through learning and conformity. Conversely, education has diminished the need for help, religiosity, and vulnerability (Immerzeel and van Tubergen 2013; Lessler et al. 2000; Langenderfer and Shimp 2001). These effects illustrate the goal attainment function of learning and empowerment. For practice, education has raised civic engagement, civility, cultural activity, distancing from others, environmental protection, exercising, health behavior, impeachment, media use, musical lifestyle, online activity, persistence, political discussion and participation, prevention, protest participation, social participation, traveling, visiting, and voting (Bull et al. 2004; Djupe and Lewis 2015; Flavin and Keane 2011; Grzywacz 2000; Guillen et al. 2011; Grasso 2014; Kerrissey and Schofer 2013; Lelli 2008; Mirowsky and Ross 2001; Norris 2011; Norris and Inglehart 2009; McCabe 2014; Papadakis 2000; Pratt et al. 2010; Tsai 2006; Van Eijck 2001; Weisberg 2005; Welzel 2013). These activating effects reflect the functions of goal attainment and integration through learning and conforming. Conversely, education has discouraged birth, deviance, discrimination, housework, intergenerational association, natural lifestyle, personal care, prostitution, recourse, resistance, and returning from migration (Backman and Nilsson 2011; Gershuny 2000; Katz-Gerro 1999; Korinek et al. 2005; Lubbers et al. 2006; Su and Feng 2013; Swader and Vorobeva 2015; Torche 2011). These effects again reflect the functions of goal attainment and integration through learning and conforming. Eventually, education has escalated social class, earnings, insurance coverage, organizational membership, wealth, and social status (Cerin and Leslie 2008; Knab et al. 2008; Pettigrew 2002; Schnittker and Behrman 2012; Straughn and Andriot 2011; Whyte and Gao 2009). Education is functional to capital acquisition and is valuable and desirable to pursue. Having inadequate education is thus worrisome.

As the core of life quality feeling, happiness typically highlights the contemporary affective aspect of the Feeling (Lydon-Staley et al. 2019; Wadsworth 2014). It is acute, discrete, and intense in drawing and demonstrating psychic energy (Cropanzano et al. 2011; TenHouten 2007). Such energy is functional to sustain attention, humor, and resilience to stress in exploration, optimism, and relaxation (Fredrickson and Losada 2005). The exploration can facilitate information processing, proactivity, and resource acquisition (Cropanzano et al. 2011; Fredrickson 2001). Such acquired resources can foster creativity, health, optimism, and relational quality (Waugh 2014). Hence, happiness performs the function of goal attainment or fulfillment to establish the self, identity, character, and social relationships (Conway et al. 2014; Kaplan 2006; Stets and Trettevik 2014). In addition, happiness has contributed to justice, judgment, patriotism, and even fighting for the country (Cropanzano et al. 2011; Turner and Stets 2005). These contributions represent the function of adaptation, which concerns the fair exchange in returning the favor. That is, feeling happy in a place generates support for the place.

Satisfaction registers the retrospective, cognitive aspect of life quality feeling (Hagerty 2003). It manifests such qualities as homeostasis and stability (Cummins et al. 2003; Heidemeier and Staudinger 2012). Homeostasis means that fluctuation in satisfaction is temporary. Satisfaction with life is a popular indicator of utility, particularly in the democracy (Ateca-Amestoy et al. 2014; Radcliff 2001; Stavrova 2014). Life involved in life satisfaction comprises 11 facets of education, employment, family, finance, friendship, health, housing, partnership, recreation, religion, and transportation (Mallard et al. 1997). Income and safety are particularly noteworthy (Burchardt 2005; Nielsen and Smyth 2008). Life satisfaction has contributed to intelligence, job commitment, marriage, political participation, social cohesion, social networking, volunteering, and voting (Chan 2014; Flavin and Keane 2011; Luhmann et al. 2013; Schaie 2013; Yoo and Jeong 2017). As such, life satisfaction demonstrates the enabling effect of the goal attainment function for social involvement. Life satisfaction has also strengthened support and trust for society and polity, such as democracy (Chan 2014; Chen and Zhong 1998). This strengthening reflects the adaptation function of fair exchange involving the society or polity.

Financial or economic satisfaction is a vital indicator of utility (Vera-Toscano et al. 2006; Yu and Chiu 2016). This satisfaction appears to be the most important to represent life satisfaction (Wan 1992). Income satisfaction is particularly crucial (Obucina 2013; Zagorski 2011). Financial satisfaction has facilitated budgeting and self-control (Sahi 2017). This facilitation manifests the goal attainment function of enabling and facilitating. Moreover, financial satisfaction has fostered political participation (Lee and Lee 2019). This influence reflects the adaptation function of returning the favor and the goal attainment function of enabling. Accordingly, financial satisfaction based on a polity contributes to support for the polity.

Autonomy or having a free choice and control over life is a crucial life quality feeling emphasized by discourses on capability, existentialism, liberalism, neoliberalism, and postmodernism. Capability discourse regards autonomy as essential for the capability to uphold democracy and well-being (Laruffa 2020). Alternatively, autonomy is an ideal in existentialism (Ryan and Deci 2006). Accordingly, existentialism idealizes autonomy because of godlessness and mortality and thus the absence of destiny and supernatural domination (Cox 2012). Similarly, liberalism and its humanist basis maintain autonomy as relevant and functional for enlightenment in the anthropocentric stance (Zimran 2020). They thus liken autonomy to humanity. Furthermore, neoliberalism highlights the relevance of autonomy to capitalism, its competitiveness, flexibility, individualism, and privatization as opposed to regulation and organization (McLean 2015). In addition, postmodernism emphasizes autonomy in terms of independence and self-help to sustain optimism because others are not trustworthy (McLean 2015). Autonomy also reflects the value of recreation to avert external pressure and alienation (Walker et al. 2001). Eventually, autonomy has contributed to effectiveness and performance in work, participation, and relatedness (Gagne and Deci 2005; Weinstein and Ryan 2010). As such, autonomy is a strength underpinning the function of goal attainment in facilitating work and social life.

Health can be a central life quality feeling covering exercising, fitness, safety, vitality, and the absence of disease, impairment, obesity, physical functioning, sleepiness, symptoms, and the risk of mortality (Baker et al. 2009; Cutler and Lleras-Muney 2008; Hagquist and Andrich 2004; Headey et al. 2001; Thiede and Traub 1997). The importance of health rests on its indication of capability conducive to achievement or functioning (Lelli 2008). Moreover, health is favorable according to discourses on healthism, capitalism, modernization, neoliberalism, pragmatism, social democracy, and utilitarianism (Albrecht 2005; Njoh 2009; Petersen 1996; Tink et al. 2020; Zweifei and Breyer 1997). Healthism treasures or yearns for bodily balance, beauty, consumption, control, fitness, flexibility, and nutrition, as opposed to risk (Arguedas 2020; Halasz 2018; Wiest et al. 2015). To achieve health, healthism advocates personal choice, control, dieting, discipline, management, moderation, and responsibility as opposed to fun and pleasure (Brown 2018; Jaye et al. 2018; MacGregor et al. 2021). Healthism also upholds individualism as opposed to hedonism (Lavrence and Lozanski 2014). Healthism moralizes health and its technology (Arguedas 2020; Brown 2018; Wiest et al. 2015). Healthism arises from anxiety about health, insecurity, risk, medicalization, and decline in religion and particularly salvation (Arguedas 2020; Brown 2018; Harrington and Fullagar 2013; Jaye et al. 2018). Accordingly, medicalization is the social force facilitating and thus raising the concern for health and healthism. Meanwhile, the decline in religion and thus salvation in the afterlife heightens personal responsibility for health. In addition, insecurity and risk uplift personal control and responsibility (Jaye et al. 2018). Healthism thus represents ethics, morality, religion, and even fear of death (Brown 2018; Kristensen et al. 2016; Pelters and Wijma 2016). What is more, healthism also rests on neoliberalism (Luna 2019; MacGregor et al. 2021). Essentially, healthism builds on such neoliberal emphases as activism, calculation, capitalism, choice, consumption, docility, individualism, management, rationality in terms of cost–benefit analysis, self-care, self-control, self-discipline, self-governing, and surveillance (Jaye et al. 2018; Lavrence and Lozanski 2014; Luna 2019; MacGregor et al. 2021; Wiest et al. 2015). The emphases require personal monitoring of health. They also champion the value of health generally (Tink et al. 2020). Relevant neoliberal tenets are accountability, activism, individualization, responsibility, self-care, self-examination, self-governance, self-improvement, and self-management (Inthorn and Boyce 2010; Petersen 1996; Tink et al. 2020). Accordingly, personal care for the personal asset or resource of health is paramount (Ashcroft 2015). In addition, health is a significant modern concern for leisure, recreation, and sport (Njoh 2009; Young et al. 2021). Health is also amenable to and compatible with modern practice, policy, and technological advancement (Albrecht 2005). Furthermore, health is valuable for production according to utilitarian discourse (Zweifei and Breyer 1997). Health has contributed to social cohesion, coping, cultural activity, environmentalist activity, financial transfer, spiritual activity, role diversification, search for meaning, self-enhancement, social activity, volunteering, and voting (Adeola 2000; Ben-Zur 2002; Mitrut and Wolff 2011; Goerres 2007; Immerzeel and van Tubergen 2013; Kazarian and Martin 2006; Scherger 2009; Stalker 2008; Tomich and Helgeson 2002). Hence, health demonstrates the function of goal attainment for activating various personal and social activities.

Analysis of World Values Survey data illustrated that current life quality feelings identified two factors, worry, and delight. Worry consisted of that about the terrorist attack, civil war, war, government wiretapping, inability to give children a good education, losing or job, or not finding a job. Worrying about the terrorist attack was the central one, relating most highly with other worries. Meanwhile, delight consisted of financial satisfaction, autonomy, and happiness. In addition, health and life satisfaction were recent life quality feelings temporally separate from the current life quality feelings.

Among the items of the worry factor, worry about education was the highest ($M = 69.0$, on the 0–100 scale). Other worries with a similarly moderate level were those about losing or not finding a job ($M = 64.4$), terrorist attacks ($M = 61.0$), and war ($M = 60.3$). Lower worry happened to civil war ($M = 55.0$) and government wiretapping ($M = 45.6$). In all, worry was substantial, reflecting various social risks.

Happiness was moderately high and highest among life quality feeling items ($M = 69.6$). Autonomy, life satisfaction, and health were the next highest ($M = 62.3$–67.7). They tended to be functional. In addition, financial satisfaction was somewhat lower at the modest level ($M = 56.4$). Life quality feelings were generally moderately high despite the equally high level of worry (Table 2.1).

Table 2.1 Means, standard deviation, and factor loadings on well-being

Item	*M*	*SD*	Worry	Delight	
Worrying about terrorist attack	61.0	34.0	0.866	0.087	Q184
Worrying about civil war	55.0	35.4	0.857	0.072	Q185
Worrying about war involving my country	60.3	33.7	0.844	0.057	Q183
Worrying about government wire-tapping or reading my mail or email	45.6	35.8	0.563	0.057	Q186
Worrying about not being able to give my children a good education	69.0	32.9	0.475	−0.070	Q182
Worrying about losing my job or not finding a job	64.4	35.1	0.453	−0.089	Q181
Being satisfied with the household financial situation	56.4	25.8	−0.054	0.675	Q59
Having free choice and control over life	67.7	25.2	0.022	0.525	Q55
Being happy	69.6	24.0	0.029	0.507	Q10
Health	62.3	29.1			Health
Life satisfaction	63.5	25.6			Satis

Note % variance explained = 56.4

Social Experiences

Based on World Values Survey data, social experiences consist of economic hardship, neighborhood nuisance, victimization, security, and familial saving. Essentially, experience means a product of learning, independent of one's self-feeling (Bowker 2016). Experience is socially crucial according to discourse on contractarianism, empiricism, feminism, foundationalism, majoritarianism, naturalism, postmodernism, pragmatism, stoicism, and theology including Christianity and Buddhism (Bowker 2016; Janack 2012). Contractarian discourse emphasizes objectivity in suppressing one's self and identity (Bowker 2016). Empiricism asserts the ability and need for one's interpretation with senses (Janack 2012). Feminism avers the preponderance of culture, language, and thus communication (Janack 2012). Foundationalism holds that experience is necessary to represent reality (Janack 2012). Majoritarian discourse downplays selfhood and creativity to uphold democracy (Bowker 2016). Naturalism regards adaptation, compliance, and internalization are natural and entail experience (Janack 2012). Postmodern discourse also downplays the self, emphasizing mediation and self-sacrifice (Bowker 2016). Pragmatist discourse treasures experience for adaptation to the environment while downplaying individualism or the self (Bowker 2016). Stoicism favors the natural as opposed to desire and emotion (Bowker 2016). What is more, Buddhism erases the self and thus buttresses experience (Bowker 2016). Similarly, Christianity deemphasizes subjectivity in favor of experience (Bowker 2016). All these discourses champion experience with nature as opposed to feeling in oneself.

Experience of economic hardship is about inability, insufficiency, maladjustment, and strain in the material, including durables, housing, and service accessibility (Carle et al. 2009; Robinaugh et al. 2016). Such experience has eroded persistence and fomented suicide (Economou et al. 2016; Mirowsky and Ross 2001). These influences reflect the negative side of the adaptation function such that the experience indicates the cost or deprivation to inhibit working and living. Moreover, the experience has undermined support and trust in social and political senses (Blomberg and Kroll 1999; Reeskens and Vandecasteele 2017; Ross and Mirowsky 2009). These influences again illustrate the adaptation function when the experience is a hurt to impede support and trust.

Experience of neighborhood nuisance reflects disorder, deprivation, or problems in the neighborhood. The problems include incivility, poverty, and stresses (Brown et al. 2004; Congdon 2010; Vartanian 1999). More specifically, the problems consist of alcoholism, discrimination, drug sale, interference, and robbery. They contradict smart growth in the neighborhood (Perren et al. 2004). Alcoholism involves binge drinking alcohol (Grzywacz and Almeida 2008). It has provoked aggression and resulted in illness, injury, hospitalization, and various pathologies (Brotchie et al. 2004; Haapanen-Niemi et al. 1999). Alcoholism thus indicates dysfunction in goal attainment due to its debilitating impacts. Discrimination reflects cultural diversity, power distance, maladjustment, and the lack of community in the neighborhood (Oppedal et al. 2004; Outlaw 1999; Petersen et al. 2003; Tsai 2006). Discrimination is justifiable with neoliberal discourse, prizes freedom and marketability (Reid 2013). Accordingly, discrimination reflects the freedom to discount demerits. Such experience has fomented deviance (Berry and Sabatier 2010). The impact suggests the dysfunction in adaptation such that a noxious experience invokes a noxious response. Drug sale or related abuse is a problem characterized by danger, immorality, obsession, compulsion, and illegality (Sussman and Ames 2001). It is also problematic because it perpetuates stress, anxiety, and illness rather than relieving them (Hathaway 2003). These impacts indicate the dysfunction of a drug sale in goal attainment, as drug abuse weakens the ability to maintain health and work. Drug abuse has been accusable for its lack of self-control (Hathaway 2003). Some religions' abuse is also unacceptable (Moiseeva and Pozniakova 2009). Hence, drug sale is dysfunction in integration or conformity to social norms. Similarly, interference and robbery represent crime, which is socially unacceptable and fearful (Waiton 2008). Crime is problematic according to discourses on communitarianism, conservatism, and risk (Waiton 2008). Communitarian discourse condemns crime for its subversion of the community or social relation, which is necessary and valuable for living. Conservative discourse detests crime for immorality or undermining established values and order. In addition, risk discourse regards crime as risky and fearful, thus failing human life. These discourses thus find crimes such as robbery to be dysfunctional in goal attainment and integration. More generally, the disorder has eroded attachment and trust in the community and society (Brown et al. 2004; Ross and Mirowsky 2009).

Experience of victimization includes that in the family as well as oneself. Victimization features arousal, negativity or noxiousness, scarring, and needs for neutralization and readjustment (Russo and Roccato 2010; Shippee 2012). The experience has fomented cynicism, neuroticism, and the valuation of violence (Kirk and Papachristos 2011; Lincoln et al. 2003; Nabi and Horner 2001). These effects indicate the dysfunctions of victimization in goal attainment and adaptation. As such, victimization is debilitating and provokes resistance. Hence, victimization has spurred doping and migration, undercut performance, healthy behavior, and even crime reporting (Hanson et al. 2010; Lineres 2004; Morenoff et al. 2008). Nevertheless, victimization has raised caring and helping (Staub and Vollhardt 2008). This raising suggests the latency or idealistic consistency function of victimization in helping others and oneself. In addition, victimization enlarges perceptions about abuse, deviance, extremity, and risk and their approval (McNeeley and Yuan 2017; Nabi and Horner 2001). These effects similarly illustrate the function of victimization in latency or generalization. Eventually, victimization has raised support for policing, prevention, and punishment but eroded social trust (Olivera 2015). These effects reflect the adaptive function of victimization to call for prevention and distrust others. Victimization invokes neoliberal and prevention discourses (Frazier and Falmagro 2014). The former highlights personal responsibility to tackle victimization, thus championing its adaptive function. Similarly, prevention discourse emphasizes agency and empowerment, focusing on vulnerability and weakness.

The experience of security or safety is functional. It has contributed to civility, postmaterialism, and social capital, and has eroded leftism (Curley 2010; Hraba et al. 2001; Sangster and Reynolds 1996; Williamson 2002). Civility means a concern for collectivity, conformity, conservation, morality, plurality, politeness, publicness, responsibility, and virtue or character (Boyd 2006; Chenoweth 2021; Labigne 2012; Shah and Scheufele 2006; Smyth and McKnight 2013). Postmaterialism means valuing the natural environment and self-expression (Norris 2011). Social capital means resources accessible from social relation (Flap and Volker 2013; Woolcock 1998). Leftism means the ideology favoring redistribution and social intervention (Alesina and Angeletos 2005; Finseraas 2010). The effects of security thus illustrate the adaptation function for fair exchange and resource acquisition. For instance, security helps build social relationships to acquire resources, thus lessening the need for redistribution. Security has also fostered legitimizing, trust, and support for law and the market rather than redistribution and tax (Grimmelikhuijsen and Meijer 2015; Hraba et al. 2001; Houtman 2000; Braithwaite 1998). These effects again reflect the adaptation function of security for fair exchange. Eventually, security has boosted the provision of social support (Pena-Lopez and Sanchez-Santos 2016). This boosting is another manifestation of the adaptation or exchange function of security.

Experience of family saving is functional. Accordingly, saving has eroded egalitarianism, which favors equality (Saunders and Wong 2012). The effect indicates the adaptation function such that saving relieves the need for redistribution to maintain equality. Thus, saving has diminished support for redistribution (Saunders and Wong 2012). In addition, saving has raised aspiration for learning and social trust (Chou 2003; Uslaner 2002). These effects reflect the goal attainment function such that saving enables aspiration and social trust and thus risking. Saving is justifiable with discourses on morality and sustainability (Ribeiro and Soares 2017). That is, saving counts as moral and helpful to sustainability.

Factor analysis of World Values Survey data revealed the four experience factors of economic hardship, neighborhood nuisance, victimization, and security. Economic hardship comprised having no medicine or medical treatment, cash income, and food. Neighborhood nuisance comprised racist behavior, military interfering, drug sale, robbery, and alcohol consumption. Victimization covered that in family as well as oneself. Security contrasted security with unsafety from crime. In addition, family saving was an experience not falling into the four factors.

Among the experiences, feeling secure in the neighborhood was the highest, at a moderately high level ($M = 67.6$). This experience tended to be functional. The next highest was family saving, which was modest ($M = 46.0$). All the others did not reach a modest level. Thus, social experience tended to be low or rather low. The lowest was being a crime victim, which was very low ($M = 6.6$). Comparably low was the experience of family as the crime victim ($M = 7.6$). These experiences did not seem to be functional (Table 2.2).

Table 2.2 Means, standard deviations, and factor loadings on social experiences

Item	*M*	*SD*	hard	Nuisance	Victim		Secure
Gone without medicine or medical treatment that you needed	22.7	30.6	0.791	0.120	0.047	0.057	0.075
Gone without a cash income	27.1	32.9	0.786	0.116	0.030	0.134	−0.005
Gone without enough food to eat	16.6	28.3	0.749	0.162	0.013	0.022	0.118
Racist behavior in your neighborhood	16.3	27.0	0.185	0.781	0.051	0.114	0.046
Police or military interfering with people's private life in your neighborhood	17.9	26.9	0.232	0.665	0.052	0.163	0.141
Drug sale in streets in your neighborhood	24.0	34.5	0.172	0.615	0.093	0.381	0.164
Robberies in your neighborhood	26.3	30.3	0.164	0.502	0.111	0.297	0.392
Alcohol consumption in streets in your neighborhood	34.3	35.3	0.140	0.434	0.083	0.764	0.169
Family saving money	46.9	34.8	0.002	−0.041	−0.029	0.002	−0.003
Family as the crime victim	7.6	26.4	0.026	0.056	0.996	0.051	0.024
You as the crime victim	6.6	24.8	0.055	0.102	0.377	0.035	0.128
Feeling secure in your neighborhood	67.6	25.9	−0.065	−0.085	−0.096	−0.073	−0.484
Felt unsafe from crime in your home	20.0	29.1	0.563	0.165	0.115	0.032	0.462

Note % variance explained = 71.7
Hard = Economic hardship, Nuisance = Neighborhood nuisance, Victim = Victimization, Secure = Security

Practices

Practices or activities consist of private and public ones done privately and publicly, respectively. Private activities include e-activity, learning, spiritual activity, risk aversion, and weapon carrying. In contrast, public activities include active organizational participation, appealing, strike participation, voting, participation in a demonstration for some environmental cause, and giving money to an ecological organization, as given in World Values Survey data.

Private activity rests on privatism, which advocates autonomy rather than openness to the public (Connor and Doan 2021). Privatism is justifiable or reasonable for realizing desire and fairness in support of the market, as facilitated by technology concerning communication and information (Hampton 2016; Pospech 2020). The ideology arises from distrusting the politics and public and colonization and politicization (Cook 2001; Pospech 2020). Privatism stands on liberalism, neoliberalism, and discourse on rights or entitlement (Huber 2012; Lokot 2020; Tapper and Kobayashi 2018). Liberal and neoliberal discourses value the market. Neoliberal discourse additional treasures commercialization, competition, deregulation, and privatization as opposed to state planning and welfare. Meanwhile, the ideology of rights prizes narcissism and selfishness (Cote et al. 2021; Zitek and Jordan 2019). Narcissism upholds grandiosity, self-absorption, and superiority (Cote et al. 2021; Hammond et al. 2014; Moeller et al. 2009). Hence, private activity and privatism realize the function of latency or ideational consistency with liberal, neoliberal, and rights ideologies.

Public activity reflects publicness, citizenship, or civicness (Evers 2009; Williamson 2002; Tomhave 2012). Publicness reflects the concern for collectivity, conformity, morality, and responsibility (Boyd 2006; Chenoweth 2021; Shah and Scheufele 2006; Smyth and McKnight 2013). Such practice is reasonable for the big society, civil society, common good, democracy, and justice to be transparent, open, and public (Coleman and Firmstone 2014; Garred 2013; Jennings and Russell 2019; White 2006). For instance, democracy entails public deliberation, mobilization, participation, and reasoning (Edyvane 2017; Jennings and Russell 2019; Uppal 2021). Publicness also reflects curiosity about public affairs and truth (Smith 2002). In addition, publicness is responsible for relationship building and peacemaking (Smith 2002). These reasons illustrate the goal attainment function of publicness for activating and enabling. Publicness also benefits from technological advancement (Coleman and Firmstone 2014). Thus, publicness again embodies the function of goal attainment or power realization by technology. Furthermore, publicness has sustained favor for fairness and trust in public services (Vera-Toscano et al. 2006). These effects reflect the function of latency or ideational consistency to align attitudes with practice. Publicness also rests on discourses on capability, Christianity, communitarianism, contractarianism, justice, and liberalism. Discourse on capability maintains that publicness realizes and nurtures agency, autonomy, and equality (Laruffa 2020). Christianity treasures the public good and social trust (Hordern 2013). Contractarian discourse presupposes interdependence and advocates common interest and consent (Gerrard 2002; Hordern 2013). Justice discourse emphasizes consent, cooperation, and publicity as opposed to discrimination, prejudice, and segregation (Mason 2012). Liberal discourse embraces sociability, moderation, open-mindedness, plurality, and tolerance (Boyd 2006). Hence, public activity has its latency function basis on some ideologies.

As a private activity, e-activity consists of using the Internet, personal computers, and email. These activities feature anonymity, globalization, immediacy, individualization, interactivity, multimedia, networking, and virtual reality (Caldwell 2020; Dutton 2013; Fuchs 2008; Fullwood 2019; Katz and Rice 2002; Kellerman 2014). Notably, they realize the logic of rhizome as characterized by connection, heterogeneity, and multiplexity (Fuchs 2008). As such, e-activity functions for differentiation, distanciation or stretching across space, globalization, individualization, mobilizing, networking, teamwork, and social capital development (Caldwell 2020; Fuchs 2008; Kellerman 2014; Livingstone et al. 2007; Mesch and Coleman 2007; Norris

2001; Wallace 2016). These functions represent goal attainment or enabling through the work of e-activity. For instance, the feature of networking of e-activity enables and thus reinforces networking at large. E-activity has thus engendered knowledge, leadership, and social capital (Karikari et al. 2017; Katz and Rice 2002; Park and Kaye 2017; Yoo and Jeong 2017). These effects reflect the enabling function of goal attainment. In addition, e-activity has fostered environmentalism, liberalism, neoliberalism, and racism, and depreciated obedience and traditionalism (Norris 2001). Such fostering indicates the latency function to maintain consistency between practice and ideology. Accordingly, e-activity involves environmentalist, liberal, neoliberal, and racist elements rather than traditional ones. Similarly, e-activity has cultivated confidence in knowledge and science, interest in public affairs, support for abortion, business, choice, civil rights, women and their rights, gay rights, pornography, homosexuality, premarital sex, and trust (Jennings and Zeitner 2003; Norris 2001; Robinson and Martin 2009; Settle 2018). The cultivation reflects the functions of latency and integration, maintaining consistency within and across people, respectively. E-activity involves those elements, including knowledge, science, and others. Moreover, e-activity has enhanced the perception of difference (Settle 2018). This enhancement also reflects the heterogeneous and plural nature of the activity, thus the latency function to maintain consistency. Furthermore, e-activity has engendered addiction, civic engagement, following of fashion, protest participation, violence, and volunteering (Chak and Leung 2004; Jennings and Zeitner 2003; Lee and Chan 2016; Miyata et al. 2008; Settle 2018; Wei 2007). These influences reflect the functions of integration and latency through learning and habituation. In addition, e-activity is advisable with communitarianism, existentialism, modernism, neoliberalism, and presentism discourses. According to communitarianism, establishing the community and norm is paramount (Dahlberg 2007). Existentialism emphasizes freedom (Toews 2018). Modernism cherishes self-determination (Toews 2018). Neoliberalism encourages individualization, liberty, networking, and self-responsibility (Fuchs 2008; Toews 2018). Presentism treasures immediacy and promptness (Kellerman 2014). Realizing these ideologies is the function of e-activity in latency or ideational consistency. This function is the functionalist view of e-activity (Fuchs 2008).

As a private practice, learning from various media rests on liberal discourse (Tanggaard 2009). Accordingly, being free to learn rather than receiving compulsion is preferable (Tanggaard 2009). Learning from media is exceptionally functional for globalization, individualization, and postindustrialization (Wood 2010). Postindustrialization notably favors competition, planning, selfhood, and subjectivity as opposed to affiliation, community, and trust (Wood 2010). The function represents that of goal attainment through activating and enabling. However, learning from media is responsible for polarization (Mendelsohn and Nadeau 1996). This polarization results from the integration or norm conforming function of social and thus media influence such that polarized media engender polarized learning. Essentially, learning from media has raised the election decision, evaluation of electoral candidates and parties, perception about issue salience, mistrust, political awareness, information, interest, and participation (Bartels 1993; Goidel and Shields 1994; Iyengar 1990; Katz-Schiavone et al. 2008; Meyer et al. 1998; Moy and Pfau 2000; Semetko and Schoenbach 1994). These effects follow the functions of integration or norm conformity.

As a component of learning from the mass media, watching television represents parasocial interaction crucial for group belonging and identity development (Derrick et al. 2009; Steele 1999). Such watching is functional in upholding enjoyment, meeting the prevailing video culture, and maintaining the status quo (Grindstaff and Turow 2006; Tukachinsky and Eyal 2018; Mutz 1998). They also register the integration function of learning for the person and social system. Specifically, watching television has nurtured authoritarianism, individualism, nationalism, neoliberalism, political knowledge, and racism (Bennett et al. 2000; Coffe and Geys 2007; Hooghe 2003; Norris and Inglehart 2009; Paterson 2008). By contrast, watching television has reduced religiousness (Norris and Inglehart 2009). Watching television has also raised perceptions about crime, violence, and harm due to social welfare (Nabi and Sullivan 2001; Scharrer 2008; Sotirovic 2000). Similarly, watching television has buttressed belief in traditional gender roles, favor for politicians, interest in politics, support for foreigners and rights, and trust in government (Fung and Ma 2000; Hooghe and Kern 2015; Kennamer 1987; Norris 2011; Pattie et al. 2004; Paxton and Knack 2012). However, watching television has raised political alienation and eroded support for censorship and welfare spending, tolerance, and trust in other people (Coffe and Geys 2007; Shah et al. 1999; Sotirovic 2001; Zanin 2017). In practice, watching television has boosted attention to news, cheating, using other media, volunteering, and worshipping idols (De Backer et al. 2007; Moy et al. 2005; Ozbay 2008; Pattie et al. 2004; Wuthnow 2004). By contrast, watching television has dampened affiliating, health behavior, participation in civic and political activities and protest, and reading (Best and Krueger 2002; Signorielli 1998; van der Meer and van Ingen 2009; Wernet et al. 2005). These influences reflect the integration function of learning from television. In addition, they reveal the goal attainment function such that watching television displaces other activities departing from the goal of watching television.

As a private practice, spiritual activity is a kind of personal development that searches for sacredness (Dalby 2006; Kalkstein and Tower 2009; Pargament and Mahoney 2009). Such activity is functional for connection, interpersonal interaction, meaning-making, meaningfulness, networking, optimism, tolerance, transcendence, and understanding (Dalby 2006; Hart and Goldenberg 2008; Hill and Pargament 2003; Kiesling et al. 2006; Miller and Thoresen 2003). This function reflects goal attainment through such activities as searching. Furthermore, spiritual activity has fostered intelligence and artistic ability with age (Wink and Dillon 2003). This growth manifests the goal attainment function such that the activity is productive and developmental. Moreover, spiritual activity has strengthened communitarianism and forgiveness. The strengthening reflects the integration function of the activity in learning about meaning and norms. Conversely, spiritual activity has dampened humor and appreciation of others (Adler and Fegley 2005; Saroglou and Anciaux 2004). Such dampening also reflects the integration function of learning about personal meaning rather than pleasing others. This reflection is because spiritual activity heightens the sense of personal superiority and worth (Shek 2010).

What is more, spiritual activity has sustained studying and volunteering (van Tienen et al. 2011; Wink and Dillon 2003). These effects reflect the latency function in maintaining consistency among the activities. Volunteering is compatible with spiritual activity, notably its search for meaning (Dovidio et al. 2006). Spiritual activity stands on humanism, which emphasizes agency rather than religious determination and fatalism (MacDonald and Friedman 2002).

Risk aversion, as another private activity, presupposes threat experience (Makhanova and Shepherd 2020). Aversion has underlain radicalism and self-defeating humor (Erickson and Feldstein 2007; Soliman et al. 2016). These influences reflect the latency function in maintaining consistency among untoward ideas. Conversely, aversion has diminished prosociality (Collins and Feeney 2004). In addition, aversion has fostered the values of avoidance and protection (Makhanova and Shepherd 2020). These influences also reflect the latency function to maintain consistency among ideas. Moreover, aversion has raised attendance at a self-help group, recourse, and vigilance (Makhanova and Shepherd 2020; Meng and Chen 2014). Conversely, aversion has reduced communication or talking, coping, shopping, and walking (Seaton and Beaumont 2008; Makhanova and Shepherd 2020). All the influences reflect the latency or idea consistency function for deactivation, demeaning, and withdrawal in oneself.

As an isolated private activity, weapon carrying has defense or protection and offense or violence perpetration functions. Protection has encouraged crime reporting (Akers and Kaukinen 2009). The influence reflects the latency function to maintain consistency between protection and crime reporting. Violence is a destructive, harmful, noxious, and unruly means of discharging anger, grievances, and sociopathy (Abrahms 2008; Eatough et al. 2008; Emjaian et al. 2018; Pinker 2011; Pulkkinen 2018; Spitzberg 2013). It stems from catharsis, individualization, media promotion, panic, and self-defense (Bufacchi 2007; Carlton 2006; Littman and Paluck 2015; Petrou and Kandylis 2016; Stott et al. 2017). Its importance rests on its lethality and occasional success (Bufacchi 2007). As such, violence has led to the experience of success (Jasper et al. 2015). This effect reflects the goal attainment function such that violence is an effective force. Meanwhile, violence has fostered tolerance for violence (Markowitz 2001). This fostering reflects the latency function to maintain consistency between practice and attitude. Moreover, violence has escalated crime (Tanner-Smith et al. 2013). This escalation is another manifestation of the latency function. Violence is controversial or even objectionable from consequentialism, conservatism, deontology, and feminism discourse. Consequentialist discourse weighs the cost and benefit of violence, with the destruction of life and resources as costs and liberation and rights assertion as benefits (Bufacchi 2007; O'Boyle 2002). Conservative discourse emphasizes the maintenance of ethics and morality as threatened by violence (Zafirovski 2010). Deontological discourse weighs conformity to duty against extremism (O'Boyle 2002; Spitzberg 2013). Feminist discourse opposes violence, coercion, militarism, oppression, and radicalism and accentuates collectivism and mutual support (Calloni 2016; Forester 2019; Harvie and Manzis 2011). These discourses thus constrain violence through the latency function of rationalization.

As a public activity, organizational participation represents civic engagement and formal social capital (Palmer et al. 2011; Wang and Graddy 2008). The participation has fostered civility, knowledge, and socialist ideology (Gilberbloom and Markham 1995; Marsh 2005; Pattie et al. 2004). The fostering reflects the integration function of learning through organizational participation. Similarly, the participation has nurtured attachment to the community, orientation to charity, support for deliberation, and political and social trust (Geys 2012; Guillen et al. 2011; Jacobs et al. 2009; Sokolowski 1996; Tak 2017). The nurturing again registers the function of learning from the organization. Moreover, organizational participation has weakened the perception of corruption in society (Morris and Klesner 2010). In practice, organizational participation has facilitated choosing, collective action, community and political participation, donation, protest, social cohesion, and voting (Boiney and Paletz 1991; Klandermans and de Weerd 2000; Letki 2008; Marsh 2005; Wang and Graddy 2008; Yip et al. 2007). These effects reflect the goal attainment function such that organizational participation strengthens abilities to enable the practices. Moreover, the integration function also applies as the participation shows the norms to learn the practices. Conversely, organizational participation has reduced alcoholism and cheating (Ozbay 2008). This reduction reflects the integration function to conform to the norm. Participation in an environmental organization, including related demonstrations and donation, arises from and reinforces environmentalism. Environmentalism centers on life from a global perspective (Borne 2009). Such ideology has its ground in the bourgeoisie to eliminate disasters to fulfill postmaterialism, preservation, reflexivity, and responsibility under individualization (Anderson 2010; Goldblatt 1996; Guneratne 2008; Humphrey 2010; Inglehart 1990). Hence, the ideology has adaptation and latency functions to preserve resources according to the rationale. The ideology has enhanced the perception of risk and environmental problems in society (Ojala 2005; Wong and Wan 2011). This enhancement manifests the latency function to maintain consistency between ideology and perception. Moreover, the ideology has sustained welfare support and eroded government trust (Goren 2000; Lubell 2003). These influences also show the latency function to maintain consistency between environmentalism and demand on government. In addition, environmentalism has sustained political participation and protest (Lee and Norris 2000; Norris 2002). This sustaining reflects the latency function as environmentalism typically involves politics (Woodrum 1997). Regarding its justifying discourse, environmentalism stands on consumerism and romanticism. Consumerism advocates the individual's right to identify with environmentalism and consume its supportive commodities (Glasson 2015). Accordingly, consumers need to be resistant the governmental regulation of the environment. Romanticism treasures aesthetics, innocence, nobility, and rights (Dryzek 1997; Foss 2009). It thus holds that the beauty of nature is paramount. Other justifying discourses emphasize cosmopolitanism, sustainability, survival, and discount progress (Dryzek 1997; Guneratne 2008; Seippel 1999). Contrariwise, discourses disputing environmentalism are those upholding anthropocentrism, intellectualism, neoliberalism, and utilitarianism. Anthropocentrism centers on humans rather than nature (Anderson 2010). Intellectualism or rationalism highlights administration, science, and technology to solve environmental problems (Dryzek 1997; Glasson 2015). Neoliberalism treasures liberalization and marketization rather than any regulation favoring environmentalism (Hultgren 2018; Maxton-Lee 2020; Vesalon and Cretan 2015). Utilitarianism is serious about environmentalism's tangible cost and benefit (Varner 2008). According to the latency function of rationalization, these discourses countering environmentalism constrain environmentalism.

Participation in a consumer organization rests on consumerism. Consumerism includes the promotion of desire and favor for capitalism, consumption conspicuously and ethically, expressionism, hedonism, materialism, and neoliberalism (Comor 2010; Glasson 2015; Higgins-Desbiolles 2010; Himes 2007; Jones 2019; Wang 2012; Yngfalk 2016). Neoliberal consumerism particularly emphasizes personal agency, control, access to information, and rights such as to safety (Yngfalk 2016). Overall, consumerism rests on conditions for affluence, competition, fashion, independence, individualization, knowledgeability, marketization, media significance, needs for gratification, identity, and rights, risk, and self-determination (Higgins-Desbiolles 2010; Himes 2007; Stehr 2008; Yngfalk 2016). These conditions and needs promote or spur consumerism. As such, consumerism arises from the workings of such functions as goal attainment based on capability and adaptation to gain utility. Consumerism has thus championed market orientation to consolidate the market economy (Murphy 2000). This consolidation reflects the latency function to maintain consistency among ideas. In addition, consumerism is justifiable with discourses on hedonism, individualism, materialism, neoliberalism, postmodernism, and romanticism (Jones 2019; Slater 2005; Soper 2007; Yngfalk 2016). Hedonism favors consumption for collective and ethical interests and personal interests (Soper 2007). Individualism detests reliance on others, including their charitable provision (Bossy 2014). Materialism values commodities (Jones 2019). More than this, neoliberalism treasures agency, contracting, freedom, transaction, and commodification (Gilbert 2008; Slater 2005; Yngfalk 2016). Postmodernism opposes self-discipline, such as that in consumption (Slater 2005). Romanticism favors the feeling of consumption and downplays the economic cost of consumption (Slater 2005). These discourses represent the rational basis for consumerism according to the latency function of rationalization. Contrariwise, consumerism is questionable in discourses on anti-imperialism, Christianity, communitarianism, leftism, and socialism (Gilbert 2008; Himes 2007; Higgins-Desbiolles 2010; Soper 2007). Anti-imperialism opposes imperialism created by capitalism and commodification (Higgins-Desbiolles 2010). Christianity treasures asceticism such as saving, frugality, and restraint rather than marketing to boost desires (Himes 2007). Communitarianism embraces mutual aid rather than consumption individually (Gilbert 2008). Leftism condemns manipulation in capitalism and commodification (Soper 2007). Similarly, socialism disfavors advertising, exploitation, and oppression (Jones 2019). These discourses constrain consumerism and its associated participation in a consumer organization according to the latency function of rationalization. Participation in a consumer organization would reduce because of the countering discourses that do not rationalize the participation.

Participation in a humanitarian or charitable organization stands on humanitarianism, based on the latency function of rationalization. Humanitarianism appears to be a virtue or deontological duty or principle (Crossley 2020). The ideology prizes caring, dignity, freedom, impartiality, protection, rights or entitlement, and self-determination (Ager and Ager 2011; Bendixsen 2018; Brigg 2018; Hoekstra 2021; Vestergaard 2013). The ideology includes Christian, factivist, pragmatist, and socialist versions. Christian or pastoralist humanitarianism treasures caring, consent, and individualism rather than discipline and responsibility (Mitchell 2017). Factivist accentuates evidence and rationality, such as that about the need for care, as bases for caring (Mitchell 2017). Pragmatist humanitarianism allows for inconsistency and selectivity in caring (Crossley 2020). Socialist humanitarianism emphasizes the state's role in caring as opposed to capitalism (Hirono 2013). Humanitarianism has been conducive to demand on government and support for affirmative action, health spending, and taxation (Barker and Tinnick 2006; Maldonado et al. 2019). These influences reflect the latency function of maintaining consistency between ideology and social attitude. Because of the demand, humanitarianism has raised political alienation or disengagement (Coffe and Geys 2007). Conversely, humanitarianism has weakened support for weaponry (Barker and Tinnick 2006). Humanitarianism has buttressed political and protest participation (Foschi and Lauriola 2014; Li and Song 1992). The ideology and participation are thus compatible, as indicated by the latency function. Discourses supportive of humanitarianism include Christianity, communitarianism, consequentialism, cosmopolitanism, feminism, and rights (Crossley 2020; Haustein 2021; Mitoma and Bystrom 2013; Vestergaard 2013). Christianity upholds universal love and even sacrifice for others (Haustein 2021; Vestergaard 2013). Communitarianism emphasizes mutual support in the community (Crossley 2020). Consequentialist discourse weighs the benefits of humanitarianism (Crossley 2020; Vestergaard 2013). Cosmopolitan discourse advocates commonality and helps across borders. Feminism treasures caring (Mitoma and Bystrom 2013). Rights discourse accentuates the right to receive care and empowerment (Mitoma and Bystrom 2013; Vestergaard 2013). These discourses justify humanitarianism with the latency function of rationalization. By contrast, discourses countering humanitarianism center on liberalism, neoliberalism, and statism (Mitchell 2017; Roepstorff 2020). Liberalism prizes accountability and self-governing (Mitchell 2017). Neoliberalism treasures the market and profit (Mitchell 2017). Statism favors state control and welfare (Mitchell 2017). These countering discourses would undercut humanitarianism and related organizational participation based on the latency function of rationalization.

Participation in a professional organization reveals adherence to professionalism. Professionalism champions its professional accountability, authority, autonomy, bargaining power, calling, collegial control, continuance, disciplining, dominance, efficiency, excellence, honesty, individuation, integrity, normativity, respect, and self-regulation (Chisholm et al. 2006; Evetts 2003; McAulay et al. 2006; Svensson 2006; Vestergaard 2013; Wiseman and Shefler 2001). They serve to enhance professional power according to the function of goal attainment. For the organization, professionalism other demands hierarchy, review of performance, standardization, and target setting (Evetts 2013). Its neoliberal version emphasizes managerialism and uniformity or universalization (Abramov 2016). As such, professionalism rests on credentialism, essentialism, individualism, and managerialism (Carollo and Solari 2019; Evetts 2003; Svensson 2006). Credentialism emphasizes credentials (Evetts 2003). Essentialism posits the centrality of science as opposed to folk knowledge (Carollo and Solari 2019). Individualism sustains the professional as an independent worker (Evetts 2003). Managerialism buttresses management and marketization and denounces any conspiracy against management (Evetts 2003; Svensson 2006). In addition to getting discursive support based on the latency function of rationalization, professionalism exhibits its merits in promoting professional accountability, autonomy, choice, civility, collaboration, complexity, confidentiality, identity, legitimacy, marketing, monopoly, motivation, stability, success, and training (Evetts 2003, 2013; Svensson 2006). As such, professionalism represents power or social status and strengthens professional effectiveness with the goal attainment function.

Participation in an art organization manifests artistic orientation. Such orientation encompasses aestheticism, expressionism, and romanticism (Habb 2011; Wilder 2007). Aestheticism emphasizes disinterest, impersonality, indirection, purposelessness, and randomness. Expressionism highlights decoration, distortion, fun, and inspiration. Romanticism prizes automaticity, autonomy, creativity, imagination, independence, individuality, irony, nature, passion, simplicity, spontaneity, subjectivity, sublimation, and wilderness. Overall, artistic orientation has led to political alienation (Coffe and Geys 2007). According to the latency function, this influence reflects the contradiction between the orientation and political involvement in maintaining consistency among ideas. As such, the function indicates consistency between artistic orientation and political alienation. In addition, artistic orientation is justifiable as a manifestation of culture (Khan et al. 2015). As such, the orientation again fulfills the latency function of cultivation.

Participation in a music organization originates from musical orientation. Such orientation has reduced consumerism (Wansink and van Itterum 2012). This reduction reflects the latency function when the orientation is incongruous with consumerism. The incongruity stems from the emphasis of consumerism on materialism as opposed to expressionism in musical orientation (Wang 2012). Meanwhile, musical orientation rests on neoliberalism, emphasizing autonomy, freedom, distinctiveness, and hedonism (Griffin et al. 2018). Moreover, musical orientation is associated with misery or material deprivation (Haynes and Nowak 2021). The orientation thus has its discursive basis to fulfill the latency function of cultivation.

Participation in an education or learning organization stands on orientation toward learning or studying. Learning or studying is crucial to erase uncertainty and fulfill rationality (Robert and Bukodi 2005). With learning or studying, attachment, commitment, political interest, and support for welfare grow (Bosma et al. 2016; Howe 2010; Schindler et al. 2010; van Riper et al. 2019). The growth reflects the integration function of learning and conformity. Moreover, learning has consolidated political knowledge and religiosity (Howe 2010; Immerzeel and van Tubergen 2013). The consolidation manifests the goal attainment function of production, such that learning produces its products. Furthermore, learning or studying has buttressed political participation and voting (Glanville 1999). Such influences register the integration function of learning. Conversely, learning or studying has impeded childbirth (Huinink and Kreyenfeld 2006). This impeding reflects the displacement of time and effort between activities. The displacement indicates the latency function, such that learning and childbirth are incongruous. Eventually, learning or studying has impeded parenthood and working (Parrado 2005; Vartanian 1999). The impedance reflects inconsistency between learning and the others, considering the latency function. Learning or studying is justifiable with liberal discourse, which opposes compulsion or domination by others (Tanggaard 2009).

Participation in a labor union is justifiable with its functions. The function transpires in the contributions of the participation to class consciousness, job evaluation, and perception of justice (Kalleberg et al. 2000; Simpson and Kaminski 2005; Western 1999). These contributions reflect the integration function of learning through participation. Conversely, the participation has impeded closedness to the supervisor and loyalty (Ervasti 2008; Hodson 1997). These impacts reflect latency function such that the participation is incongruous with closeness and loyalty. Furthermore, the participation has fostered civic and protest activism, political involvement, social cohesion, strike participation, studying, and voting (Bills 2005; Dixon and Roscigno 2003; Hodson 2001; Norris 2002; Rosenfeld 2010; Sing 2004). These effects test on both integration and latency functions in learning and consistency maintenance. Conversely, labor union participation has diminished organizational mobility and turnover (Kapur 1998; Miller and Mulvey 1991). Integration and latency functions again apply to the bonding. Eventually, the participation has strengthened employment as opposed to unemployment, earnings, and party membership (Mincer 1993; Norris 2002; Yankow 2006). The influences reflect production and consistency maintenance's goal attainment and latency functions. Labor union participation rests on socialist discourse, which seeks to heighten labor power (McIlroy 2014).

Participation in a political party embodies partisanship. Partisanship is justifiable as an intermediary in democracy, an exceptionally liberal democracy free of religious influence (Tracy and Hughes 2014; Weber 2021). Moreover, partisanship has strengthened egalitarianism, political knowledge, and values for the family and voting (Goren 2005; Richey 2009; Straughn and Andriot 2011; Urbatsch 2014). Such strengthening reflects the integration function of learning through participation in the party. Furthermore, partisanship has fostered belief in conspiracy, liking for the party, favor for affirmative action, immigrants, rights, and weaponry, political interest, tolerance for immorality, and trust in government (Enders 2022; Goren 2005; Kravitz and Klineberg 2004; Marcus et al. 2000; Paterson 2018; Pearson-Merkowitz and Dyck 2017; Pattie et al. 2004; Prior 2019; Suh et al. 2012). These influences also reflect the integration of learning. Partisanship has furthermore raised attention, choice, civic activity, donation, political awareness, discussion, identification, and voting (Claassen and Povtak 2010; Djupe and Lewis 2015; Echabe et al. 1988; Gil de Zuniga et al. 2017; Hutchings 2003; Marcus et al. 2000; Mcclurg 2006; Soler-i-Marti 2015). These influences reveal the latency function in maintaining consistency. Partisanship is also justifiable with liberal, nationalist, and pluralist discourses (Herman

2021; Weber 2021; Whigham 2019). Partisanship is contributory and integral to liberalism, nationalism, and pluralism.

Participation in a sports organization necessarily involves sport. Sport represents training for dexterity, self-esteem, and skills in playing balls, running, static balance, and dynamic balance (Durbin 2020; Stafford 2000). Such training is enjoyable, typically organized, complying with and fitting norms, and related to career (Hendry et al. 1993; Jodl et al. 2001; Prins et al. 2014; Simpkins et al. 2006). As promoted by the mass media, it is valuable and even virtuous for discipline, entertainment, regulation, and teamwork (Jaeger 2004; Mauro 2020; Tink et al. 2020). Furthermore, sports involvement is treasurable for building achievement, character, communities, efficacy, fairness, popularity, social relations, social status, and visibility (Baron 2007; Crosnoe 2001; Eccles and Barber 1999; Eitle and Eitle 2002; Kavussanu and Roberts 2001; Larson et al. 2006; Shields and Bredemeier 2008). Achievement in sport appears in emotion regulation, goal setting, persistence, time management, and public recognition (Larson et al. 2006). Sport involvement has sustained social trust (Brown et al. 2014; Zanin 2017). This influence reflects the latency function regarding consistency between sport and trust in partners and teammates. Conversely, sports involvement has eroded support for foreigners (Gries et al. 2010). This erosion again reflects the latency function such that sport involves competition with foreigners. Sports involvement has raised bonding, cohesion, and organizational activity (Apinunmahakul and Devlin 2008; Bonaiuto et al. 1999; Guillen et al. 2011). This raise manifests the latency function of sport as a prosocial activity. Conversely, sports involvement has diminished smoking (Luschen et al. 1996). This diminishment reflects the latency function regarding inconsistency between sport and smoking or social disengagement. Smoking is noxious to health and social relationships (Meng and Chen 2014). In addition, sports involvement is justifiable with discourses on Christianity, consumerism, neoliberalism, and Olympism. Christianity favors competition through sports involvement (Tink et al. 2020). Consumerism highlights enrichment and prestige from sports involvement (Moscoso-Sanchez et al. 2015). Neoliberalism treasures achievement, profitability, and utility through sports involvement (Hovden 2012; Darnell 2012). Olympism envisions that sports involvement realizes egalitarianism and other virtues (Darnell 2012). Other discourses consider sports involvement affordable, loyal to the nation, mediatized, mentally sound, natural, and rewarding (Hovden 2012; Shor and Yonay 2010; Stevenson et al. 2008). These discourses establish the basis for sports involvement with the latency function of rationalization.

Participation in a recreational organization embodies leisure or recreational involvement. Such involvement features personal freedom (Wu, Liu, and Wang 2010). It encompasses affiliation, agency, conspicuousness, identity work, self-discipline, self-expression, and status making (Blackshaw 2017; Kyle and Chick 2004). Particularly, individualist recreation emphasizes choice, flexibility, and spontaneity (Rojek 2005). Recreation for liquid modernity features consumption, performance, pleasure, precarity, and self-realization as opposed to compliance and being ethical (Blackshaw 2017). Alternatively, transcendentalist recreation treasures ecstasy, inspiration, and miracles (Blackshaw 2017). Recreation is instrumental to community building, health planning, self-development, or personal enhancement such as identity development, status making, stress reduction, and well-being (Arai and Pedlar 1997; Gershuny 2000; Iwasaki et al. 2005; Kuentzel 2000; Roberts 2004). Hence, recreation realizes the goal attainment function of production with mental and physical energy. Recreation also stands on functionalism, humanism, liberalism, neoliberalism, and post-work discourses. Functionalist discourse maintains that recreation is civilizing and conservative in sustaining adjustment, citizenship, health, self-realization, and social cohesion (Rojek 1995). Humanist discourse posits that recreation realizes freedom and solidarity (Rojek 1995). Liberal discourse states that recreation embodies equality and participation (Tink et al. 2020). Neoliberal discourse emphasizes personal responsibility in recreation. Post-work discourse treasures choice and social capital from recreation (Rojek 2005). In addition, discourse on health promotion and illness prevention extols recreation (Tink et al. 2020). These discourses thus justify recreation with the latency function of rationalization. However, recreation is vulnerable to discourses on cost, efficiency, and industrialism, which champion work and success (Tink et al. 2020).

Participation in a self-help group represents empowerment, social capital, and social connection (Flogheraiter and Pasini 2009; Wituk et al. 2000). The group operates with principles of altruism, analogic thinking, balance or non-leading, commonality, coordination with professionals, community or integration, consensus, consent getting, continuity, decentralization, democracy, encouragement, exchange, flexibility, inclusion, mutuality, non-hierarchy, praising, sharing, self-determination, spontaneity, stability, and strength capitalization (Carlsen 2003; Corrigan et al. 2005; Finn 1999; Gitterman 2005; Glicken 2004; Jagendorf and Malekoff 2000; Laudet et al. 2003; Litwak and Meyer 1966; Steinberg 2004). Among the principles, the principle of strength eliminates stigma, blame, and victimhood (Glicken 2004). Self-help group participation arises from the sharing of problems, the complementarity of mutual help, deinstitutionalization, low cost, economic or financial constraint, and strengths available in participants (Chatwin and Tovey 2004; Hatzidimitriadou 2002; Jagendorf and Malekoff 2000; Lorenz 1998; Wing 2000). This rise illustrates the adaptive response according to the adaptation function. Participation is also a response to demands for community, empowerment, self-acceptance, and self-reliance instead of reliance on elites (Riessman and Carroll 1995). Following the latency function, this is a response to maintain consistency among ideas and practices. The self-help group thus substitutes for familial and community networking, which are declining (Hatzidimitriadou 2002). Moreover, the participation is adequate, such as in empowerment and stigma reduction (Hatzidimitriadou 2002; Lorenz 1998; Norcross 2006; Pistrang et al. 2008). This adequacy verifies the goal attainment function of production. Specifically, the participation has lessened disorder and raised power and skills (Anderson-Butcher et al. 2004; Hatzidimitriadou 2002; Peterson et al. 2001). These effects illustrate the goal attainment function of the participation. The participation has also sustained concern for the group, confidence in coping, enthusiasm, and evaluation of caring, coping, and controllability (Kondo and Wada 2009; Schiff and Bargal 2000). Conversely, the participation has eroded trust in professionals (Mechanic and Meyer 2000; Salzer et al. 1999). In practice, the participation has diminished substance or alcohol abuse, smoking, and reliance on professionals (Cameron 2002; Devine et al. 1997; Hanewinkel and Wiborg 2006; Humphreys et al. 1996). Eventually, participation has reduced homelessness (Devine et al. 1997). These impacts further demonstrate the goal attainment function and latency function in respectively realizing the aim of the self-help group and maintaining consistency with practice. In addition, participation in the self-help group is justifiable with discourses on liberalism, pluralism, and non-hegemony, all emphasizing democracy in problem resolution (Jakimow 2009; Young and Reynolds 2017). These discourses furnish the latency function to rationalize such participation.

Attendance at a religious organization manifests religiosity or religiousness. Religiosity features authoritarianism, community, ethics, ritualism, sacredness, solidarity, strictness, and the supernatural (Donnelly 2013; Grayling 2013; Kalkstein and Tower 2009; Peifer 2010; Stavrova and Siegers 2014). In practice, religiosity functions socially as an axiom and identity through inculcation (Demerath 2002; Gay and Lynxwiler 2009; Wuthnow 2011). Religiosity is valuable for belonging, binding, character building, disciplining, educating, meaning-making, moralizing, regulating, and sharing (De Graaf 2013; Demerath 2002; Haidt 2012; Medvedovski and Allison 2017; Skerkat and Ellison 1999). The values illustrate the integration function of religion for learning and norm conformity. As such, religiosity has cultivated authoritarianism, civility, conservativism, egalitarianism, empathy, familism, hawkishness, knowledge about politics, optimism, patriotism, progressivism, pronatalism, racism, radicalism, responsibility, traditionalism, and values for conformity, helping, marriage, and world betterment (Devos et al. 2002; Diez-Nicolas 2002; Saunders and Wong 2012; Furnham 1997; Harris 1994; Hooghe 2003; Ishio 2010; James and Luo 1999; Jost 2020; Jones and Brayfield 1997; Keyes 2002; Kim and Wilcox 2013; McCright and Dunlop 2008; Pedahzur and Canetti-Nisim 2004; Wuthnow 2004). Such cultivation illustrates the integration function of learning and norm conformity through spiritual activity. Conversely, religiosity has discounted hedonism, humanitarianism, humor, individualism, leftism, liberalism, materialism, nationalism, Postmaterialism, and values for comfort, freedom, money-making, studying, and survival (Barker and Tinnick 2006; Coffe and Geys 2007; Devos et al. 2002; Dy-Liacco et al. 2009; Flouri 2003; Gill 2004; Kunovich 2009; James and Luo 1999; Jou 2011; Saraglou 2004; Shmueli 1999; Wuthnow 2004). These influences show the other side of the integration function in religious learning. Religiosity has sustained perceptions about legitimacy, security, and social harmony (Clemence 2001; Urbatsch 2014). Furthermore, religiosity has buttressed moral judgment, party identification, racial identification, retributive attribution, sexual restrictiveness, support for abortion, benevolence, censorship, charity, civility, compatriots, corporations, euthanasia, freedom, generativity, government, immigrants, marriage, military action, norms, parties, police, punishment, recourse, redistribution, and tradition, and trust in institutions and people (Barker and Tinnick 2006; Brown and Ferris 2007; Devos et al. 2002; Gibson 2013; Hakhverdian and Mayne 2012; Jost 2020; Letki 2006; Nagayoshi and Sato 2014; Saucier and Skrzypinska 2006; Shuman et al. 1992; Sullivan 2001; Wink and Dillon 2003; Woodrum 1992; Zanin 2017). These pervasive influences reveal the integration function in learning from spiritual activity. Conversely, religiosity has weakened support for affirmative action, divorce, gender equality, gun control, homosexuality, highbrow culture, premarital sex, public pensions, universal healthcare, welfare, and women's rights, tolerance, and volunteering motives (Barker and Tinnick 2006; Chappell and Prince 1997; Gilberbloom and Markham 1995; Inglehart and Norris 2003; James and Luo 1999; Jost 2020; Katz-Gerro and Shavit 1998; Lynch and Myrskyla 2009; Saucier and Skrzypinska 2006; Sullivan 2001; Urbatsch 2014). Religiosity has raised civic activism and engagement, cohesion, compliance, coping, donation, emotional expression, environmental protection, forgiveness, health behavior, helping, political participation, role-taking, volunteering, and voting. (Claassen and Povtak 2010; Marien and Hooghe 2011; Kim and Wilcox 2013; Myers and Weeney 2008; Perks and Haan 2011; Phalet et al. 2010; Ravanera et al. 2003; Saroglou and Anciaux 2004; Sherkat and Ellison 2007; Stalker 2008; Wiepking and Maas 2009; Wuthnow 2004). Conversely, religiosity has dampened collective action, consumption, criminal activities, deviance, doping, gambling, protest participation, sexual activity, social interaction, and suicide (Andrews et al. 2015; Ayalon et al. 1993; Corcoran et al. 2011; Duberstein et al. 2004; Guo et al. 2008; Hatch 2007; Skerkat and Ellison 1999; van de Werfhorst and Kraaykamp 2001). The influences mark the integration function of learning from religious attendance. Religiosity is justifiable with discourses on communitarianism, enlightenment, existentialism, teleology, traditionalism, and religionism (Friedman 1992; Grayling 2013; Perlin 2011; von Stuckrad 2013). These discourses affirm the functions of religiosity for community, enlightenment, meaning-making, enacting intelligent designs, and tradition. Existentialism notably emphasizes the ego, freedom, identity, meaning, spontaneity, wonder, awe, reverence, humility, surrendering, and worship toward greatness (Friedman 1992). Teleological discourse holds religion as an intelligent design for the goal attainment function (Grayling 2013). In addition, religiosity is discursively functional for aestheticization, moralizing, recovery, relaxation, solidarity, and understanding of the cosmos (Grayling 2013; Marks 2004; von Stuckrad 2013). These discourses justify religiosity with the latency function of rationalization. However, religiosity is problematic in discourses on behaviorism, feminism, humanism, materialism, modernization, neutrality, scientification, secularization, and socialism (Ager and Ager 2011; Browning and Cooper 2004; Grayling 2013; Haddorff 2000; Schrijvers and Wiering 2018; von Stuckrad 2013). Accordingly, religiosity is antithetical to behavioral, material, modern, and scientific reality. Humanism cherishes autonomy, community, curiosity, intelligence, reasoning, kindness, and responsibility (Grayling 2013). Conversely, humanism denounces the afterlife, myth, and ritual. Alternatively, modernization discourse emphasizes individualization and self-regulation (von Stuckrad 2013). Feminism detests patriarchy underpinning religion (Schrijvers and Wiering 2018). Similarly, socialism prizes working and reject domination (Browning and Cooper 2004; Hjelm 2014). These discourses constrain religiosity with the latency function of anti-religion rationalizing.

Appealing or protest participation is a collective, direct or outright, mobilized, somewhat organized action targeting the authority (Barker et al. 2021; Berman and Wittig 2004; de Costa 2006; Morgan and Chan 2016; Stewart et al. 2012). The action involves dissenting, identification, labeling, persuading, politicizing, and voicing to create a public image (Armony and Armony 2005; DeLuce and Peeples 2002; Pfaff and Kim 2003; Stewart et al. 2012; Wulff et al. 2015). Appealing reflects and reinforces polarization and anti-institutionalization (Stewart et al. 2012). Appealing is functional for democracy, justice, and liberalization because of its immediacy (de Costa 2006; Mooijman et al. 2018; Owen 2017). This function represents the goal attainment function of planned production. Appealing emanates from counter-hegemonic ideology, smartphone technology, urbanization, and the decline in state power, without other opportunities (Bosi and Della Porta 2012; de Costa 2006; Owen 2017). Conversely, appealing diminishes with proletarianization, depriving the material basis for appealing (de Costa 2006). That is, affluence enables appealing. Appealing has fostered flexibility, knowledge, skills, and susceptibility (Opp 1989; Vestergren et al. 2017). The influences reflect the integration function of learning and training through appealing. Conversely, appealing has diminished religiousness (Skerkat 1998). This effect reflects the latency function of the incongruity between appealing and religiousness. Appealing has also raised perceptions about its legitimacy, incentive, and opportunity (Opp and Kittel 2009). These effects reflect wishful thinking with the latency function of rationalization. Similarly, appealing has bolstered appraisal for collective efficacy and injustice, belief in a benevolent and just world, commitment, and favor for radicalization and politicization. These impacts also champion the latency function of rationalization. Furthermore, appealing has escalated attention to politics, impulsive expression, organizing, and political participation (Baumann et al. 2015; Lee and Chan 2008; Vestergren et al. 2017). These escalations again manifest the latency function in maintaining consistency among the practices. Conversely, appealing has eroded religious attendance (Skerkat 1998). The erosion indicates the latency function regarding incongruity between the practices. In addition, appealing is justifiable with discourses on anarchism, cosmopolitanism, humanitarianism, liberalism, populism, radicalism, realism or Machiavellianism, and social justice (Chaitin et al. 2017; Gans 1992; Mantena 2012; Parson 2015; Stewart et al. 2012). Anarchism advocates autonomous criticism against consent, duty, gratitude, and obligation (Gans 1992). Cosmopolitanism fuels appealing by treasuring equality and denigrating differences, exclusion, and hegemony (Rojo 2014). Humanitarianism champions appealing to concerns about disease, hunger, and refugees (Chaitin et al. 2017). Liberalism prioritizes the right to protest due to conscience freedom to remove domination (Drury 2002; Gans 1992; Stewart et al. 2012). Populism also popularizes the right to protest (Kohn 2013; Parson 2015). Radicalism encourages radical action in appealing (Stewart et al. 2012). Realism denied agreement, ideals, and morality, which constrains appealing (Mantena 2012). Social justice discourse emphasizes empowering and violence and downplays cooperation and dialogue (Chaitin et al. 2017). Nevertheless, appealing is questionable according to discourses on conflict resolution, conservatism, familialism, pathology, and statism (Chaitin et al. 2017; Drury 2002; Mantena 2012; Parson 2015; Stewart et al. 2012). These discourses favor the family and state as opposed to conflict and revolution. Notably, pathology discourse chastises appealing as an atavism, regression or barbarism, hysteria, irrationality, mob rule, opportunism, and self-defeating rather than normalcy and peace (Drury 2002). These discourses constrain appealing with the latency function of anti-protest rationalization.

Joining strikes means activism to sabotage work. It is functional as negotiation and support for the labor union (Litor 2019). It is justifiable with constitutionalist discourse, which asserts the right to strike (Litor 2019). However, the strike is objectionable to economic, institutionalist, managerialist, and neoliberal discourses (Litor 2019; Greenberg 2004). These discourses treasure bureaucracy, efficiency, and management and demean cost, labor, and unemployment.

Voting arises in a competitive, politicized situation (Chaney 2014). It is an individual political action rather than a collective one (Aldrich 1993). Voting arises from citizenship, civil society, and democracy (Abelson et al. 1992; Bynner and Ashford 1994; Persell 1997). Notably, democracy emphasizes accountability, citizen empowerment, and legitimacy based on voting (Bennett and Resnick 1990; Joslyn and Cigler 2001). Thus, voting realizes citizenship, civil society, and democracy through the goal attainment function. Voting has contributed to political activism and knowledge (Chaffee et al. 1994; Martinelii and Chaffee 1995; Straughn and Andriot 2011). The contributions manifest the latency function in maintaining politically consistent ideas and practices. Voting has been conducive to the perception of government responsiveness (Mattes and Southall 2004). This influence also stems from the latency function. Likewise, voting has sustained belief in government efficacy, favor for politicians, polarization, support for democracy and urban renewal, and trust in institutional and political sectors such as the government (Ahlfeldt 2011; Beasley and Joslyn 2001; Donovan and Karyn 2006; Finkel 1995; Hakhverdian and Mayne 2012; Marion 2006; Mattes and Southall 2004; Nimmo and Savage 1976). These impacts emanate from the latency function to consistency between practice and attitudes. Furthermore, voting has generated civic, community, political, protest participation, and violence (Djupe and Lewis 2015; Dorff 2017; McVeigh and Smith 1999; Ozbay 2008). Such generation unfolds the latency function in maintaining consistency among practices. Voting draws support from discourses on collectivism or statism, communitarianism, consequentialism, egalitarianism, egoism, liberalism, paternalism, populism, proceduralism, and republicanism (Brennan 2011; Malone 2005; Nyenhuis 2020). Accordingly, voting satisfies personal and collective interests in equal, free, instrumental ways. As such, communitarianism praises voting for consolidating bonding (Brennan 2011). Consequentialist discourse finds voting to contribute to welfare (Brennan 2011). Liberalism states that voting realizes equality, individualism, justice, partnership, privacy, and self-interest (Brennan 2011). Paternalist discourse endorses voting for checking and watching the government (Malone 2005). Proceduralist maintains voting as a necessary procedure in democracy (Brennan 2011). Republican discourse advocates political participation as opposed to subjugation to domination (Brennan 2011).

World Values Survey data reveals four private activity factors: e-activity, learning, spiritual activity, and risk aversion from factor analysis. E-activity comprised using the Internet, personal computer, and email. Learning comprised reading printed magazines, reading daily newspapers, listening to radio news, using the mobile phone, talking with friends or colleagues, and watching TV news. Spiritual activity comprised praying, religious attendance, and thinking about the meaning and purpose of life. Risk aversion comprised preferring not to go out at night and not carrying much money. In addition, weapon carrying did not fall into the four factors.

Among private activities, watching TV news was the highest at a very high level ($M = 81.5$). The next highest activity was not carrying much money, which approached a very high level ($M = 72.6$). Thinking about the meaning and purpose of life, talking with friends or colleagues, and preferring not to go out at night were at a moderate level ($M = 61.9$–65.1). These activities tended to be functional. By contrast, weapon carrying was the lowest and at a very low level ($M = 11.0$). Also close to the very low level were using the email, using the Internet, and reading printed magazines ($M = 22.0$–26.2). These activities did not seem normative or functional to the social system (Table 2.3).

Regarding public activities, World Values Survey Data revealed four major factors: active organizational participation, appealing, strike participation, voting, and two isolated activities, participating in a demonstration for some environmental cause and giving money to an ecological organization. Active organization participation comprised that in an environmental organization, consumer organization, humanitarian or charitable organization, professional association, art, music, or education organization, labor union, political party, sport or recreational organization, self-help group, and religious organization. Appealing encompassed joining

Table 2.3 Means, standard deviations, and factor loadings on private practice

Item	*M*	*SD*	E-activity	Learn	Spirit	Avoid
Using the Internet	24.6	40.5	0.960	0.242	−0.052	−0.025
Using the personal computer	36.9	42.1	0.755	0.231	−0.096	−0.064
Using the email	22.0	36.0	0.729	0.384	0.034	−0.028
Reading printed magazines	26.2	38.3	0.200	0.680	0.021	0.005
Reading daily newspapers	46.9	46.3	0.128	0.616	0.117	−0.003
Listening to radio news	38.6	42.2	0.129	0.444	0.188	0.024
Using the mobile phone	49.2	45.2	0.273	0.425	0.100	0.031
Talking with friends or colleagues	62.3	44.4	0.200	0.419	0.159	−0.018
Watching TV news	81.5	32.1	0.075	0.405	−0.135	0.066
Praying	49.9	40.5	−0.091	0.057	0.952	0.014
Religious attendance	47.1	37.2	−0.089	0.018	0.816	0.013
Thinking about the meaning and purpose of life	65.1	30.6	0.080	0.207	0.297	0.040
Preferring not to go out at night	61.9	48.6	−0.093	−0.050	0.018	0.830
Not carry much money	72.6	44.6	−0.012	0.003	−0.042	0.579
Carrying a knife, gun, or other weapon	11.0	31.3	0.012	0.077	0.077	0.121

Note % variance explained = 57.6
Computer = e-activity; Learn = Learning; Spirit = Spiritual activity; Avoid = Risk aversion

boycotts, attending peaceful demonstrations, and signing a petition. Strike participation combined having joined strikes and joining strikes. Voting comprised that in a local election and national election.

Among public activities, voting in a national election and local elections was the highest, at a very high level (*M* = 88.4 and 86.4). Voting thus tended to be functional or normative. By contrast, all other public activities were very low. The lowest was joining strikes (*M* = 0.1). Other lower public activities were joining boycotts (M = 4.2), attending peaceful demonstrations (M = 6.1), participating in a demonstration for some environmental cause (*M* = 7.1), having joined boycotts (*M* = 8.0), being active in a self-help group (*M* = 8.0), having joined strikes (*M* = 9.2), and giving money to an ecological organization (*M* = 9.4). These activities did not seem normative or functional to the social system (Table 2.4).

Feelings, Experiences, and Practices

Factor analysis of feelings, experiences, and practices in World Values Survey data revealed four second-order factors: well-being, public engagement, stress, and informational activity. Well-being comprised delight, life satisfaction, and health. Delight was a first-order factor comprising financial satisfaction, autonomy, and happiness. Public engagement comprised appealing, strike participation, organizational participation, participation in green demonstrations, spiritual activity, and green donation. Stress comprised insecurity (i.e., the reverse of security), economic hardship, and neighborhood nuisance. Informational activity comprised e-activity and learning. In addition, family saving, voting, weapon carrying, victimization, worry, and risk aversion did not fall into the four second-order factors. Hence, the feelings, experiences, and practices primarily consisted of four major second-order factors and six detached first-order factors.

Among the factors, voting was highest at the very high level (*M* = 86.4). Security, (*M* = 73.6), risk aversion (M = 67.3), delight (M = 66.3), life satisfaction (*M* = 63.5), family saving (*M* = 63.5), and health (*M* = 62.3) were moderately high. These factors tended to be functional, normative, popular, prominent, or sustainable. By contrast, victimization (*M* = 7.1), participation in green demonstrations (*M* = 7.1), strike (*M* = 9.2), and green donation (*M* = 9.4) were extremely low. Additionally, weapon carrying (*M* = 11.0) and organizational participation (*M* = 14.8) were very low. Economic hardship (*M* = 22.2), e-activity (*M* = 23.9), and neighborhood nuisance (*M* = 24.3) were close to the very low level. These low levels signify low functionality or at least normativity or popularity (Table 2.5).

Table 2.4 Means, standard deviations, and factor loadings on public practices

Items	*M*	*SD*	Organ	Appeal	Strike	Vote
Being active in an environmental organization	11.4	26.4	0.791	0.107	0.029	0.014
Being active in in a consumer organization	9.5	23.9	0.766	0.083	0.043	−0.016
Being active in a humanitarian or charitable organization	12.8	28.5	0.763	0.117	0.015	0.027
Being active in a professional association	12.1	27.4	0.715	0.146	0.036	0.027
Being active in an art, music, or education organization	15.0	30.2	0.669	0.144	0.036	0.008
Being active in a labor union	13.0	27.9	0.633	0.135	0.092	0.031
Being active in a political party	15.4	30.2	0.624	0.211	0.080	0.064
Being active in a sport or recreational organization	17.6	32.4	0.612	0.144	0.033	0.001
Being active in a self-help group	8.0	24.1	0.535	0.025	0.076	0.040
Being active in a religious organization	25.4	38.0	0.485	0.164	0.113	0.048
Participating in a demonstration for some environmental cause	7.1	25.7	0.270	0.173	0.191	0.065
Giving money to an ecological organization	9.4	29.2	0.214	0.164	0.076	0.023
Joining boycotts	4.2	20.0	0.116	0.704	−0.026	−0.055
Attending peaceful demonstrations	6.1	23.9	0.166	0.621	0.159	−0.038
Signing a petition	11.2	31.4	0.148	0.586	−0.001	0.018
Having joined boycotts	8.0	27.1	0.117	0.540	0.218	0.048
Having attended peaceful demonstrations	13.6	34.3	0.142	0.494	0.339	0.072
Having signed a petition	20.9	40.7	0.141	0.474	0.145	0.074
Having joined strikes	9.2	28.9	0.140	0.203	0.968	0.045
Joining strikes	0.1	0.4	0.047	0.210	0.705	−0.083
Voting in a local election	86.4	22.2	0.052	0.001	0.007	0.846
Voting in a national election	88.4	21.1	0.029	0.035	−0.026	0.842

Note % variance explained = 52.6
Organ = Active organizational participation, Appeal = Appealing

Summary

Factor analysis of World Values Survey data reveals life quality feelings factors about worry and delight, social experience factors about economic hardship, neighborhood nuisance, victimization, and family saving, private activity factors about e-activity, learning, spiritual activity, risk aversion, and weapon carrying, and public activity factors about organizational participation, appealing, strike participation, voting, and environmental participation, and green donation. Among the factors, voting was the

Table 2.5 Means, standard deviations, and factor loadings on well-being, public engagement, private activity, and stress

Factor	*M*	*SD*	Well-being	Public engage	Stress	Inform
Delight	66.3	19.6	0.820	0.148	−0.057	−0.030
Life satisfaction	63.5	25.6	0.708	0.013	−0.024	0.043
Health	62.3	29.1	0.450	0.104	−0.025	0.117
Family saving	63.5	32.2	0.218	−0.061	−0.158	0.209
Appealing	14.1	26.6	0.013	0.613	0.062	0.188
Strike	9.2	28.9	−0.017	0.579	0.041	−0.012
Organizational participation	14.8	21.5	0.014	0.512	0.129	0.052
Green demonstration	7.1	25.7	0.029	0.481	0.128	0.030
Spiritual activity	56.5	28.7	0.097	0.372	0.257	−0.108
Green donation	9.4	29.2	0.052	0.354	0.020	0.124
Voting	86.4	21.1	0.056	0.225	−0.072	−0.166
Weapon carrying	11.0	31.3	0.015	0.176	0.141	0.002
Security	73.6	22.5	0.204	0.054	−0.676	−0.084
Economic hardship	22.2	26.5	−0.259	0.182	0.570	−0.175
Neighborhood nuisance	24.3	24.6	−0.104	0.290	0.540	−0.016
Victimization	7.1	21.5	−0.001	0.073	0.265	0.076
Worry	59.5	25.9	0.036	0.091	0.213	−0.047
Risk aversion	67.3	40.3	0.040	−0.040	0.130	−0.087
E-activity	23.9	38.0	0.123	0.084	−0.059	0.732
Learning	48.1	30.6	0.148	0.339	0.021	0.499

Note KMO = 0.724, 41.9% variance explained

highest and a very high level, and tended to be normative and functional. Security, risk aversion, delight, life satisfaction, family saving, and health were moderately high, thus appearing to be normative and functional. By contrast, victimization, participation in green demonstration, and green donation were extremely low. Weapon carrying, organizational participation, economic hardship, e-activity, and neighborhood nuisance were also very low. The low level suggests low normativity or functionality.

Chapter 3
Life Quality Production: Theory

For millennia, a person's quality of life or well-being has been a crucial aim for explanation, prediction, and promotion (Howell and Howell 2008). Essentially, life quality is a marker of civilization (Ng et al. 2003), which is, in turn, vital because it is the center for human meaning, identity, dignity, and social order (Collins 2001). As a civilization marker, life quality is personal and socially meaningful to the focus of ethics (Veenhoven 1984). Specifically, clarifying life quality or the good life for promotion has been the mission of ethics. Ethics is essentially an enterprise to develop the good in humans (de Bruin 2016; Koven 2015; Kleinig et al. 2015). Moreover, life quality is an ultimate motivator that induces actions to generate changes (Lai et al. 2007) and is an ultimate and universal goal (Helliwell and Putnam 2005; Lane 2000). For these reasons, life quality focuses on public policy and politics (Diener et al. 2009; Marks and Shah 2005). Such a policy has informed education, development—including sustainable development—and democratization, among others, for advancing life quality (Popovic 2014; Thin 2012). Hence, life quality is the social indicator representing the yardstick for development (Andrews and Withey 1976; Diener et al. 1999). At the same time, well-being or life quality needs advancement because of its inadequacy due to social dysfunction, individualization, risk, and crisis (Cummins et al. 2009; Diener and Suh 1999; Lane 2000). The need also arises from human longevity, which demands quality of life (Veenhoven 2005, 2008). Hence, the value and need for life quality call for research to clarify the predictors or determinants of life quality.

Briefly outlined, life quality refers to a changeable state rather than a stable trait (Haller and Hadler 2006; Luo and Kao 2001). Nevertheless, it is applicable and of concern universally or everywhere and to everyone (Cummins 2000; Meulemann 2010). Accordingly, everyone is conscious and concerned about life quality. Essentially, life quality is not a need, an opportunity (Cummins 2005), or economic welfare (Lane 1991; Sirgy 2001).

Given its nature, life quality has generally been predictive of or influential on actions such as academic performance, decision making, donation, and various activities (Coffey et al. 2016; Guven 2012; Lane 2000; Lyubomirsky et al. 2005, 2006;

C. Cheung, *Production Dynamics for Life Quality in the Incipient 21st Century*,
https://doi.org/10.1007/978-981-19-3827-6_3

Wang and Graddy 2008). It also has had a curvilinear effect on political engagement in terms of increasing and reducing engagement with growth in life quality in lower and higher ranges, respectively (Oishi and Koo 2008). All these actions are socially relevant and generate impacts on society. First, academic performance is crucial to socialization and human development (de Bruyn et al. 2003; Wilson et al. 1997). Socialization is functional for maintaining order and continuity in society (Taylor et al. 2000). Meanwhile, human development is undoubtedly the basis for societal development (Yuan and Han 2003). Donation is likewise crucial for building social capital and civil society (Foster et al. 2001). Social capital, meaning social connection for accessing resources, is laudable for democracy, provision of public goods, social control, and norm observance (Coleman 1988; Holliday and Tam 2001; Narayan and Cassidy 2001). It is also a cornerstone of civil society, which sustains mutual aid without economic incentive and political coercion (Wnuk-Lipinski 2007). Civil society is crucial because it is functional for the protection and integration of people and society (Alexander 1997; Wnuk-Lipinski 2007).

In addition, life quality facilitates the experiences of success, relationships, and family functioning (Oishi and Koo 2008; Lyubomirsky et al. 2005, 2006; Smith and Hamon 2012). These experiences can reflect the proper operation of society. The experiences of success can indicate a societal environment conducive to personal success, relationship building, and family functioning (Buechler 2011; Fingerman et al. 2011; Jasper et al. 2015; Kingsbury and Scanzoni 1993). This environment, in turn, indicates openness, opportunities, support, and good order available in society.

In addition to the rationale based on the value of and need for research on the causes of life quality, prevalent issues in the formation of life quality provide a reason for the research. These issues center on the unpredictability of life quality because of its indeterminate and fuzzy conceptualization (Clark et al. 2008; Veenhoven 2008). Further research is necessary to build on a solid framework about life quality.

Wave 6 of the World Values Survey indicated that the four major concepts of life quality are health and life satisfaction in the past and delight and worry in the present. Delight, in turn, is a combination of happiness, the experience of free choice and control, and financial satisfaction. First, health registers the capability or functioning aspect of life quality, highlighting the power to live and act (Nevariz 2011; Phillips 2006; Tomer 2002). It also upholds the hedonist aspect of life quality, emphasizing normalcy or pleasure as opposed to pain (Ryff 1989). Furthermore, it reflects the humanist aspect of life quality in fulfilling the integral human nature (Kurtz 1988). Similarly, as a basic need to fulfill, health is a component of the need fulfillment approach to life quality (Naverez 2011; Phillips 2006). Second, life satisfaction represents hedonist and eudemonic or perfectionist approaches to life quality to uphold pleasure and fulfillment, respectively (Huta 2017; Keyes 2014; Lewinsohn et al. 1991; Sirgy 2012). In addition, life satisfaction represents the prudential dimension of life quality, which emphasizes deliberate engagement (Sirgy 2012). Life satisfaction also indicates the utilitarian conception of life quality, which emphasizes satisfaction (Peffer 1990; Sirgy 2001). Third, as a component of or antecedent to life satisfaction, financial satisfaction is an indicator of the hedonist dimension of life quality (Ryff 1989). By contrast, control, mastery, or autonomy registers the capability conception of life quality (Phillips 2006; Huta 2017) and indicates the eudemonic or perfectionist dimension of life quality to fulfill human nature (Hounknatin et al. 2014; Huta 2017; Ryff and Singer 1998; Sirgy 2012). Fourth, worry is a negative affect representing hedonist life quality (Huta 2017). It is a negative indicator of the absence of agency emphasized in the prudential dimension of life quality (Phillips 2006). In addition, worry is a negative indicator of a technocratic life quality, which urges creativity, science, and work (Nevarez 2011).

Health, life satisfaction, worry, and delight in happiness, mastery, and financial satisfaction cover a broad spectrum of life quality, including hedonist, utilitarian, prudential, eudemonic, perfectionist, humanist, and capability forms. The most rudimentary traditional form of life quality is the hedonist one, emphasizing good mood and satisfaction (MacLeod 2015; Son and Wilson 2012). Desire or need fulfillment is also a marker of a hedonist good life. Hedonism emphasizes the hot system in the person to enjoy, relax, and feel safe and good (Huta 2017). It treasures affective, emotional, attitudinal, and experiential aspects of life quality, encompassing carefreeness, comfort, consumption, ease, pleasure, enjoyment, relaxation, satisfaction, and freedom (Armon 1984; Huta 2017; MacLeod 2015; Phillips 2006; Sirgy 2012). Conversely, a hedonist life quality means the absence of pain, depression, anxiety, stress, and strain (Huta 2017). Hedonism emphasizes momentary present, real-time, and tangible life quality (Huta 2017; Sirgy 2012). It is also egocentric in enhancing oneself (Huta 2017; Phillips 2006). The utilitarian perspective of life quality is a refinement of the hedonist one, highlighting the satisfaction of desire or preference (Carson 2000; Haybron 2008). Income, consumption, purchasing power, material acquisition, life satisfaction, and happiness are utilitarian life quality elements (Nevarez 2011; Peffer 1990; Phillips 2006; Sirgy 2001). More advanced or sophisticated life quality is prudential life quality, which presupposes deliberation and rationality (Phillips 2006; Sirgy 2012; Tomer 2002). Emphasized in prudential life quality are accomplishment, autonomy, self-determination, engagement, agency, liberty, flow, relation, self-aspect, aspiration, and understanding, including self-knowledge, knowledge about the world, and being in touch with reality (Phillips 2006; Sirgy 2012; Tomer 2002). Eudemonic life quality presumes good personal functioning to be prosocial in living (Haybron 2008; Ryan et al. 2008). It treasures a cold system in the person that does not build on pleasure (Haybron 2008; Hute 2017). Cherished in eudemonia is accomplishment, aliveness, authenticity, autonomy, mastery, growth, relation, purpose, self-acceptance, awe, balance, competence, connection, contemplation, creativity, curiosity, elevation, engagement, excellence, expressiveness, integration, justice, meaningfulness, mindfulness, moderation, rightness, self-actualization, virtue, and vitality (Hounknatin et al. 2014; Hute 2014; Kimiecik 2011; McDowell 2010; Phillips 2006; Ryff 2013; Ryff and Singer 1998; Waterman 2008). More than fulfilling human functioning is the perfectionist desire to achieve the best in the person (Sirgy 2012). The perfectionist strand emphasizes autonomy, capacity, cognitive complexity, development, effectiveness, morality, meaningfulness, productivity, purpose, control, relation, and self-esteem (Sirgy 2012). Eudemonia and perfectionism also build on the humanist dimension of life quality, which presupposes personal responsibility and prioritization of needs (Kurtz 1988; Nevarez

2011). Unfolded in humanism is the life quality of accommodation, appreciation, affirmation, atheism, benevolence, community, creativity, fairness, growth, philosophy, health, integrity, intelligence, intimacy, learning, meaningfulness, motivation, rationality, self-actualization, self-discipline, tolerance, trustworthiness, and understanding (Hightower 1988; King 2001; Kurtz 1988; Nevarez 2011; Sheldon and Kasser 2001). Humanist good life also emphasizes being, which includes beauty, honesty, completion, grace, justice, self-sufficiency, self-validity, simplicity, truthfulness, and wholeness (Maslow 1999). Sprouting from eudemonia, perfectionism, and humanism is the capability or functioning view of life quality, highlighting human potentiality (Nevarez 2011; Phillips 2006; Tomer 2002). This view includes affiliation, health, control, play, practical reasoning, imagination, choice, engagement, work, freedom, mobility, nourishment, self-help, and education (Nevarez 2011; Phillips 2006; Sirgy 2001; Tomer 2002). The view also highlights an advanced form of capability or functioning in accomplishment, balance, clarity, commitment, discipline, harmony, integrity, purpose, serving, and wisdom (Tomer 2002). Hence, the various strands of life quality are not mutually exclusive. They overlap and converge to specify life quality elements for gratification, fulfillment, perfection, humanizing, and functioning. Health, life satisfaction, delight, and no worry are among the elements.

Health covers fitness, vitality, and physical functioning (Headey et al. 2001; Uchino et al. 2001; Yanez et al. 2009). Conversely, health means the absence of symptoms, impairment, disease, obesity, and mortality risk (Cutler and Lleras-Muney 2008; Svebak et al. 2004; Thiede and Traub 1997). It applies to the person's various parts or aspects, including the heart, mouth, and weight (Hadden et al. 2003; Halvari and Halvari 2006; Uchino et al. 2001). Health also implies healthy behavior or practice, including exercising and healthcare for preventive or curative purposes (Culter and Lleras-Muney 2008). Conversely, health means the absence of alcoholism, cigarette smoking, drug abuse, and dieting (Culter and Lleras-Muney 2008). Health can depend on perception or subjective judgment (Farone et al. 2008; Staudinger et al. 1999). Such a health self-assessment has become more popular and essential as it negatively predicts morality (Sullivan 2003). Health is not purely an objective, technical measure (Staudinger et al. 1999).

Health is undoubtedly important considering the rationale of capability (Lelli 2008). It is a basic capability for human living, action, and functioning. Furthermore, health is justifiable with the utilitarian concerns for consumption and production (Zweifel and Breyer 1997). Hence, it is also a primal utility for maintenance and pursuit. In this connection, health has shown many contributions to other aspects of life quality. Accordingly, it has contributed to or constituted hedonist and eudemonic life quality (Son and Wilson 2012). Health has contributed to positive affect and satisfaction, including life satisfaction, financial satisfaction, marital satisfaction, and family satisfaction (Cramm et al. 2012; Guo and Huang 2005; Koromeckyj-Cox et al. 2007; Plagnol 2011; Zotti et al. 2016). Health has also contributed to mastery, self-esteem, social life quality, and a sense of community (Carr and Friedman 2005; Jorgensen et al. 2010; Schieman 2001; Son and Wilson 2012). Conversely, health has prevented anxiety, depression, and loneliness (Koromeckyj-Cox et al. 2007;

Young et al. 2001; Yu and Chiu 2016). It has likewise affected many behaviors. Notably, health has facilitated voting, volunteering, social cohesion, environmentalist activism, social activity, cultural activity, spiritual activity, and search for meaning (Adeola 2000; Goerres 2007; Immerzeel and van Tubergen 2012; McClelland 1982; Scherger 2009; Son and Wilson 2012; Tolsma et al. 2009; Tomich and Helgeson 2002). Nevertheless, health has also been a risk factor for alcoholism (Chumbler et al. 2000). It has discouraged medical service use, including visiting physicians (Headey and Grabka 2007; Kirby and Kaneda 2005). Nevertheless, it has also discouraged civic engagement (Groot et al. 2007). Moreover, health has shown more fundamental impacts, such as contributions to socioeconomic status, saving, insurance coverage, and the number of children (Chakrabarty et al. 2008; Gross and Brammli-Greenberg 2004; Mulatu and Schooler 2002). Conversely, health has prevented poverty, divorce, and welfare reception (Dekkers 2008; Gao et al. 2009; Yang and Yen 2012). Indeed, health has numerous implications for the person and society through behaviors.

Life satisfaction implicitly encompasses satisfaction with life domains, including health, friendship, education, transportation, religion, living partnership, employment, housing, finance, family, and recreation (Mallard et al. 1997). Hence, it is associated with health and financial satisfaction owing to the part–whole relationship. Moreover, satisfaction is inherently associated with goal attainment, hope, and optimism (Pavot et al. 1998).

Life satisfaction has myriad implications for oneself and society. Undeniably, it has been conducive to life quality, including health, outlook, and self-efficacy (Celso et al. 2003; Corcoran et al. 2011; Oishi et al. 2000; Rocke and Lachman 2008). Conversely, life satisfaction has eroded loneliness (Neto and Barros 2003). It has also activated political participation, Internet use, social cohesion, volunteering, and voting (Bengtson et al. 1994; Chan 2014; Plavin and Keane 2011; Yoo and Jeong 2017) while discouraging civic engagement and collective action (Corcoran et al. 2011; Sonderskov 2011). Life satisfaction has also prepared for political interest, support for democracy and foreigners, and trust in government and other people (Chan 2014; Chen and Zhong 1998; Rochelle 2015). However, it has raised prejudices (McLaren 2003). Life satisfaction has consolidated intelligence, leftism, and radicalism (Plutzer 1997; Schaie 2013) but has discouraged divorce (Yang and Yen 2012). All these impacts on oneself and society are crucial.

The sense of control, controllability, or mastery overlaps with or is synonymous with agency and competence (Ohmer 2007; Gan et al. 2004; Lu and Kao 2002). It is associated with empowerment, learning, and resource availability (Itzhaky and York 2000; Papadopoulos et al. 2013; Sargent-Cox et al. 2015). Its importance lies in its contribution to adaptation (Sargent-Cox et al. 2015). Essentially, the contributions of mastery are myriad. To the person, mastery has sustained happiness, health, mental health, and life satisfaction (Helson and Srivastava 2001; Judge et al. 2002; Sargent-Cox et al. 2015). Notably, mastery has raised the perception of quality in the neighborhood (Greenberg 1999) and has sustained physical activities (Sargent-Cox et al. 2015). It has also prepared for commitment and social trust (Burke and Stets 1999). Meanwhile, it has discouraged leftist support (Helson and Srivastava 2001). Notably, mastery has buttressed functioning, studying, and acquiring economic resources (Conger and Conger 2002; Hostetler et al. 2007; Sargent-Cox et al. 2015).

Worry is a negative emotion that falls into hedonist life quality. It is conceptually like agitation (Higgins 1998). It represents arousal and signifies danger, uncertainty, irrationality, and vigilance (Alonso-Arbiol et al. 2007; Zeidner and Matthews 2011). Thus, worry is physiologically indicatable or detectable (Zeidner and Matthews 2011). The danger is likely to be unspecified, diffused, uncertain, formless, distal, and future. Worry is of concern because of the danger and signal for disorders and social problems (Bouton et al. 2001; Cheng and Cheung 2005). Hence, it can target various problems, such as crime, death, illness, cancer, inequality, unemployment, unsafety, violence, missing out, and loss of self-esteem (Blackwell et al. 2017; Faunce 2003; Fridberg and Kangas 2008; Kuper and Nicholl 2004; McCabe et al. 2016; Rothstein and Uslaner 2005; Ruiter et al. 2004; Vuori 2015; Wilson et al. 2012; Zhong 2010). Worry can also apply to various life domains, including the environment, finance, government, health, job, school, interpersonal relations, reality, and sexuality (Best and Krueger 2010; Cichy et al. 2007; Cyranowski and Andersen 1996; Hellevik 2003; Young et al. 2001; Zeidner and Matthews 2011). Qualities or experiences such as attachment, attractiveness, competence, dating, interest, and other people can also be targets for worry (Nielsen et al. 2017; Peter and Valkenburg 2007; Reed and Selbee 2003; Rossi 2004a; Wilson et al. 2012). Moreover, worry is noteworthy because of its susceptibility to social construction or a shallow form of socialization, which may exaggerate risks, usually through mass media (Hubbard 2003).

Worry is notable because of its consequences on the person and society. It is detrimental to life quality (Baumeister et al. 2013; Dobewall et al. 2013). Specifically, it raises depression and loneliness (Gillath et al. 2005; Linares et al. 2016) and impairs health, life satisfaction, marital quality, and social life quality (Litman et al. 2017; Pfattheicher et al. 2017). Fundamentally, worry engenders psychopathology, valuation of threat, and curiosity (Christian et al. 2017; Litman et al. 2017; Mogg and Bradley 1998). Conversely, it impedes humor and intelligence (Ackerman and Wolman 2007; Kuiper and Nicholl 2004). In addition to affecting the predispositions, worry raises support for police spending, prison spending, treatment spending, and redistribution (Cohen et al. 2006) while weakening liking and strengthening prejudice (Harwood et al. 2005). In practice, worry breeds avoidance, blaming, dysregulation, prevention, Internet use, protection, recourse, violence, and even suicide (Atkeson and Maestas 2012; Blackwell et al. 2017; Bish and Michie 2010; Dutton et al. 2016; Lee-Baggley et al. 2001; Leung et al. 2005; Meng and Chen 2014; Nielsen et al. 2017; Pulkkinen et al. 2009). However, it likewise encourages commitment and volunteering (Faunce 2003; Reed and Selbee 2003). Conversely, worry inhibits donation, political choice, political participation, prosocial behavior, and sexual activity (Best and Krueger 2010; Marcus and MacKuen 2001; Piliavin and Callero 1991; Rossi 2004a; Zhong 2010). All these practices make a difference in society.

Functionalist Explanation for Life Quality

Functionalist theorizing based on the Parsonsian analytical scheme is helpful to understand life quality. The analytical scheme breaks down every entity into four constituents corresponding to the four functions of goal attainment or fulfillment, adaptation, integration, and pattern maintenance or latency (Parson 1968; Munch 1987). These functions result from the conjunction of two dimensions, namely, internal/external and instrumental/consummatory ones. Essentially, any function is to sustain the whole or system through internal and external and instrumental and consummatory workings. Fulfillment is the consummatory and external function to discharge energy or drives to attain goals. Adaptation is the instrumental and external function to be calculative to reap benefits. Integration is the consummatory and internal function to consolidate components. Latency is the instrumental and internal function to fit ideals. In the social context, fulfillment is to exert power and drive to realize potentialities. Adaptation involves calculation to optimize gains. Integration highlights conformity to social norms or other people. Latency is to maintain consistency with ideas, ideals, ideologies, beliefs, values, attitudes, and the mind or consciousness.

Life quality is composed of four components corresponding to the four functions of adaptation, fulfillment, integration, and latency. The adaptation component of life quality is present in hedonist and utilitarian life quality to optimize benefits, pleasure, fun, consumption, satisfaction, income, wealth, security, and safety (Huta 2017; Son and Wilson 2012; Waterman 2003). Hence, happiness, life satisfaction, health, and worry belong to the adaptation component. Meanwhile, the fulfillment component corresponds to humanist, eudemonic, and perfectionist life quality, emphasizing autonomy, benevolence, fairness, mastery, and self-actualization (Kurtz 1988; Nevarez 2011; Ryff et al. 2003; Tomer 2002). Hence, control, mastery, autonomy, and freedom represent the fulfillment component. In addition, life quality has the integration components of social integration, conformity, assimilation, harmony, and connectedness, which define social life quality (Giddens 1984; Huta 2017). Life quality also consists of the latency component to maintain cognitive or conceptual integration or self-connectedness, as preached in existentialist life quality (Hightower 1988; Huta 2017; Thin 2012).

The analytical-functionalist approach represents a mega theory for expounding life quality as well as numerous psychosocial elements (Fararo 2001; King 2011; Lackey 1987; Munch 1987, 1988; Parsons 1968; Savage 1991; Seidl and Normann 2014; Turner 2013). To be complete, the meta-theory comprises voluntaristic and deterministic parts. The voluntaristic part specifies internal forces for meeting the four requisite functions of goal attainment or fulfillment, adaptation, integration, and pattern maintenance or latency. These functions involve the four causal mechanisms of realization, optimization, conformity, and consistency maintenance or rationalization. Meanwhile, the deterministic parts specify external forces to influence through coercion, manipulation, channeling, and structuring.

Voluntaristic Mechanism of Realization

The voluntaristic mechanism of realization highlights the internal forces of power, energy, drive, habit, inclination, need, motive, and resources to exert influences for attaining goals or fulfilling one's nature or trait (Munch 1987). For instance, aggressive power, motive, or aggressiveness drives aggression. A more general example is that resources afford or facilitate actions. The causal mechanism thus relies on an internal driving or propelling force mechanically or hydraulically. The mechanism incorporates explanations based on power, resources, drive, motivation, need, personality, emotion, and arousal. It depicts the processes of discharging, venting, driving, predisposing, precipitating, enabling, and affording. Notably, the mechanism incorporates the conflict view, highlighting power and its differential and struggle as determinants. Generally, the mechanism posits that resources, power, and traits facilitate consumption, stress relief, attainment of desirable goals, and fulfillment of potentialities, with all these constituting life quality (Diener and Fujita 1995; Malinowski 2014; Parks et al., 2014; Sirgy 2012; Stavrova 2014). The most obvious driving force is the trait of life quality, happiness, or health to maintain or perpetuate life quality (Haller and Hadler 2006; Lindenberg 2001; Luo and Kao 2001). Another way is to translate one resource into another resource, which is life quality, consisting of happiness, satisfaction, and health. This manner just obeys the principles of conservation, displacement, and hydraulic action. For example, the simple logic suggests that income leads to spending for consumption to maintain health and gratification (Ackerman et al. 1997; Clark et al. 2008).

The realization mechanism posits that life quality results from internal forces, habits, traits, needs, drives, and resources oriented toward or facilitating life quality. These internal forces include activity factors such as interesting hobbies, exhilarating activities, and volunteering, which are rewarding to oneself (Sirgy 2012). The forces also include those stemming from attachment, which provides security and, in turn, is gratifying (Mikulincer and Shaver 2014). Moreover, the forces spring from pleasant emotions that broaden and build thinking and thus the ways to achieve life quality. (Malinowski 2014; Nickerson 2007; Parks et al. 2014). Specifically, positive emotions sustain adaptive coping, savoring, and resource acquisition to enjoy life and attain life quality. The forces also include capabilities, such as health, income, and knowledge to constitute or translate into broader life quality (Sirgy 2012). Specifically, cognitive capability includes positive thinking and realization of reward (Diener and Lucas 1999). Other cognitive capabilities include attention, computation, coping, knowledge acquisition, and self-regulation (Matthews 1997; Tyron 1997). Conversely, having irrational beliefs is cognitive incapability that drives life quality (Sirgy 2012). Capability also includes the construction of a good life consisting of pleasant life events (Leonardi et al. 2005). Moreover, the capability to control, select good experiences, and compensate for loss is helpful (Frazier et al. 2007). Similarly, developing or finding life chances is another realization force (Sirgy 2012). The dialectic capability of synthesis, compromising, and transcendence is relevant (Galtung 2005). Accomplishment consists of realization forces, such as those about life tasks and roles (Sheldon and Kasser 2001). Knowledge and the ability to achieve clarity and meaningfulness and avoid ambiguity represent epistemological, knowledge-based, or conceptual power to realize life quality (Demerath 2012). Adaptability to maintain financial, nutritional, healthy, intimate, safe, and successful conditions is another realization force (Hill and Buss 2008). Realization force for maintaining a set point or equilibrium for life quality includes extraversion, non-neuroticism, income, control, and self-esteem (Cummins 2010; Sirgy 2012). Accordingly, the force of the set point maintains life quality at a level after fluctuation. From the production perspective, realization forces or resources are human capital, social capital, and their combination (Islam et al. 2006). From the humanist perspective, human capital includes responsibility, striving, acceptance, authenticity, autonomy, creativity, humility, humor, intentionality, sympathy, uniqueness, and vision (Rowan 2001; Sheldon and Kasser 2001). Conversely, the perspective maintains that antagonism, defensiveness, and egocentrism are negative human capital indicators. The perspective underlies the realization mechanism that self-actualization determines life quality. Meanwhile, social capital covers friendship or relationship success, which rests on friendliness, extraversion, sociability, vigor, and conflict resolution skill (Bishop 2015; Kroll 2011). Professional or academic success also indicates human and social capital, which rests on perseverance, optimism, and extraversion (Bishop 2015). Essentially, extraversion and optimism are temperaments conducive to life quality (Diener et al. 1999). From the psychoanalytic perspective, realization forces include catharsis, adaptive ego defense, conscious control, and control over arousal (Greene 1999; Solomon et al. 1991). Specifically, discharge of noxious emotion is salutary. Achieving consciousness about realization to fulfill the reality principle in the psychoanalytic view is crucial. Relatedly, investing in reality in creative fantasy, mental rehearsal, planning, problem-solving, resting and refreshing, self-motivation, and self-improvement are relevant realization forces (Baylis 2005). Conversely, minimizing the evasion of reality through denial, escapism, isolation, procrastination, and substance abuse is salutary (Baylis 2005). Similarly, self-determination is a basis for life quality, in line with the realization logic (Chirkov et al. 2003; Deci and Ryan 2008; Gountas et al. 2012; Niemiec and Ryan 2014; Sirgy 2012). Self-determination hinges on the satisfaction of needs, comprising those for autonomy, competence, and relatedness. The influence of self-determination is thereby an influence of habit. Generally, resources such as age, education, income, wealth, homeownership, and physical functioning are also realization forces. Conversely, deprivation, including its absolute and relative forms, propels ill-being or impedes well-being (Stavrova 2014). Furthermore, personality is the general predisposing, realizing force shaping life quality (Lakey 2014). The realization mechanism hinges on the production of life quality with resources and endowments (Lindenberg 2001).

According to the realization mechanism, health, specifically, is a realization or a resource and endowment. A realization or driving force stems from material resources associated with a socioeconomic class (Muntaner and Lynch 2002). Conversely, exploitation and deprivation are forces that impair health. Relative deprivation arising from social comparison is the driving force that produces ill-health (Pham-Kanter

2009). Meanwhile, whereas resources sustain health, resource loss particularly jeopardizes health (Hobfoll and Schumm 2002; Vincens et al. 2018). Biological or physiological resources or capabilities are bases for health realization (Kiecolt-Glaser et al. 2002). In this junction, stress, illness, and age are driving forces that weaken health, given the deterioration of the immunological function. The realization mechanism also posits that health maintenance depends on the maintenance ability. Hence, skills in processing and handling health information and executing health behaviors are important driving forces for health maintenance (Fisher and Fisher 2002).

Life satisfaction has its driving forces according to the realization mechanism. The most fundamental of these forces are genetic and personality factors that predetermine life satisfaction (Richards 2016). From the evolutionary perspective of adaptation, the capabilities to meet needs and take opportunities are driving forces to realize life satisfaction (Welzel and Inglehart 2010). Alternatively, livability, including income, comfortable living conditions, and fulfillment of basic needs, is a realization force for life satisfaction (Diener and Biswas-Diener 2002; Saris 2001; Schyns 2001). Such needs concern food, water, housing, work, environment, healthcare, security, relationship, and education (Camfield and Guillen-Royo 2010). The social-democratic regime that facilitates livability helps construct life satisfaction (Radcliff 2001). Conversely, deprivation, notably relative deprivation, including that in income and status, drives life satisfaction downward (Brockmann et al. 2009; Firebaugh & Schroeder 2009). Unemployment and inflation underlying deprivation are driving forces countering life satisfaction (Zotti et al. 2016). Additional resources relevant to life satisfaction include marriage or partnership and cognitive, emotional, and social ones (Rettig et al. 1999; Soons et al. 2009). Social capital, involving the social connection for accessing resources, is a social resource sustaining life satisfaction (Kroll 2011).

Worry has its specific realization forces. It results from stress, pressure, (over)stimulation experienced, power imposed, and uncertainty (Forte 2001; Pollio et al. 1997; Zeidner and Matthews 2011; Ungar 2001). These pressing forces also emanate from loss, separation, and insecurity concerning resources or other valuable things (Nielsen et al. 2017; Rosen and Schulkin 1998; Zeidner and Matthews 2011). Social integration, conversely, provides security and resources to avoid worry (Vuori 2015). Physically and mentally, relaxation reduces tension or worry (Zeidner and Matthews 2011). Cognitive (executive) functioning is a driving force to inhibit worry (Degnan and Fox 2007). Inability in the cognitive functioning or information processing that creates biases or distortions engenders worry (Hogg and Bradley 1998; Zeidner and Matthews 2011). Conversely, the cognitive ability to simplify, restructure, and decenter drive out worry (Beck and Emery 1985; Zeidner and Matthews 2011). In turn, cognitive ability sustains behavioral techniques, including those for relaxation, self-regulation, coping, and graduated tolerance or acceptance, to inhibit worry (Zeidner and Matthews 2011). Psychic conflict involving sex or libido, mortality, and other drives is a driving force for worry (Baumeister et al. 2013; Pollio et al. 1997; Zeidner and Matthews 2011). Conversely, psychic repression and other defenses drive out worry. Physiological factors are critical driving forces for worry (Neal et al. 2002). Notably, smiling and verbalizing drive out worry (Neal et al.

2002). Conversely, illness impairs physical functioning and fuels worry (Bouton et al. 2001). The experiences of threat, hindrance, humiliation, and impairment are apparent driving forces for worry (Zeidner and Matthews 2011).

Voluntaristic Mechanism of Optimization

The voluntaristic mechanism of optimization serves the adaptation function to gain from the external environment (Munch 1987; Parsons 1968). This mechanism upholds the utilitarian goal to achieve desires and satisfy needs. The characteristic force of the mechanism is that of gravitation, attraction, pulling, fascination, infatuation, or incentive. Nevertheless, the force stems from calculation, rational thinking, or rationality, in appraisal according to personal standards. The mechanism thereby highlights the influence of gain expected or realized. Gain that is more valuable or required is more influential. Such value or requirement declines with existing gain or endowment. That is, (additional) income is less valuable, required, or influential in the presence of high income or wealth. Hence, gain can be material or non-material based on appraisal. Generally, the optimization mechanism posits that perceived or expected gain from life attracts commitment to and enjoyment of life in terms of health maintenance, life satisfaction, and delight as opposed to worry, thus maintaining life quality. Such commitment and maintenance are worthwhile for perpetuating the gain. In other words, maintaining life quality represents support for life as a reciprocation to gain, to gain continuously from life (Yamaoka 2008).

The optimization mechanism suggests that life quality results from the utility of life quality or gain or benefit minus cost in life. Essentially, life quality due to gain is higher when the gain is more valuable. In terms of the value of life quality, the utility has buttressed life quality appraisal (Welzel 2013). Meanwhile, gain can happen from an increase in food, income, reward, power, intimacy, sexual activity, marriage, offspring, security, safety, knowledge, capability, success, fitness, life chance, friendship, social support, and resources (Bishop 2015; Cummins 2010; Guven and Sorensen 2012; Hill and Buss 2008; Malinowski 2014; Mikulincer and Shaver 2014; Namini et al. 2010; Sirgy 2012; Turner 2013). Security, in turn, stems from attachment, love, relief, and gratitude (Mikulincer and Shaver 2014; Parks et al. 2014). Receiving support has notably been a typical gain to lift life quality (Deci et al. 2006). Perception about a benevolent or fair world is also gainful and salutary (Oishi et al. 2011; Tomich and Helgeson 2002). Conversely, loss or cost transpires in the experiences of an accident, risk, opposition, divorce, and widowhood (Jasso 2001; Lane 2000; Sabelli and Carlson-Sabelli 1991; Sirgy 2012). Notably, loss is more influential than gain, according to the prospect formulation (Diener and Biswas-Diener 2002). That is, one cares more about loss than about gain. Hence, deprivation, notably the relative form, has been detrimental to life quality (Guillen-Royo 2008' Wang and VanderWeele 2011). Cost has also arisen from incivility, aggression, victimization, and unfair treatment experienced (Andrews and Withey 1976; Graham et al. 2010; Jones et al. 2014; Posel and Casale 2011). Meanwhile, gain crucially hinges on appraisal, which depends on the standard of comparison (Lakey 2014; Schwarz and Strack 1999). Herein, when the comparison standard is high, gain is small, indicating the importance of relative gain (Hagerty 2000; Parducci 1995). When the average or maximum gain of others is higher, one's gain is less valuable. Notably, gain is more valuable when novel and unique (Demerath 2012). More concretely, gain arises from consumption, savoring, and absorption or the experience of flow (Baylis 2005; Parks et al. 2014; Sirgy 2012). Gain also means loss prevention through compensation (Frazier et al. 2007). Need satisfaction or fulfillment, goal attainment, desire fulfillment, and expectation matching also register gains (Arthaud-Day and Near 2005; Bartsch and Oliver 2017; Diener and Biswas-Diener 2002; Nabi and Prestin 2017; Sirgy 2012). Gain is less valuable when it is more abundant. Thus, whereas income is salutary, income squared is demoralizing in the presence of income (Arthaud-Day and Near 2005). Specifically, the linear effect of income is positive, but its quadratic effect is negative. All these gains and related characteristics are conducive to life quality. According to the optimization mechanism, they generate the attraction, gravitation, or pulling force to draw life quality. Gain motivates and justifies the action to maintain life quality.

According to the optimization mechanism, health mainly benefits from several gains, including the experiences of advantage and fairness (Jasso 2001; Scambler 2002). Specifically, reception or experiences of support and health promotion have been salubrious (Halvari and Halvari 2006; Shi 1993), whereas experiences of loss in terms of exploitation and resource loss are debilitating (Hobfoll and Schumm 2002; Muntaner and Lynch 2002) and experiences of earning reduction and deprivation have impaired health (Aytac et al. 2008; Kondo et al. 2008). According to the optimization mechanism, gain from life is encouraging for health maintenance. More relevantly, gain from health maintenance is the attraction force for the maintenance (Blalock 2007; Kasparian et al. 2009; Smith and Stasson 2000). The gain is higher when health problems are more severe and likely because of greater vulnerability and susceptibility (Brewer et al. 2007; Floyd et al. 2000; Smith and Stasson 2000).

The optimization mechanism also indicates that life satisfaction is contingent on several forces of attraction or gravitation. These forces identify the utility or gain from life in terms of justice, livability, including income from various sources and material supplies, economic development, and marriage or partnership (Hagerty 1998; Radcliff 2001; Saris 2001; Schyns 2001; Soons et al. 2009; Tyler et al. 1997). In terms of hedonism and the value of self-esteem, the utility has sustained life satisfaction (Crocker et al. 1994; Datler et al. 2013). Hence, gain in food, water, housing, work, environment, and education is satisfying (Camfield and Guillen-Royo 2010; Salinas-Jimenez et al. 2011). Essentially, the value of gain matters, such that more valuable gain engenders greater life satisfaction (Oishi et al. 1999). Similarly, the need for gain enhances the satisfying effect of the gain (Namini et al. 2010). Importantly, loss exerts a greater impact on life satisfaction than gain (Richards 2016). Loss is particularly dissatisfying, not compensable by satisfaction raised by gain. Moreover, loss or deprivation in a relative sense is dissatisfying (Brockmann et al. 2009). The deprivation can be relative to aspiration and the development or progressive trend (Tyler et al. 1997). Thus, high aspiration or expectation leads to low life satisfaction (Schyns 2000). Alternatively, when the standard for comparison is high, life satisfaction is low (Rampichini and D'Andrea 1998). A comparison with the upper level impairs life satisfaction (Kongarchapatara et al. 2014). Conversely, the relative gain is attractive and satisfying (Firebaugh and Schroeder 2009). In all, gain and its determinants are attraction forces for life satisfaction according to the optimization mechanism.

Considering the optimization mechanism, worry also has its specific attraction or gravitation forces. Such forces emanate from loss in the self, goal, and health (Bouton et al. 2001; Mogg and Bradley 1998; Zeidner and Matthews 2011). The loss can be in terms of risk, danger, threat, interruption, and uncertainty (Mogg and Bradley 1998; Ungar 2001; Zeidner and Matthews 2011). Conversely, experiences of security, hope, good relationships, and social status indicate gains to lessen worry (Arnau 2018; Forte 2001; Nielsen et al. 2017; Pollio et al. 1997). Experiences of gain in terms of social harmony and support have prevented worry (Lee and Robbins 1998; Schwartz and Melech 2000).

Voluntaristic Mechanism of Conformity

The voluntaristic mechanism of conformity hinges on the normative influence or assimilating force to make responses meet social demands or expectations (Munch 1987). This mechanism rests on the premise of the importance and operation of the normatively shared lifeworld. Conformity is socially valuable and indicates social desirability (Willmann et al. 1997). It is typically a virtue (Ulbig 2002) and is instrumentally valuable because it is conducive to social functioning (Opp 2002). Conformity in society thereby pervasively takes the forms of obedience, acceptance, abiding, submissiveness, receiving regulation, community involvement, and even social contribution (Alnsour and Meaton 2009; Ball 2004; Dickson et al. 2009; Hogg and Adelman 2013; Tyler 1998; Ulbig 2002). Hence, perceiving the social norm, requirement, or expectation and conforming to or assimilating with it are the critical factors of the conformity mechanism, which importantly fulfills the integration function. Generally, the conformity mechanism regards life quality because of receiving social influence, persuasion, pleasing, flattering, and guidance for learning and conforming to the norm, request, demonstration, or modeling for life quality (Diener and Lucas 1999; Schuessler and Fisher 1985; Stavrova 2014; Yan 1995). The simplest way to conform is through social contagion when pleasure or life quality transmits among people.

When applied to life quality, the conformity mechanism emphasizes the assimilating forces. The most evident force is the salutary effect of social norm conformity or matching (Stavrova 2014). These forces consist of socializing or social involvement, in which one interacts and shares with others (Bishop 2015; Sirgy 2012). Socializing is salutary because it meets the function of social integration (Son and Wilson 2012). Generally, any attempt to maintain social relationships, harmony, or integration is enjoyable (Baylis 2005). Another assimilating force stems from the reception of psychotherapy, which maintains life quality through conformity to ideas provided (Parks et al. 2014). More generally, matching others' expectations is salutary in fulfilling social integration (Bartsch and Oliver 2017). Similarly, imitation represents an assimilating force for life quality because it pleases others and their support (Diener and Lucas 1999). Additional assimilating forces that are salutary include acceptance, humility, respect, intimacy, openness, sympathy, friendliness, attachment, social networking, and identification (Bishop 2015; Phillips 2006; Rowan 2001). Likewise, performing in socially desirable ways is enjoyable (Schwarz and Strack 1999). Similarly, conflict resolution is pleasurable (Bishop 2015). Conversely, antagonism, egocentrism, defensiveness, and resistance are anti-assimilating forces and demoralizing (Rowan 2001). Discrepancy and deviation from others' expectations or the social norm are also discomforting (Park 2010). One instance is deviance from the norm about the life course, such as late marriage (Clausen 1986). Hence, conformity to or assimilating with others or the social norm typically upholds life quality because it fulfills the function of social integration.

According to the conformity mechanism, health depends particularly on several assimilating forces. Such forces or conformity factors have resided in meeting with kin and/or friends, attending organizations, and religious involvement (Helliwell and Putnam 2005; Mayer 2017; Thoits and Hewitt 2001). Moreover, interpersonal and institutional trust and religiosity have been constituents of conformity to maintain health (Helliwell and Putnam 2005; Hourtado et al. 2011; Mayer 2017). Fundamentally, perception of the social norm for maintaining health has fostered health maintenance (Smith and Stasson 2000). Herein, the perception antedates conformity to the norm. Conversely, deviance (from social norms) and risky behavior have been detrimental to health or its maintenance (Spohn and Kaplan 2000; Umeh 2004). Essentially, conformity and deviance happen to social norms that are wholesome.

Life satisfaction also has its assimilating forces to illustrate the conformity mechanism for buttressing the integration function. These forces have generally applied to communication, socializing, organizational or religious attendance, civic engagement, cultural activity, social networking, social cohesion, and social involvement (Dittman and Goebel 2010; Kroll 2011; Lim and Putnam 2010; Taormina and Gao 2010; Thoits and Hewitt 2001; Winkelmann 2009). These activities essentially presuppose learning and conformity to social norms, which are generally satisfying. Fundamentally, agreeableness, patriotism, and religiosity indicate conformity to social norms and satisfaction (Ambrey and Fleming 2014; Kroll 2011; Selim 2008). Trust in the organization, government, institution, people, and others are precursors to conformity and satisfaction (Abbott et al. 2011; Gehring 2013; Rozer and Kraaykamp 2013; Yamaoka 2008).

Worry also has its assimilating forces concerning the conformity mechanism. Such forces transpire in comments and shaming received and threats to ego from others (Starrin et al. 2009; Zeidner and Matthews 2011). Worry is learnable, depending on learning from and modeling after others (Bouton et al. 2001; Zeidner and Matthews 2011). That is, one's worry can stem from others' worry. The peer norm is particularly influential (Zeidner and Matthews 2011). Networking with optimistic and normal figures has prevented worry, whereas networking with immature figures has fomented worry (Cichy et al. 2007). Hence, the peer norm can shape one's worry through the conformity or contagion mechanism.

Voluntaristic Mechanism of Consistency

he voluntaristic mechanism of consistency (maintenance) emphasizes rationalizing forces to sustain consistency among ideas, cognitions, attitudes, values, beliefs, and/or behaviors. It fulfills the latency or pattern maintenance function to stabilize a deep structure in the mind or the society. Its emphasis is on substantive or value rationality developed through deliberation and reflection. Personality is the typical structure requiring consistency or stabilization (Zhou 2008). With its consistency and stability, personality has been a determinant of life quality (Dy-Liacco et al. 2009). The consistency mechanism, exemplified by personality, maintains rationality in the person (Munch 1988). Generally, it regards life quality because of rationalizing to maintain consistency with beliefs, values, attitudes, behaviors, habits, and conscious personality traits (Maslow 1999; Milbraith 1982; Park 2010; Sirgy 2012). The mechanism suggests that the belief of maintaining life quality, such as health and happiness, is good to make life quality happen. That is, one performs what one believes to be desirable or virtuous. Pro-health and pro-life attitudes are rationalizing forces to maintain life quality. More broadly, ethical ideologies such as hedonism, eudemonism, perfectionism, humanism, and prudentialism are generators of life quality (Diener and Lucas 2000; Guillen-Royo 2008). Apart from the idea of goodness or virtue, ideas about truth, naturalness, value or importance, necessity, and oneself or identity are also constituents of rationalization (Cantor and Sanderson 1999; Demerath 2012; Diener and Fujita 1995; Ferssizidis et al. 2010; Sirgy 2012; Son and Wilson 2012; Suh 2002; Veenhoven 1998). One maintains health because one believes in the goodness, importance, naturalness, and/or meaningfulness of health and/or one regards health to represent oneself. Essentially, the mechanism states that once one finds maintaining health or life quality to be consistent or compatible with one's belief, one will maintain health or life quality.

The consistency mechanism highlights rationalizing forces to sustain life quality to fulfill the latency function. These forces consist in habituation or adaptation, engagement in life including, hobby or interesting activity, learning, planning, mindfulness or awareness, problem-solving, theorizing, working, consumption, and creative activity (Baylis 2005; Cummins et al. 2009; Milbraith 1982; Niemiec and Ryan 2014; Sirgy 2012; van Bruggen 2000). Specifically, ideas or beliefs in resilience, optimism, positive thinking, self-regulation, growth, social order, or the tendency to maintain life quality lead to life quality (Diener and Lucas 1999; Dweck 2012; Matthews 1997; Napier and Jost 2008; Stavrova 2014). For instance, having a stable attribution of success is salutary (Sirgy 2012). That is, endurance and tolerance in life help rationalize life quality. Hence, life quality can grow with time (Sirgy 2012). In addition, holding a positive identity is salutary (Demerath 2012). As a belief in the supernatural and social support, religiosity is also a rationalizing force for life quality

(Stavrova 2014). Holding the personality traits of agreeableness, hardiness, openness, internal control, and emotional stability has been a force to maintain life quality, maintaining consistency between the traits and life quality (DeNeve and Cooper 1998; Hounknatin et al. 2014; Webster et al. 2014). Similarly, holding the ideologies of conservatism or rightist thought has been conducive to life quality because the ideologies support life and the status quo (Borgonovi 2008; Selim 2008). Specifically, favor for various aspects of life, including the community, market, nation, partner, and studying, has introduced a rationalizing force to maintain life quality (Banse and Kowalick 2007; Graham and Pettinato 2002b; Schulz 1995; Selim 2008; Stanley et al. 2011). Likewise, trust in various people and institutions, including the family, bank, government, neighbors, police, healthcare, and people in general, has been conducive to life quality (Abbott and Sapsford 2006; Berry and Welsh 2010; Helliwell and Putnam 2005; Leung et al. 2011). Conversely, having feelings about deficiency and ambiguity generates a rationalizing force that impedes life quality (Demerath 2012; Sirgy 2012). Moreover, engaging in deviance, escapism, procrastination, and drug abuse is detrimental to life quality (Baylis 2005). Holding the traits of psychoticism and neuroticism has eroded life quality given that these traits are contradictory to life quality (Bauer et al. 2005; Furnham and Cheng 2000; Webster et al. 2014). The tendency or preference for rationalization is a rationalizing force to maintain life quality (Napier and Jost 2008).

The consistency mechanism applied to health or its maintenance includes the following factors to illustrate rationalizing forces. Holding the trait of internal control is conducive to health maintenance in maintaining consistency between the trait and the behavior (Smith and Stasson 2000). Similarly, holding an autonomous motivation is consistent with health maintenance (Halvari et al. 2010). Holding the ideology of conservatism is a rationalizing force to sustain health (Borgonovi 2008). Conversely, risking is contradictory and thus detrimental to health maintenance (Umeh 2004).

The consistency mechanism suggests the following factors specifically for sustaining life satisfaction. Favor for modernity, nationality, religion and other life aspects has sustained life satisfaction to rationalize or maintain consistency among the attitudes and satisfaction (Kedem-Friedrich and Maged Al-Atawneh 2004; Selim 2008; Zotti et al. 2016). Life satisfaction has also increased with the values of tolerance, tradition, and self-transcendence, which are not demanding (Appleton and Song 2008; Datler et al. 2013). Similarly, trust in various people and institutions in social, political, government, interpersonal, and organizational aspects has displayed the rationalizing function (Abbott et al. 2011; Brockmann et al. 2009; Kroll 2011; Rozer and Kraaykamp 2013; Yamaoka 2008). The ideologies of conservatism and rightist thought provide rationalizing forces for life satisfaction (Groot et al. 2007; Selim 2008). The traits of appreciation, openness, hedonism, and optimism or positivity have likewise been conducive to life satisfaction (Adler and Fegley 2005; Hahn et al. 2013). Conversely, the traits of neuroticism and pessimism have contradicted and weakened life satisfaction (Ambrey and Fleming 2014; Extremera et al. 2007). Critical belief has been antithetical to life satisfaction (Kluegel and Smith 1986). Moreover, egalitarianism has been discouraging to life satisfaction as society is unlikely egalitarian and is thus dissatisfying (Rozer and Kraaykamp 2013).

For worry, the consistency mechanism suggests the following rationalizing factors. The cognitive factors of exaggeration, uncertainty, vigilance, sensitivity, and prevention focus are consistent with, and thus conducive, to worry (Higgins 1998; Mogg and Bradley 1998; Neal et al. 2002; Zeidner and Matthews 2011). Taking responsibility also contributes to worry (Pollio et al. 1997). Support for the authority has relieved worry, possibly due to the rationalizing process involving trust in and help expected from the authority, which is also a notable source of worry. The practices of avoidance, monitoring, and hygiene maintenance are consistent with and conducive to worry (Cheng and Cheung 2005; Meiser et al. 2000). Conversely, simplification relieves worry (Beck and Emery 1985). The traits of agreeableness, hardiness, humor, and optimism have been rationalizing forces against worry (Beasley et al. 2003; Becker et al. 1997; Kelly 2002).

Deterministic Mechanism

The deterministic mechanism focuses on causal forces external to the person, without emphasis on the person's consciousness and voluntarism. Possibly, the external forces can impinge on the person without the person's awareness and deliberation in conformity or compliance. The forces represent social or structural determinism (Piven and Cloward 2005) to be germane to structural-functionalism. According to the analytical-functionalist view, these social forces comprise the political, economic, community, and cultural (Scholte 1993). Political determinism highlights authoritarian controlling forces by the authority, law, and powerful sources (Munch 1987; Turner 2013). Through coercion, monitoring, channeling, structuring, and arranging, it is forceful. Related to economic determinism is technological determinism or technocratism, as technology is part or based on resources, notably the economic one (Wood 2003). Such determinism also exerts its impacts through facilitation, enabling, empowerment, channeling, and structuring. In addition, it can exert forces indirectly through hiring powerful forces, including political or authoritarian ones (Carlton 2006; Steel et al. 2012). Determinism arising from the community is situational determinism (Billett 2011). Situations can be the home, school, restaurant, washroom, stadium, and foreign country. They are influential through social pressure, guidance, framing, and rules. Generally, social interaction is the key to situation determinism or interactive determinism (White et al. 2008). Apart from the physical field of the community, the symbolic or idealistic field of culture is a source of determinism, that is, cultural determinism. Such determinism or structuralism comprises religious, linguistic, and historical determinism (Carlton 2006; Fall et al. 2004; Lowndes and Roberts 2013; Moller and Skaaning 2013; Ramone 2011). It exerts influences through social construction and, therefore, symbolic or idealistic structuring. All the various forms of determinism exert their influences according to functionalist logic, which maintains that the influences happen because they are functional to the whole system. Accordingly, all the political, economic, community, and cultural establishments and determinism are requisite operations for society.

When applied to life quality, the deterministic mechanism has the following external forces. Among those forces, those closest come from parents, with parental marital discord and parent–child tension impairing one's life quality (Amato and Chendle 2005). Hence, contagion from parents represents the operation of situational determinism. Similarly, sickness and risk within the family have impaired life quality, again manifesting contagion (Kingston and Knight 2006; Lee et al. 2006). At the community level, noise, pollution, and crime are external forces harmful to life quality (Inglehart 1990; van Praag and Ferrer-I-Carbonell 2004; Kingston and Knight 2006). Conversely, social cohesion, societal quality, morale, and safety in the community are external forces facilitating life quality (Cheung and Leung 2011; Wen et al. 2010). At the national level, association, social capital, tolerance, and voluntary work are external forces buttressing life quality (Kim and Kawachi 2007; Veenhoven 2008). All these forces may manipulate or forge life quality even without personal awareness. Concerning cultural determinism, cultural factors include complexity versus simplicity, individualism versus collectivism, and tightness versus looseness (Triandis 2000). Individualist, theistic and Protestant, and national cultures have sustained life quality (Diener and Suh 1995; Inglehart and Klingemann 2000; Suh and Koo 2008), whereas collectivist national culture has impeded life quality (Suh and Koo 2008). Moreover, national-level education has maintained life quality (Lane 2000), which may reflect the support of education for sustaining life quality in the country, as life quality is a desirable goal of education (Izquierdo and Minguez 2003; Vanderstraeten 2003). Specifically, as education promotes life quality, it manipulates and eventually raises life quality. Moreover, the national government, polity, or state has boosted life quality through its governance quality and stability (Della Fave 2014; Helliwell and Putnam 2005). Accordingly, the stable and effective state may be capable of manipulating life quality. Conversely, democracy, liberalism, and openness in the national regime have impeded life quality (Inglehart and Klingemann 2000; Muffels and Fouarge 2004; Veenhoven 2000; Welzel 2013). This outcome is attributable to the low intervention of the state to promote life quality.

The deterministic mechanism wields the following external forces precisely to sustain health. Social class or its arrangement affects health through exploitation and other manipulations (Muntaner and Lynch 2002). The job or productive relation, particularly those in the lower class or manual or menial occupations, is exhausting, wearing, and even debilitating. Residence in the city has also enhanced health maintenance (Lin et al. 2008), suggesting the benefits of urban facilities and other resources. Beyond the individual, the spouse, marriage, or partnership is influential on health through the work and health of the spouse (Stolzenberg 2001). Remarkably, the spouse's education has buttressed health maintenance (Lin et al. 2008). Some contagion or pressure is available in such a context. Physical and sentimental proximity between the couple provides the basis for mutual influence. Family income, assets, or socioeconomic status have promoted health in the broader family context (Beaudoin 2009; Pham-Kanter 2009; Zarychta 2015). Such promotion may be due to facilitation by economic and related resources, including the hiring of healthcare services (Zarychta 2015). Trust within the family has also enhanced health, possibly because trust reflects and invites help to sustain health (Zarychta 2015). Conversely, illness and disability found in the family have impaired health (Chen et al. 2008; Zarychta 2015). Contagion and burden within the family are likely responsible for the influence. At the community level, community development, education, environmental quality, health services, social capital, social cohesion, organizational membership, voting, and trust have shown their benefits to health (Franzini et al. 2005; Fujisawa et al. 2009; Hadden et al. 2003; Lavis and Stoddart 2003; Stafford et al. 2005; Sundquist and Yang 2007). These community factors may provide resources and help for health promotion. Conversely, crime, disorder, unemployment, and racism within the community have been deleterious to health (Franzini et al. 2005; Staffford et al. 2005). These community factors may constrain resources and assistance available for health promotion. The number of physicians and nurses has been conducive to health maintenance (Vargas-Lagos 1991). Education, religiosity, household income, organizational membership, social capital, voter turnout, and trust have displayed their contributions to health (Blakely et al. 2001; Herian et al. 2014; Kim and Kawachi 2007; Helliwell and Putnam 2005). These national factors indicate the resources, motivation, and assistance for advancing health nationally, including compatriots. These deterministic social forces suggest that aggregate resources, motivation, and effort shape personal health, even without personal awareness and voluntarism. Herein, altruism, citizenship, civic orientation, and philanthropy may play critical roles in helping one another to advance health. Biological determinism, emphasizing immunological and genetic factors, is crucially applicable to health (Kiecolt-Glaser et al. 2002). Such determinism, nevertheless, is beyond the scope of social determinism.

The deterministic mechanism applies to life satisfaction considering the following specific external forces. At the interpersonal level, including marriage and partnership, the sense of modernity and life satisfaction have been helpful to personal life satisfaction (Kedem-Friedrich and Maged Al-Atawneh 2004). Contagion and mutual support may be responsible for the interpersonal influence. A sense of modernity means the orientation to maintain health, economic prosperity, and life quality (Davis and Robinson 2001). Conversely, depression has been detrimental to life satisfaction (Groot and Van Den Brink 2003). Similarly, family assets, income, economic condition, and education have been conducive to life satisfaction (Ambrey and Fleming 2014; Christoph 2010; Evans and Kelley 2004; Rampichini and D'Andrea 1998). At the community level, socioeconomic status, trust, particularly social trust, and volunteering have shown benefits to life satisfaction (Dittman and Goebel 2010; Frey and Stutzer 2005; Pattie et al. 2004; Yip et al. 2007). These community forces reflect community support to raise life satisfaction, even bypassing voluntaristic factors. Conversely, deprivation in the community has been deleterious to life satisfaction (Cramm et al. 2012). Resource constraints in the community will thus hinder life satisfaction. In the community at the national level, civic participation, voluntary organization membership, and social capital generally have been satisfying (Helliwell 2006; Wallace and Pichler 2009). Meanwhile, in the cultural aspect of the country, religiosity, civility, and trust, particularly social trust, have upheld life satisfaction (Bjornskov 2003; Bond and Lun 2014; Helliwell 2006; Rozer and Kraaykamp 2013). They may facilitate resource sharing to sustain satisfaction. National demographics characterized by health and youth have contributed to life satisfaction (Helliwell 2006; Rampichini and D'Andrea 1998). They are national resources underlying the satisfaction through sharing and mutual help. In the economic aspect of the country, economic development or condition, employment, and income have exhibited their contributions to life satisfaction (Castles 2000; Gehring 2013; Okulicz-Kozaryn 2012; Rampichini and D'Andrea 1998). Conversely, deprivation, inflation, and unemployment at the national level have been dissatisfying (Bjornskov 2003; Bohnke 2008; Pacek and Radcliff 2008). In the national polity, welfare provision and generosity, government effectiveness, social expenditure, and socialism have been conducive to life satisfaction (Bohnke 2008; Pacek and Radcliff 2008; Radcliff 2001, 2008). Hence, external resources and support are satisfying, and external constraints are dissatisfying because they exert direct impacts to boost or weaken life satisfaction.

When applied to worry, the deterministic mechanism has the following specific external forces. From the dyadic or interpersonal perspective, the imminent external forces stem the parents, partner, spouse, and other relatives. Parents exert forces to control or forbid through protection, parenting, and other rearing practices (Watt and Stewart 2003). Conversely, parents create an atmosphere conducive to worry (Watt and Stewart 2003). Similarly, the partner's worry and control have been external determinants of worry (Cump and Kulk 1997; Cundiff et al. 2015). As such, the partner serves as the source of contagion and manipulation. Such contagion has also stemmed from relatives (Meiser et al. 2000). The ritual has appeared to prohibit worry (Homer et al. 2007). Herein, the ritual serves as a family forced to restrain worry and other emotions. Specifically, it stipulates manners and emotional expressions for dining, gathering, and other activities. At the neighborhood or community level, poverty, disorder, and instability have been external forces creating worry (Ross et al. 2000). A straightforward way is a contagion within the community, such that one worries along with others. Alternatively, the disorder means the absence of other people to prevent worry in the community. Similarly, inflation has increased worry at the national level, whereas economic development has lowered worry (Schwartz and Melech 2000). Improved national conditions would mean that more services are available to prevent worry. Herein, worry is a target for prevention at any level (Bouton et al. 2001; McNally 1990).

Predictors of Life Quality

The predictors of personal life quality include personal and national factors. Personal factors include sociodemographic characteristics, experiences, and practices. Predicting the current quality of life of delight and worry can predict the recent life quality of health and life satisfaction. National factors include those indicating modernization, globalization, and basic living conditions. The effects of these life quality factors represent the statics of life quality production. To reveal the dynamics of life quality production, the effects of time (i.e., the wave of the survey) and its interactions with personal and national factors are additionally essential (Table 3.1).

Table 3.1 Hypothesized functionalist effects on personal life quality

Predictor	FA	AA	IA	LA	D
Wave					+
Personal					
Irreligious				+	
Family income	+				
Female				+	
Age	–				
Age squared		+			
Married	+				
Cohabited	+				
Divorced	–				
Separated	–				
Widowed	–				
Kid	+				
Mother immigrant	(–)				
Father immigrant	(–)				
Education	+				
Graduation age	+				
Interest	+				
Living with parents	+				
Full-time employment		+			
Part-time employment		+			
Self-employment		+			
Retired		(–)			
Homemaking		(–)			
Student		(–)			
Unemployed		–			
Public employment			+		
Private business employment			–		
Nonprofit organization employment			–		
Intellectual work		+			
Creative work		+			
Independent work		+			
Supervision		+			
Earner		(+)			
Earner employed		(+)			
Economic hardship		–			

(continued)

Table 3.1 (continued)

Predictor	FA	AA	IA	LA	D
Neighborhood nuisance		–			
Victimization		–			
Security		+			
Family saving		+			
E-activity			–		
Learning			–		
Verbal involvement		+			
Television watching		+			
Spiritual activity			+		
Risk aversion		+			
Weapon carrying		+			
Organizational participation			–		
Appealing				–	
Strike				–	
Voting				–	
Green demonstration				–	
Green donation				–	
Health	+				
Life satisfaction	+				
National					
Population size					+
Phone per capita					+
Land per capita					+
Technology: scientific and technical journals per capita					+
Credit: domestic credit to the private sector (% of GDP)					+
Prosperity: GPD per capita					+
Income inequality					–
Globalization					+
Government effectiveness					+
Democracy					+
Liberty					+
Human development					+
Human capital					+
CO_2					+

Notes FA = Fulfillment-voluntaristic, AA = Adaptation-voluntaristic, IA = Integration-voluntaristic, LA = Latency-voluntaristic, D = Deterministic

Sociodemographic Characteristics

Sociodemographic characteristics are preexisting and stable attributes, including age, gender, education, parental immigration, marriage, employment, work status or quality, and religiosity. They are likely to shape personal life quality through the voluntaristic mechanisms of power realization, utility rationalization, norm conformity, and idea consistency. Accordingly, the characteristics engender resources, expectations, social experiences, and ideas for the voluntary development of life quality. Notably, age is likely to unfold a quadratic effect on life quality, composed of those from age and its square. In other words, the relationship between age and life quality is likely to manifest a U-curve.

Age. Age is likely to erode life quality, mainly according to the voluntaristic mechanism of power realization. Here, age signifies the decline in resources, power, energy, capability, vitality, controllability, and human capital (Charles and Carstensen 2009; Frazier et al. 2007; Von Krogh and Wallin 2011). Old age means high inadequacy, deficit, disengagement, disconnection, and unfavorable experience (Frazier et al. 2007; Marcum 2013; O'Rand 1996). These have been dissatisfying experiences (Barber et al. 2010; Baumeister et al. 2013). Conversely, age signifies vulnerability, which has been detrimental to life quality (Charles 2010). Hence, age has negatively affected marriage, income, and other social status indicators (Goerres 2007; Plagnol and Easterlin 2008). Low status has induced low life quality (Carrieri 2012; Wen et al. 2010). Meanwhile, the older adult has tended to have low education (Goerres 2007). Moreover, age has weakened abilities and resources, including those about thinking, memorizing, and functioning, affecting stability (Chow et al. 2007; Gerstorf et al. 2006; Herd et al. 2008). Such dysfunction is debilitating (Abbott and Sapsford 2006; Carrieri 2012). Age has likewise increased illness and unsafety and has reduced friendship, social connection, and social integration (Goerres 2007; Schaie 2013; Ziersch et al. 2005). This finding means that older persons receive less support and fewer resources, probably due to stratification by age in society (Carr 2004). This lack of external support or resources has impaired life quality (Abbott and Sapsford 2006; Chan and Lee 2006). Loneliness and helplessness impede life quality. Moreover, age has diminished extrinsic and intrinsic motivation, tolerance, and evaluation of government (Ferssizidis et al. 2010; Goerres 2007). This diminished motivation and evaluation have weakened life quality (Ferssizidis et al. 2010; Moller 2005). In practice, age has also reduced communication, eating, consumption, sleeping, studying, cooperation, gaining, traveling, community activity, cultural activity, leisure activity, political activity, personal care, and pursuit of goals (Frazier et al. 2007; Graham and Pettinato 2002b; Marcum 2013; Tilley 2002). This finding reflects low energy in old age. Consequently, age has bred distress and negative affect and reduced health, identity, self-regard, and self-efficacy (Alea et al. 2004; Caplan and Schooler 2007; Goerres 2007; Sheldon and Kasser 2001). Specifically, age has dampened personal growth and purpose in life (Ryff et al. 2004). That is, the older person has been lower in life quality.

Mid-age. Mid-age is vital as a separate factor because the effect of age may not be a linear one. Life quality can be different between mid-age and older or younger age. Specifically, mid-age is likely to reduce life quality. Life quality is likely to be lower in mid-age than in younger or older. Conversely, the square of age is likely to sustain life quality, primarily according to the voluntaristic mechanism of optimization, which suggests the mid-age person finds or expects a lower gain than the younger or older person. Concerning socioeconomic status, the mid-age person has had lower savings, wealth, and family income than has the other (Anderseon and Nevitte 2006; Keister 2003; van Praag and Ferrer-I-Carbonell 2004). This lower status has decreased life quality (Veenhoven 1984; Obucina 2013). Regarding experience, the mid-age person has had lower affordability, friendship, and social interaction than the younger or older person (Glaeser and Gottlieb 2006; Hallerod 2006; Prouteau and Wolff 2008). Such weakened relationships have eroded life quality (Barrett 1999; Helliwell et al. 2010). Meanwhile, the mid-age person has had higher aspirations and political alienation than the others (Coffe and Geys 2007; Plagnol and Easterlin 2008). A higher aspiration means a greater difficulty to gain and thus a lower gain. Meanwhile, alienation means powerlessness (Coffe and Geys 2007). Hence, aspiration and alienation have impaired life quality (Galtung 2005; Nickerson et al. 2007; Stutzer 2004). Conversely, the mid-age person has had lower social trust, political trust, political appraisal, and support for the market (Hayo 2004; Marien 2011; Traunmuller 2011; Shi 2000) than the others. Mistrust has diminished life quality (Berry and Welsh 2010). For instance, mistrust would lead to worry, thus impairing life quality. In practice, the mid-age person has been less socially cohesive than has the younger or older person (Wilkinson 2008). The lack of social cohesion has eroded life quality (Kahneman et al. 2010). For instance, the lack of social cohesion would mean a lack of achievement in serving society, thus hindering life quality. All these results indicate lower gain from life as expected by the mid-age person. Consequently, the mid-age person has had lower life quality, including health, housing quality, housing satisfaction, leisure satisfaction, financial satisfaction, environmental satisfaction, life satisfaction, and social quality, than has the others (Distante 2013; Fridberg and Kangas 2008; Logan et al. 1999; van Praag and Ferrer-I-Carbonell 2004; van Praag et al. 2003).

Gender. The woman is likely to have higher life quality than the man, primarily due to the voluntaristic mechanism of consistency maintenance. This gender difference is attributable to the socialization or sociocultural influence that promotes gentleness, tranquility, endurance, and complacency in the woman (Guimond et al. 2013; Rundman and Glick 2008). Fundamentally, evolutionary processes have implanted the traits or habits of agreeableness, endurance, deference, and even longevity rather than competition in the woman (Conway and Schaller 2002; Guimond et al. 2013; Hopcroft 2016). In addition, the subordination or oppression perspective suggests that the woman smiles more frequently than does the man (Fischer and Evers 2013). These traits or habits have been conducive to life quality (Cheung and Leung 2011; DeNeve and Cooper 1998; Hounknatin et al. 2014; Webster et al. 2014). For instance, this reflects the case of a more optimistic person being happier. Accordingly, the woman has supported others, including the market and government and its policy, as does the man (Lindh 2015; Morris and Klesner 2010; Rentziou et al. 2011; Wang et al. 2011). Similarly, the woman is more trustful of the government, education, police, medicine, and others (Ahern and Hendryx 2003; Feingold 1994; Hooghe et al. 2015; Moy and Pfau 2000; Sun et al. 2013) and more religious than the man is (Baker and Smith 2009; Immerzeel and van Tubergen 2013). Moreover, the woman has had lower perceptions about problems and risks than has the man (Niemi et al. 1999; Trumbo et al. 2008). All these orientations have been salutary (Graham and Pettinato 2002b; Mattes and Christie 1997; Oishi et al. 2011). Consequently, the woman is higher than the man in life quality indicators such as mastery, self-efficacy, and satisfaction with government, democracy, and life (Dyck and Lascher 2009; Hansen et al. 2012; Tiliouine et al. 2006; Norris 2011; van der Toorn et al. 2010). In all, maintaining consistency among happy and tolerant attitudes, behaviors, and life quality underlies the greater life quality in the woman than in the man..

Education. Education or age at graduation (i.e., an older graduate has higher education) is likely to contribute to life quality considering the voluntaristic mechanism of power realization. Accordingly, education is power in terms of human capital (Dolton et al. 2004; Izquierdo and Minguez 2003). Education can crucially generate great benefits with its explosive and transformative processes and effects (Yair 2003). It enhances discovery, creativity, choice, competition, and confrontation to ensure gains. Specifically, education has upgraded intelligence, memory, general knowledge, political knowledge, and civic skill (Pratt et al. 1996; Verba et al. 1995; Shin 2012; Stevens et al. 2001; Wilson et al. 2012). Abilities and knowledge have been conducive to life quality (Cheng 2003; Diener and Fujita 1995). Possibly, in this case, one knows how to boost happiness. Education has also reduced the experiences of threat, victimization, discrimination, and social exclusion (Backman and Nilsson 2011; Kaukinen 2004; Kessler et al. 1999; Raijman et al. 2003). These experiences have impaired life quality or life satisfaction (Graham et al. 2010; Kirmanoglu and Baslevent 2014). For instance, one feels unhappy when excluded from joining a rejoicing social activity. The moment of exclusion, discrimination, or victimization is also likely to inflict pain on the maltreated person. Conversely, education has facilitated the reception of social support and networking (Cerin and Leslie 2006; Miyata et al. 2008), and the experiences have been salutary (Helliwell and Putnam 2005; Michalos et al. 2005). Conceivably, one rejoices at friendly support from others. Education has also facilitated making choices, exercising, civic engagement, political participation, and preventive action (Chan 2014; Kim and Wilcox 2013; Leung et al. 2005; Morenoff et al. 2008; Stone and Buttice 2010), all of which are demonstrations of power or strength. These practices have also shown their contributions to life quality (Barber et al. 2010; Yang et al. 2012). Specifically, exercising one's power is rejoicing. Education has further enhanced socioeconomic status regarding class and earnings (Pettigrew 2002; Schnittker and Behrman 2012; Whyte and Gao 2009). The status has sustained life quality (Haller and Hadler 2006; Jones et al. 2014; Wang and VanderWeele 2011). Eventually, education has advanced life quality in terms of health, self-efficacy, self-esteem, living standards, and satisfaction, including that with life, safety, and security (Cerin and Leslie 2008; Corcoran et al. 2011;

Emler and Frazer 1999; Jmes and Amato 2013; Whyte and Gao 2009; Yienprugsawan et al. 2010). Conversely, education has prevented distress and depression, thus safeguarding life quality (Al-krenawi et al. 2011).

Parental immigration. Concerning the voluntaristic mechanism of realization or power, parental immigration is likely to lower life quality because of the lack of resources. Such immigration status typically represents a financial deficit, welfare dependency, and marginalization by natives (Boeri et al. 2002; Clune 1998; Portes and Rumbaut 2001). This status also breeds personal harm and inadequacy in skills and earnings (Borjas 1999). Hence, it has engendered functional limitations (Herd et al. 2008), consistent with the immigrant's difficulty in living and adapting to the host society. The status has also resulted in low social capital and a high level of social exclusion (Bask 2005; Fanning et al. 2001). Moreover, it has impeded civic engagement, political participation, social cohesion, and volunteering (Ravanera et al. 2003; Sonderskov 2011; Stromblad and Myrberg 2013). These are manifestations of low power or capability, and they all register the immigrant's adaptation difficulty. Eventually, the status has resulted in unemployment, poverty, and lack of marriage (Kurz et al. 2005; Posthumus et al. 2013; Ravanera et al. 2003; Thornton et al. 2007). All these indicate inadequate resources or capability, which are the bases for life quality (Diener and Fujita 1995; Sirgy 2012). Consequently, the status has generated depression, psychosis, and lower health and life satisfaction (Ambrey and Fleming 2014; Islam et al. 2006; Lofors and Sundquist 2007).

Marriage. Marriage or cohabitation is likely to bring higher life quality than divorce, separation, widowhood, or singleness. This result follows the voluntaristic mechanism of power realization, which states that resources buttress life quality. Crucially, marriage counts as a vital resource to solve social problems (Lichter et al. 2002). Similarly, cohabitation counts as a functional resource (Barlow 2004). Hence, marriage has prevented functional limitations (Li and Chung 2008; Smith et al. 2006), and impairs life quality (Abbott and Sapsford 2006). Meanwhile, it has increased social closeness, friendship, social capital, social networking, social interaction, social integration, and social support (Apinunmahakul and Devlin 2008; Cornwall 2009; Lizardo 2006; Mata and Pendakur 2014; Sampson 1991; Volker et al. 2007). Social capital and related resources have been salutary (Jones et al. 2014; Oshio and Kobayashi 2010). Conversely, marriage has reduced the experiences of discrimination, social exclusion, and victimization (Carr and Friedman 2005; Ross and Mirowsky 2009; Wojcieszak and Mutz 2009). Cohabitation has also reduced social deprivation (Rijken and Groenewegen 2008). These experiences have been debilitating (Delbosc and Currie 2011; Graham et al. 2010). Furthermore, marriage has facilitated such practices as civic engagement, community involvement, consumption, donation, family functioning, neighboring, and political participation (Bednell et al. 2013; Dressler 1991; Flavin and Keane 2011; Kerrissey and Schofer 2013; Magee 2008; Smith and Hamon 2012; Swaroop and Morenoff 2006). These practices have reflected resource abundance or affordability and have shown their benefits to life quality (Appleton and Song 2008; Helliwell et al. 2010; Kroll 2011). Marriage has also led to homeownership and reduced welfare receipt (London 2003; Manturuk et al. 2010). Homeownership and exemption from welfare receipt indicate the resource basis for life quality (Granzin and Haggard 2000; Veenhoven 2005). Consequently, marriage has contributed to health, financial adequacy, self-esteem, relationship quality, and satisfaction with achievement, family, finance, friendship, health, living standards, and life (Bellani and D'Ambrosio 2011; Hou et al. 2015; Koromeckyj-Cox et al. 2007; Lelli 2008; Louis and Zhao 2002; Marks 1996; McMullin and Cairney 2004; Mitrut and Wolff 2011; Yienprugsawan et al. 2010). Cohabitation has also championed life satisfaction (Evans and Kelley 2004; Gudmundsdottir 2013). Marriage or cohabitation is likely to provide support to enhance life quality. Conversely, marriage has prevented depression, fear, loneliness (Akiyama and Antonucci 2002; Koromeckyj-Cox et al. 2007; Moore and Shepherd 2006), and depression (Johnson and Wu 2002; Silverstein and Ruiz 2006).

Employment. Full-time or part-time employment or earning, as opposed to unemployment, homemaking, retirement, and studying, is likely to raise life quality considering the voluntaristic mechanism of optimization. Accordingly, experience or expectation of gain is the gravitational force on life quality. In other words, employment is an intentional way to earn money or other benefits, including social inclusion (Graham et al. 2002; Ravanera et al. 2003). Moreover, employment by an able-body person is socially normative (Clark et al., 2008) and, as such, can gain social approval. The norm tends to apply to women and men (Pfau-Effingere 2012; Sanchez 2007). This application stems from equalizing life chances for women and men (Giele 2008). Meanwhile, expansion of the labor market requires female employment (Barnett and Hyde 2001). Female employment can withstand the economic crisis and concomitant layoff (Sanchez 2007). Regardless of gender, gain from employment has been evident. Indeed, employment has raised personal income (Growiec and Growiec 2010), which has prevented poverty (Fan et al. 2004). Moreover, employment has facilitated insurance and marriage (Anderson and Eamon 2004; de Graaf and Kalmijn 2003) and fostered experiences of friendship, social capital, social support received, and cohesion found in the community (Anciaes et al. 2017; Chang 2009; Groot et al. 2007; Tsai 2006). These are gainful experiences conducive to life quality (Gudmundsdottir 2013; Kim and Kawachi 2007; Michalos et al. 2005; Wen et al. 2010). Conversely, employment has reduced the experiences of stress, social exclusion, arrest, and criminal contact (Allwood and Widom 2013; Brayne 2014; Myer et al. 2008; Ross and Mirowsky 2009). Reduction in such experiences has restored life quality (Baumeister et al. 2013; Delbosc and Currie 2011; Kingston and Knight 2006). Employment has also sustained skill and functional ability rather than vice versa (Kerrissey and Schofer 2013; Li and Chung 2008). For instance, it provides training or practice chances to maintain, refresh, or upgrade skills. These traits are instrumental in attaining life quality (Diener and Fujita 1995; Zotti et al. 2016). Hence, employment contributes to life quality, including health, purposiveness, mastery, personal growth, relationship quality, satisfaction with finance and life, self-acceptance, and self-efficacy (Abucina 2013; Corcoran et al. 2011; Distante 2013; Hansen et al. 2012; Ryff et al. 2004). This outcome illustrates the humanist and neoliberal value of employment in self-realization or demonstrating one's competence and contribution (Walkerdine and Bansel 2010). Conversely, employment has prevented depression, distress, dysfunction, loneliness, powerlessness, and psychosis

(Goldberg and Perry-Jenkins 2004; Keyes 2002; Koromeckyj-Cox et al. 2007; Lofors and Sundquist 2007; Myer et al. 2008; Ross and Mirowsky 2009).

Public employment. Employment in the public or state sector is likely to fare better in life quality than is employment in the business or nonprofit sector or non-employment. Conversely, employment in the nonprofit sector is likely to have lower life quality than the other employment or non-employment. Such variation is explicable by the voluntaristic mechanism of conformity. Accordingly, the nonprofit sector creates a social environment or norm about social problems, inadequacy, failure, and suffering in society and people (Fric 2008; Milligan and Fyfe 2005; Perotin 2001). This sector is thus prone to take a conflict perspective to reveal problems in society (Fric 2008). Moreover, employees in this sector are likely to locate and work with disadvantaged people, thus witnessing adversity and distress (Milligan and Fyfe 2005). Hence, employment in the nonprofit sector takes the norm to redress problems in society (Freund 2005). By contrast, the public sector creates a social environment or norm about order, security, prosperity, progress, and success in society (de Jonge 2012; Knittila and Kubit 2000; Spicker 2013). Moreover, public employment is more rewarding in job security and others than employment in another sector (Kurz et al. 2005; Tung and Yang 2006). This difference relies on the voluntaristic mechanism of optimization. Hence, public employment has buttressed optimism and trust (Atkinson 2013; Brewer and Sigelman 2002), which are conducive to life quality (Abbott and Sapsford 2006; Magalette and Oliver 1999) and are also likely to lead to the public employee's higher caring, volunteering, and civic engagement (Sarasa 2008; Rosenfeld and Richman 1997; Wilson and Musick 1997). These practices foster or reflect life quality (Chang 2009; Kroll 2011; Muffels and Fouarge 2004).

Work quality. The quality of working conditions in terms of independence, creativeness, intellectuality, and status is likely to be salutary because of its gainfulness. This effect follows the voluntaristic mechanism of optimization. Work independence reflects individualization as a feature of work quality (Bauman 2001). It has contributed to life satisfaction and pride (Hodson 1996; Kelly and Kelly 1994), which are parts of life quality (Huta 2017; Khattab and Fenton 2009). As another feature of work quality, creativeness at work has been pleasurable (Henderson 2004). Intellectuality at work, as opposed to manual work, represents a higher class (Layte et al. 2000). Such a working condition has higher earnings, upward mobility, and life satisfaction (Blanchflower and Oswald 2000; Dieckhoff 2007; Knight and Song 2005). Conversely, intellectuality at work has reduced work stress, control imposed, and social isolation (Bian et al. 2005; Gallie et al. 1998; Jones 2001). Thus, intellectuality at work is gainful. As another work quality indicator, occupational status or class has facilitated social support reception, social capital, and friendship (Lennartsson 2010; Wuthnow 2004). These experiences have been salutary (Borgonovi 2008; Kim and Kawachi 2007; Michalos et al. 2005). Conversely, intellectuality at work has prevented stress, social exclusion, illness, insomnia, economic hardship, and deprivation (Green et al. 2014; Pettigrew 2002; Muhlau 2014; Stansfeld and Marmot 1992). These experiences have been debilitating (Baumeister et al. 2013; Carrieri 2012; Gudmundsdottir 2013; Oshio et al. 2011). Hence, the status or class has secured life quality, including health, financial adequacy, hope, and satisfaction with distribution, finance, life, and welfare (Davis and Davenport 1999; Haller and Hadler 2006; Kangas 2003; Hadjar and Samuel 2015; Peterson and Seligman 2004; Vera-Toscano et al. 2006; Yamaoka 2008). Conversely, the status or class has prevented depression and death (Burke 2008; Dahl 1993). As an indicator of social class, the supervisory role has sustained social capital, friendship, and social status (Whyte and Gao 2009; Wuthow 2002). These experiences have been conducive to life quality (Gudmundedottir 2013; Kim and Kawachi 2007; Salinas-Jimenez et al. 2011). It has also safeguarded life satisfaction and self-efficacy (Corcoran et al. 2011; Rampichini and D'Andrea 1998). Work quality has generally contributed to satisfaction with the job, friendship, leisure, and social status (Sirgy et al. 2001). All these factors manifest the gain from work quality or status.

Religiosity. Sociodemographic characteristics are preexisting and stable attributes, including age, gender, education, parental immigration, marriage, employment, work status or quality, and religiosity. They are likely to shape personal life quality through the voluntaristic mechanisms of power realization, utility rationalization, norm conformity, and idea consistency. Accordingly, the characteristics engender resources, expectations, social experiences, and ideas for the voluntary development of life quality. Notably, age is likely to unfold a quadratic effect on life quality, composed of those from age and its square. In other words, the relationship between age and life quality is likely to manifest a U-curve.

Age. Age is likely to erode life quality, mainly according to the voluntaristic mechanism of power realization. Here, age signifies the decline in resources, power, energy, capability, vitality, controllability, and human capital (Charles and Carstensen 2009; Frazier et al. 2007; Von Krogh and Wallin 2011). Old age means high inadequacy, deficit, disengagement, disconnection, and unfavorable experience (Frazier et al. 2007; Marcum 2013; O'Rand 1996). These have been dissatisfying experiences (Barber et al. 2010; Baumeister et al. 2013). Conversely, age signifies vulnerability, which has been detrimental to life quality (Charles 2010). Hence, age has negatively affected marriage, income, and other social status indicators (Goerres 2007; Plagnol and Easterlin 2008). Low status has induced low life quality (Carrieri 2012; Wen et al. 2010). Meanwhile, the older adult has tended to have low education (Goerres 2007). Moreover, age has weakened abilities and resources, including those about thinking, memorizing, and functioning, affecting stability (Chow et al. 2007; Gerstorf et al. 2006; Herd et al. 2008). Such dysfunction is debilitating (Abbott and Sapsford 2006; Carrieri 2012). Age has likewise increased illness and unsafety and has reduced friendship, social connection, and social integration (Goerres 2007; Schaie 2013; Ziersch et al. 2005). This finding means that older persons receive less support and fewer resources, probably due to stratification by age in society (Carr 2004). This lack of external support or resources has impaired life quality (Abbott and Sapsford 2006; Chan and Lee 2006). Loneliness and helplessness impede life quality. Moreover, age has diminished extrinsic and intrinsic motivation, tolerance, and evaluation of government (Ferssizidis et al. 2010; Goerres 2007). This diminished motivation and evaluation have weakened life quality (Ferssizidis et al. 2010; Moller 2005). In practice, age has also reduced communication, eating, consumption, sleeping, studying, cooperation, gaining, traveling, community activity, cultural activity, leisure activity, political activity, personal care, and pursuit of goals (Frazier et al. 2007; Graham and Pettinato 2002b; Marcum 2013; Tilley 2002). This finding reflects low energy in old age. Consequently, age has bred distress and negative affect and reduced health, identity, self-regard, and self-efficacy (Alea et al. 2004; Caplan and Schooler 2007; Goerres 2007; Sheldon and Kasser 2001). Specifically, age has dampened personal growth and purpose in life (Ryff et al. 2004). That is, the older person has been lower in life quality.

Mid age. Mid-age is vital as a separate factor because the effect of age may not be a linear one. Life quality can be different between mid-age and older or younger age. Specifically, mid-age is likely to reduce life quality. Life quality is likely to be lower in mid-age than in younger or older. Conversely, the square of age is likely to sustain life quality, primarily according to the voluntaristic mechanism of optimization, which suggests the mid-age person finds or expects a lower gain than the younger or older person. Concerning socioeconomic status, the mid-age person has had lower savings, wealth, and family income than has the other (Anderseon and Nevitte 2006; Keister 2003; van Praag and Ferrer-I-Carbonell 2004). This lower status has decreased life quality (Veenhoven 1984; Obucina 2013). Regarding experience, the mid-age person has had lower affordability, friendship, and social interaction than the younger or older person (Glaeser and Gottlieb 2006; Hallerod 2006; Prouteau and Wolff 2008). Such weakened relationships have eroded life quality (Barrett 1999; Helliwell et al. 2010). Meanwhile, the mid-age person has had higher aspirations and political alienation than the others (Coffe and Geys 2007; Plagnol and Easterlin 2008). A higher aspiration means a greater difficulty to gain and thus a lower gain. Meanwhile, alienation means powerlessness (Coffe and Geys 2007). Hence, aspiration and alienation have impaired life quality (Galtung 2005; Nickerson et al. 2007; Stutzer 2004). Conversely, the mid-age person has had lower social trust, political trust, political appraisal, and support for the market (Hayo 2004; Marien 2011; Traunmuller 2011; Shi 2000) than the others. Mistrust has diminished life quality (Berry and Welsh 2010). For instance, mistrust would lead to worry, thus impairing life quality. In practice, the mid-age person has been less socially cohesive than has the younger or older person (Wilkinson 2008). The lack of social cohesion has eroded life quality (Kahneman et al. 2010). For instance, the lack of social cohesion would mean a lack of achievement in serving society, thus hindering life quality. All these results indicate lower gain from life as expected by the mid-age person. Consequently, the mid-age person has had lower life quality, including health, housing quality, housing satisfaction, leisure satisfaction, financial satisfaction, environmental satisfaction, life satisfaction, and social quality, than has the others (Distante 2013; Fridberg and Kangas 2008; Logan et al. 1999; van Praag and Ferrer-I-Carbonell 2004; van Praag et al. 2003).

Gender. The woman is likely to have higher life quality than the man, primarily due to the voluntaristic mechanism of consistency maintenance. This gender difference is attributable to the socialization or sociocultural influence that promotes gentleness, tranquility, endurance, and complacency in the woman (Guimond et al. 2013; Rundman and Glick 2008). Fundamentally, evolutionary processes have implanted the traits or habits of agreeableness, endurance, deference, and even longevity rather than competition in the woman (Conway and Schaller 2002; Guimond et al. 2013; Hopcroft 2016). In addition, the subordination or oppression perspective suggests that the woman smiles more frequently than does the man (Fischer and Evers 2013). These traits or habits have been conducive to life quality (Cheung and Leung 2011; DeNeve and Cooper 1998; Hounknatin et al. 2014; Webster et al. 2014). For instance, this reflects the case of a more optimistic person being happier. Accordingly, the woman has supported others, including the market and government and its policy, as does the man (Lindh 2015; Morris and Klesner 2010; Rentziou et al. 2011; Wang et al. 2011). Similarly, the woman is more trustful of the government, education, police, medicine, and others (Ahern and Hendryx 2003; Feingold 1994; Hooghe et al. 2015; Moy and Pfau 2000; Sun et al. 2013) and more religious than the man is (Baker and Smith 2009; Immerzeel and van Tubergen 2013). Moreover, the woman has had lower perceptions about problems and risks than has the man (Niemi et al. 1999; Trumbo et al. 2008). All these orientations have been salutary (Graham and Pettinato 2002b; Mattes and Christie 1997; Oishi et al. 2011). Consequently, the woman is higher than the man in life quality indicators such as mastery, self-efficacy, and satisfaction with government, democracy, and life (Dyck and Lascher 2009; Hansen et al. 2012; Tiliouine et al. 2006; Norris 2011; van der Toorn et al. 2010). In all, maintaining consistency among happy and tolerant attitudes, behaviors, and life quality underlies the greater life quality in the woman than in the man.

Education. Education or age at graduation (i.e., an older graduate has higher education) is likely to contribute to life quality considering the voluntaristic mechanism of power realization. Accordingly, education is power in terms of human capital (Dolton et al. 2004; Izquierdo and Minguez 2003). Education can crucially generate great benefits with its explosive and transformative processes and effects (Yair 2003). It enhances discovery, creativity, choice, competition, and confrontation to ensure gains. Specifically, education has upgraded intelligence, memory, general knowledge, political knowledge, and civic skill (Pratt et al. 1996; Verba et al. 1995; Shin 2012; Stevens et al. 2001; Wilson et al. 2012). Abilities and knowledge have been conducive to life quality (Cheng 2003; Diener and Fujita 1995). Possibly, in this case, one knows how to boost happiness. Education has also reduced the experiences of threat, victimization, discrimination, and social exclusion (Backman and Nilsson 2011; Kaukinen 2004; Kessler et al. 1999; Raijman et al. 2003). These experiences have impaired life quality or life satisfaction (Graham et al. 2010; Kirmanoglu and Baslevent 2014). For instance, one feels unhappy when excluded from joining a rejoicing social activity. The moment of exclusion, discrimination, or victimization is also likely to inflict pain on the maltreated person. Conversely, education has facilitated the reception of social support and networking (Cerin and Leslie 2006; Miyata et al. 2008), and the experiences have been salutary (Helliwell and Putnam 2005; Michalos et al. 2005). Conceivably, one rejoices at friendly support from others. Education has also facilitated making choices, exercising, civic engagement, political participation, and preventive action (Chan 2014; Kim and Wilcox 2013; Leung et al. 2005; Morenoff et al. 2008; Stone and Buttice 2010), all of which are demonstrations of power or strength. These practices have also shown their contributions to life quality (Barber et al. 2010; Yang et al. 2012). Specifically, exercising one's power is rejoicing. Education has further enhanced socioeconomic status regarding class and earnings (Pettigrew 2002; Schnittker and Behrman 2012; Whyte and Gao 2009). The status has sustained life quality (Haller and Hadler 2006; Jones et al. 2014; Wang and VanderWeele 2011). Eventually, education has advanced life quality in terms of health, self-efficacy, self-esteem, living standards, and satisfaction, including that with life, safety, and security (Cerin and Leslie 2008; Corcoran et al. 2011; Emler and Frazer 1999; Jmes and Amato 2013; Whyte and Gao 2009; Yienprugsawan et al. 2010). Conversely, education has prevented distress and depression, thus safeguarding life quality (Al-krenawi et al. 2011).

Parental immigration. Concerning the voluntaristic mechanism of realization or power, parental immigration is likely to lower life quality because of the lack of resources. Such immigration status typically represents a financial deficit, welfare dependency, and marginalization by natives (Boeri et al. 2002; Clune 1998; Portes and Rumbaut 2001). This status also breeds personal harm and inadequacy in skills and earnings (Borjas 1999). Hence, it has engendered functional limitations (Herd et al. 2008), consistent with the immigrant's difficulty in living and adapting to the host society. The status has also resulted in low social capital and a high level of social exclusion (Bask 2005; Fanning et al. 2001). Moreover, it has impeded civic engagement, political participation, social cohesion, and volunteering (Ravanera et al. 2003; Sonderskov 2011; Stromblad and Myrberg 2013). These are manifestations of low power or capability, and they all register the immigrant's adaptation difficulty. Eventually, the status has resulted in unemployment, poverty, and lack of marriage (Kurz et al. 2005; Posthumus et al. 2013; Ravanera et al. 2003; Thornton et al. 2007). All these indicate inadequate resources or capability, which are the bases for life quality (Diener and Fujita 1995; Sirgy 2012). Consequently, the status has generated depression, psychosis, and lower health and life satisfaction (Ambrey and Fleming 2014; Islam et al. 2006; Lofors and Sundquist 2007).

Marriage. Marriage or cohabitation is likely to bring higher life quality than divorce, separation, widowhood, or singleness. This result follows the voluntaristic mechanism of power realization, which states that resources buttress life quality. Crucially, marriage counts as a vital resource to solve social problems (Lichter et al. 2002). Similarly, cohabitation counts as a functional resource (Barlow 2004). Hence, marriage has prevented functional limitations (Li and Chung 2008; Smith et al. 2006), and impairs life quality (Abbott and Sapsford 2006). Meanwhile, it has increased social closeness, friendship, social capital, social networking, social interaction, social integration, and social support (Apinunmahakul and Devlin 2008; Cornwall 2009; Lizardo 2006; Mata and Pendakur 2014; Sampson 1991; Volker et al. 2007). Social capital and related resources have been salutary (Jones et al. 2014; Oshio and Kobayashi 2010). Conversely, marriage has reduced the experiences of discrimination, social exclusion, and victimization (Carr and Friedman 2005; Ross and Mirowsky 2009; Wojcieszak and Mutz 2009). Cohabitation has also reduced social deprivation (Rijken and Groenewegen 2008). These experiences have been debilitating (Delbosc and Currie 2011; Graham et al. 2010). Furthermore, marriage has facilitated such practices as civic engagement, community involvement, consumption, donation, family functioning, neighboring, and political participation (Bednell et al. 2013; Dressler 1991; Flavin and Keane 2011; Kerrissey and Schofer 2013; Magee 2008; Smith and Hamon 2012; Swaroop and Morenoff 2006). These practices have reflected resource abundance or affordability and have shown their benefits to life quality (Appleton and Song 2008; Helliwell et al. 2010; Kroll 2011). Marriage has also led to homeownership and reduced welfare receipt (London 2003; Manturuk et al. 2010). Homeownership and exemption from welfare receipt indicate the resource basis for life quality (Granzin and Haggard 2000; Veenhoven 2005). Consequently, marriage has contributed to health, financial adequacy, self-esteem, relationship quality, and satisfaction with achievement, family, finance, friendship, health, living standards, and life (Bellani and D'Ambrosio 2011; Hou et al. 2015; Koromeckyj-Cox et al. 2007; Lelli 2008; Louis and Zhao 2002; Marks 1996; McMullin and Cairney 2004; Mitrut and Wolff 2011; Yienprugsawan et al. 2010). Cohabitation has also championed life satisfaction (Evans and Kelley 2004; Gudmundsdottir 2013). Marriage or cohabitation is likely to provide support to enhance life quality. Conversely, marriage has prevented depression, fear, loneliness (Akiyama and Antonucci 2002; Koromeckyj-Cox et al. 2007; Moore and Shepherd 2006), and depression (Johnson and Wu 2002; Silverstein and Ruiz 2006).

Employment. Full-time or part-time employment or earning, as opposed to unemployment, homemaking, retirement, and studying, is likely to raise life quality considering the voluntaristic mechanism of optimization. Accordingly, experience or expectation of gain is the gravitational force on life quality. In other words, employment is an intentional way to earn money or other benefits, including social inclusion (Graham et al. 2002; Ravanera et al. 2003). Moreover, employment by an able-body person is socially normative (Clark et al., 2008) and, as such, can gain social approval. The norm tends to apply to women and men (Pfau-Effingere 2012; Sanchez 2007). This application stems from equalizing life chances for women and men (Giele 2008). Meanwhile, expansion of the labor market requires female employment (Barnett and Hyde 2001). Female employment can withstand the economic crisis and concomitant layoff (Sanchez 2007). Regardless of gender, gain from employment has been evident. Indeed, employment has raised personal income (Growiec and Growiec 2010), which has prevented poverty (Fan et al. 2004). Moreover, employment has facilitated insurance and marriage (Anderson and Eamon 2004; de Graaf and Kalmijn 2003) and fostered experiences of friendship, social capital, social support received, and cohesion found in the community (Anciaes et al. 2017; Chang 2009; Groot et al. 2007; Tsai 2006). These are gainful experiences conducive to life quality (Gudmundsdottir 2013; Kim and Kawachi 2007; Michalos et al. 2005; Wen et al. 2010). Conversely, employment has reduced the experiences of stress, social exclusion, arrest, and criminal contact (Allwood and Widom 2013; Brayne 2014; Myer et al. 2008; Ross and Mirowsky 2009). Reduction in such experiences has restored life quality (Baumeister et al. 2013; Delbosc and Currie 2011; Kingston and Knight 2006). Employment has also sustained skill and functional ability rather than vice versa (Kerrissey and Schofer 2013; Li and Chung 2008). For instance, it provides training or practice chances to maintain, refresh, or upgrade skills. These traits are instrumental in attaining life quality (Diener and Fujita 1995; Zotti et al. 2016). Hence, employment contributes to life quality, including health, purposiveness, mastery, personal growth, relationship quality, satisfaction with finance and life, self-acceptance, and self-efficacy (Abucina 2013; Corcoran et al. 2011; Distante 2013; Hansen et al. 2012; Ryff et al. 2004). This outcome illustrates the humanist and neoliberal value of employment in self-realization or demonstrating one's competence and contribution (Walkerdine and Bansel 2010). Conversely, employment has prevented depression, distress, dysfunction, loneliness, powerlessness, and psychosis (Goldberg and Perry-Jenkins 2004; Keyes 2002; Koromeckyj-Cox et al. 2007; Lofors and Sundquist 2007; Myer et al. 2008; Ross and Mirowsky 2009).

Public employment. Employment in the public or state sector is likely to fare better in life quality than is employment in the business or nonprofit sector or non-employment. Conversely, employment in the nonprofit sector is likely to have lower life quality than the other employment or non-employment. Such variation is explicable by the voluntaristic mechanism of conformity. Accordingly, the nonprofit sector creates a social environment or norm about social problems, inadequacy, failure, and suffering in society and people (Fric 2008; Milligan and Fyfe 2005; Perotin 2001). This sector is thus prone to take a conflict perspective to reveal problems in society (Fric 2008). Moreover, employees in this sector are likely to locate and work with disadvantaged people, thus witnessing adversity and distress (Milligan and Fyfe 2005). Hence, employment in the nonprofit sector takes the norm to redress problems in society (Freund 2005). By contrast, the public sector creates a social environment or norm about order, security, prosperity, progress, and success in society (de Jonge 2012; Knittila and Kubit 2000; Spicker 2013). Moreover, public employment is more rewarding in job security and others than employment in another sector (Kurz et al. 2005; Tung and Yang 2006). This difference relies on the voluntaristic mechanism of optimization. Hence, public employment has buttressed optimism and trust (Atkinson 2013; Brewer and Sigelman 2002), which are conducive to life quality (Abbott and Sapsford 2006; Magalette and Oliver 1999) and are also likely to lead to the public employee's higher caring, volunteering, and civic engagement (Sarasa 2008; Rosenfeld and Richman 1997; Wilson and Musick 1997). These practices foster or reflect life quality (Chang 2009; Kroll 2011; Muffels and Fouarge 2004).

Work quality. The quality of working conditions in terms of independence, creativeness, intellectuality, and status is likely to be salutary because of its gainfulness. This effect follows the voluntaristic mechanism of optimization. Work independence reflects individualization as a feature of work quality (Bauman 2001). It has contributed to life satisfaction and pride (Hodson 1996; Kelly and Kelly 1994), which are parts of life quality (Huta 2017; Khattab and Fenton 2009). As another feature of work quality, creativeness at work has been pleasurable (Henderson 2004). Intellectuality at work, as opposed to manual work, represents a higher class (Layte et al. 2000). Such a working condition has higher earnings, upward mobility, and life satisfaction (Blanchflower and Oswald 2000; Dieckhoff 2007; Knight and Song 2005). Conversely, intellectuality at work has reduced work stress, control imposed, and social isolation (Bian et al. 2005; Gallie et al. 1998; Jones 2001). Thus, intellectuality at work is gainful. As another work quality indicator, occupational status or class has facilitated social support reception, social capital, and friendship (Lennartsson 2010; Wuthnow 2004). These experiences have been salutary (Borgonovi 2008; Kim and Kawachi 2007; Michalos et al. 2005). Conversely, intellectuality at work has prevented stress, social exclusion, illness, insomnia, economic hardship, and deprivation (Green et al. 2014; Pettigrew 2002; Muhlau 2014; Stansfeld and Marmot 1992). These experiences have been debilitating (Baumeister et al. 2013; Carrieri 2012; Gudmundsdottir 2013; Oshio et al. 2011). Hence, the status or class has secured life quality, including health, financial adequacy, hope, and satisfaction with distribution, finance, life, and welfare (Davis and Davenport 1999; Haller and Hadler 2006; Kangas 2003; Hadjar and Samuel 2015; Peterson and Seligman 2004; Vera-Toscano et al. 2006; Yamaoka 2008). Conversely, the status or class has prevented depression and death (Burke 2008; Dahl 1993). As an indicator of social class, the supervisory role has sustained social capital, friendship, and social status (Whyte and Gao 2009; Wuthow 2002). These experiences have been conducive to life quality (Gudmundedottir 2013; Kim and Kawachi 2007; Salinas-Jimenez et al. 2011). It has also safeguarded life satisfaction and self-efficacy (Corcoran et al. 2011; Rampichini and D'Andrea 1998). Work quality has generally contributed to satisfaction with the job, friendship, leisure, and social status (Sirgy et al. 2001). All these factors manifest the gain from work quality or status.

Religiosity. Religiosity or having religious faith is likely to weaken life quality regarding the voluntaristic mechanism of idealistic consistency. Accordingly, religious faith imparts a belief in personal weakness, powerlessness, guilt, sinfulness, humility, inferiority, fatalism, and uncontrollability (Turner 2009). Religious faith can make one lazy, inactive, and dependent rather than hardworking (Davidson 2008). Hence, religiosity is a source of anxiety and conflict, struggle, or battle (Davidson 2008; Thorson 1998). This finding stems from the psychoanalytic view that religiosity reflects illness or neurosis (Myers 2014). These are rationalizing forces that sustain illness and unhappiness. Religiosity thus encounters criticism from existentialist, humanist, and individualist thoughts (Friedman 1992; Turner 2009), maintaining that the personal pursuit of meaning, identity, responsibility, autonomy, choice, and satisfaction is necessary and desirable. These thoughts presume that the person is intelligent and thoughtful. The thoughts thus support secularization as a way of modernization (De Graaf 2013). Consistent with the idealistic consistency mechanism, religiosity has sustained authoritarianism, conservatism, rightism, racism, and radicalism (Barker and Tinnick 2006; Finseraas 2010; Hall et al. 2010; Hooghe 2003; Pedahzur and Canetti-Nisim 2004). These are ideas contradicting personal life quality. Conversely, religiosity has attenuated hedonism, liberalism, and humor (Devos et al. 2002; Gill 2004; Saraglou 2004). The attenuation reflects the idea to denounce life quality. Such attenuation has also eroded life quality (Gattino et al. 2015; Welzel and Inglehart 2010). Moreover, religiousness has bred favors for punishment, restriction, and censorship (Saucier and Skrzypinska 2006; Woodrum 1992). The favors are antithetical to enjoyment. Conversely, religiosity has impeded tolerance (Saucier and Skrzypinska 2006). Reduced tolerance has led to reduced satisfaction (Appleton and Song 2008). A person with high tolerance would be less likely to find something to be dissatisfying and worrying. In practice, religiosity has discouraged consumption and sexual activities (Ayalon et al. 1993; Cochran et al. 2004). Reduced consumption and sexual activities have led to reduced life quality (Schulz 1995; Wadsworth 2014; Wang and VanderWeele 2011). Insufficient food consumption would reduce one's health and make one distressed. Religion has displayed a negative effect (Parker 1985). Notably, it has induced dissatisfaction with the neighborhood (Ayalon et al. 1993). Religiosity has also impaired health (Yamaoka 2008). For instance, religiously stipulated dieting may erode one's health.

Experiences

According to the voluntaristic mechanism of optimization, the experiences of economic hardship, neighborhood nuisance, victimization, security, and family saving are likely to affect life quality. The experiences represent gains or losses from life to attract or repel satisfaction, commitment, and other excitements with life.

Economic hardship. Economic hardship, financial hardship, financial difficulty, economic stress, or economic pressure is an adverse experience (Robila 2006). It typically involves material hardship in consumption, housing, living environment, meeting needs, and service reception (Carle et al. 2009). Hardship is likely to impair life quality, considering the voluntaristic mechanism of optimization. Accordingly, hardship means the experience of loss rather than the gain in life to foment life dissatisfaction and lower life quality. Hence, economic hardship has directly diminished life quality, including health (Ahnquist et al. 2012; Gudmundsdottir 2013). Conversely, economic hardship has raised depression, distress, strain, and normlessness (Ahnquist et al. 2012; Akiyama and Antonucci 2002; Aytac and Rankin 2009; Ross and Mirowsky 2009) and led to suicide (Economou et al. 2016). Suicide is generally a concomitant of anxiety, depression, hopelessness, loneliness, and lower life quality (Dutton et al. 2016; Economou et al. 2016; Henry et al. 1993).

Neighborhood nuisance. Neighborhood nuisance is likely to erode life quality, considering the voluntaristic mechanism of optimization. Specifically, the nuisance represents a loss rather than a gain to generate dissatisfaction and unhappiness in response. Hence, it has directly diminished life quality (van Praag and Frijters 1999). Conversely, the nuisance has bred depression and normlessness (Pei and Kim 2017; Ross and Mirowsky 2009). Moreover, the nuisance has attenuated attenuated community attachment and social trust (Brown et al. 2004; Marschall and Stolle 2004). The attenuation has led to the erosion of life quality (Berry and Welsh 2010) and to the experiences of economic hardship, victimization, and neighborhood unsafety (Kanan and Pruitt 2002; Like 2011; Whelan and Maitre 2013), experiences that impair life quality (Graham et al. 2010; Gudmundsdottir 2013; Ziersch et al. 2005). For instance, victimization is harmful physically and mentally, thus weakening life quality. Conversely, the nuisance has weakened social capital and networking (Congdon 2010; Ross and Mirowsky 2009), diminishing life quality

(Helliwell and Putnam 2005; Kim and Kawachi 2007). The nuisance has also been responsible for poverty and lowered earnings and income in the person and family (Vartanian 1999). For instance, it would worsen one's sleep, energy, and performance, thus lowering earnings. These outcomes have weakened life quality or satisfaction (Baumeister et al. 2013; Guven and Sorensen 2012). For instance, the poor person would encounter great difficulty satisfying one's needs in life.

Victimization. Victimization is likely to impair life quality because it is a loss needed to avoid, considering the voluntaristic mechanism of utility optimization. Hence, victimization is likely to be discouraging and generate a force of resentment. It has eroded life quality, including satisfaction and intimacy (Graham et al. 2010; Hanson et al. 2010; Sun et al. 2013). Conversely, it has fomented depression, distress, fear, and posttraumatic syndrome (Kanan and Pruitt 2002; Lineres 2004; Wager 2012). Furthermore, victimization has fomented cynicism and eroded social trust (Kirk and Papachristos 2011; Olivera 2015). Herein, the victim would be more likely to be wary and defensive than others. These effects have lowered life quality, such as self-esteem (Lai et al. 2007; Oishi et al. 2011). Victimization has also raised perception about risk (Mesch 2000), detrimental to life quality (Schoon 2006; Zotti et al. 2016). Victimization has consolidated the experience of unsafety in the neighborhood (Kanan and Pruitt 2002), an experience that has eroded life quality (Ziersch et al. 2005). In practice, victimization has instigated doping (Lineres 2004). Herein, the victim is likely to take doping to cope with victimization or as relief from its stress. Victimization has also stabilized neuroticism (Lincoln et al. 2003), which has weakened life quality (Webster et al. 2014).

Security. Security, as an experience, is likely to raise life quality, according to the voluntaristic mechanism of optimization. Herein, security represents the gain from various aspects of life, such as work, food, and economic aspects (Sacks and Levi 2010; Urbatsch 2014). According to the voluntaristic mechanism, the gain generates a gravitational force for living actively and happily. Hence, security has contributed to life quality, including health (Chen et al. 2008; Muffels and Fouarge 2004) and induced attitudes such as trust and support for democracy, law, and the market (Braithwaite 1998; Hraba et al. 2001; Schwartz et al. 2010). Thus, one would attribute the cause of security to the institutions. These attitudes have been salutary (Berry and Welsh 2010; Mattes and Christie 1997), manifesting the contribution of security to support for living. Security has also prevented the ideology of leftism (Hraba et al. 2001; Inglehart 1997; Plutzer 1997). One who has a higher sense of security would be more willing to redistribute one's resources to others. Security has facilitated marriage and prevented poverty (Kieffer et al. 2005; Muffels and Fouarge 2004). For instance, having secure housing is a contributor to marriage. Marriage has been conducive to life quality, whereas poverty has been detrimental to life quality (Baumeister et al. 2013; Carrieri 2012).

Family saving. The experience of saving money in the family is likely to elevate life quality, considering the voluntaristic mechanism of utility optimization. Experience indicates a gain in life to justify satisfaction with and commitment to life. Hence, the saving experience has contributed to satisfaction with finance and life (Obucina 2013; Vera-Toscano et al. 2006) and has also clearly promoted financial adequacy and health (van Praag and Ferrer-I-Carbonell 2004; van Praag et al. 2003). Conversely, the experience has prevented anomie or normlessness (Zhao and Cao 2010). Anomie represents maladjustment with society or life (Brockmann et al. 2009). Herein, family saving represents a social norm. Moreover, the experience has been conducive to social trust and learning aspirations (Uslaner 2002). Herein, the experience of saving would enhance one's confidence. These attitudes have been salutary (Berry and Welsh 2010; Linssen et al. 2011). The experience has also prevented the experience of social exclusion (Lin et al. 2013). In this connection, family saving tends to be normative and socially attractive, thus lessening social exclusion. Such prevention has also been salutary (Delbosc and Currie 2011).

Practices

The practices of E-activity or surfing, learning, verbal involvement, television watching, risk aversion, weapon carrying, organizational participation, appealing, voting, and environmentalist or green activism are likely to affect life quality according to some voluntaristic mechanisms. These practices are influential, possibly because of the attractive force of gain, the assimilating force of conformity or learning, and the rationalizing force of ideological consistency maintenance. The logic underlying the influence is that one feels satisfied, healthy, or well by doing something.

E-activity. Cyber involvement or information and communication technology (ICT) use is likely to impede life quality regarding the voluntaristic mechanism of norm conformity. The use is likely to lead to exposure to norms in cyberspace that are challenging, criticizing, demanding, and dissatisfying to generate assimilating forces to induce discontent or weaken life quality. Such exposure crucially normalizes critical comments, aspirations, and disgust depicted in cyberspace (Norris 2001). Conformity to such normalizing is typical, known as the externality (Katz and Rice 2002). The normative influence on conformity is potent because of the technological capability of speedy communication and expression with ICT (Fuchs 2008). The use fits the popular social norm for self-expression, networking, globalization, information sharing, knowledge advancement, postindustrialism, and postmodernism (Dan et al. 2011; Fuchs 2008; Katz and Rice 2002; Livingstone et al. 2007; Norris 2001; Wallace 2016). These norms favor flexibility, efficiency, freedom, democracy, and argumentation. They obtain ideological support from the individualist, liberal, neoliberal, critical, deliberative, romantic, and postmodern perspectives (Dahlberg 2007; Fuchs 2008; Norris 2001), ideologies that hail technology, individualization, rights, self-expression, competition, criticism, and contestation. Conversely, the ideologies or norms discourage friendliness, cooperation, solidarity, respect, tolerance, and support for the elite and whole, such as society and satisfaction (Dalberg 2007; Fuchs 2008). Generally, such norms are antithetical to satisfaction, contentment, and life quality (Bishop 2015; Chuang 2005; Hightower 1988; Phillips 2006; Veenhoven 2005; Waterman 2008). Hence, E-activity has led to the experiences of impairment in social, vocational, and financial aspects (Shapira et al. 2000). Such experiences, according to the conformity mechanism, would be the results of social construction, which raises awareness about and identification with dire conditions. When one sees poor people on the Web, one sympathizes with them and finds oneself falling into their conditions. The use has also diminished traditional values, fostered newer, confrontational values (Norris 2001), and buttressed support for personal rights, choice, and freedom (Norris 2001). These individualist or liberal attitudes have been dissatisfying (Oishi 2000; Radcliff 2001). When one becomes more egocentric, one is more likely to find unsatisfied personal desires. The use has thus fomented depression and distress (Shapira et al. 2000; Yoo and Jeong 2017). Furthermore, it has provoked protest and violence (Lee and Chan 2016; Wei 2007). Specifically, one learns to protest from protestors viewed in cyberspace. These practices have reflected or bred injuries and unhappiness (Galtung 2005). That is, one's violence can invoke others' violence in return to hurt oneself.

Learning. Reading newspapers, books, and others is likely to diminish life quality, considering the utilitarian mechanism of norm conformity. This diminishment is likely to occur because of the norms for reporting bad news and changes or something stressful in various reading materials (Mutz 1998). The norms also endorse criticism, argumentation, and dissent for truth-seeking (Kiousis 2001). Hence, reading has raised the experience and perception of risk (Harda-Rapp 2003; Norton and Duck 2001). The risk has covered inequality, unemployment, and welfare dependency (Sotirovic 2001; Taylor-Gooby et al. 2003). Such perception and experience have eroded life quality or satisfaction (Lee et al. 2006; Schoon 2006). If one found adverse conditions in society, one would worry about one's conditions. Reading has also buttressed leftist orientation (Paterson 2008), which is detrimental to life quality (Kluegel and Smith 1986). Herein, the orientation is associated with the adverse appraisal of society, leading to discontent. Consequently, reading newspapers has bred protest (Norris and Inglehart 2009) because newspapers expose injustice and grievances as the reason for one to engage in protest. Protesting has provoked worry, anger, dissatisfaction, and discontent, thus weakening life quality (Boehnke and Wong 2011; Gomez-Roman and Sabucedo 2014; Opp and Kittel 2009). For instance, participation in protest would instigate opposition harmful to the protester.

Verbal involvement. Verbal involvement as a learning component, comprising talking and listening, is likely to enhance life quality through the voluntaristic mechanism of utility optimization. The involvement is likely to be gainful in acquiring or conveying information for adaptation and securing gains (Giles and Soliz 2015). This adaptation can happen in involvements such as persuasion, justification, and information seeking (Afifi and Robbins 2015; Braaten 1991; Dillard 2015). Hence, verbal involvement is gainful in building social capital or gainful social connection (Narayan and Cassidy 2001). The contribution of social capital to life quality has been evident (Jones et al. 2014). In reaping social gains, verbal involvement has thereby sustained social trust, political interest, and political appraisal (Austin and Pinkleton 1999; Rothstein and Uslaner 2005; Tsfati et al. 2009). Specifically, one can gain from the polity and community. Essentially, one needs communication to develop trust in others. Such social gain tends to be salutary (Berry and Welsch 2010;

Sirgy 2012). Gain from verbal involvement has also appeared to increase political knowledge (Valentino and Sears 1998). Knowledge has been satisfying (Diener and Fujita 1995). Verbal involvement has been beneficial in strengthening one's leadership (Lee and Chan 2016), which tends to be a basis for life quality (Hute 2017; Peterson et al. 2008). Hence, gain in life quality from verbal involvement has been evident (Kahneman et al. 2010; Schulz 1995). This gain has happened in meaningfulness and satisfaction with life and the partner (Baumeister et al. 2013; Knies 2012; Schulz 1995). Conversely, verbal involvement has prevented depression (Simon and Lively 2010).

Television watching. Television watching as a learning component is likely to enhance life quality following the voluntaristic mechanism of utility optimization. Television watching is gainful in that it is simply entertaining and thus salutary. Such gain arises from the function of television to maintain the status quo rather than create trouble (Mutz 1998). The gain is prominent because of the dominance of video culture nowadays (Grindstaff and Turow 2006). Notably, the viewing has promoted rather than impeded social capital (Beaudoin and Thorson 2006). For instance, the viewing provides shared information for conversation and socializing to build social capital. Social capital has been gainful and salutary (Jones et al. 2014). The viewing has also raised trust in people and the government, including the legislature (Hooghe and Kern 2015; Moy and Pfau 2000; Pattie et al. 2004). Possibly, it provides visualized images to build trust in people and government. Furthermore, it has sustained political interest and favor for politicians (Norris 2011). The interest and favor are compatible with or indicative of life quality or satisfaction (Moller 2005; Sirgy 2012). Meanwhile, the viewing has reduced protest and reading (Best and Krueger 2002); van der Meer and van Ingen 2009). Reading has fueled protest, which has, in turn, led to worry (Boehnke and Wong 2011; Norris and Inglehart 2009). Hence, television viewing can bolster life quality indirectly. Conversely, the viewing has fostered volunteering (Wuthnow 2004), which has been, in turn, gainful in championing life quality (Borgonovi 2008; Chang 2009). The viewing has also been gainful in advancing political knowledge (Bennett et al. 2000; Chaffee et al. 1994). Eventually, television viewing has buttressed satisfaction with democracy (Norris 2011).

Risk aversion. According to the voluntaristic mechanism of utility optimization, risk aversion is likely to sustain life quality. The aversion would reduce risks or costs, thus advancing gains relatively. According to the mechanism, the gains are encouraging, satisfying, or salutary. Essentially, risk aversion has encouraged the reception of counseling and led to the experience of success (Meng and Chen 2014; Ullrich et al. 2007), which are undoubtedly functional bases for life quality (Meng and Chen 2014; Oettingen and Chromick 2018; Scabini and Cigoli 1997). Counseling aims to bolster life quality (Fawcett 2012). The experiences have also been associated with recourse and attendance at a self-help group, a kind of social capital (Fine 2010; Meng and Chen 2014). These practices have been conducive to life quality (Jones et al. 2014; Van Haaften et al. 2004). Eventually, risk aversion promotes life quality by reducing arousal and distress (Alonso-Arbiol et al. 2007; Linares et al. 2016). It is likely to promote life quality through mediation by receiving counseling, help from the self-help group, and other forms of social support or social capital.

Weapon carrying. Carrying weapons is likely to bolster life quality regarding the voluntaristic mechanism of utility optimization. Herein, carrying weapons is gainful because it is likely to lead to expectation and experience of effectiveness in securing safety. The gain would stem from protection and defense, which relate to safeguarding and are salutary. Notably, the gain has evolved from the increase of affiliative and self-enhancement humor (Erickson and Feldstein 2007), which has, in turn, been conducive to life quality (Gattino et al. 2015). A humorous one is likely to feel happy. Moreover, carrying weapons would sustain the gain in safety. Such gain has been directly salutary (Jones et al. 2014; Wen et al. 2010). Specifically, the gain has sustained health, neighborhood quality perception, and satisfaction with the country, neighborhood, and life (Cummins et al. 2003; Frey et al. 2007; Olson et al. 2016). Conversely, the gain has lowered fear of crime (Chiricos et al. 2000).

Organizational participation. Civic organizational participation is likely to erode life quality, considering the voluntaristic mechanism of norm conformity. Accordingly, such an organization is likely to hold the norms of empowerment, challenge, contention, agonistic, competition, and criticism (Alexander 1997; Howell 2012). The norms favor organizational surveillance over society (Howell 2012). Therefore, participation in civic organizations is likely to internalize the norms through the conformity mechanism or assimilating force. Hence, organizational participation has fueled protest and collective action (Klandermans and de Weerd 2000; Yip et al. 2007). This fueling is likely a result of empowerment in knowledge acquisition (Marsh 2005). Moreover, protest and collective action are the commonly organized activities of civic organizations. Protest, in turn, has been detrimental to life quality through the elevation of worry (Boehnke and Wong 2011), possibly because the protestor would suffer in the protest.

Appealing. Appealing, protesting, complaining, or unconventional political participation is likely to diminish life quality due to the voluntaristic mechanism of idea consistency. Accordingly, appealing reflects a need, deficit, deprivation, grievance, challenge, voicing, experiences of oppression and victimization, and dissatisfaction (Pfaff and Kim 2003; Stewart et al. 2012). These features of rationalizing forces undermine life quality (Graham et al. 2010; Guillen-Royo 2008). Notably, appealing has been conducive to radicalization and extremism (Claassen 2008; Vestergren et al. 2017), both associated with emotional maladjustment (Besic and Kerr 2009). For instance, the radical or extremist would be furious and agitated and connect to revenge, blaming, and a spiral of retribution (Davies 2008). Furthermore, they indicate competition, risk, and segregation (Davies 2008; Veugelers 2000). Maladjustment is a negative indicator of life quality, and revenge and others have been deleterious to life quality (Baumeister et al. 2013; Delbosc and Currie 2011; Zetti et al. 2016). Moreover, appealing has helped acquire knowledge (Price et al. 2006). Knowledge, in turn, has bred suspicion and mistrust of various institutions and policies (Bernstein 2001; Kabakian-Khasholian et al. 2000; McGraw et al. 2002; Scholz and Lubell 1998; Yang and Tang 2010; Zhu and Ke 2001). These attitudes have been impediments to life quality (Abbott and Sapsford 2006; Mattes and Christie 1997).

Voting. Political voting in a political election is likely to diminish life quality given the voluntaristic mechanism of idea consistency. Herein, voting reflects concern, dissatisfaction, deficiency, the need for help, and the wish to change or control political policy and practice (Rose and Pettersen 2000). That is, voting is likely a response to problems, crises, and calamities (Bennett and Resnick 1990). Such dire conditions and discontent are consistent with weakened life quality. For instance, voting suggests feelings about personal weakness and the demand to rationalize inadequate life quality. It has predicted activism, protest, extremism, and violence (Beasley and Joslyn 2001; McVeigh and Smith 1999; Ozbay 2008; Straughn and Andriot 2011). These activities have been dissatisfying and noxious to health or life quality (Boehnke and Wong 2011; Krahe 2001). Meanwhile, voting does not bring appreciable gains to raise life quality (Aldrich 1993).

Green activism. Green or environmentalist activism, including donation and participation in the environmentalist demonstration, is likely to impede life quality regarding the voluntaristic mechanism of idea consistency. Herein, green activism opposes practice that harms the environment and involves a desire to change, counteract, and curtail the practice (Lee and Norris 2000). Hence, the contribution implies dissent, cynicism, subversion, and deviance from conventional views (Taylor 2000). Obviously, the contribution has eroded perceived life quality in the environment or the community (Wulfhorst and Kranich 1999). Possibly, it leads to the exposure of information about environmental degradation and, therefore, eroding life quality. Green activism has also led to the perception about risk and problems in the environment (Ojala 2005; Wong and Wan 2011). Such perception has impaired life quality (Van Haaften et al. 2004). Furthermore, green activism has predisposed to protest rather than conventional political participation (Lee and Norris 2000; Norris 2002). Protesting has agitated worry (Boehnke and Wong 2011). Hence, green activism exerts demands to weaken life quality because of the rationalizing process of consistency maintenance.

Spiritual activity. Rather than religious faith, spiritual activity is likely to secure life quality given the voluntaristic mechanism of utility optimization. Spiritual activity is likely to be gainful and attract feelings about life quality. Such gain tends to accrue from social interaction, integration, support received, enjoyment in the atmosphere with music or serenity, receiving blessed food, tutoring, caring, counseling, and other blessings (Katz-Gerro and Shavit 1998; Schwadel 2012; Wuthnow 2011). Attendance can gain meanings, belongingness, and religious interpretations of reality (Demerath 2002; Skerkat and Ellison 1999). Hence, it is salutary by maintaining personal coherence and social cohesiveness (Levin and Chatters 1998). The salutary contribution of spiritual activity has been evident (Helliwell and Putnam 2005; Wuthnow 2004). Specifically, attendance has been conducive to health, mastery, and satisfaction with life, democracy, and police (Helliwell and Putnam 2005; Kwak et al. 2010; Marx 2014; Ng and Fisher 2016; Schieman 2001). Conversely, spiritual activity has prevented depression (Ellison et al. 2001; Hao 2000). The salutary contribution of spiritual activity is attributable to the contribution of the attendance to health behavior, civic engagement, social cohesion, volunteering, and prosocial behavior (Kim and Wilcox 2013; Myers 2008; Perks and Haan 2011; Ravanera et al.

2003; Wuthnow 2004). These practices have been salutary, satisfying, or salubrious, such as maintaining health (Borgonovi 2008; Caprara and Steca 2005; Dittman and Goebel 2010; Kroll 2011; Yang et al. 2012; Harter and Arora 2010). Conversely, attendance has prevented suicide, doping, and other deviant behaviors (Cochran et al. 2004). Some religious activities or interventions aim to prevent such sinful practices. Prevention of these behaviors would safeguard life quality, notably health (Hathaway 2003). Moreover, spiritual activity has boosted the perceptions or experiences of security and social capital (Chang 2009; Urbatsch 2014). That is, religious fellows would constitute one's social capital. Conversely, attendance has prevented illness (Muennig et al. 2013). Some religious activities may have healing or illness preventive functions, which can be the selling point of religion. Illness has impeded life quality (Carrieri 2012; Linssen et al. 2011). The attendance has also fostered civility, tolerance, and trust in people, institutions, and government (Gibson 2013; Hakhverdian and Mayne 2012; Keyes 2002; Stoyan et al. 2016; Zanin 2017). This fostering is the aim of some religious activities. Such attitudes or orientations have been conducive to life quality (Abbott et al. 2011; Gehring 2013; Napier and Jost 2008; Rozer and Kraaykamp 2012). Notably, spiritual activity is different from religious faith in that attendance represents a social action to gain social experience, whereas the faith may not be so (Rip et al. 2012; Schwadel 2012). As such, the gainful experience from spiritual activity triggers the mechanism of optimization.

Life Quality

Life quality in terms of health and life satisfaction before can predict life quality of delight and worry currently. The World Values Survey measured health and life satisfaction these days, implying that they preceded delight and worry, which referred to current states. The prediction of life quality with life quality is apparent, reflecting stability or consistency in life quality. This consistency reflects the voluntaristic mechanism of idealistic consistency. Hence, health has been a predictor of life quality (Baumeister et al. 2013; Webster et al. 2014). Conversely, health problems have eroded life quality (Harter and Arora 2010; Jones et al. 2014). Moreover, life satisfaction has been a predictor of life quality in general (Rocke and Lachman 2008). Specifically, autonomy has depended on satisfaction (Chang et al. 2009; Gayne and Deci 2005). Mastery has also arisen from health and satisfaction (Andreoletti et al. 2001; Schieman 2001). Financial satisfaction has benefited from health (Mitrut and Wolff 2011; Plagnol 2011). Worry has also been lower when health has been better (Young et al. 2001).

National Indicators

Essential national indicators include the six elements of PISTOL and those representing modernization. Based on the social entropy view, PISTOL encompasses population, information, space, technology, organization, and living (Bailey 1994). Essentially, the entropy views maintain that society is not in equilibrium when resources and energy are draining to increase disorder or entropy. Thus, PISTOL represents the essential elements or energy forms to prop life, the world, and society. Except for population, the other five elements have their proxies in terms of phones per capita for circulating information, land per capita, technology export per capita, bank credit to the private sector to represent the organization, and GDP per capita to represent living in the country. Whenever an indicator involves monetary terms, it is in real, internationally comparable terms, such as the currency of the United States. Besides these entropy bases, modernization indicators include income inequality, globalization, government effectiveness, democracy, liberty, human development, human capital, and environmental risk (Dahlberg et al. 2018). These indicators are also in comparable terms, such as per capita, to minimize their correlations with population.

Population. The size of the national population is likely to buttress life quality according to the deterministic mechanism. Specifically, a large national population enables the provision of additional resources and support to raise life quality. Notably, national population size has sustained government spending per capita, including social and educational aspects (Pattie et al. 2004). More people may exert greater pressure to urge the government for additional spending. National population size has also increased wages (Glaeser et al. 2009). Population size may generate a synergistic effect to raise the worker's productivity and thus the wage. Moreover, national income has been conducive to personal life quality by enhancing nationwide support (Diener and Biswas-Diener 2002; Diener et al. 2010; Ram 2010). For instance, people around one another can help maintain one another's health. Moreover, national population size has been conducive to capitalism or its support (Bjornskov and Paldam 2012). More people can generate a larger amount of capital for the development of capitalism. The larger amount of capital can provide more resources to satisfy people's immediate needs and thus enable their support for investment or capitalism. In this connection, capitalism is justifiable for boosting economic development and providing support, resources, and a free environment to people (Rubinstein 1993; Schram 2015). Meanwhile, national population size has facilitated welfare provision or its support (Iida and Matsubayashi 2010). For instance, more people can pay more taxes for the specific use of welfare spending on needy people. National welfare availability and generosity have provided economic and other resources to raise life quality (Muffels and Fouarge 2004)..

Information: phone per capita. According to the deterministic mechanism, information available in society, such as through the phone, represents an external resource that shapes behaviors and feelings indicative of life quality. Such a national resource is practical because of its speed and low cost (Hossain and Cheng 2003). Nowadays, information can be powerful and valuable because of its global circulation. The power of information hinges on ICT (information and communication technology), which establishes the cyber or virtual world for information accumulation and circulation. Thus, information is multifarious and rich in content. Information is the source or target of learning and creativity, particularly value creation (Hossain and Cheng 2003). It is undoubtedly the basis for functioning in education, work, business, and government (Hossain and Cheng 2003). Hence, information has been a resource enabling life quality, including satisfaction and self-efficacy (Norris 2011; Dyck and Lescher 2009). For example, when one suffers from an acute illness, the availability of information on the illness and emergency health services can prompt others to call for help to maintain one's health. The information available in society can also facilitate support, interest, and favor for societal conditions, including policies, rights, and politicians (Koch 1998; Rose and Pettersen 2000). These attitudes have been indicative or conducive to life quality (Gramham and Pettinato 2002b; Mattes and Christie 1997; Stanley et al. 2011). Similarly, information has sustained social trust (Pattie et al. 2004), and salutary (Helliwell and Putnam 2005). Information has also raised aspiration (Norris 2011). For example, the availability of information on ways to maintain health can enable one to maintain health and, therefore, boost one's aspiration for health. Aspiration has been reflective or conducive to life quality (Frazier et al. 2007; Linssen et al. 2011). Moreover, information has buttressed the perception about government performance (Uslaner 2008). For example, information on government performance can lead one to realize the performance. The realization has been satisfying (Bjornskov et al. 2013; Liao et al. 2005). Information has also propelled health behavior, prevention, cooperation, and social cohesion (Blalock 2007; Lepkowski and Couper 2002; Volker et al. 2007). For example, health information can enable people to help their family members maintain health. These practices have safeguarded life quality, including health and satisfaction (Baumeister et al. 2013; Chang 2009; Dittman and Goebel 2010; Myers 2008). Information has likewise facilitated the reception of social norms (Morgan et al. 2003). For instance, information on social norms can enable people to teach others about the norms. Such reception has been conducive to life quality by avoiding anomie (Muffels and Fouarge 2004). Information has also contributed to power and leadership, including opinion leadership (Nunkoo 2015; O'Cass and Pecotich 2005; Stokman et al. 2013). For example, the availability of information on a leader's merit can raise the willingness of others to follow the leader and recognize his or her power. Such statuses are constituents of life quality (Farran et al. 1991; Peterson et al. 2008; Huta 2017). Conversely, information has prevented vulnerability (Langenderfer and Shimp 2001). For example, information on a disease can allow people, such as health professionals, to prevent others from being vulnerable or susceptible to the disease. The vulnerability would weaken life quality (Charles 2010).

Information circulation facilitated by phone is likely to enhance life quality through the deterministic mechanism. The phone represents an external resource optimizing communication and information sharing, which are salutary. Communication has demonstrated its contribution to life quality, including meaningfulness and satisfaction with life and the partner (Baumeister et al. 2013; Knies 2012; Schulz 1995).

Conversely, communication has diminished depression (Simon and Lively 2010). For instance, when one encounters a traumatic accident, others can use the phone to call for emergency services. Similarly, people can use phones to communicate amusing messages to others.

Space: land per capita. Space in terms of land per capita in a country is likely to sustain life quality, according to the deterministic mechanism. Herein, land is a resource for production, dwelling, and leisure or refreshing activities. It consists of private space mainly in housing and public space predominately located in parks and the countryside. For housing, housing size or space is the principal constituent of housing quality (Day 2013; Logan et al. 1999; Zhou and Suhomlinova 2001). Housing size, space, or quality has been conducive to life quality (Jiang et al. 2011). Housing size has facilitated health, need fulfillment, and satisfaction with housing and the neighborhood (Day 2013; Guardiola and Garcia-Munoz 2011; Walder and He 2014). For instance, larger housing would have a lower risk of infection, an external source that impairs health. Larger housing also implies less pressure and control from others to constrain one's life quality. Housing size has also reduced the experience of crowdedness (Chen 1999), which has, in turn, engendered depression (Riad and Norris 1992). Furthermore, housing quality has prevented violence (Farrington 2007). Better housing quality implies better housing security and, consequently, a lower risk of violence. Violence has eroded life quality to raise depression (Wright et al. 2015). Alternatively, exposure to or living in the countryside has been salutary in reducing illness and anxiety (Fridberg and Kangas 2008). The countryside would prevent infection among people who are scattering there. Generally, public space is a supposed determinant of life quality (Nevarez 2011). Conversely, crowdedness in various aspects has been detrimental to life quality as the opposite of spaciousness. Apart from raising depression, crowdedness has raised blood pressure and created behavioral problems (Evans and Saegert 2000). For instance, crowdedness may heighten the threat among people to foment behavioral problems. Crowdedness has also led to racism and migration (Biggs and Knauss 2012; Crowder et al. 2006). This effect is simply the crowding-out effect, which has been indicative of dissatisfaction (Kleinhans 2009; Menahem 2001; Pardos-Prado 2011; van Vugt et al. 2003). Notably, crowdedness would impose pressure and demands on people and agitate worrying and stressful competition.

Technology: technology export per capita. Technology is a resource external to the person (Schroeder and Swedberg 2002; Welzel 2013). It is very likely to advance personal life quality at the national level considering the deterministic mechanism. This advancement has characterized industrialization or capitalism (Schroeder and Swedberg 2002). Essentially, the advancement benefits from the spillover effect of technology on society (Fukuyama 2003). In this connection, technology provides the infrastructure or base structure for societal progress (Schofer 2004). The principal contribution of technology is to work, productivity, and thus employment (Goetz et al. 2011). As such, technology safeguards economic life quality, notably including income (Florida 2005; Welsch 2002). Technology heightens productivity and its economic reward to raise economic life quality. Crucially, technology has championed quality in society, including environmental quality (Welzel 2013). For instance, technology has helped prevent and protect against environmental or natural hazards, such as storms. Technology has sustained self-efficacy and satisfaction with democracy (Norris 2001). For instance, mastering technology can give one a sense of self-efficacy. Moreover, technology has facilitated people's emancipation, including its value and expression (Welzel 2013; Welzel and Inglehart 2010). Accordingly, it gives one freedom and thus the enjoyment and valuation of freedom. Technology has also enhanced interest in and support for public policy (Jennings and Zeitner 2005; Norris 2001). Herein, technology helps the government raise people's interest in and support for the government. It has facilitated the acquisition of social capital, including that from family and friends (Katz and Rice 2002; Yoo and Jeong 2017). Technology helps people provide support to their family members and facilitates leadership, thus raising social status (Park and Kaye 2017). That is, technology helps one lead, monitor, and control others.

Organization: bank credit rate. Organization in terms of the ratio of bank credit to the private sector to prosperity or economic development (GDP) in a country is likely to enhance life quality considering the deterministic mechanism. Herein, the organization represents a resource to engage, maintain order, and sustain belongingness (Jacobs et al. 2009; Wang and Graddy 2008). It also consolidates social capital to convey resources to people through transforming various forms of capital (Carpiano 2008; Palmer et al. 2011). Acquiring financial resources from various sources, including banks, is a basis for the organization. Organization exerts external, deterministic forces through its collective and concentrated power in commanding, controlling, scheming, scheduling, coordinating, and unifying (Demers 2007; Foss and Klein 2013; Furnham 1997; Seidl 2014). Organizational involvement or membership of various kinds has contributed to personal life quality (Carrieri 2012; Jones et al. 2014; Posel and Casale 2011; Wang and VanderWeele 2011). Specifically, the contribution has happened to health, happiness, quality perception, self-efficacy, social integration, and satisfaction with life, friendship, police, city, and society (Hooghe 2003; Logan et al. 1999; Paxton 1999; Sun and Wang 2012; Vincens et al. 2018; Wallace and Pichler 2008). For instance, an organization such as a clinic represents a facility to maintain people's health and other aspects of life quality. Organizational involvement has also fostered feelings of attachment to, commitment to, favor for, and support for society or its institutions or policies (Marx 2014; Shi 2000; Stolle 2001; Tak 2017; Whitham 2012). In addition, organizational involvement has championed tolerance for and trust in various people and institutions, including the government (Bekkers and Boisman 2009; Coffe and Geys 2007; Goren 2005; van Ingen and Bekkers 2015; Welzel 2013). At least, the organization would foster people's trust in their fellow members. Conversely, organizational involvement has diminished feelings of political alienation (Coffe and Geys 2007) and buttressed the perceptions or experiences of security, social capital from various sources, and social support (Erickson 2004; Coffe and Geys 2007; Mata and Pendakur 2014; Pena-Lopez and Sanchez-Santos 2016; Wuthnow 2002). This finding simply reflects the mutual support among organizational members. More essentially, organizational involvement has strengthened leadership, prosociality, and charity (Mata and

Pendakur 2014; Park and Keye 2017; Sokolowski 1996). For instance, within an organization, members should help one another. Conversely, organizational involvement has eroded egoism (Kitts 2003). The organization requires and raises its members' allegiance to itself. Furthermore, organizational involvement has raised education, income, and class position (Growiec and Growiec 2010; Li and Walder 2001; Zhou and Suhomlinova 2001). Eventually, it has boosted consumption, donation, neighboring, and volunteering (Cattell 2004; Grootaert and van Bastelaer 2002; Kerrissey and Schofer 2013; Sobieraj and White 2004; Taniguchi 2013). For instance, the organization would mobilize people to perform volunteering. Conversely, organizational involvement has discouraged suicide (Helliwell 2006). In this connection, organizational members are likely to help one another prevent suicide.

Living standard: economic development. The national living standard, typically in terms of economic development or GDP per capita, is likely to facilitate personal life quality regarding the deterministic mechanism. Accordingly, economic development provides economic resources that can transform into different resources to buttress life quality. Economic development is valuable and reflective of modernity (Peet and Hatwick 2009). It is also conducive to democracy by raising personal dignity and receiving recognition (Fukuyama 1995). Moreover, national economic development is vital to provide compensation of loss (Bourguignon et al. 2007). Economic development has the meanings of good life, need fulfillment, and emancipation (Peet and Hatwick 2009). From the utilitarian view, economic development represents life quality (Peet and Hatwick 2009). Hence, the contribution of national economic development to personal life quality has been evident (Inglehart 2010; Wallace and Pichler 2009). This contribution is the central thesis of modernization (Inglehart 2010). Specifically, national economic development has raised relationship quality, self-efficacy, and satisfaction with life and democracy in the person (Corcoran et al. 2011; Fridberg and Kangas 2008; Helliwell et al. 2010; Norris 2011). Accordingly, national wealth provides facilities for citizens to live, perform, and relate to other people well. For instance, wealthy neighbors would be helpful and pleasing. National economic development has likewise been conducive to the woman's survival (Williamson and Bochmer 1997). The woman would possibly benefit from environmental resources and support (Guo et al. 2008; Wuthnow 2004). Conversely, national economic development has diminished illness and economic hardship experienced personally (Fridberg and Kangas 2008). Herein, national wealth affords public welfare and healthcare to prevent citizens' illness and economic hardship. These experiences have jeopardized life quality (Carrieri 2012; Gudmundsdottir 2013). Similarly, national economic development has dampened perceptions about anomie, risk, and threat in society (Schneider 2007; Schwartz and Melech 2000). That is, national wealth affords the maintenance of peace and harmony. Such perceptions have been detrimental to life quality (Deaton et al. 2010). National economic development has also advanced knowledge in the person (Norris 2011; Booth and Richard 1998). Conceivably, national wealth affords public education and information circulation to raise citizens' knowledge. Furthermore, national economic development has fostered tolerance and trust in institutions, government, and people (Marien 2011; Norris 1991; Tov and Diener 2008). At this juncture, national wealth facilitates supportive institutions to earn citizens' trust. Such attitudes have been conducive to life quality (Berry and Welsh 2010; Mattes and Christie 1997). National economic development has also encouraged volunteering (Inglehart 2003; Salamon and Sokolowski 2003). Herein, national wealth would afford to sponsor or organize citizens' volunteering. Essentially, volunteering hinges on institutional organizing. Volunteering has contributed to life quality (Borgonovi 2008; Piliavin 2008).

Income inequality. National income inequality means that national income concentrates on a minority of people. It gauges the difference in income between the high-income few and the low-income majority. National income inequality is likely to erode personal life quality due to the deterministic mechanism. Accordingly, the inequality deprives resources and foments problems, including conflict, antagonism, pressure, and crime to hurt the person and thus impair his or her life quality (Jencks 2002; Neckerman and Toche 2007). These problems represent external forces impinging on the person and impairing his or her life quality. The inequality also reflects exploitation, unfairness, and injustice (Fein 2012; Godoy et al. 2004; Suchweh 2012). Hence, it is the source of or ground for injustice, struggle, protest, crisis, and unhappiness (Goldberg 2012; Grover, 2011; Jencks 2002; Jordahl 2009). Income inequality has fomented crime and violence (Ousey and Lee 2013; van Wilsem 2007). Crime in society has impeded life quality (Inglehart 1990; Kingston and Knight 2006). Certainly, the victim of a crime would feel unhappy. Moreover, violence has been a source of depression (Wright et al. 2015). More importantly, the victim of violence would feel depressed. Conversely, income inequality has reduced volunteering (Lipford and Yandle 2009; Musick and Wilson 2008). Income inequality would fuel segregation and boundaries among people to hinder their volunteering. Volunteering in society has nurtured life quality (Veenhoven 2005). Income inequality has weakened life quality (Napier and Jost 2008; Oshio and Kobayashi 2010). Specifically, income inequality has impaired health and satisfaction with life and finance (Kim and Kawachi 2007; Meulemann 2010; Winkelmann and Winkelmann 2010). The impairment has been attributable to stress, frustration, invidious social comparison, social disintegration, social distrust, and material and relative deprivation caused by income inequality (Blakely et al. 2001; Eibner and Evans 2004; Subramanian and Kawachi 2006). Moreover, income inequality would obstruct sharing and helping among people, making their life unsatisfactory. Conversely, income inequality has increased the risk of anxiety and death (Kawachi et al. 1997; Schwartz and Melech 2000) and led to illness, social exclusion, and other disadvantages experienced (Jones et al. 2015; Portes and Vickstrom 2011). For instance, income inequality would discourage people's concern for public hygiene, thus fomenting their illness. These experiences have undermined life quality (Carrieri 2012; Guillen-Royo 2008; Sonderlund et al. 2017). Conversely, income inequality has weakened social capital (Portes and Vickstrom 2011). Income inequality would entrench barriers among people to erode social capital. Weakened social capital has weakened life quality (Jones et al. 2014; Oshio and Kobayashi 2010). Income inequality has also diminished perceptions about fairness and justice in society (Eriksson et al. 2015; Oishi et al. 2011). Income inequality causes people to treat each other unequally and possibly unfairly. Such diminished perceptions have diminished life quality (Liao et al. 2005; Oishi et al. 2011). Conversely, income inequality has bolstered perceptions about anomie and corruption in society (Teymoori et al. 2016; Uslaner 2008). Specifically, it has impeded the formation of common social norms, which can discourage corruption. Corruption in society has reduced life quality, including satisfaction with life, democracy, and police (Helliwell et al. 2010; Norris 2011; Sun and Wang 2012; Veenhoven 2005). Income inequality also has lower trust, including institutions, government, and people (Lundasen et al. 2013; Oishi et al. 2011; van Oorschot and Arts 2005; Zmerli and Castillo 2015). People would hold the government and other institutions responsible for income inequality and its harm. The lowered trust has lowered life quality (Abbott and Sapsford 2006; Berry and Welsh 2010; Hommerich and Tiefenbach 2018). Furthermore, income inequality has weakened self-direction (Bond and Lun 2014). Income inequality suggests power inequality, which popularizes domination and submission and dampens personal self-direction. Such orientation has been favorable to life quality (Veenhoven 1998). Conversely, income inequality has bred functional disability, poverty, and single parenthood (Kim and Kawachi 2007; Nilson 1981; Portes and Vickstrom 2011). Income inequality represents poverty in relative terms, which would fuel many adversities. These conditions have been detrimental to life quality (Baumeister et al. 2013; Carrieri 2012). Meanwhile, income inequality has discouraged homeownership (Martin 2000), possibly because it impedes building decent common living environments and housing for sale. Essentially, a good common living environment is necessary for the value of good housing. Homeownership has been conducive to health, financial adequacy, life quality in the neighborhood and family, and satisfaction with housing and the neighborhood (Harris 2001; Mirowsky and Ross 1999; Ng et al. 2005; Roy and Chaudhuri 2008; Wilson and Hammer 2001). Conceivably, the owned home provides a better environment and facilities to champion life quality than the other home.

Globalization. Globalization in a country means heightening its exposure to, connection with, communication with, marketing with, and diffusion of information, materials, capital, services, and people with the world (Axford 2013; Dryzek 2006; Sirgy et al. 2004; Walker 2005). According to the deterministic mechanism, such globalization is likely to boost personal life quality. Globalization would provide resources, opportunities, and various forces to facilitate life quality, forces that have consisted in those raising national commonality, rights, freedom, equality, revenue, social welfare, and technology (Brady et al. 2007; Dreher et al. 2008; Hunter 2016; Langman 2005; Tsai 2006; Welzel 2013). For instance, globalization has facilitated the transmission of ideas of resources worldwide. These conditions have been salutary or satisfying (Napier and Jost 2008; Radcliff 2008; Ram 2010; Veenhoven 2005). For example, social welfare can safeguard citizens' utility and thus life quality. Specifically, commonality has prevented depression (Riad and Norris 1992) by, for instance, fostering mutual support, which can be preventive against depression. Moreover, commonality has bred liking and trust (Riemer et al. 2014; Stokman et al. 2013). Such attitudes have been salutary (Oishi et al. 2011; Stanley et al. 2011). Similarly, receiving liking from others is delightful. Commonality has also facilitated relation formation and prevented relation dissolution (Kossinets and Watts 2009). Such facilitation and prevention have been salutary (Gudmundsdottir 2013; Harter and Arora 2010). Commonality has buttressed social interaction and social cohesion (Carley and Krackhardt 1996; Granzin and Olsen 1998). These practices have been salutary, such as preventing depression (Baumeister et al. 2013; Kawachi and Berkman 2001). For example, social interaction can reduce loneliness. Notably, globalization has championed life quality reasonably by enhancing revenue, profit, and resource availability (Sirgy et al. 2004).

Government effectiveness. Government effectiveness is likely to enhance personal life quality considering the deterministic mechanism. Accordingly, it means providing practical resources to people through social welfare, national security, infrastructure, and public services to facilitate the advancement of life quality. Typically, the government needs or aspires to effectively tackle aging, disability, crime, drug abuse, migration, poverty, risks, and crises (Janoski and Wang 2005; Karger et al. 2007; Nolan 2009; Scourfield and Welsh 2003; Walker 2005). The effectiveness also consists in facilitating cooperation, education, employment, health, peace, virtue, rights such as human rights, life quality, resources, welfare, security, and development (Brooks 2013; Cairney 2012; Gaus 2011; Karger et al. 2007; Koven 2015; Martinez 2009; Roy 2007; Seymour and Pincus 2008; Shortall and Warner 2010; Smart 2001; Walters 2012; Wuthnow 2006. Yanagisawa 2011). This result means that effective government performance would provide resources and benefits in various aspects to champion people's life quality. Government effectiveness has contributed to personal life quality (Bohnke 2008). Specifically, it has raised satisfaction with democracy and the police (Bratton and Mattes 2001; Murphy 2009) and reduced the experience of environmental problems (Wong and Wan 2011). This experience has been detrimental to life quality (Carrieri 2012; van Haaften et al. 2004). Instead, the effectiveness has sustained perceptions about harmony, justice, and high living standards in society (Mizrahi 2016; Taylor et al. 2015; Wong and Shik 2011). These perceptions have buttressed life quality, including reduced anxiety (Oishi et al. 2011; Schwartz and Melech 2000). Government effectiveness has advanced economic development or prosperity (Guisan 2009). Furthermore, the effectiveness has sustained support for or legitimized the government and its policy (Shin 2012; Grimes 2006; Wolfe et al. 2016). Government effectiveness has also raised trust in institutions, government, political agencies, and people (Grimes 2006; Guisen 2009 Heatherington and Globetti 2002; Nunkoo and Smith 2013). All these findings suggest that an adequate government benefits the citizen and thus earns his or her trust. Government effectiveness has also prevented suicide (Helliwell 2006). Effective government services, including medical and emergency ones, can save lives.

Democracy. Democracy typically refers to the liberal, representative form of democracy. Such a form emphasizes assertiveness, reaction, association, participation in the election, and equality in citizens' freedom (Dryzek and Dunleavy 2009; Ringen 2007; Shin 2012). It strives to maintain the check and balance, neutrality, tolerance, non-interference, liberty, protection of rights, the rule of law and majority, and economic and political competition (Ceva and Zuolo 2013; Dryzek and Dunleavy 2009; Fairfield 2008; Moller and Skaaning 2013; Pettit 2012; Ringen 2007; Shin

2012). Hence, democracy provides resources and channels for people to optimize their life quality. Democracy as such is likely to champion personal life quality, considering the deterministic mechanism. In support of this, democracy has enhanced life quality in life satisfaction and self-efficacy (Corcoran et al. 2011; Frey and Stutzer 2000; Meulemann 2010). Notable reasons include fairness and the minimization of corruption in democracy (Frey and Stutzer 2000). Democracy is also likely to sustain life quality through maintaining peace because of its emphasis on and features of sympathy and negotiation rather than fighting (Moller and Skaaning 2013). Peace or nonviolence has been salutary (Wright et al. 2015). Democracy has facilitated alliances in society (Hausermann 2006), possibly because it heightens the freedom of association, which builds alliances. Alliances have been salutary (Baumeister et al. 2013; Lane 2000). Moreover, democracy has fostered people's knowledge (Shin 2012). It encourages citizens to be knowledgeable to become independent and helpful to governance. Knowledge has been a basis of satisfaction and self-efficacy (Dyck and Lascher 2009; Norris 2011). Democracy has engendered perceptions about freedom and institutional legitimacy (Gilley 2009; Moller and Skaaning 2013), fostering life quality, notably satisfaction with life and democracy (Abbott et al. 2011; Mookerjee and Beron 2004; Norris 2011). Democracy has facilitated support, favor, and trust in institutions, government, law, democracy, and politicians (Norris 1999a, 1999b; Remmer 2012; Shin 2012). These attitudes have been salutary (Abbott and Sapsford 2006; Mattes and Christie 1997).

Liberty. Liberty musters significant value from the ideology of liberalism (Rasmussen and Den Uyl 2005). Such ideology advocates for people's rights to be free. Concerning the deterministic mechanism, liberty at the national level is likely to geminate personal life quality. Accordingly, national liberty provides opportunities for people to optimize their life quality. At least, liberty reduces the risk of depriving people's resources. Hence, liberty has facilitated personal well-being, including satisfaction with life and democracy (Abbott et al. 2011; Mookerjee and Beron 2004; Norris 2011). Liberty has also undergirded support and trust in government, democracy, and the market (Magalhaes 2014; Mishler and Rose 1997; Wong et al. 2016). Herein, as people enjoy their liberty facilitated by the government, democracy, and/or other institutions, they naturally feel indebted to and trustful in the institutions. These attitudes have been conducive to life quality (Abbott and Sapsford 2006; Graham and Pettinato 2002b; Mattes and Christie 1997). Conversely, liberty has prevented perceptions about the democracy deficit (Norris 2011). Democracy has been a basis for personal life quality or satisfaction (Frey and Stutzer 2000; Meulemann 2010; Veenhoven 2008).

Human development. Human development is the composite of education, life expectancy, and prosperity or national income. It hinges on the capability for development or life quality (Inglehart and Welzel 2005). National human development is likely to lift personal life quality. From the deterministic view, national human development represents the availability of physical, economic, and educational resources and support for optimizing each other's life quality. National human development has championed personal life quality (Eikemo et al. 2008; Meulemann 2010; Napier and Jost 2008). Specifically, national human development has safeguarded health and life satisfaction (Basabe et al. 2002; Eikemo et al. 2008). Accordingly, healthy, wealthy, and educated people can help one another be healthy and satisfied. National development has raised national civility (Bond and Lun 2014). Possibly, educated people can help others be civilized. National civility would reflect the case that citizens help one another to boost their life quality. Similarly, national human development has fostered people's donation (Fridberg and Kangas 2008b), possibly because it can create a donation opportunity. Donation has led to life quality (Chang 2009). Moreover, national human development has strengthened people's knowledge (Norris 2011). For instance, educated people can teach or put knowledge into others. Knowledge has been a basis for life quality (Dyck and Lascher 2009; Norris 2011). National human development has also elevated people's social trust, support, and responsibility (Kangas 2008b), possibly because they become more trustworthy as people have higher education. These attitudes have been conducive to life quality (Hommerich and Tiefenbach 2018).

Human capital per capita. Human capital consists of ability, education, training, and skill inalienable from the human (Blair 2011). Specifically, according to the data source, it comprises education and returns to education or meritocracy (Dahlberg et al. 2018). Human capital at the national level is likely to facilitate personal life quality, reflecting the deterministic mechanism. People's human capital provides resources for each person to develop life quality. Hence, one's life quality can benefit from others' human capital through their help. National human capital has raised personal income (Florida 2005), which has sustained life quality (Gattino et al. 2015; Wang and VanderWeele 2011). More specifically, education in a country has sustained personal health (Herian et al. 2014). Conversely, education in a country has reduced illness in the person (Jones et al. 2015). Illness has weakened life quality (Carrieri 2012; Linssen et al. 2011), possibly because educated people can maintain personal hygiene, prevent disease transmission, and help others avoid health concerns. Similarly, education in a country has reduced personal obesity and smoking (Herian et al. 2014). For instance, health professionals, who typically have high education, can help others maintain healthy habits. Obesity has generated anxiety and eroded self-esteem and satisfaction in life and weight (Frederick et al. 2016; Hintsanen et al. 2010; Kahneman et al. 2010). Moreover, it has impaired health (Ferraro and Farmer 1999). Similarly, smoking has impaired health (Michalos et al. 2005; Veenstra et al. 2005). One's smoking can endanger the health of others nearby, such as one's family members. Conversely, education in a country has buttressed employment and income and diminished poverty in the person (Goetz et al. 2011; Lipford and Yandle 2009; Robert and Bukodi 2005). Notably, meritocracy in the country would encourage people's employment because they regard employment as rewarding and fair. Another possibility is for educated people, such as human service and career guidance professionals, to help others gain employment and avoid poverty. Employment has been conducive to life quality (Carrieri 2012; Wang and VanderWeele 2011), whereas poverty has eroded living quality and life quality (Clark et al. 2008; Lever et al. 2005). Education in a country has also raised the social capital accessed by the person (Portes and Vickstrom 2011). That is, the more educated person would be more obliging and trustworthy. Social capital has been a basis for life quality (Jones et al. 2014;

Oshio and Kobayashi 2010). Moreover, education in a country has lowered personal perception about corruption in society and sustained personal perception about institutional legitimacy (Collier 2002; Gilley 2009), possibly because educating people can help curb corruption, thus buttressing the perceptions. Perception of corruption has undermined life quality, including satisfaction with life, democracy, and police (Helliwell et al. 2010; Hwang et al. 2005; Norris 2011; Veenhoven 2005). Education in a country has also fostered personal trust in government and people and support for democracy (Cohen and Bolt 2005; Uslaner and Brown 2005). These attitudes have been salutary (Abbott and Sapsford 2006; Hommerich and Tiefenbach 2018; Mattes and Christie 1997). Education in a country has likewise boosted volunteering by the person (Lipford and Yandle 2009), possibly because educated people can help establish organizations that mobilize volunteering. Volunteering has been salutary (Borgonovi 2008; Chang 2009).

Environmental risk: CO_2 emission per capita. Environmental risk includes degradation, deterioration, destruction, depletion, crowding, poor housing, and harmful emission in the environment, such as CO_2 (Esaisason 2014; Fisher and Freudenburg 2004; Riad and Norris 1992; Swanson et al. 1992; Van Haaften et al. 2004). It also means poor quality, cleanliness, and sanitation in the environment (Scruggs 2003). Notably, the risk represents a postindustrial risk of overdevelopment, technological dominance, and loss of humanity (Baum et al. 2002; Pujol 1999). Environmental risk is likely to impair personal life quality regarding the deterministic mechanism. Accordingly, the risk deprives resources and support for people to maintain their life quality. It also creates traps, impediments, risks, and harm to erode personal life quality. Such harm arises because of contagion among people and objects within the environment (Settersten and Andersson 2002). Hence, environmental risk has dampened personal life quality, including health and life satisfaction (Stafford et al. 2005; Tiliouine et al. 2006; Van Haaften et al. 2004). Environmental pollutants are detrimental to people's health. Moreover, environmental risk has weakened attachment and liking toward the environment (Mesch and Manor 1998). People would like to avert environmental risks, but dampening these attitudes has led to reduced life quality (Berry and Welsh 2010; Leung et al. 2011; Stanley et al. 2011). Environmental risk has also provoked protest (Scafuto and La Barbera 2016), which has eroded life quality by raising worry (Boehnke and Wong 2011). Furthermore, environmental risk has reduced social capital (Cummins et al. 2003), possibly because environmental risk would discourage people's commitment to the environment or community. Reduced social capital has reduced life quality (Jones et al. 2014; Oshio and Kobayashi 2010).

Time

The passage of time reflects something more than modernization and social change. More generally, it reflects denaturalization, humanization, or anthropologization.

Nature is dwindling, eroding, and losing with humans' presence, activity, and footprinting. Notably, such features of the passage of time do not necessarily lead to development or destruction and can have no bearing on civilization. Even for people in primitive or uncivilized societies, their presence, living, and subsistence drain natural resources and change the natural landscape and ecology. Nevertheless, such change in nature inclines toward denaturalization because such change results from human presence and/or interference or intervention. For example, even when a person steps on the grass in the wild, natural conditions and ecology begin to change not naturally but responsively to the person's action. Apart from the change in nature, change in society or social change is a prominent component of the passage of time. Hence, the passage of time comprises social change and natural change, which are primarily denaturalization or humanization as a response to human presence and/or action. Essentially, natural, environmental, and social changes do not mean improvement or deterioration. The crux, anyhow, is the increasing presence of people and, subsequently, their modification of the world. This modification can include greening and de-greening, such as reforestation and deforestation. Change in nature can include increased plantation and greenery, which are nevertheless artificial. The change in time includes individualization, humanization, and civilization and the aspects of modernization, such as globalization, economic development, technological development, and human development (Harper and Leicht 2011).

Individualization is demonstrably a social change, such that the passage of time maintains a significant positive correlation with independence in work (partial $r = 0.315$, after partialling out effects of countries) and a significant negative correlation with full-time employment (partial $r = -0.345$). Specifically, engagement or embeddedness in regular and controlled work diminishes with time. The passage of time in terms of individualization is likely to raise personal life quality, considering the deterministic mechanism. Accordingly, individualization relieves external control and constraints and thus facilitates personal freedom and life quality. Essentially, individualization encompasses disintegration, deregulation, and enhancement of the self (Bauman 2001; Beck and Beck-Gernsheim 2002). On the one hand, disintegration, detachment, disembeddedness, or disconnection primarily happens in work, production, and/or class, institution, and familial and communal roles (Burgess 2018). It also means disconnection in production, leading to independence at work. Disintegration can happen spatially with dissociating from a place (Bauman 2001) and means erosion in habit and commitment. On the other hand, deregulation means competition, polarization, and emphasis on the free market, thus downplaying the community (Burgess 2018). This outcome signifies the loss of power of institution and authority. Hence, individualization maintains personal choices (Burgess 2018), implying the plurality of lifestyles, alternatives, and even seductions without an absolute standard. Furthermore, it embraces the enhancement of the self, including self-orientation, self-interest, self-culture, self-determination, self-referentiality, personal rights, and individual therapy. The self becomes the standard, without reference to others. The three main features of individualization thus buttress personal independence, freedom, choices, and resources for personal interest. Personal independence has been conducive to life quality in terms of health and mastery (Papadopoulos et al. 2013; Roy and Chaudhuri 2008). Freedom perceived in society has also been salutary (Abbott and Sapsford 2006; Haller and Hadler 2006). Specifically, freedom has maintained health, self-esteem, and life satisfaction (Gehring 2013; Glendinning et al. 2003). Conversely, it has prevented depression and symptoms (Glendinning et al. 2003). Similarly, personal choice has been conducive to life quality (Abbott and Sapsford 2006); it has championed self-determination and satisfaction with life and neighborhood (Day 2013; Gagne and Deci 2005; Helliwell et al. 2010). Notably, self-determination is a humanist form of life quality, representing living (Gagne and Deci 2005; Wehmeyer et al. 2009) and signifies societal progress (Kagitcibasi 2005). Personal choice has also facilitated intrinsic motivation, effort, and performance (Patall et al. 2008). These attitudes and practices have contributed to life quality (Ferssizidis et al. 2010; Mattes and Christie 1997). Furthermore, personal choice has elevated personal income (Growiec and Growiec 2010), while personal resources and conservation have bolstered life quality (Jones et al. 2014; Martin and Westerhof 2003).

Individualization is likely to reduce the influences of the deterministic mechanism and the voluntaristic mechanism of social conformity. Conversely, it is likely to accentuate the influences of the voluntaristic mechanisms of power realization, utility optimization, and idealistic consistency. The attenuation of the influence of the deterministic mechanism means that the influences of the national factors of PISTOL and modernization dwindle with time. That is, national or external resources are likely to be less conducive to personal life quality with time. Conversely, national constraints or deprivations are likely to be less harmful to personal life quality with time. Meanwhile, the diminution of the influence of socially induced voluntaristic mechanism purports that the influences of the Internet, media, organization, and work sector decline with time. This decline means that association with such social factors has less interference with personal life quality with time. Conversely, personal resources, perceived gain, and idealistic consistency are likely to be more salutary with time. The key to these possible influences of individualization is the increase in personal influence and the reduction in social and national influences. Such reduction in social and national influences has happened in social sensitivity due to independence (Bekker et al. 2011). This finding suggests that the independent person is less susceptible to social influence.

The passage of time signifies development in population and material. The latter includes prosperity or living standard, organization, globalization, government effectiveness, human development, and human capital. Hence, progress or modernization characterizes the passage of time. The contribution of progress or development to personal life quality is evident because they are virtually synonymous (Bell 2010; Galtung 2005). In addition, modernization or development increases national resources and their availability to citizens (Johnson 2009). Resource availability is a deterministic force to raise personal life quality. Hence, national modernization has championed personal life quality by enhancing autonomy (Delhey 2010). Accordingly, autonomy has been a cornerstone of life quality (Gayne and Deci 2005). Resources are also accessible from social capital, social cohesion, assistance, helpfulness, or social support from other people in the country. Such access has been salutary (Wen et al. 2010) and has been salubrious or beneficial to health (Franzini et al. 2005; Fujisawa et al. 2009; Helliwell and Putnam 2005). In addition, access has contributed to satisfaction with life and neighborhood (Cramm et al. 2012; Sampson 1991). Similarly, it has been conducive to success (Furstenberg and Hughes 1995). Conversely, the access has diminished distress and depression (Gary et al. 2007; Wright et al. 2015) and has prevented illness (Wen et al. 2010). In addition, the access has fostered trust in government and medicine and favor for the community (Ahern and Hendryx 2003; Han et al. 2017; Whitham 2012). Trust and favor have engendered life quality (Abbott and Sapsford 2006; Mattes and Christie 1997; Stanley et al. 2011).

Development, progress, or modernization in economic, material, social, or simply demographic aspects is likely to increase external or social influences according to the deterministic and socially oriented voluntaristic mechanisms. Availability or access to social resources or support in the country has sustained regulatory quality there (Lee et al. 2011). This result suggests that national influence grows with the availability or access. In addition, the access has raised personal trust or favor in the community, government, and other institutions (Ahern and Hendryx 2003; Han et al. 2017; Whitham 2012). This raising suggests the growth in receptivity or susceptibility to social influence with the access. Similarly, national economic development or prosperity has elevated personal trust in people and institutions, including the government (Marien 2011; Norris 1999a; Traunmuller 2011). This outcome also suggests increased susceptibility to social influence with national prosperity. Moreover, national prosperity has buttressed government effectiveness and legal quality (Bjornskov 2005; Guisan 2009), which suggests increasing governmental influence with prosperity.

Change in the environment or nature has the characteristics of humanization, anthropologization, artificialization, or denaturalization. These characteristics, in turn, rest on population growth with time. Specifically, the presence of people changes the natural environment, either increasing or reducing plantation, vegetation, desertization, atmospheric temperature, and/or natural beauty. National population growth is likely to reduce external or social influences, which reflect the deterministic and socially induced voluntaristic mechanisms. Conversely, national population size is likely to elevate the influence based on the utilitarian voluntaristic mechanism of optimizing. In this connection, national population size has championed personal support for capitalism and distrust of government (Bjornskov and Paldam 2012; Eldersveld et al. 1995). Capitalism, in turn, means egoism, encompassing self-actualization, private ownership, rationalization, utilitarianism, and profit-making, and discourages collectivism, socialism, and statism (Bernstein 2012). As such, capitalism would attenuate external and social influences and raise the influence of personal rational choice or perceived gain. Moreover, distrust of government would reduce the governmental influence.

A more general social change is postmodernization, which is likely to increase unpredictability or diminish the effects on life quality with time. Postmodernization is excessive modernization that goes beyond modernization to create qualitative changes (Alvarado 1996; Cote 2000; Inglehart 1997). Culturally, postmodernization rides on hyperdifferentiation to produce diversity and variety (Martinelli 2005; Venkatesh 1999). For example, it is less predictable when life quality takes more forms and emerges in more ways. Postmodernization mostly features consumerism, including choice, specialization, fashioning, commodification, and uniqueness (Crook et al. 1992; Glennie 1998; Leonard 1997; Ritzer 1997; Venkatesh 1999). It is less predictable when life quality is more individually unique or idiosyncratic. When people develop and treasure their tastes more intensely, their life quality is less predictable. Other prominent cultural-postmodern elements include art, aestheticization, arationality, ephemerality, superficiality, eclecticism, and liberalization (Blackshaw 2005; Gartman 1998; Martinelli 2005; Ritzer 1997; Tester 2004). When life quality is less reliant on rational and standard thinking, it is less predictable. Furthermore, postmodern culture emphasizes uncertainty and indeterminacy (Boje 1995; Tester 2004). Economically, consumption, mediatization, and flexibilization are the most salient features in postmodernization (Gartman 1999; Heaphy 2007; Turner 2003). Hence, the material and real economy shrinks with postmodernization. When life quality stands more intensely on virtual reality, it is less predictable. Postmodernization accentuates democratization, privatization, and denationalization (Crook et al. 1992; Inglehart 2000; Scambler 2002). Specifically, when life quality is less reliant on the stable structure of polity, it is less predictable. Hence, the polity becomes less important and influential with postmodernization. Individualization, defamilialization, destandardization, and fragmentation are prominent (Heaphy 2007; Jacques 1998). Similarly, it is less predictable when life quality has fewer standards and connections to a stable structure. Again, uncertainty, indeterminacy, ambiguity, contingency, and chaos increase in various aspects of postmodernization (Heaphy 2007). If life quality does not have a standard form, it will not be predictable. Eventually, unpredictability is the common theme of postmodernization (Tester 2004).

The underlying logic of the postmodernization thesis about increasing unpredictability with time is the decentering and deconstruction of concepts, factors, and phenomena (Alvesson 2002; Ritzer and Goodman 2001). Accordingly, all those observed are fickle, unstable, chancy, fragmented, liquid, unstructured, and groundless. Hence, variables are idiosyncratic, fictional, unrealistic, and thus not comparable, estimable, and analyzable (Mommaas 2004; Rosenau 1992). According to the postmodern logic, deterministic and voluntaristic mechanisms and any grand theory collapse and are inapplicable (Alvesson and Deetz 2000).

Chapter 4
Life Quality Production: Findings

Evidence on the statics and dynamics of production of life quality evolved from the statistical analysis of World Values Survey data. The unit of analysis was the person. To present the person in the world population, the weighting of data was necessary to equalize the representative data from each country because cases from a larger country had greater weight while those from a smaller country had smaller weight. Eventually, the weighted sample represented the distribution of people from different countries in the world population.

Statistical Analysis of Life Quality

The principal statistical analysis of life quality was the linear regression analysis of four life quality indicators: health, life satisfaction, delight, and worry, following some preliminary analyses using correlation or partial correlation analysis and factor analysis. Worry was available only at Wave 6, so no time effect on worry was estimable. Delight was the composite of happiness, the experience of free choice and control, and financial satisfaction. The regression analysis focusing on personal predictors had five steps to include predictors cumulatively. Step 1 entered time (i.e., the wave of the survey) and significant country indicators in terms of dummy variables as fixed predictors. Step 2 added personal background characteristics and response characteristics such as acquiescence (i.e., rating everything highly) as predictors. Step 3 added personal experiences and practices as predictors. To analyze health or life satisfaction, Step 4 added significant interactions with time as predictors to examine time differentials in the effects of personal background characteristics, experiences, and practices. By contrast, for the delight analysis, Step 4 added health and life satisfaction, measured these days, as predictors. Step 5 only for the analysis of delight, added significant interactions with time to scrutinize differentials in the effects of personal background characteristics, experiences, practices, health, and life satisfaction. For the analysis of worry, Step 4 added health and life satisfaction. The

C. Cheung, *Production Dynamics for Life Quality in the Incipient 21st Century*,
https://doi.org/10.1007/978-981-19-3827-6_4

analysis of worry had no Step 5 because time was not a variable in the analysis. For selecting significant predictors in regression analysis, the criteria for each predictor were the p-value below 0.01 and the tolerance above 0.3 to avoid the problem of multicollinearity. Meanwhile, the regression analysis focused on national indicators as the predictors proceeded in three steps. The first step selected significant national indicators as predictors. Significant interactions between time and national indicators entered the regression model in the second step. Lastly, the third step added significant country indicators to control for their fixed effects. If the regression analysis entered country indicators first, it would preclude other national indicators from entering the regression model. To minimize the problem of multicollinearity, each interaction term took the standard scores of its constituents for forming the product.

Partial correlation analysis controlled for the wave displayed significant national life quality differences. Health was notably higher than the average in Nigeria (partial $r = 0.088$) and the United States (partial $r = 0.063$). The better health in Nigeria reflected the greater proportion of the young population there (Falola and Paddock 2012; Lewis 2007). Meanwhile, better health in the United States might reflect the greater prosperity and resources (Shortall and Warner 2010). Conversely, health was notably lower than the average in Russia (partial $r = -0.113$) and Japan (partial $r = -0.061$). The poorer health in Russia is consistent with the higher malnutrition and mortality there (Gavrilova et al. 2000), while the poorer health in Japan might be due to the older population there (Pilling 2014; Targgort Murphy 2014). Life satisfaction was notably higher than the average in Mexico (partial $r = 0.122$) and Brazil (partial $r = 0.101$), reflecting the greater happiness in Latin America (Minkov 2011). Conversely, satisfaction was notably lower than the average in India (partial $r = -0.152$) and Egypt (partial $r = -0.090$). Life satisfaction was lower in India probably because poverty is more likely there (Basu and Mallick 2008). Accordingly, poverty has reduced life satisfaction (Firebaugh and Schroeder 2009). Delight was notably higher than the average in Mexico (partial $r = 0.122$) and the United States (partial $r = 0.079$). Again, the higher delight reflects the greater happiness in Latin America (Minkov 2011). The higher delight or happiness in the United States is consistent with the findings in previous work (Phillips 2006). Conversely, it was notably lower than the average in Egypt (partial $r = -0.106$) and Russia (partial $r = -0.081$). Worry was notably higher in Mexico (partial $r = 0.168$) and the Philippines (partial $r = 106$). The higher worry in Mexico might be due to the welfare retrenchment there (Marier and Mayer 2007), while the higher worry in the Philippines might be due to the fatalism there (Tuason 2008). Conversely, worry was notably lower in the United States (partial $r = -0.187$) and Germany (partial $r = -0.131$). These countries have been happier than have others (Fukuyama 1995; Phillips 2006) (Table 4.1).

Factor analysis presented a 2-D space to approximate relationships between life quality and the countries. The two dimensions appeared to contrast with cognitive life quality, consisting of life satisfaction, delight, and health, with emotional life quality consisting of worry on the one hand and India with China on the other hand. This space depicted that Mexico, Brazil, and the United States had closer or more positive relationships with cognitive life quality than did other countries. Conversely, Russia,

Table 4.1 Partial correlations between life quality and countries

Country	Health	Life satisfaction	Delight	Worry
Brazil	0.023**	0.101**	0.064**	0.028**
China	−0.003	0.027**	−0.033**	−0.073**
Egypt	−0.035**	−0.090**	−0.106**	0.068**
Ethiopia	−0.003	−0.067**	−0.038**	
Germany	0.005	0.033**	−0.006	−0.131**
India	0.005	−0.152**	−0.038**	0.013*
Indonesia	0.016**	0.025**	0.036**	
Iran	−0.003	−0.006	−0.008	
Japan	−0.061**	0.019**	−0.033**	0.086**
Mexico	0.006	0.122**	0.122**	0.168**
Nigeria	0.088**	−0.037**	0.012**	0.074**
Pakistan	0.037**	0.044**	0.037**	0.042**
Philippines	−0.025**	0.022**	0.027**	0.106**
Russia	−0.113**	−0.049**	−0.081**	−0.012
Turkey	−0.010*	0.037**	0.022**	0.015*
Vietnam	−0.027**	0.023**	0.009*	
US	0.063**	0.078**	0.079**	−0.187**

Note The partial correlations resulted from controlling for the wave
* $p < 0.05$, ** $p < 0.01$

Egypt, India, and China had remote, weak, or negative relationships with cognitive life quality. Meanwhile, China also had a weak relationship with worry (Fig. 4.1).

Predicting Health

The first step of regression analysis focused on personal predictors showed that health was significantly lower in Russia, Egypt, and the Philippines ($\beta = -0.111$ to -0.025) and higher in Nigeria and Pakistan ($\beta = 0.036 - 0.086$). These national differences, nevertheless, were weak or trivial. Variation in health due to other countries was insignificant and smaller.

The second step of regression analysis focused on personal background characteristics that significantly predicted health. Among these characteristics, age exhibited the strongest and most negative effect on health ($\beta = -0.216$). This effect reflected the voluntaristic mechanism of power realization. That is, the older person is less powerful and thus less healthy. Nevertheless, the square of age did not display a significant effect on health. In addition, education showed a relatively strong and positive effect on health ($\beta = 0.092$). The effect again registered the voluntaristic mechanism of power realization. That is, higher education means higher power to

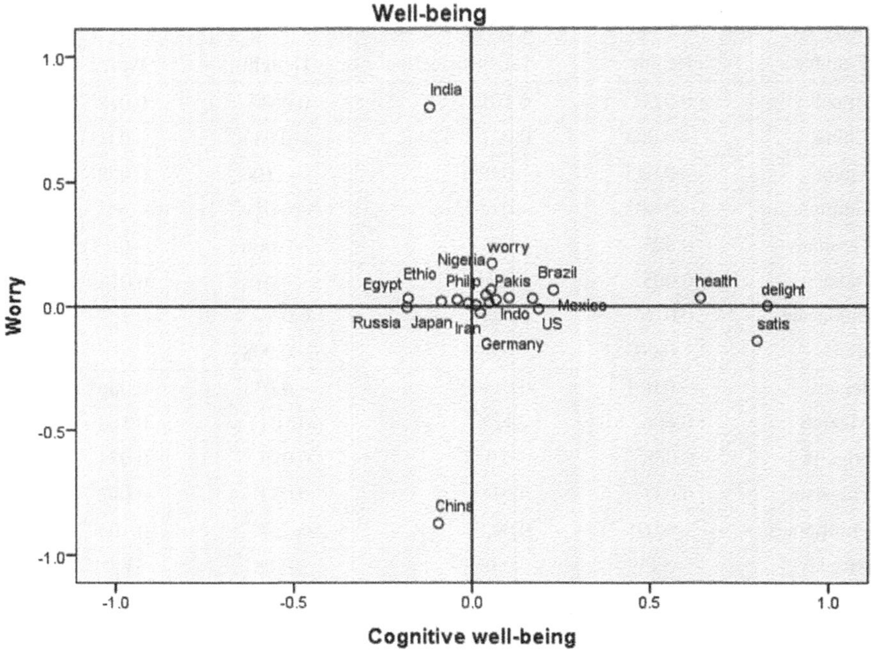

Fig. 4.1 Factor loadings on the two dimensions of life quality. Ethio = Ethiopia, Indo = Indonesia, Pakis = Pakistan, Philip = Philippines, satis = life satisfaction

maintain better health. The other significant effects of background characteristics were trivial ($\beta < 0.05$). Time emerged to have a significant positive effect on health ($\beta = 0.055$) after controlling for significant background characteristics. The time effect implied the deterministic mechanism of external resources or guidance.

The third step of regression analysis added personal experiences and practices as predictors of health. Most of these predictors presented significant effects on health. The strongest and negative effect was due to economic hardship ($\beta = -0.132$). This effect reflected the voluntaristic mechanism of utility optimization. Accordingly, economic hardship means a loss in life, which would be detrimental to life quality, such as health or its maintenance. Simply speaking, losing is dissatisfying and discouraging. The effect buttressed the voluntaristic mechanism of power realization as well. Economic hardship meant the shortage of financial resources to afford health maintenance. The effect of family saving was the second strongest and positive one ($\beta = 0.098$). This effect also endorsed the voluntaristic mechanism of utility optimization. Accordingly, family saving represents a gainful experience, which justifies health maintenance. Simply speaking, gaining is satisfying. Moreover, the effect suggested the voluntaristic mechanism of power realization. At this juncture, family saving provided financial resources affording health maintenance. The third strongest and negative effect was from the experience of neighborhood nuisance ($\beta =$

-0.082). The effect again purported the voluntaristic mechanism of utility optimization. Accordingly, the nuisance means a perceived loss in life and thus dissatisfaction with life, including health. By contrast, security displayed a significant positive effect on health ($\beta = 0.050$). This effect also implied the voluntaristic mechanism of utility optimization. Security means gaining from life and thus the willingness to support life in terms of health maintenance. Moreover, the contribution of security suggested the voluntaristic mechanism of power realization. Specifically, security represents power or resources to afford health maintenance. The other effects of experiences and practices were very trivial ($\beta = 0.05$).

The fourth step of regression analysis revealed significant differential health effects due to time, involving the interactions between time and background characteristics, experiences, and practices. Among these effects, the interaction between time and voluntary organizational participation maintained the strongest and positive effect on health ($\beta = 0.248$). This interaction effect showed that the negative effect of organizational participation on health became a positive effect at Wave 6. That is, organizational participation became less influential in diminishing health. Earlier, the negative effect of participation on health reflected the voluntaristic mechanism of norm conformity. The organization tended to be concerned with various problems, including health problems, and this organizational concern likely drew the participant's concern for health problems. This organizational concern likely drew the participant's concern for health problem. Similarly, the positive effect of being irreligious on health became a negative effect with time ($\beta = -0.063$). That is, being irreligious became less influential in sustaining health. The contribution of being irreligious to health may reflect the voluntaristic mechanism of idea consistency. Accordingly, being irreligious is associated with the belief in personal power and thus personal health maintenance. Another case was the diminishing negative influence of children on health such that the influence became positive with time ($\beta = 0.061$). The negative effect of children on health may be due to the children's burden, which is stressful and debilitating. This effect reflects the deterministic mechanism of external force. Furthermore, the positive effect of education on health declined with time to become a negative effect ($\beta = -0.055$). The positive effect of education on health registers the voluntaristic mechanism of power realization. That is, education is a resource facilitating health maintenance. Living with parents also reduced its negative influence on health with time to hold a positive effect ($\beta = 0.052$). The negative effect of living with parents reflects the deterministic mechanism of external constraint. Accordingly, living with parents poses a constraint to impede health. The positive effect of e-activity also shrank to maintain a negative effect with time ($\beta = -0.050$). Earlier, the positive effect of e-activity endorsed the voluntaristic mechanism of power realization. The use means acquiring knowledge and, therefore, the power to maintain health. In contrast to the decline in influence, verbal involvement increased its positive effect on health with time ($\beta = 0.096$). The contribution of verbal involvement to health endorsed the voluntaristic mechanism of utility optimization. Accordingly, the involvement tends to be gainful, rejoicing, and salubrious. Age also increased its negative effect with time ($\beta = -0.053$). In all, most of the effects on health became weaker rather than stronger, meaning that health became more unpredictable. This finding is consonant with the postmodernization thesis. Notably, the reduction in most effects, including those from social and personal sources, suggested that it was unlikely to reflect individualization only (Table 4.2).

In the first step of regression analysis focused on the national predictors of health, land (per capita) emerged to be the most influential predictor exerting a significant negative effect on health ($\beta = -0.089$). This effect represented the deterministic mechanism of external influence. The influence, nevertheless, was adverse in this case, showing the diffuseness, insufficiency, and/or inaccessibility of resources to sustain health. When the space is larger, resources such as clinics are farther away and less accessible. Importantly, land itself may not be salubrious. Rather, other health maintenance resources, including healthcare professionals and even neighbors, are beneficial to health. The wave, national liberty, and national globalization also had significantly positive but trivial effects on health.

The third step of regression analysis focused on the national predictors of personal health revealed significant effects from four interactions with time with the control of country indicators. Among them, the strongest and negative effect on health was the interaction between time and national government effectiveness ($\beta = -0.112$). National government effectiveness was less beneficial to health with time. The effect reflected the deterministic mechanism of external influence. Herein, government effectiveness might entail urges for effectiveness or productivity harmful to health. The next strongest and positive effect on health was the interaction between time and national liberty ($\beta = 0.066$). That is, the benefit for national liberty increased with time. Notably, time strengthened the effect of national liberty, which departed from the individualization and postmodernization theses. Nonetheless, the effect of liberty purported the deterministic mechanism of external influence. In this case, national liberty means reducing external control, which is stressful and debilitating. A comparable effect on health was from the interaction between time and national income inequality ($\beta = -0.067$). Accordingly, the inequality was increasingly detrimental to health. Nevertheless, the significant positive effect of interaction between time and national population size was trivial ($\beta = 0.018$). This effect showed that national population size slightly increased its benefit to health with time. The effect endorsed the deterministic mechanism of external influence. With this, other people in the country are increasingly helpful in safeguarding one another's health. Such an increase may be because of the greater knowledge and more effective aid from people (Table 4.3).

Predicting Life Satisfaction

The first step of regression analysis of life satisfaction showed the significant effects of the wave and some country indicators. Accordingly, the wave indicated a positive effect ($\beta = 0.066$), indicating that life satisfaction increased with time. Among the country indicators, India showed the strongest and negative effect on life satisfaction

Table 4.2 Standardized effects on health

Predictor	(1)	(2)	(3)	(4)
Wave	0.015	0.055^{***}	0.049^{***}	0.148^{***}
Russia	-0.111^{***}	-0.098^{***}	-0.071^{***}	-0.046^{***}
Nigeria	0.086^{***}	0.050^{***}	0.063^{***}	−0.009
Pakistan	0.036^{***}	0.021***	0.035^{***}	0.016^{*}
Egypt	-0.036^{***}	−0.038***	-0.022^{**}	-0.024^{**}
Philippines	-0.025^{**}	-0.042^{***}	-0.030^{***}	-0.052^{***}
Acquiescence		0.183^{***}	0.239^{***}	0.347^{***}
Irreligious		0.041^{***}	0.032^{**}	-0.044^{***}
Family income		0.005	0.070^{***}	0.069^{***}
Female		−0.003	−0.004	−0.010
Age		-0.216^{***}	-0.241^{***}	-0.265^{***}
Age squared		0.006	0.000	0.004
Married		0.018	0.012	0.000
Cohabited		0.002	0.011	0.022^{**}
Divorced		0.000	0.003	−0.004
Separated		−0.016	−0.006	−0.002
Widowed		−0.007	−0.007	−0.013
Kid		-0.032^{**}	−0.005	0.013
Father immigrant		0.017^{*}	0.037^{***}	0.050^{***}
Education		0.092^{***}	0.022^{*}	-0.029^{**}
Graduation age		0.011	0.032^{***}	0.038^{***}
Interest		0.036^{***}	0.035^{***}	0.044^{***}
Living with parents		-0.021^{*}	−0.010	0.008
Full-time employment		0.017	0.021^{*}	0.005
Part-time employment		−0.001	0.016	0.011
Self-employment		0.006	0.001	−0.006
Retired		−0.007	0.007	−0.007
Homemaking		0.003	0.004	0.005
Student		−0.004	0.014	0.042^{***}
Public employment		0.017	0.004	−0.009
Private business employment		0.021^{*}	0.020^{*}	0.029^{**}
Nonprofit organization employment		0.017^{*}	0.003	−0.005
Creative work		−0.013	0.003	0.031^{**}
Independent work		0.035^{**}	0.015	−0.015
Supervision		0.017	0.005	−0.002
Earner		−0.012	0.006	0.017

(continued)

Table 4.2 (continued)

Predictor	(1)	(2)	(3)	(4)
Earner employed		0.031^{***}	0.002	−0.004
Economic hardship			-0.132^{***}	-0.273^{***}
Neighborhood nuisance			-0.082^{***}	-0.263^{***}
Security			0.050^{***}	-0.023^{**}
Family saving			0.098^{***}	0.045^{***}
E-activity			0.029^{**}	-0.030^{**}
Learning			-0.022^{*}	-0.031^{**}
Spiritual activity			0.039^{***}	-0.039^{**}
Risk aversion			-0.046^{***}	-0.041^{***}
Weapon carrying			0.035^{***}	−0.015
Organizational participation			-0.042^{***}	0.122^{***}
Appealing			0.003	0.023^{**}
Voting			−0.010	-0.112^{***}
Green demonstration			0.003	-0.167^{***}
Wave × Organizational participation				0.248^{***}
Wave × Irreligious				-0.063^{***}
Wave × Learning				0.096^{***}
Wave × Education				-0.055^{***}
Wave × Living with parents				0.052^{***}
Wave × Kid				0.061^{***}
Wave × Age				-0.053^{***}
Wave × E-activity				-0.050^{***}
Wave × Self-employed				-0.029^{***}
Wave × Cohabited				0.026^{**}
Wave × Family income				-0.031^{**}
Wave × Divorced				-0.022^{**}
R^2	0.024	0.154	0.202	0.230

* $p < 0.05$, ** $p < 0.01$, *** $p < 0.001$

($\beta = -0.143$). The second strongest and positive effect on life satisfaction was from Mexico ($\beta = 0.105$). In addition, Egypt and Russia exhibited lower life satisfaction ($\beta = -0.098$ and -0.061), whereas Brazil displayed higher life satisfaction ($\beta = 0.079$). The other differences due to countries were trivial ($\beta < 0.05$).

The second step of regression analysis primarily based on personal predictor focused on personal background characteristics as predictors of life satisfaction. Among the characteristics, independent work showed the strongest and positive effect on the satisfaction ($\beta = 0.106$). The contribution of independent work to life satisfaction registered the voluntaristic mechanism of utility optimization. Accordingly,

Table 4.3 Standardized effects of national characteristics on health

Predictor	(1)	(2)	(3)
Wave	0.022***	0.023***	0.035***
Land	−0.089***	−0.094***	−0.119***
Liberty	0.037***	0.033***	0.111***
Globalization	0.027***	0.020***	−0.040***
Wave × Government effectiveness		−0.125***	−0.112***
Wave × Income inequality		−0.081***	−0.067***
Wave × Liberty		0.082***	0.066***
Wave × Population		0.034***	0.018**
Japan			−0.102***
India			−0.109***
Philippines			−0.051***
Egypt			−0.042***
R^2	0.009	0.015	0.028

* $p < 0.05$, ** $p < 0.01$, *** $p < 0.001$

such work is gainful and satisfying. Education was the second strongest background characteristic for predicting life satisfaction positively ($\beta = 0.070$). The contribution of education on life satisfaction represented the voluntaristic mechanism of power realization. In this regard, education is power sustaining life satisfaction. The effects of other personal characteristics were trivial ($\beta < 0.05$).

The third step of regression analysis revealed that several experiences and practices make a significant difference in life satisfaction. Economic hardship exerted the strongest and most negative effect on life satisfaction ($\beta = -0.181$). This negative effect registered the voluntaristic mechanism of utility optimization. The hardship represents a loss, which is dissatisfying. The next strongest predictors were family saving and security, both displaying positive effects on life satisfaction ($\beta = 0.123$ and 0.101, respectively). The contribution again manifested the voluntaristic mechanism of utility optimization. Herein, the saving is gainful and is therefore satisfying. Civic organizational participation and neighborhood nuisance experienced followed, both delivering negative effects on life satisfaction ($\beta = -0.070$ and −0.065, respectively). The effects of these experiences were adverse, considering the voluntaristic mechanisms of norm conformity and utility optimization. On the one hand, as the civic organization is concerned with problems, it forges a norm for dissatisfaction for the participant to follow. On the other hand, the nuisance represents a loss, which is dissatisfying. The effects of other experiences or practices were insignificant or trivial ($\beta < 0.05$).

The fourth step of regression analysis revealed four significant effects from interactions with time. Among them, the strongest and most positive was the interaction between civil organizational participation and time ($\beta = 0.297$). This effect neutralized the negative effect of organizational participation ($\beta = -0.070$). Thus, the effect of organizational participation was weaker and became positive with time. The second strongest and negative effect was from the interaction between time and irreligiousness ($\beta = -0.124$). This effect negated the positive effect of irreligiousness ($\beta = 0.041$). Hence, the effect of irreligiousness was weaker and became negative with time. The contribution of being irreligious reflected the voluntaristic mechanism of idea consistency. Accordingly, being irreligious indicated the belief in the personal power to sustain life satisfaction. Both interaction effects supported the postmodernization thesis about weakening the effect with time. The two other significant interaction effects were trivial ($\beta < 0.05$) (Table 4.4).

The final step of regression analysis of life satisfaction primarily based on country-level predictors showed several significant predictors, including some country indicators and time. These country indicators manifested that life satisfaction was lower in Egypt ($\beta = -0.092$) and higher in the Philippines and Pakistan ($\beta = 0.060$ and 0.020). Time had a trivial positive effect on life satisfaction, showing a slight increase in satisfaction with time. The strongest and most positive effect was from national human development ($\beta = 0.225$), which reflected the deterministic mechanism of external influence. In this case, national human development represents external resources or aid to elevate one's life satisfaction. Following this was the negative effect of national government effectiveness ($\beta = 0.068$), which registered the deterministic mechanism of external constraint. Herein, the government imposes an external constraint on the person to restrain his or her freedom and thus life satisfaction. The more effective the government, the stronger will be the constraint. In addition, the interaction between national human development and time had a negative effect on life satisfaction ($\beta = -0.049$). This effect weakened the main effect of national human development. Thus, national human development was less conducive to life satisfaction with time. This weakening supported both postmodernization and individualization theses. The interaction between democracy and time also displayed a positive effect on life satisfaction ($\beta = 0.050$). That is, the contribution of democracy to life satisfaction increased with time. The contribution embodied the deterministic mechanism of external support or opportunity. Accordingly, democracy provides liberty and respect to the citizen and raises his or her life satisfaction. Once significant in the second step of the analysis, the interaction between income inequality and time was not significant in the third step with the control for significant country indicators (Table 4.5).

Predicting Delight

As a composite of happiness, free choice, and financial satisfaction, delight displayed some significant national differences in the first step of regression analysis. Among the difference, the greater difference emerged from Mexico, which had higher delight than the others ($\beta = 0.118$). The second strongest difference happened in Egypt, with lower delight than the others ($\beta = -0.105$). In addition, delight was lower in Russia

Table 4.4 Standardized effects on life satisfaction

Predictor	(1)	(2)	(3)	(4)
Wave	0.066***	0.087***	0.084***	0.148***
India	−0.143***	−0.215***	−0.194***	−0.092***
Mexico	0.105***	0.094***	0.124***	0.148***
Egypt	−0.098***	−0.107***	−0.083***	−0.073***
Brazil	0.079***	0.091***	0.090***	0.112***
Russia	−0.061***	−0.048***	−0.023**	0.005
Nigeria	−0.047***	−0.076***	−0.051***	−0.097***
Pakistan	0.031***	0.018*	0.035***	0.048***
Turkey	0.026**	0.015	0.000	−0.008
Germany	0.022**	0.027***	0.003	−0.007
Acquiescence		0.253***	0.327***	0.437***
Irreligious		0.041***	0.022	−0.045***
Family income		0.028***	0.111***	0.136***
Female		0.030**	0.026**	0.027**
Age		−0.009	−0.041***	−0.064***
Age squared		0.046***	0.038***	0.042***
Married		0.046***	0.020	0.001
Cohabited		0.012	0.018*	0.027**
Divorced		−0.015	−0.009	−0.015
Separated		−0.030***	−0.020**	−0.016*
Widowed		0.004	−0.002	−0.011
Kid		0.010	0.038***	0.048***
Father immigrant		0.000	0.027***	0.044***
Education		0.070***	−0.005	−0.049***
Graduation age		−0.014	0.023**	0.037***
Interest		0.033***	0.039***	0.048***
Living with parents		−0.009	−0.007	0.000
Full-time employment		0.005	0.005	−0.017
Part-time employment		0.001	0.016	0.004
Self-employment		0.005	−0.009	−0.015
Retired		0.005	0.019*	0.011
Homemaking		0.041***	0.045***	0.038***
Student		−0.010	0.017	0.032***
Public employment		−0.024**	−0.025**	−0.029**
Private business employment		−0.008	0.007	0.031**
Nonprofit organization employment		−0.003	−0.019*	−0.040***

(continued)

Table 4.4 (continued)

Predictor	(1)	(2)	(3)	(4)
Creative work		-0.035^{**}	0.002	0.028^{**}
Independent work		0.106^{***}	0.065^{***}	0.038^{**}
Supervision		0.033^{***}	0.024^{**}	0.009
Earner		-0.031^{**}	−0.002	0.018
Earner employed		0.015	-0.021^{*}	-0.034^{***}
Economic hardship			-0.181^{***}	-0.307^{***}
Neighborhood nuisance			-0.065^{***}	-0.271^{***}
Security			0.101^{***}	0.014
Family saving			0.123^{***}	0.103^{***}
E-activity			−0.015	-0.040^{***}
Learning			−0.017	-0.023^{**}
Spiritual activity			0.030^{**}	-0.052^{***}
Risk aversion			0.006	0.019^{*}
Weapon carrying			0.014	-0.042^{***}
Organizational participation			-0.070^{***}	0.100^{***}
Appealing			−0.008	0.013
Voting			−0.012	-0.124^{***}
Green demonstration			0.005	-0.176^{***}
Wave × Organizational participation				0.297^{***}
Wave × Irreligious				-0.124^{***}
Wave × Age				-0.041^{***}
Wave × Part-time employment				0.022^{**}
R^2	0.063	0.148	0.227	0.262

* $p < 0.05$, ** $p < 0.01$, *** $p < 0.001$

($\beta = -0.079$) and higher in Brazil ($\beta = 0.060$). The other national differences were trivial ($\beta = 0.05$).

The second step of regression analysis focused on predicting delight by personal characteristics and revealed several significant effects. The strongest and most positive effect was from independent work ($\beta = 0.122$). This contribution endorsed the voluntaristic mechanism of utility optimization. Accordingly, independent work is free and gainful, thereby delighting. The second strongest and positive effect was from education ($\beta = 0.084$), which represented the voluntaristic mechanism of power realization. Herein, education provided power to sustain and satisfy one's life. Following this was the positive effect of marriage ($\beta = 0.067$). Again, the voluntaristic mechanism of power realization applied to the contribution of marriage. One finds support and other resources from marriage to delight one's life. Due to personal background characteristics, the other effects were trivial ($\beta < 0.05$).

Table 4.5 Standardized effects of national characteristics on life satisfaction

Predictor	(1)	(2)	(3)
Wave	0.036***	0.037***	0.024***
Human development	0.212***	0.200***	0.225***
Government effectiveness	−0.065***	−0.052***	−0.068***
Wave × Human development		−0.076***	−0.049***
Wave × Democracy		0.054***	0.050***
Wave × Income inequality		−0.035***	−0.009
Egypt			−0.092***
Pakistan			0.060***
Philippines			0.020***
R^2	0.030	0.032	0.047

* $p < 0.05$, ** $p < 0.01$, *** $p < 0.001$

The third step of regression analysis focused on person-level predictors that revealed experiences and practices significantly predictive of delight. Economic hardship showed the strongest negative effect on delight ($\beta = -0.307$). This effect reflected the voluntaristic mechanism of utility optimization. Accordingly, economic hardship represented a loss, which is frustrating and prevents one from delight. In other words, it is illogical to feel delighted due to a loss. The second strongest predictor was the experience of neighborhood nuisance, whose effect was again negative ($\beta = -0.173$). The negative effect also manifested the voluntaristic mechanism of utility optimization. Accordingly, the experience of neighborhood nuisance means a loss to prevent delight. Following this was the experience of family saving, which positively affected delight ($\beta = 0.097$). The contribution of family saving endorsed the voluntaristic mechanism of utility optimization again. Herein, family saving means a gain in life to warrant delight. Another notable predictor was the practice of strike, which negatively affected delight ($\beta = -0.054$) and registered the voluntaristic mechanism of consistency. The strike represents discontent and is dissonant with delight or consonant with non-delight. The effects of other experiences or practices were trivial ($\beta < 0.05$).

The fourth step of regression analysis focused on predicting delight by health and life satisfaction showed their significant effects. Accordingly, both health and life satisfaction introduced positive effects on delight ($\beta = 0.162$ and 0.413, respectively). These effects realized the voluntaristic mechanism of consistency. All health, life satisfaction, and delight indicate life quality and maintain consistency with one another. These effects substantially mediated the effects of economic hardship, neighborhood nuisance, family saving, and strike. The effects of these experiences or practices dwindled remarkably in the presence of the effects of health and life satisfaction.

The fifth step of regression analysis added interactions between time and other person-level predictors that displayed significant effects on delight. Among the interactions, that between verbal involvement and time exhibited the strongest positive effect ($\beta = 0.110$), indicating that the contribution of verbal involvement to delight strengthened with time. Such an increase lent support to the individualization thesis, which suggests the increasing importance of personal predictors. Essentially, the contribution of verbal involvement rests on the voluntaristic mechanism of utility optimization. At this juncture, verbal involvement is gainful and thus delighting. The second strongest interaction was that between e-activity and time, which manifested a negative effect on delight ($\beta = -0.092$). This interaction showed that the negative effect of e-activity strengthened with time. Again, this effect supported the individualization thesis about the increasing influence of personal predictors. The negative effect of e-activity registered the voluntaristic mechanism of norm conformity. Accordingly, the cyber world engaged in E-activity installs a norm of discontent to lessen delight. The third important interaction was that between irreligiousness and time, which exerted a negative effect on delight ($\beta = -0.081$). This interaction showed that the positive effect of irreligiousness weakened with time and became negative with time. This result could support the individualization thesis because irreligiousness is a traditional and social factor exerting an influence on the person externally. Hence, individualization would dampen the external influence. Based on the voluntaristic mechanism of consistency, irreligiousness would affirm the personal power to foster delight. However, such an empowering role of irreligiousness declined with time. Another interaction was between creative work and time, which delivered a positive effect on delight ($\beta = 0.052$). The interaction effect appeared to diminish the negative effect of creative work on delight. This diminution again supported the individualization thesis, which suggests the weakening of external influence. Herein, creative work represented an external influence from the work setting. This external influence was detrimental to delight in the voluntaristic mechanism of utility optimization. Creative work is demanding and thus stressful and represents a loss to restrain delight. Hence, the principal interaction effects championed the individualization thesis that posits the strengthening of personal influence and the weakening of external influence (Table 4.6).

The first step of regression analysis focused on predicting delight through a national indicator revealed some significant effects. Among the effects, the strongest was the negative effect of land per capita ($\beta = -0.085$), which remained significant in the final analysis step ($\beta = -0.182$). This effect reflected the deterministic mechanism of external deficiency. Specifically, the larger space means the lower availability and accessibility of resources, including people and their aid at a spot, thus weakening personal delight. The second strongest effect was the positive effect of national human development ($\beta = 0.083$). This effect remained significant in the final analysis step ($\beta = 0.142$). The contribution realized the deterministic mechanism of external support. That is, greater national human development means more resources and higher quality for delighting each other. The third strongest effect

Table 4.6 Standardized effects on delight

Predictor	(1)	(2)	(3)	(4)	(5)
Wave	−0.077***	−0.040***	−0.029**	−0.070***	−0.008
Mexico	0.118***	0.105***	0.151***	0.094***	0.116***
Egypt	−0.105***	−0.118***	−0.101***	−0.057***	−0.045***
Russia	−0.079***	−0.064***	−0.012	0.002	0.030***
Brazil	0.060***	0.070***	0.071***	0.028***	0.060***
Pakistan	0.037***	0.018*	0.046***	0.023***	0.008
India	−0.029**	−0.133***	−0.081***	−0.008	0.008
Philippines	0.027**	−0.015*	0.018*	0.018**	0.013*
Turkey	0.021**	0.005	−0.018*	−0.012	−0.022***
Acquiescence		0.343***	0.486***	0.297***	0.384***
Irreligious		0.027**	−0.013	−0.023*	−0.048***
Family income		−0.016*	0.067***	0.013*	0.011
Female		0.007	0.001	−0.008	−0.018**
Age		−0.008	−0.051***	0.002	−0.026**
Age squared		0.046***	0.037***	0.021**	0.027**
Married		0.067***	0.037**	0.025**	0.021***
Cohabited		0.015	0.022**	0.013	0.018**
Divorced		−0.007	−0.003	0.000	−0.006
Separated		−0.026**	−0.016*	−0.006	−0.004
Widowed		−0.003	−0.012	−0.010	−0.011
Kid		−0.023*	0.013	−0.001	0.014
Father immigrant		−0.006	0.032***	0.013*	0.020**
Education		0.084***	−0.022*	−0.021*	−0.049***
Graduation age		−0.015	0.034***	0.023**	0.027***
Interest		0.027**	0.038***	0.014*	0.019**
Living with parents		−0.020*	−0.012	−0.009	0.003
Full-time employment		0.018	0.021*	0.017*	−0.003
Part-time employment		0.003	0.036***	0.026***	0.019**
Self-employment		0.025**	0.008	0.012	−0.019**
Retired		0.003	0.017*	0.012	0.012
Homemaking		0.026**	0.035***	0.015*	0.030***
Student		−0.006	0.025**	0.016*	0.013
Public employment		−0.022*	−0.047***	−0.032***	−0.033***
Private business employment		−0.008	−0.009	−0.012	0.014
Nonprofit organization employment		0.011	−0.056***	−0.038***	−0.050***

(continued)

Table 4.6 (continued)

Predictor	(1)	(2)	(3)	(4)	(5)
Creative work		−0.054***	0.003	−0.001	0.018
Independent work		0.122***	0.080***	0.048***	0.033**
Supervision		0.033***	0.015*	0.007	0.004
Earner		−0.030**	0.008	0.006	0.015*
Earner employed		0.034***	−0.010	−0.003	−0.007
Economic hardship			−0.307***	−0.184***	−0.273***
Neighborhood nuisance			−0.173***	−0.108***	−0.253***
Security			−0.020**	−0.015*	−0.013*
Family saving			0.097***	0.034***	0.019**
E-activity			−0.028**	−0.026**	−0.081***
Learning			−0.040***	−0.033***	−0.022**
Risk aversion			−0.036***	−0.027***	−0.014*
Weapon carrying			0.017*	0.004	−0.013*
Organizational participation			−0.047***	−0.011	0.049***
Appealing			0.015	0.008	0.097***
Strike			−0.054***	−0.028***	−0.178***
Voting			−0.037***	−0.031***	−0.104***
Green demonstration			0.001	−0.004	−0.089***
Health				0.162***	0.148***
Life satisfaction				0.413***	0.376***
Wave × Appealing					0.144***
Wave × Mother immigrant					0.077***
Wave × Irreligious					−0.081***
Wave × E-activity					−0.092***
Wave × Verbal involvement					0.110***
Wave × Health					−0.044***
Wave × Creative work					0.052***
Wave × Unemployed					0.028***
Wave × Earner working					−0.026***
Wave × Self-employment					−0.027***
Wave × Married					−0.026***
Wave × Kid					0.021**
R^2	0.044	0.181	0.299	0.478	0.498

* $p < 0.05$, ** $p < 0.01$, *** $p < 0.001$

was the negative effect of national population size ($\beta = -0.070$), which turned out to be the strongest effect in the final step of analysis ($\beta = -0.220$). The negative effect of national population size manifested the deterministic mechanism of an external hindrance. Herein, the larger number of people around imposes a greater constraint on resources and thus personal delight. Another notable effect was the positive effect of income inequality ($\beta = 0.062$). This effect remained significant in the final step of analysis ($\beta = 0.142$). The effect of inequality represented the deterministic mechanism of external constraint. That is, such a constraint discouraged mutual help and thus delight. Another significant effect was the trivial positive effect of national liberty ($\beta = 0.033$). This contribution endorsed the deterministic mechanism of external opportunity. National liberty facilitates people to maximize their delight in their ways, rather than to exploit or to drain personal resources.

The second step of regression analysis focused on national predictors revealed that four interactions between the indicators and time showed significant effects on delight. Among the interactions, the one involving globalization exhibited the strongest and negative effect on delight ($\beta = -0.116$). Globalization was increasingly unfavorable to delight with time. The negative effect of globalization manifested the deterministic mechanism of external constraint (Axford 2013). Accordingly, globalization constrains national cohesion and related mutual and localized support (Kunovich 2009). Moreover, it imposes stress on people by requiring them to adapt to global conditions (Arnett 2002). Another notable interaction was involving technology, which unfolded a positive effect on delight ($\beta = 0.060$). Technology was increasingly beneficial to delight with time. The contribution of technology manifested the deterministic mechanism of external support. That is, technology represents a resource to facilitate personal delight. The other two interactions had only trivial effects on delight ($\beta < 0.05$). These interaction effects remained significant in the third step of analysis, which found significantly lower delight in Egypt and Japan than in other countries (Table 4.7).

Predicting Worry

In the first step of regression analysis of worry, significant country indicators were the focus of examination. Mexico had the highest worry ($\beta = 0.181$). In addition, worry was notably higher in the Philippines ($\beta = 0.116$), Nigeria ($\beta = 0.087$), Egypt ($\beta = 0.083$), India ($\beta = 0.061$), Pakistan ($\beta = 0.057$), and Brazil ($\beta = 0.051$). Conversely, worry was lower in Germany ($\beta = -0.113$).

The second step of regression analysis focused on personal background predictors of worry revealed several significant effects. The strongest effect was the negative effect of creative work on worry ($\beta = -0.096$), which reflected the voluntaristic mechanism of utility optimization. Herein, creative work is gainful and satisfying, thus relieving worry. The second strongest effect was the negative effect of self-employment ($\beta = -0.083$). This negative effect again reflected the voluntaristic mechanism of utility optimization. Herein, self-employment provides freedom and

Table 4.7 Standardized effects of national characteristics on delight

Predictor	(1)	(2)	(3)
Wave	−0.083***	−0.080***	−0.088***
Liberty	0.033***	0.034***	−0.045***
Human development	0.083***	0.068***	0.142***
Land	−0.085***	−0.091***	−0.182***
Population	−0.070***	−0.084***	−0.220***
Income inequality	0.062***	0.053***	0.142***
Wave × Globalization		−0.116***	−0.100***
Wave × Technology		0.060***	0.043***
Wave × Credit		0.035***	0.023**
Wave × Democracy		0.019***	0.017**
Egypt			−0.179***
Japan			−0.077***
R^2	0.017	0.022	0.049

* $p < 0.05$, ** $p < 0.01$, *** $p < 0.001$

gains, which impede worry. By contrast, the effect of independent work on worry was positive ($\beta = 0.063$), suggesting the voluntaristic mechanism of utility optimization. In this case, independent work burdens the worker and gathers little external support to induce a loss, which activates personal worry. Other notable negative effects on worry were age ($\beta = -0.062$) and education ($\beta = -0.056$). These negative effects reflected the voluntaristic mechanism of power realization. Accordingly, both age and education offer power to resist worry. By contrast, another positive effect on worry was from irreligiousness ($\beta = 0.065$). This positive effect reflected the voluntaristic mechanism of utility optimization. Specifically, irreligiousness draws less support, notably from religious fellows, to maintain a gain and thus leads to worry. Other personal background effects were trivial ($\beta < 0.05$).

The third step of regression analysis focused on personal factors revealed significant personal experiences and practices predictive of worry. Among the factors, risk aversion indicated the strongest positive effect on worry ($\beta = 0.105$), which reflected the voluntaristic mechanism of consistency. That is, risk aversion and worry are cognate or consonant. The second strongest effect was the negative effect of the experience of family saving ($\beta = -0.102$). This negative effect registered the voluntaristic mechanism of utility optimization. Herein, the saving means a gain, which is preventive of worry. The third strongest effect was the negative effect of carrying weapons ($\beta = -0.094$). Other negative effects were from civic organizational participation and voting ($\beta = -0.053$), which reflected the voluntaristic mechanism of consistency. That is, the participation represents active involvement rather than worry. Conversely, withdrawal rather than participation is consonant with worry. Other effects from personal experiences or practices were trivial ($\beta < 0.05$).

The fourth step examined the additional effects of health and life satisfaction on worry. Both effects were significant and negative ($\beta = -0.043$ and -0.085, respectively) and represented the voluntaristic mechanism of idea consistency. That is, health and life satisfaction are positive indicators of life quality, whereas worry is a negative indicator of worry. The former is dissonant with the latter. Nevertheless, they were very weak, indicating that worry was largely independent of health and life satisfaction (Table 4.8).

In the first step of regression analysis focused on national indicators as predictors of worry, four national indicators emerged as significant. The strongest predictor was bank credit to the private sector per capita, which exerted a negative effect on worry ($\beta = -0.137$). This predictor remained significant with the control of country indicators in the second analysis step ($\beta = -0.036$). The negative effect on worry reflected the deterministic mechanism of external support. Accordingly, credit in the private sector reflects the work of the organization, which provides support to people to relieve their worry. Nevertheless, much of the credit effect was due to the variation in worry among countries. The second strongest predictor was national CO_2 emission, which presented a negative effect on worry ($\beta = -0.126$). This effect remained significant with the control of country indicators in the second step ($\beta = -0.170$). The negative effect reflected the deterministic mechanism of external support. Herein, CO_2 emission indicates national development (Scruggs 2003), which provides support to lessen personal worry. The third predictor was income inequality, which also yielded a negative effect on worry ($\beta = -0.079$). This predictor remained significant in the second analysis step ($\beta = -0.143$). The negative effect registered the deterministic mechanism of external opportunity. That is, income inequality is reflective of national economic development (Alessio 2011). Such development provides external support to dampen personal worry. The fourth predictor was technology export per capita, which indicated a negative effect on worry ($\beta = -0.045$) and demonstrated the deterministic mechanism of external resources. That is, technology facilitated people to prevent their worry. With the control of significant country indicators in the second step, the effect became stronger ($\beta = -0.234$) (Table 4.9).

Summary

Analysis of personal data from the World Values Survey and national data revealed several significant and relatively important personal and national factors for predicting life quality appraisals in the average person in the world. Notably, life quality appraisals involve health, life satisfaction, delight, and worry. These factors characterize the statics of life quality production. In addition, variations due to time in the appraisals and their susceptibility to the factors indicate the dynamics of life quality production. The statics and dynamics are explicable with the analytical-functionalist framework, which comprises voluntaristic and deterministic mechanisms.

Table 4.8 Standardized effects on worry

Predictor	(1)	(2)	(3)	(4)
Mexico	0.181^{***}	0.156^{***}	0.161^{***}	0.173^{***}
Germany	-0.113^{***}	-0.094^{***}	-0.079^{***}	-0.078^{***}
Philippines	0.116^{***}	0.066^{***}	0.069^{***}	0.069^{***}
Nigeria	0.087^{***}	0.040^{***}	0.030^{***}	0.029^{***}
Egypt	0.083^{***}	0.052^{***}	0.044^{***}	0.035^{***}
Pakistan	0.057^{***}	0.005	−0.007	−0.002
India	0.061^{***}	-0.104^{***}	-0.052^{***}	-0.066^{***}
Brazil	0.051^{***}	0.049^{***}	0.059^{***}	0.068^{***}
Turkey	0.029^{***}	0.005	0.002	0.001
Acquiescence		0.371^{***}	0.423^{***}	0.465^{***}
Irreligious		0.065^{***}	0.054^{***}	0.057^{***}
Family income		0.027^{***}	−0.010	0.001
Female		0.000	−0.012	−0.010
Age		-0.062^{***}	-0.051^{***}	-0.065^{***}
Age squared		-0.020^{*}	−0.018	−0.015
Married		0.030^{**}	0.019	0.021
Cohabited		0.017^{*}	0.014	0.016
Divorced		−0.005	−0.006	−0.007
Separated		0.023^{**}	0.020^{**}	0.018^{*}
Widowed		0.004	−0.004	−0.005
Kid		0.030^{**}	0.027^{**}	0.030^{**}
Father immigrant		0.023^{**}	0.034^{***}	0.039***
Education		-0.056^{***}	-0.038^{***}	-0.038^{***}
Graduation age		-0.033^{***}	-0.020^{*}	-0.017^{*}
Interest		0.018^{*}	0.025^{**}	0.030^{***}
Living with parents		0.003	0.005	0.005
Full-time employment		−0.005	−0.018	−0.017
Part-time employment		-0.045^{***}	-0.051^{***}	-0.048^{***}
Self-employment		-0.083^{***}	-0.090^{***}	-0.091^{***}
Retired		0.017	0.011	0.012
Homemaking		0.005	0.006	0.010
Student		0.028^{**}	0.029^{**}	0.031^{***}
Public employment		0.033^{***}	0.042^{***}	0.039^{***}
Private business employment		0.042^{***}	0.059^{***}	0.059^{***}
Nonprofit organization employment		0.048^{***}	0.041^{***}	0.037^{***}
Creative work		-0.096^{***}	-0.062^{***}	-0.061^{***}

(continued)

Table 4.8 (continued)

Predictor	(1)	(2)	(3)	(4)
Independent work		0.063***	0.049***	0.056***
Supervision		−0.034***	−0.023	−0.021**
Earner		−0.015	−0.014	−0.014
Earner employed		−0.021**	−0.020*	−0.022**
Economic hardship			0.005	−0.021*
Neighborhood nuisance			−0.061***	−0.076***
Security			0.014	0.013
Family saving			−0.102***	−0.088***
E-activity			−0.019*	−0.019*
Learning			−0.006	−0.008
Spiritual activity			−0.013	−0.008
Risk aversion			0.105***	0.102***
Weapon carrying			−0.094***	−0.102***
Organizational participation			−0.053***	−0.052***
Appealing			−0.008	−0.013
Voting			−0.053***	−0.054***
Green demonstration			−0.007	−0.006
Health				−0.043***
Life satisfaction				−0.085***
R^2	0.074	0.207	0.241	0.250

* $p < 0.05$, ** $p < 0.01$, *** $p < 0.001$

Table 4.9 Standardized effects of national characteristics on worry

Predictor	(1)	(2)
Credit	−0.137***	−0.036***
CO_2	−0.126***	−0.170***
Income inequality	−0.079***	−0.143***
Technology	−0.045***	−0.234***
Mexico		0.184***
Japan		0.162***
Egypt		0.064***
Nigeria		−0.061***
Philippines		0.035***
Brazil		0.033***
R^2	0.065	0.202

* $p < 0.05$, ** $p < 0.01$, *** $p < 0.001$

Statics in Life Quality Production

The statics of life quality production maintains that some personal and national factors affect personal life quality, according to the voluntaristic and deterministic mechanisms of the analytical-functionalist framework. The personal factors include education, family saving, economic hardship, neighborhood nuisance, age, marriage, religious faith, self-employment, independent work, creative work, security, verbal involvement, weapon carrying, civic organizational participation, strike, and voting. Among these personal factors, education, young age, marriage, and religious faith sustain life quality with the voluntaristic mechanism of power realization. Meanwhile, self-employment, independent work, creative work, family saving, security, and weapon carrying tend to represent gains to champion life quality with the voluntaristic mechanism of utility optimization. Conversely, economic hardship, neighborhood nuisance, and strike participation tend to involve losses to weaken life quality according to the voluntaristic mechanism of utility optimization. In addition, risk aversion seems to represent an adverse practice that impedes life quality or invokes worry according to the voluntaristic mechanism of idea consistency. Conversely, voting reflects a normative action that maintains life quality through the voluntaristic mechanism of idea consistency. Civic organizational participation also seems to enhance learning about social problems, which erodes life satisfaction according to the voluntaristic mechanism of norm conformity. Nevertheless, according to the voluntaristic mechanism of power realization, civic organizational participation may also gather social support to dispel worry. Meanwhile, the national factors include national human development, liberty, government effectiveness, population, land, and income inequality. In addition, life quality varies among countries. Notably, life quality is higher in Mexico, Brazil, Nigeria, and Germany and is lower in Russia, Egypt, India, Pakistan, and the Philippines. These national factors realize the deterministic mechanism in producing life quality (Table 4.10).

The person's education showed contributions to all four aspects of personal life quality, health, life satisfaction, delight, and no worry. These contributions reflect the voluntaristic mechanism of power realization. That is, education, as a human resource, enables one's pursuit of life quality (Dolton et al. 2004; Izquierdo and Minguez 2003). Specifically, education is influential in raising a person's choice, discovery, creativity, authenticity, learning, rationality, and even excitement (Yair 2003). Such raising is conducive to personal life quality (Abbott and Sapsford 2006; Baylis 2005; Bettencourt and Sheldon 2001; Helliwell et al. 2010; Mikulincer and Shaver 2014; Napier and Jost 2008; Rowan 2001). The pervasive contribution of education lends support to the advocacy for education in Confucianism, structural-functionalism, pragmatism, and critical theory (Izquierdo and Minguez 2003; O'Dwyer 2003; Vanderstraeten 2002). These discourses emphasize the roles of education in exemplifying the good, showing ways to achieve goals, integrating with people, acquiring norms, and deliberation on and selection of the good. The advocacy is also compatible with the exaltation of education of its contribution to rationalization, civilization, and progress (Teodoro 2003).

Table 4.10 Hypothesized and observed main static and dynamic effects on life quality (notable effect: $|\beta| > 0.10$; other significant effect: $|\beta| > 0.05$)

Predictor	Hypothesized	Observed			
		Health	Life satisfaction	Delight	No worry
Wave	+			(-)	
Russia		-	-	-	
Nigeria		+			-
India		⊖	-		-
Mexico			+	+	⊖
Egypt			-	⊖	-
Brazil			+	+	-
Germany					+
Philippines					-
Pakistan					-
Japan		⊖			⊖
National land	+	(-)		(-)	
National liberty	+	+			
National human development	+		⊕	+	
National government effectiveness	+	↓	(-)		
National population	+			(-)	
National Income inequality	-			(+)	
National globalization	+			↓	
National credit	+				⊕
National CO_2	-				◇+
Age	-	⊖			(+)
Education	+	+	+	+	+
Married	+			+	
Irreligious	+		↓		(-)
Self-employment	+				+
Independent work	+		⊕	⊕	(-)
Creative work	+				+
Economic hardship	-	⊖	⊖	-	
Neighborhood nuisance	-	-	-	⊖	(+)
Family saving	+	+	⊕	+	⊕
Security	+		⊕		
Learning	+				(-)
Risk aversion	+				◇-
Weapon carrying	+				+
Appealing	-			(+)↑	
Organizational participation	-	↓	-↓		(+)
Strike	-			-	
Voting	-				(+)

Note: Circle: notable and agreeing with the hypothesis; Diamond: notable but contrary to the hypothesis; Bracket: contrary to hypothesis; upward arrow: notably more positive with time; downward arrow: notably more negative with time

Family saving also delivered pervasive contributions to all four aspects of life quality. The contributions reflect the voluntaristic mechanisms of utility optimization and power realization. The former mechanism holds family saving to create a gainful experience or expectation, whereas the latter regards family saving as an accessible resource. A gainful experience is social inclusion afforded by savings (Lin et al. 2013). Meanwhile, gainful experiences have consisted in aspiration for achievement and trust in others (Uslaner 2002). In addition, family saving clearly reflects the resource of family income (Chakrabarty et al. 2008). The contribution of family saving endorses the significance of the family (Kiecolt 2003; Rossi 2001). For instance, sharing and altruism within the family are the sources of gain and resources (Bahr and Bahr 2001).

Neighborhood nuisance is another influential experience, but it shows adverse effects on health, life satisfaction, and delight. These effects reflect the voluntaristic mechanism of utility optimization. In this case, neighborhood nuisance represents a loss in utility. Specifically, it indicates a threat or intimidation (Melton 2000). Threat is a vital determinant of various outcomes, including prejudice, social exclusion, and withdrawal of support and volunteering (Gaines and Garand 2010; Laurence 2011; Stephan and Stephan 2000; Yzerbyt 2010). The determination operates through identification, forming the senses of insecurity and uncertainty and negative stereotypes and anxiety (Leong 2008; Stephan and Stephan 2000). Hence, threat is likely to involve anxiety and thus weakens life quality. Notably, a neighborhood threat such as nuisance is particularly influential, reflecting the neighborhood's or residential area's importance (Kearney 2006). Accordingly, the neighborhood imposes persistent and proximate influences due to the fixed housing conditions, environment, and residential stability. The resident is unlikely to evade the neighborhood influence after settling down in a place. However, neighborhood nuisance showed a negative effect on worry. This finding may be due to the contribution of the neighborhood as a source of social availability or support. Neighborhood nuisance indicates the availability of people to reduce personal worry. It may become a resource to operate according to the voluntaristic mechanism of power realization. Herein, the social resource, or social capital or social networking, has dampened personal worry (Cichy et al. 2007; Frank et al. 2014).

Economic hardship is another major impediment to life quality. Accordingly, one's health, life satisfaction, and delight suffer under economic hardship. The suffering reflects the voluntaristic mechanism of utility optimization. As such, the gloomy loss condition of economic hardship is debilitating and saddening. With economic hardship, losses can happen in victimization, social exclusion, and the unavailability of social support (Lennartsson 2010; Ross and Mirowsky 2008). The pervasive influence of economic hardship illustrates the significance of the economic dimension (Taylor et al. 2011). The significance embodies economism or economic rationality. That is, people realize the importance of economic conditions in life. Such conditions uphold utility (Braun 2011; Shaw 1999).

National human development is another influential predictor of personal life satisfaction and delight. It helps strengthen capability and motivation for securing life quality in the country (Inglehart and Welzel 2005). The development would embrace the deterministic mechanism by facilitating national or external support for personal life quality. Notably, national human development has buttressed civility in the country (Bond and Lun 2014). Civility fosters social cohesion and social support to help people secure their life quality (Letki 2008; Sonderlund et al. 2017).

National land per capita is another important predictor of life quality but inversely. The prediction reflects the deterministic mechanism of external support. Accordingly, land per capita indicates the lack of proximal support. The larger the area per capita, the fewer the people available and the less their support or facilities available. Hence, the land diffuses, dilutes, and weakens resources or support. This weakening effect illustrates the importance of spatial proximity such that closer resources are more helpful. It likewise suggests the importance of support from other people and/or their establishments.

National population size also appears to impair delight, composed of happiness, autonomy, and financial satisfaction. This impairment contradicts the expectation that population size represents an external resource bringing in human capital and support to champion life quality (Turner 2010). The impairment buttresses the view that population represents congestion to dilate resources and heighten competition (Glaeser et al. 2002). Population size thus foments disintegration, distrust, protest, and even violence (Dodson 2016; Eldersveld et al. 1995; Fridberg and Kangas 2008b; Tadjoeddin 2013). Hence, compatriots are likely to be competitors rather than helpers.

National income inequality, by contrast, displayed a contribution to personal delight. This contribution contradicts the expectation that income inequality erodes social solidarity and social capital and foments social conflicts, thus withdrawing support from one another's life quality (Alessio 2011; Jordahl 2009). Instead, the contribution accords with the functionalist view that income inequality fits the nature and requirements of society, thus sustaining each person's life quality (Alessio 2011). Specifically, income inequality maintains rather than disrupts social order, thus stabilizing people's roles and contributions to life quality. Hence, income inequality has sustained rather than undermined social capital (Rupasingha et al. 2006). This sustaining reflects the deterministic mechanism in the functionalist framework, such that national income inequality is functional to society, including its economic and social production, to generate social capital to enrich people's life quality. Notably, national income inequality fulfills the requirement of capitalism for boosting societal development (Alessio 2011).

Other personal factors that displayed a salutary effect included marriage and security. The effect commonly reflects the voluntaristic mechanism of utility optimization. On the one hand, marriage is gainful and fulfills the needs for intimacy and emotional and other support (Carbery and Buhrmester 1998; Solomon 2006). Marriage has thus contributed to the experiences of closeness, affiliation, bonding, social capital, social networking, social integration, and social support received (Apinunmahakul and Devlin 2008; Angelusz and Tardos 2001; Cornwall 2009; Lizardo 2006; Mata and Pendakur 2014; Volker et al. 2007). These experiences have been salutary (Baumeister et al. 2013; Jones et al. 2014; Oshio and Kobayashi 2010). Moreover, according to the voluntaristic mechanism of power, marriage conveys resources to champion life quality. It is, therefore, both enjoyable and empowering. The salutary role of marriage probably persists due to the support from institutions and policy and the related discourse and advocacy (Byrd 2009; Lichter et al. 2004). On the other hand, security is gainful because it has facilitated the acquisition of social capital and its accessibility (Curley 2010; Pena-Lopez and Sanchez-Santos 2016). This result indicates that security is the basis for gainful exploration (Braithwaite 1998; La Guardia et al. 2000). Meanwhile, the salutary effect of security reflects the need for security (La Guardia et al. 2000).

Dynamics in Life Quality Production

The main effect of time (i.e., the survey wave) indicates the simple dynamic of life quality, which reveals the decline of personal delight, including happiness, autonomy, and financial satisfaction, with time. The decline is compatible with that in financial and marital satisfaction and quality (Hays and Seifert 2003; Umberson et al. 2005) and is consistent with that in receiving celebration, social integration, and social capital (Grenier and Wright 2006; Logan and Cobb 2013; McPherson et al. 2006). The latter decline has predicted a decline in life quality (Berry and Welsh 2010; Jones et al. 2014; Suh 2002). Furthermore, the decline in delight is consistent with the decline in religiosity (Norris and Inglehart 2009). The latter decline has led to a decline in life quality (Kroll 2011; Lim and Putnam 2010). Furthermore, the decline in delight is partly attributable to the decline in marriage (Ellwood and Jencks 2004; South and Crowder 2000). The latter decline has been responsible for diminishing life quality (Carrieri 2012; Wang and VanderWeele 2011). Hence, life quality has diminished with time (Sarracino 2010).

The decline in delight is explicable with the dynamics of modernization. Accordingly, modernization has heightened stress, narcissism, and violence in society (Dioale and Seda 2001; Gutmann 1987). These conditions have eroded life quality (Baumeister et al. 2013; Posel and Casale 2011; Sirgy 2012). Moreover, modernization features anomie, crimes, risks, and identity crisis (Frosh 1991; Hilbert 1986; Messner 1986; Sorensen and Christiansen 2013). These features have been detrimental to life quality (Brockman et al. 2009; Helson and Srivastava 2001; Kingston and Knight 2006; Zotti et al. 2016). Specifically, social problems invoked by modernization would weaken personal life quality. The problems would be corrosive according to the deterministic mechanism of external force.

The decline in delight also reflects some features of postmodernization dynamics. These features include social conflict, distrust, de-embeddedness, unavailability, insecurity, fragmentation, incompleteness, and perversity (Gibbins and Reimer 1999; Heaphy 2007; Inglehart 2000; Jacques 1998; Pilisuk et al. 1996). The features, reflecting social problems, have been harmful to personal life quality (Abbott and Sapsford 2006; Murrell and Norris 1991; Navarez 2011; Oishi et al. 2011; Rettig et al. 1999). Disintegration in society would diminish life quality (Berry and Welsh 2010; Piliavin 2008). Others' rejection would be saddening, following the deterministic mechanism of external force.

Similarly, the decline in delight accords with some features or concomitants of individualization, including anomie, antisociality, narcissism, conflict, disembeddedness, disintegration, uncertainty, insecurity, and risk (Bauman 2001; Beck and

Beck-Gernsheim 2002; Burgess 2018; Frank and Meyer 2002; Fuchs 2015). Their harm to personal life quality has been evident (Abbott et al. 2011; Delbosc and Currie 2011; Moller 2005; Murrell and Norris 1991; Richards 2016; Sirgy 2012; Soons et al. 2009; Zotti et al. 2016). Social problems imposed on and/or experienced by a person would be inimical to personal life quality. The imposition represents the deterministic mechanism of external force.

The dynamics of life quality production also transpire in the significant and notable interaction effects of time on health and life satisfaction. Essentially, the effects support the dynamics of modernization, postmodernization, and individualization in producing life quality. In the beginning, the dynamics maintain the hypotheses about the strengthening or weakening of various effects with time. In brief, the dynamics of modernization maintain the strengthening of the rationality effect and the weakening of the non-rationality effect with time. Herein, rationality comprises instrumental and substantive rationality underlying adaptation and latency functions, respectively. The dynamics of postmodernization suggest the weakening of all effects with time. This weakening means increasing unpredictability with time. Meanwhile, the dynamics of individualization hold that the effects of individual-based factors strengthen with time, and conversely, the effects of other factors weakened with time. Notably, the three dynamics are not mutually exclusive. Findings on the strengthening or weakening accorded with the hypothesized effects showed support, which arose from most of the interaction effects. Hence, except for one effect, all the other effects reflected the dynamics of modernization, postmodernization, and/or individualization. Essentially, most of the effects exhibited weakening with time. This outcome accorded mostly with the dynamics of postmodernization and modernization. By contrast, the two effects that manifested strengthening accorded with the dynamics of individualization. The only exception not reflecting any of the dynamics of modernization, postmodernization, and individualization was strengthening the positive effect of national liberty on health. In all, the support for the dynamics of postmodernization slightly outperformed that for the other two dynamics (i.e., 8 effects supported vs. 6 effects supported) (Table 4.11).

The exceptional strengthening of the contribution of national liberty to health with time is consistent with the emancipation or liberalization thesis in social change, generally modernization, postmodernization, or individualization (Bauman 2001; Beck and Beck-Gernsheim 2002; Heaphy 2007; Martinelli 2005; Welzel 2013; Yeganeh 2017). According to the thesis, emancipation, liberalization, or freedom from restriction becomes increasingly valuable and influential, possibly attributable to the rise of personal knowledge and skill in using technology. Such an increase tends to override the increase in unpredictability with postmodernization. Specifically, an increase in the influence of national liberty or emancipation is consistent with the growing expressivism under postmodernization (Gibbins and Reimer 1999; Heinz 2002; Yeganeh 2017). This increase is also consistent with evolutionary modernization as an alternative to postmodernization (Inglehart 2018). Moreover, national liberty is consistent with the personal freedom emphasized in individualization. National liberty implies personal freedom, whose influence would rise with

Table 4.11 Observed and hypothesized dynamics in life quality production ($|\beta| > 0.05$)

Predictor	Observed main effect	Observed interact-ion effect with time	Observed time effect on the main effect	Hypothe-sized modern-ization effect	Hypothe-sized post-modern-ization effect	Hypothe-sized individua-lization effect
Organizational participation	–	+	–	–	–	–
Irreligious	+	–	–	+	–	+
Education	+	–	–	–	–	+
Living with parents	–	+	–	–	–	–
Kid	–	+	–	–	–	–
E-activity	+	–	–	–	–	+
National human development	+	–	–	–	–	–
Creative work	–	+	–	+	–	+
Verbal involvement	+	+	+	–	–	+
Age	–	–	+	–	–	+
National liberty	+	+	+	–	–	–
Support				6	8	6

individualization. Hence, the voluntaristic mechanism tends to outstrip the deterministic mechanism in national liberty. Similarly, national liberty can enable personal choice, optimization, and rationalization emphasized in modernization. Thus, the voluntaristic mechanism predicated on rationality tends to be dominant in national liberty.

Implications

The findings on life quality appraisal generate implications for theory and policy about life quality. The theory concerns the statics and dynamics of life quality production.

The statics of life quality production principally embodies the voluntaristic mechanisms of power realization and utility optimization and the deterministic mechanism of empowerment. On the one hand, the voluntaristic mechanisms are evident in the contributions of education, independent work, family saving, security, and marriage to life quality appraisal and the reduction of the appraisal by economic hardship, neighborhood nuisance, and strike. On the other hand, the deterministic mechanism raises life quality appraisal by national human development, liberty, and even income inequality, and the adverse effects of national land per capita, population size, and national government effectiveness on the appraisal. Notably, according to the functionalist explanation, the salutary effect of national inequality is because the inequality is functional to society to empower the quality of life. Meanwhile, according to the deterministic mechanism, the adverse effect of government effectiveness is due to the external regulation of government. Conversely, national liberty is conducive to life quality when the liberty sounds emancipatory and empowering. Similarly, the salutary effect of independent work also reflects personal power and freedom, thus endorsing the mechanism of power. These effects primarily highlight the vitality of internal and external power or resources for procuring life quality. Specifically, internal and external empowerment, as opposed to competition for and dilution of resources, are salutary. Land, population, and government effectiveness are not resources producing life quality, and income inequality does not drain away resources for production. The mechanisms of power realization and empowerment are more prominent than the mechanisms of utility optimization, norm conformity, and idea consistency.

The dynamics of life quality production exhibit the declines of life quality and its predictability with time. Notably, the decline in life quality or delight was not attributable to any personal and national factors included in the analysis. The decline contradicts the expectation predicated on modernization because its factors are growing. Hence, the decline is compatible with the expectation of postmodernization that life quality increasingly disconnects from modernization and other factors. Moreover, the decline possibly registers the noxious impact of denaturalization or environmental deterioration or depletion. Meanwhile, the decline in the predictability of life quality champions the postmodernization thesis, which is more plausible than those of modernization and individualization in that the decline happens in some rational and individual-based factors and non-rational and external factors. Accordingly, rational factors such as irreligiousness and creative work declined in their influences on life quality appraisal. Individual-based factors such as irreligiousness, education, E-activity, and creativity work also diminished their influences. The influence of postmodernization as such reflects the deterministic mechanism of culture. Possibly, cultural determinism arises due to the declining marginal utility of economic determinism (Inglehart 1997a). As the economic level is high, its determinism would diminish to give way to cultural determinism. The significance of postmodernization and its cultural determinism may build on technological advancement (Best and Kellner 2001; Morrow with Brown 1994). In other words, the cultural determinism of postmodernization incorporates technological determinism.

The findings imply the viability of the production approach to life quality. This approach prioritizes using resources, capability, strengths, and other forms of power to produce life quality in a realistic or material form rather than an imaginary or ideal form. Such prioritization rests on findings pinpointing the significance of the mechanisms of internal and external power and gain. The approach is thus compatible with those emphasizing production, capability, education, democratization, conservatism, realism, and utility or utilitarianism (Bell 2010; Jordan 2005; Popovic 2014; Thin 2012; White 2014). Essentially, the approach highlights making efforts to furnish resources and apply strengths to produce life quality. Education is paramount to strengthening capability. Democratization is also vital to enhance personal freedom and power as opposed to external control by the authority. Additionally, maintaining a gainful economy and environment more generally in terms of realistic and tangible utility is favorable. The approach favors conservatism in strengthening social solidarity, capital, and support to represent external power as opposed to fomenting competition and conflicts. As such, maintaining social order to boost production is permissible.

Chapter 5
Life Experience Production: Theory

The social experiences of economic hardship, neighborhood nuisance, victimization, security, and family saving represent life quality, with the former three reflecting negative quality and the latter two indicating positive quality. Such quality experiences are essential for an explanation for promoting and impeding their positive and negative quality, respectively (Cummins 2016; Veenhoven 1984). The positive quality experience realizes civilization to sustain morality and societal functioning. Hence, the explanation can rest on the analytical-structural framework.

Functionalist Explanation for Social Experiences

The analytical-functionalist framework specifies the four requisite functions for goal attainment or fulfillment, adaptation, integration, and latency. These functions operate to procure instrumental and consummatory achievements internally and externally. Herein, instrumental achievement means getting something valuable, whereas consummatory achievement means the value of the getting itself. Internal achievement means achievement within the system or subsystem, whereas external achievement means achievement outside the system or subsystem or in the external environment. Specifically, fulfillment is for external consummatory achievement, adaptation for external instrumental achievement, integration for internal consummatory achievement, and latency for internal instrumental achievement. To explain experience, one's repertory represents the fulfillment function for external consummatory achievement, one's shared understanding or learning represents the integration function for internal consummatory achievement, one's desire and thus valuation of reward represents the adaptation function of external instrumental achievement, and one's guilt feeling or moral belief represents the latency function of internal instrumental achievement (Bowker 2016; Henricks 2012). Specifically, repertory means the ability to procure something from the external environment, learning implies integrating with others within the system or social sphere, desire means the

C. Cheung, *Production Dynamics for Life Quality in the Incipient 21st Century*,
https://doi.org/10.1007/978-981-19-3827-6_5

valuation of reward from the external environment, and moral belief provides the guide to demonstrate one's internal value. Moreover, such analytical functions work at voluntaristic or personal and deterministic or extrapersonal levels.

The voluntaristic level of analytical functioning hinges on the person's consciousness or voluntarism. For the function of fulfillment, the voluntaristic mechanism is power realization or driving, such as by repertory. That is, repertory represents power for realizing and driving toward the goal. The function of adaptation relies on the voluntaristic mechanism of utility optimization or gravitating, such as through desire. That is, desire defines utility for optimization through gravitation or response to attraction. For the function of integration, the voluntaristic mechanism is norm conformity or assimilating through learning. That is, learning undergirds conformity to or assimilating with the social norm. For the function of latency, the voluntaristic mechanism is idea consistency or rationalizing, such as through guilt feeling or moral belief. Moral belief is an idea drawing consistency or is the basis for rationalizing.

The deterministic level of analytical functioning starts with the extrapersonal or collective determinants, which can be the aggregate forms of experience, repertory, desire, learning, and moral belief from the person to the collectivity. As such, these determinants are beyond one's immediate consciousness and voluntarism. Determinism thus means influence without personal consciousness and voluntarism (Dafoe 2015; Pleasants 2018, 2019). Deterministic functioning works directly and/or indirectly. Its direct path originates from collective experience determining personal experience through sharing privately and/or publicly. Private sharing means taking and owning the shared experience, whereas public sharing means taking the shared experience vicariously. Alternatively, the indirect paths of deterministic functioning comprise empowering, incentivizing, standardizing, and framing, corresponding to the functions of fulfillment, adaptation, integration, and latency, respectively. Empowering means giving power such as collective repertory to activate personal power realization or driving. Incentivizing means giving an incentive such as that defined by collective desire to attract personal utility optimization or gravitating. Standardizing means offering a social norm through collective learning to trigger personal norm conformity or assimilating. Framing means portraying a frame such as collective moral belief to induce personal idea consistency or rationalizing. At the very beginning, empowering, incentivizing, standardizing, and framing exert their collective, extrapersonal influences without personal awareness or voluntarism.

Explaining Social Experiences

The social experiences of economic hardship, neighborhood nuisance, victimization, security, and family saving are explainable with the voluntaristic and deterministic mechanisms of analytical functionalism. This framework incorporates various theories and research findings on explaining or predicting social experiences.

Economic Hardship

At the personal level based on voluntaristic mechanisms, economic hardship results from inadequate power, utility, norms, and ideas. Conversely, adequate power, utility, norms, and ideas can sustain economic abundance, comfort, or well-being.

Based on voluntaristic mechanisms, economic hardship results from inadequate power, utility, norms, and ideas at the personal level. Conversely, adequate power, utility, norms, and ideas can sustain economic abundance, comfort, or well-being.

The voluntaristic mechanism of power realization affords power to avoid economic hardship. A notable power source emanates from social class, which means productive power, capital, or resources to achieve economic adequacy (Whelan et al. 2016). In a lower-class position, unemployment or idleness has deprived economic resources and resulted in economic hardship (Fridberg and Kangas 2008; Muhlau 2014). Likewise, the unemployment of one's partner has added to one's economic hardship (Muhlau 2014). The deprivation is manifest in debt, mortgage, and other credit problems. Mainly, material deprivation has engendered economic hardship (Whelan et al. 2016). Deprivation in consumption has also induced economic hardship (Whelan and Maitre 2013). Similarly, loss of employment or earnings has culminated in economic hardship (Robinaugh et al. 2016). Conversely, income and its multiple sources have prevented economic hardship (Muhlau 2014; Whelan et al. 2016). Power or resources also evolve from education, full-time employment, homeownership, living with parents, and working time, diminishing economic hardship (Muhlau 2014; Robinaugh et al. 2016). Living in the countryside has also lessened economic hardship (Fridberg and Kangas 2008). Such a living condition has relieved economic and spatial pressure (Keister 2003; Krishman and Krotki 1993). Economic pressure from the family is also a cause of personal economic hardship (Donnellan et al. 2013). Moreover, per capita family income has cushioned economic hardship (Robinaugh et al. 2016). Power in terms of social capital, which anticipates social support, has also reduced economic hardship (Brisson 2009). Social capital has been higher in one living in the countryside (Erickson 2004; Rupasingha et al. 2006). Conversely, social exclusion has bred economic hardship (Robila 2006). Herein, social exclusion signifies deprivation and the unavailability of social welfare (Gallie 2004; Wacquant 2008). Furthermore, age, female gender, and minority status have underlain economic hardship (Fridberg and Kangas 2008). These characteristics have weakened power or resources acquired through education and employment (Aral and Walker 2012; Ross and Mirowsky 2009; Verschuur et al. 2010). Physical and cognitive disabilities have also resulted in economic hardship (Dekkers 2008; Fischer et al. 1996).

The voluntaristic mechanism of utility optimization explains economic hardship as a lack of incentive or motivation to avoid the hardship or maintain economic adequacy or livelihood (Curley 2005; Donnellan et al. 2013). Such motivation has arisen from the role of parenthood or childcare (Peterson and Klohnen 1995). Hence, having children has lessened economic hardship (Muhlau 2014), Herein,

The voluntaristic mechanism of norm conformity emphasizes the influence of the social norm of economic hardship. Hence, such a norm or popularity of economic hardship has bolstered personal economic hardship (Leu et al. 2016).

The deterministic mechanism works directly through the collective experience of economic hardship at the community and national levels. The hardship at collective levels has determined personal economic hardship (Fridberg and Kangas 2008; Robila 2006). Hence, the person shares collective hardship privately or vicariously. Either way, the person takes the experience from others.

The deterministic mechanism of empowerment indicates that contextual power or opportunity indirectly facilitates personal avoidance of economic hardship. Hence, employment opportunity in the context, notably its manufacturing industry, enables the avoidance (Brady 2006). Furthermore, economic growth, public health spending, and wages in the context have lessened personal economic hardship (Brady 2005; Gundersen and Ziliak 2004). Education, employment, and its growth in the context have also diminished personal economic hardship (Clain 2007; Fan et al. 2004; Gundersen and Ziliak 2004). Moreover, unionization, urbanization, volunteering, and development in science and engineering in the context of empowerment have impeded personal economic hardship (Clain 2007; Goetz et al. 2011; Lipford and Yandle 2009). Conversely, spatial diffusion of jobs disempowers personal employment to avoid economic hardship (Curley 2005). Similarly, unemployment in the context has determined personal economic hardship (Corcoran and Adams 1997; Vartanian and McNamara 2004). Conversely, population growth in the neighborhood and broader context is disempowering and has underlain personal economic hardship (Delang and Lung 2010). In addition, the elderly and youth populations in the context have sustained personal economic hardship (Brady 2006; Moller et al. 2003). Such populations would consume resources that empower personal work.

The deterministic mechanism of incentivizing determines personal economic hardship indirectly through national or other collective or contextual conditions. An incentive to avoid economic hardship is free-market capitalism in the contest, while a disincentive is the welfare state (Brady 2005; Palmer 2010). The welfare state induces personal dependency, inactiveness, single parenthood, and unemployment (Brady 2005). Similarly, welfare receipt in the neighborhood has determined personal economic hardship (Gundersen and Ziliak 2004; Vartanian 1999). Welfare available in the context has also championed personal economic hardship (Lipford and Yandle 2009; Muffels and Fouarge 2004). Inequality and the tax rate in the context have also been disincentives impeding personal striving to prevent economic hardship (Gundersen and Ziliak 2004; Lipford and Yandle 2009; Portes and Vickstrom 2011). Conversely, children in the context incentivize efforts to avoid economic hardship personally (Clain 2007).

The deterministic mechanism of framing maintains that contextual ideas determine personal economic hardship through framing. A frame that evolves from neighborhood quality has reduced economic hardship, possibly indirectly (Vartanian 1999). That is, personal economic hardship looks incongruous with the contextual quality frame. Reduction in the incongruity would result in a reduced sense of personal economic hardship. Conversely, marriage has raised personal economic hardship (Sanders 1990). At this juncture, marriage in the context creates a frame for marriage, home life, leisure, welfare, and reliance on government rather than work to alleviate economic hardship (Brown and Ferris 2007; Tedin et al. 2001).

Neighborhood Nuisance

At the personal level, based on voluntaristic mechanisms, the experience of neighborhood nuisance means the inability to find order and quality in the neighborhood. Meanwhile, the deterministic mechanisms regard the personal experience as inadequacy stemming from collective or contextual forces.

The voluntaristic mechanism of power realization states that neighborhood disorder results from one's inability or lack of power or resources to avoid neighborhood nuisance or improve neighborhood quality. Such resources are lower in the woman than in the man and in those with younger age or more children (Aral and Walker 2012; Conley 2001; Parrado 2005). As such, neighborhood nuisance has been higher in the woman than in the man and one with younger age or more children (Wilson and Hammer 2001; Villarreal and Silva 2006). Similarly, divorce has weakened neighborhood quality experienced (Sampson and Raudenbush 2004). Divorce has deprived resources to facilitate the quality experience (Ross and Mirowsky 2009). Conversely, age, education, civic membership, family income, and urbanity have boosted the experience of neighborhood quality (Whitham 2012; Woldoff and Ovadia 2009). These characteristics have been bases for power or resources (Flores and Telles 2012; Hallerod 2006; Keltener et al. 2008; Ross and Mirowsky 2009). In addition, social capital has enhanced the experience of neighborhood quality (Sampson and Raudenbush 2004). Essentially, such capital has enabled quality maintenance (Yetim and Yetim 2014).

The voluntaristic mechanism of idea consistency or rationalizing rests on the influences of feelings, beliefs, and practices consistent with the experience of neighborhood nuisance or quality. Hence, such ideas about mastery, optimism, trust, and belief in science have fostered the experience of neighborhood quality (Greenberg 1999). These ideas have represented the quality assessments of oneself and others (Diener and Tov 2012; Nevarez 2011; Thin 2012; Watkins 2016). Meanwhile, one's socioeconomic status has raised one's demand for quality or standard of quality (Mortimer and McLaughlin 2014). This challenging and demanding idea contradicts and thus has eroded one's quality assessment (Nickerson et al. 2007). Similarly, socioeconomic status has impaired quality assessment (Becchetta 2010). Therefore, socioeconomic status has raised the experience of neighborhood nuisance (Villarreal and Silva 2006).

The direct deterministic mechanism operates such that neighborhood or contextual nuisance determines the personal experience of neighborhood nuisance through private or public sharing. This direct determination has been evident in neighborhood disadvantage, instability, and poverty (Villarreal and Silva 2006). Conversely, neighborhood safety and cohesion have contributed to the personal experience of neighborhood quality (Olson et al. 2016). Conversely, neighborhood decay, poverty, unemployment, and violence have impeded the personal experience of neighborhood quality (Sampson and Raudenbush 2004; Whitham 2012).

The indirect deterministic mechanism of empowering envisions that contextual resources enables people to reduce neighborhood nuisance or strengthen neighborhood quality. Such contextual resources include social capital in the neighborhood (Lee et al. 2011; Milner 2002). As such, neighborhood social capital has maintained the personal experience of neighborhood quality (Crowe 2010; Whitham 2012). More generally, social capital in the context has buttressed contextual quality (Crowe 2006; Fromhold-Eisebith 2004). Conversely, population size and particularly minorities in the neighborhood have eroded the personal experience of neighborhood quality (Sampson and Raudenbush 2004; Whitham 2012). Such contextual factors dilute resources and thus disempower people (Cotter et al. 1998; Kwan and Chiu 2018). Notably, minority people have fewer resources than others (Verschuur et al. 2010). Similarly, ethnic fractionalization in the context has been detrimental to contextual quality (Kwan and Chiu 2018). Such fractionalization has obstructed enculturation and thus concentration and consolidation of power, such as social capital or solidarity (Birman et al. 2005; Putnam 2007). Empowerment also emanates from collective technology, such as computer, Internet, and phone use, and innovation and prosperity or economic development, which have improved contextual quality (Gani and Clemes 2006; Kwan and Chiu 2018). In addition, investment or financial capital and natural capital have championed contextual quality (Crowe 2006; Frey et al. 1997). All these factors represent resources or power.

The indirect deterministic mechanism of framing can influence the personal experience of neighborhood quality through collective influence on contextual quality. As such, collective religiosity has impeded contextual quality (Norris 2002). This impeding happens as collective religiosity has perpetuated tradition, thus weakening collective orientation toward collective development or modernization (Campbell et al. 2018; McDowell and Brown 2009).

Victimization

At the personal level, based on voluntaristic mechanisms, the experience of victimization means one's failure to avoid victimization or protest oneself. By contrast, victimization at the collective level comprises collective perpetration and collective victimization, as victimization entails perpetration, including self-perpetration. Thus, deterministic mechanisms apply to both perpetration and victimization collectively and personally. As necessary for victimization, perpetration is also a relevant outcome subject to voluntaristic mechanisms.

The voluntaristic mechanism of power realization emphasizes the lack of power or resources to avoid or protect against victimization (Migliaccio 2002; Sedziafa and Tenkorang 2016). Such a lack can stem from a deficiency in social support or guardianship received, dependency, deprivation, early-life detachment from parents or caretakers, inferiority, leaving or running away from home or conventional social spheres, underclass status, threat, and vulnerability generally (Bornstein 2006; Doerner and Lab 2012; Hicks and Brown 2013; Kaukinen 2004; Jacobs and Carmichael 2002; Makarios and Sams 2013; Madero-Hernandez and Fisher 2013; Ponti and Tani 2019). Notably, dependency reflects personal disorder, deprivation, and susceptibility through feelings of exaggeration, guilt, ingratiation, and submissiveness (Bornstein 2006). Dependency can stem from rewards from others, such as the spouse (Bornstein 2006; Kaukinen 2004). Nevertheless, others' support or guardianship adds to one's power to prevent victimization. Meanwhile, early-life detachment from parents or caretakers is crucial for disrupting one's internal working model to build social relationships and resources (Ponti and Tani 2019). Inferiority implies domination by others to become dependent and helpless (Doerner and Lab 2012). Leaving or running away from social networks, exemplified in rebellious people, loses social protection (Bell et al. 2007). Underclass status signifies the lack of human and financial capital for production and livelihood (Jacobs and Carmichael 2002). Threat impedes or interrupts power or resources, including those for avoiding or protecting against victimization (Chongatera 2013). Vulnerability refers to physical or mental weakness or disability (Hicks and Brown 2013).

The voluntaristic mechanism of power realization operates with the personal driving forces of self-control and social capital. These forces have prevented victimization (Hansen-Nord et al. 2014; Zavala and Guadalupe-Diaz 2019). The forces have evolved from such background characteristics as age, education, income, marriage, religious faith, residency, social class, and wealth (Angelusz and Tardos 2001; Benton 2016; Chang 2009; Tulin et al. 2018; Wuthnow 2004). Therefore, the characteristics have hindered victimization (Barnawi 2017; Chongatera 2013; Emery and Wu 2020; Hope and Morgan 2011; Reese et al. 2021; Yount and Carrera 2006). Notably, social class does not need to be high to prevent victimization, as the employed person already has had lower victimization than the student (Hansen-Nord et al. 2014; Hope and Morgan 2011). Relationship durability has also diminished victimization (Kaukinen 2004). Such durability is a social resource or impetus (Gountas et al. 2012; Schwartz 2012). Conversely, such characteristics as disability, illness, retirement, single parenthood, poverty, studying, unemployment, and welfare reception have been predictive of victimization (Barnawi 2017; Hansen-Nord et al. 2014; Kaukinen 2004; Knab et al. 2008; Pratt et al. 2010; Tseloni et al. 2004). These characteristics represent a deficiency in power or resources (Keltener et al. 2008; Langenderfer and Shimp 2001). In addition, homemaking has protected against victimization (Tseloni et al. 2004). The home is a resource that protects one from outside victimizers. Conversely, the use of the Internet has raised victimization (Pratt et al. 2010). The use tends to expose one to the risk of victimization as the Internet is not a safe space (Gunter 2013). The experiences of abuse, control, economic hardship, perpetration, and violence have been conducive to victimization (Emery and Wu 2020; Patel et al. 2012; Reese et al. 2021; Ross and Mirowsky 2009; Thompson et al. 2003). The former experiences represent the exertion of force to produce victimization. The force has likely emanated from the parent or father particularly, partner, or spouse (Emery and Wu 2020; Reese et al. 2021; Sedziafa and Tenkorang 2016).

The voluntaristic mechanism of power realization also underlies one's perpetration, causing another's victimization. Notably, the partner or spouse is likely to be the perpetrator. In this regard, power or resources, such as employment, particularly in the military, have facilitated perpetration (Barnawi 2017). Conversely, lack of power or resources inhibiting perpetration has stemmed from abusing alcohol or drugs, doping, and smoking (Barnawi 2017; Rashad et al. 2019; Walton-Moss et al. 2005). A perpetrator has been likely to be abusing substances (Thompson et al. 2003). Notably, a controlling or substance-abusing husband has been likely to victimize his wife (Sedziafa and Tenkorang 2016). Alternatively, substance abuse fuels perpetration. In addition, age, education, social class, and mental health have diminished perpetration, illustrating their restraining power (Walton-Moss et al. 2005; Rashad et al. 2019; Reese et al. 2021).

The voluntaristic mechanism of utility optimization encompasses the logic of exchange, rational choice or instrumental rationality, and utility generally (Munch 1987). According to exchange logic, victimization is a price paid for reward or dependency (Bornstein 2006; Kaukinen 2004). The logic stresses reciprocity and fairness for sustaining exchange. Hence, the pair of victimization and rewarding counts as a transaction (Doerner and Lab 2012). This exchange involves power and others such that victimization manifests power by the victimizer (Bell et al. 2007). Similarly, according to the instrumentally rational perspective, victimization counts as an investment (Brown and Brown 2006).

The voluntaristic mechanism of norm conformity identifies social factors to influence victimization or its avoidance or prevention. One's experiences of disorder and homelessness have sustained one's victimization (Like 2011; Ross and Mirowsky 2009). The neighborhood provides a norm for disorder, victimization, or its acceptance rather than avoidance. Moreover, one's witness of victimization has also maintained one's victimization (Thompson et al. 2003). The witness is likely to generate a social norm for victimization or its acceptance. In addition, victimization in one's mother has led to one's victimization (Jewkes et al. 2002). The former is likely to provide a lesson or norm for victimization or its acceptance.

The voluntaristic mechanism of idea consistency maintains that one's dispositions, attitudes, and practices shape one's experience of victimization or its acceptance, avoidance, or prevention. Attitudinally, one's detachment from parents or partners through anxiety or avoidance has raised one's experience of victimization (Ehrensuft et al. 2003; Ponti and Tani 2019). Such anxiety or avoidance is likely to underlie avoidance or dislike of others by regarding them as victimizers. Favor for alcohol drinking has also led to the experience of victimization (Jewkes et al. 2002). Similarly, alcohol drinking, conduct disorder, and criminal behavior have been conducive to the experience of victimization. Herein, alcohol drinking has engendered risks such as illness and injury and resulted in hospitalization (Haapanen-Niemi et al. 1999). These risks are compatible with victimization. Meanwhile, favor for marianismo has engendered the experience of victimization (Klein et al. 1997). Similarly, conduct and criminal behavior are risky and thus accompany victimization. At this juncture, marianismo implies submissiveness and vulnerability (Franzosi 1998). Herein, vulnerability chimes with victimization (Zavala and Guadalupe-Diaz 2019).

Furthermore, resistance has fomented the experience of victimization (Emery and Wu 2020). Resistance presupposes risks or something undesirable (Gamble 2019). Such undesirability characterizes victimization (Shippee 2012).

The direct deterministic mechanism means sharing collective victimization and perpetration privately and vicariously to induce personal victimization. Perpetration engenders victimization because the latter necessitates the former. That is, collective perpetration and victimization go together. Hence, collective crime or violence and torture have resulted in the personal experience of victimization (Jacobs and Carmichael 2002; Sullivan 2014).

The direct deterministic mechanism also works for the impact of collective perpetration on personal perpetration, which is a necessary condition for personal victimization. As such, collective perpetration has raised personal perpetration (Fagan et al. 2007; Poveda 2011; Silverman and Miller 2011). Similarly, state perpetration as securitization is a cause of personal perpetration (Ahmad and Monaghan 2019). This cause reflects the contagion of perpetration (Fagan et al. 2007). More generally, the impact can happen privately or vicariously through sharing perpetration among people. Privately, one's perpetration can cause another's victimization and perpetration in return (Berger 2005; Markowitz 2001). The latter testifies the reciprocity of coercion (Eddy et al. 2018). Vicariously, one witnesses others' perpetration and takes it as one's perpetration. Such a collective or contagious impact characterizes the risk society (Ahmad and Monaghan 2019).

The deterministic mechanism of empowering can prevent victimization or produce victimization through disempowering. In the neighborhood, collective efficacy and public control for controlling crimes or disorder to sustain order and safety have prevented personal victimization (Zhang et al. 2007). The efficacy and control register collective power to forestall victimization personally and collectively. Meanwhile, residential stability in the neighborhood has increased personal victimization (Zhang et al. 2007). The stability is likely to raise interpersonal contact and thus the opportunity and risk of victimization. This raising is also an empowering mechanism for victimization and perpetration. Similarly, population size and urbanization have raised personal victimization (Jacobs and Carmichael 2002; Tseloni et al. 2004). Such city characteristics are likely to boost interpersonal contact and thus the risk of victimization. Urbanization has also raised personal victimization (Nepal et al. 2011). Conversely, residential segregation, mainly ethnic segregation, in the city has reduced personal victimization (Jacobs and Carmichael 2002; Like 2011). Such segregation would diminish interpersonal contact, thus disempowering victimization or perpetration. Power or resources stemming from national consumption, such as on energy, education, employment, and trade, have also diminished personal victimization (Nepal et al. 2011; Schutte 2015). The power is thus protective of victimization. Conversely, national poverty indicated a disempowering factor bolstering personal victimization (Nepal et al. 2011). Moreover, diversity in the language in the country has dampened personal victimization (Schutte 2015). Such diversity would lessen interpersonal contact and thus the risk of victimization. Conversely, nativity and population concentration in the country have raised personal victimization (Nepal et al. 2011; Schutte 2015). This raising is again due to the increase in interpersonal contact when most people are natives. In addition, when a country has occupied another country, the latter has lower personal victimization (Schutte 2015). This lowering would happen when the occupying country exerts control over interpersonal contact, perpetuation, and victimization. By contrast, rebellion, particularly its power in a country, has generated personal victimization (Schutte 2015). Such rebellious factors are forces producing perpetration and victimization. Meanwhile, state force has also been conducive to personal victimization (Schutte 2015). Perpetration and victimization are simply the results of collective forces.

The deterministic mechanism of empowering also indicates that collective power affects personal perpetration, which is a necessary condition for personal victimization. Collective power or coercion is evident in collective competition, conflict, division, oppression, and pressure (Ahmad and Monaghan 2019; Hattery and Smith 2012; Hoffman and Edwards 2004; Schinkel 2004; White et al. 2015). They activate personal perpetration as a reaction (Collins et al. 2007; Felson and Outlaw 2007; Santoro and Broidy 2014). Conversely, collective police power preempts personal perpetuation (Kivimaki 2012; Pinker 2011). Similarly, collective incarceration, which represents the state as a Levitan, contains and disempowers personal perpetration (Pinker 2011). Such control is weaker when the context is poorer, and collective poverty thus triggers personal perpetration (Lee and Dusey 2011). Personal perpetration also arises from advancements in technology to popularize weapons collectively (Pinker 2011). Conversely, collective control has suppressed personal perpetration (Benson et al. 2004). The collective disadvantage, resulting in lower collective control, has bolstered personal perpetration (Benson et al. 2004). Population size in the country has also boosted personal perpetration (Cohn et al. 2004). The size heightens interpersonal contact and thus perpetration. Similarly, temperature and single parenthood in the country have bred personal perpetration (Brown 2016; Cohn et al. 2004). This breeding is likely due to stress provoked by the national features to fuel perpetration (Cano and Vivian 2003). Conversely, ethnic segregation in the country has prevented personal perpetration, possibly due to reduced contact (Bhavnani et al. 2014).

The deterministic mechanism of incentivizing suggests that the adequacy of the legal system as a collective factor discourages personal perpetration and thus victimization (Collins 2008). Such adequacy lessens the need for personal perpetration to resolve disputes. Essentially, the legal system suppresses the honor code underlying perpetration (Collins 2008). By contrast, rewards for success or profit-making even through competition and perpetration in the context incentivizes personal perpetration (Messner et al. 2008). Remarkably, the national culture of honor has bred personal perpetration (Triandis and Suh 2002). As such, perpetration would be a way to achieve honor in the country. In addition, economic inequality in the country has raised personal perpetration (van Wilsem 2007). Inequality can be an incentive for the perpetration of lower-class people. Conversely, employment and collective insurance or security in the country have discouraged personal perpetration (Brown 2016; Poveda 2011). These features provide disincentives to perpetration for compensation or reward (Krahe 2001; Stogner et al. 2014). National price or inflation has also raised personal perpetration (Poveda 2011). The price would incentivize perpetration as a gainful way of subsistence (Stott et al. 2017; Van Knippenberg et al. 2007).

The deterministic mechanism of framing maintains that collective strain is the idea or experience consonant with personal victimization or perpetration. Such strain transpires in collective inequality or polarization and marital breakdown, as they have provided personal victimization (Jacobs and Carmichael 2002; Like 2011; Nepal et al. 2011; van Wilsem 2007). Mainly, inequality or polarization underlies the disparity between perpetration and victimization. That is, people treat their unequal differently and even violently. Moreover, then a country has had an atmosphere of the cold war, personal victimization has been higher (Schutte 2015). As such, the atmosphere creates a frame for provoking perpetration and victimization. Herein, perpetration is consonant with war. Likewise, collective anomie or normlessness determines personal perpetration (Messner et al. 2013). Such anomie frames competition, dominance, individualism, and inequality instead of civilizing, generosity, integration, normativity, and regulation. This frame or its framed orientations tempts one's perpetration (Bjarnegard et al. 2019; Pauwels and De Waele 2014; Pulkkinen et al. 2009; Stogner et al. 2014). A similarly provocative collective frame publicizes the civilization clash and thus conflict, failure, and frustration (McDonald 2013). Herein, civilization is the broadest and most pervasive value and lifestyle guiding or constraining people (Huntington 1993). Civilization is vital as the center of loyalty and social identification (Collins 2001). A prominent civilization is the materialist one emphasizing art, building, capital, class, city, government, labor, literature, science, technology, and trade (Dant 2006; Nevarez 2011). By contrast, the developed world highlights education, employment, environment, goods and services, health, leisure, and safety in its civilization (Horn 1993). A civilization clash is evident in orientalism, which regards Western civilization, which embraces democracy, liberalism, and pluralism, as superior to Eastern civilization (Bottici and Chall 2010). Another frame concerns social disintegration, which features individualization and polarization (Heitmeyer and Anhut 2008). Such a frame discourages sympathy and thus permits or encourages perpetration (Gelles 2007; Twenge and Campbell 2003). Another provocative frame, based on social construction, is brutalization (Grasner 2013). In addition, donation, education, social cohesion, and social interaction at the collective level have discouraged personal perpetration (Brown 2016; Lansford and Dodge 2008; Poveda 2011). These features are incongruous with perpetration. Conversely, national anomie, minority population, punishment, and the men-to-women ratio or competitiveness have induced personal perpetration (Fagan et al. 2007; Fei and Zakrzewski 2021; van Wilsem 2007). These competitive and punitive features have encouraged perpetration at the personal level (Collins et al. 2007; Farrington 2018).

Security

At the personal level based, on voluntaristic mechanisms, the experience of security stems from one's protection or other mental or physical work in creation, perception, or even appreciation. By contrast, deterministic mechanisms share the experience directly or activate voluntaristic mechanisms to produce the experience indirectly.

The voluntaristic mechanism of power realization specifies power or resources to afford the experience of security or its underlying action. Power notably rests on social class as opposed to vulnerability, such as a disadvantaged position (Rader et al. 2012; Taylor-Gooby 2001). As such, social class sustains security, whereas vulnerability hampers security. Power also arises from competence, which has been conducive to the experience of security (Valera and Guardia 2014). Competence, in turn, has benefitted from one's age, control, and reception of support (Valera and Guardia 2014). Thus, age has upheld the experience of security (Carter and Wolfe 2021). Meanwhile, education, employment, organizational membership, possession, and social capital or networking have buttressed security (Brisson 2009; Coffe and Geys 2007; Gaitan-Rossi and Shen 2018; Sacks and Levi 2010). They have been the sources of power or resources (Hofstetter et al. 1999; Keltener et al. 2008; Ross and Mirowsky 2009). Conversely, female gender, minority, rural residence, being a victim, and the experience of others' influence have weakened the experience of security (Carter and Wolfe 2021; Fernandes 2018; Gaitan-Rossi and Shen 2018; Urbatsch 2014; Valera and Guardia 2014). These characteristics have indicated a lack of power or resources (Aral and Walker 2012; Flores and Telles 2012; Mapelli 1993). In addition, religious attendance has sustained the experience of security (Urbatsch 2014). This sustaining indicates the production of security through empowerment from religious attendance.

The voluntaristic mechanism of utility optimization posits that the experience of security results from protective work needed. Such a need stems from having children, particularly in the family. Having children thus has sustained the experience of security (Coffe and Geys 2007; Urbatsch 2014). That is, work to buttress security is exceptionally gainful or valuable in the presence of children.

The voluntaristic mechanism of norm conformity proposes that the experience of security results from learning from the social environment. Thus, watching television has weakened the experience of security (Coffe and Geys 2007). Watching television indicates learning about social insecurity commonly portrayed on the screen (Riddle 2010). Moreover, security experience depends on other people's appraisal of one's security (Hintsanen et al. 2010). This dependence reflects learning and conformity, given that one regards others as a mirror.

The voluntaristic mechanism of idea consistency maintains that the experience of security results from rationalizing to maintain consistency with various experiences, dispositions, perceptions, attitudes, and practices. Alternative experiences that have sustained the security experience are ease, equality, police performance, and protection by law (Gaitan-Rossi and Shen 2018; Sacks and Levi 2010). Mainly, experiences in crime control and prevention in the neighborhood have been conducive to the experience of security (Kanan and Pruitt 2002; Fernandes 2018). Conversely, the experiences of aggression, conflict, deprivation, vandalism, and victimization of various kinds have eroded the experience of security (Fernandes 2018; Gaitan-Rossi and Shen 2018; Peruzzi 2014; Sacks and Levi 2010; Valera and Guardia 2014; van der Bracht et al. 2017). As such, the experience of getting social support and cohesion have weakened the experience of security (Carter and Wolfe 2021; Valera and Guardia 2014). These experiences have raised the experience of insecurity based on rationalizing the experiences. Particularly, experiences of disorder, incivility, and policing in the neighborhood have eroded the experience of security (Fernandes 2018; Kanan and Pruitt 2002). Thus, police performance has impaired the experience of security (Carter and Wolfe 2021). In addition, such dispositions as agreeableness, conscientiousness, and extraversion have sustained the experience of security (Becker et al. 1997). This sustaining happens as agreeableness sustains solidarity, conscientiousness has secured attachment and relatedness, and extraversion has strengthened social networking (Fraley et al. 2011; Graziano and Tobin 2009; Hounkpatin et al. 2015). Such perceptions as those about government fairness and police legitimacy have also contributed to the experience of security (Carter and Wolfe 2021; Sacks and Levi 2010). Furthermore, talking with neighbors has eroded the experience of security (Fernandes 2018). Such talking is likely about recourse, providing help, or protection, as thus consonant with the experience of insecurity (Hays and Kogl 2007).

The direct deterministic mechanism indicates that sharing collective experience privately or publicly is the determinant of the personal experience. As such, homicide in the city, as a collective experience of insecurity, has eroded the personal experience of security (Gaitan-Rossi and Shen 2018).

The deterministic mechanism of empowering emphasizes collective power or resources for maintaining personal security. Such collective power or resources include income and infrastructure in the context. These contextual resources have safeguarded personal security (Kanan and Pruitt 2002; Sacks and Levi 2010). Conversely, poverty in the city has eroded personal security (Gaitan-Rossi and Shen 2018). This erosion reflects the reverse mechanism of disempowering. More broadly, technology in the context is a basis for power to enable or erode personal security (Asogwa 2020). That is, protective technology is empowering, whereas invasive technology is disempowering. Furthermore, national inequality and ethnic or other forms of diversity in the neighborhood have sustained personal security (Gaitan-Rossi and Shen 2018; Kanan and Pruitt 2002). This sustaining is due to the collective force of division to reduce contact, competition, and conflict (Dodson 2016; Solt 2015). The reduction has upheld security (van der Bracht et al. 2017). In addition, socioeconomic status in the context has buttressed collective security (Frohlich et al. 2002). The status is the power to afford the maintenance of security.

The deterministic mechanism of framing maintains that the personal experience of security results from consistent or incongruous experiences in the context. Such contextual experiences are incivility and living standards in the city, discouraging the personal experience of security (Gaitan-Rossi and Shen 2018; Taylor-Gooby 2001).

Such contextual experiences would create a frame of relative deprivation (Taylor-Gooby 2001). Meanwhile, the experiences of deprivation and incivility have been conducive to the experience of insecurity (Kanan and Pruitt 2002; Peruzzi 2014). Moreover, contextual stability or durability shapes collective security (Norris 2012). Stability and security are consonant.

Family Saving

At the personal level, based on voluntaristic mechanisms, the experience of family saving reflects one's contribution to or support for family saving. Hence, family saving reflects personal saving and family income or wealth. By contrast, deterministic mechanisms share the experience of personal or family saving or wealth directly or trigger voluntaristic mechanisms to produce the experience indirectly.

The voluntaristic mechanism of power realization posits that personal or family saving results from power originating from the goal set for the saving (Curney and Gale 2001). This goal, in turn, relies on financial resources, such as income, and thus does not hold under poverty (Curney and Gale 2001; Obben and Waayer 2011; Wolff and Resnick 2012). Particularly, saving is likely when income is stable (Obben and Waayer 2011). Family income has also contributed to personal saving (Chakrabarty et al. 2008). Moreover, physical power or health has been conducive to saving (Chakrabarty et al. 2008). In this connection, health has produced financial resources (Mulatu and Schooler 2002). Meanwhile, saving has been lower in older age, retirement, female gender, and minority status (Anderson and Nevitte 2006; Brisson 2009; Obben and Waayer 2011). Likewise, family income has been lower when one has been higher in age, being a minority member, poor, receiving welfare, or in school (Bellair and Roscigno 2000; van Praag and Ferrer-I-Carbonell 2004; Vartanian 1999). These conditions have had lower power or resources to facilitate saving (Aral and Walker 2012; Ross and Mirowsky 2009; Verschuur et al. 2010). Power in terms of social capital has also buttressed saving (Brisson 2009). Conversely, family income has been higher when one's education, income, or work engagement has been higher (Angelusz and Tardos 2008; Guardiola and Garcia-Munoz 2011; Vartanian 1999). Furthermore, family income has increased with one's social capital (Angelusz and Tardos 2008). As such, one's power or resources contribute to the family's resources. In addition, family resources in terms of family members' adulthood, education, employment, possession, or social class have contributed to family income (Guardiola and Garcia-Munoz 2011; Walder 2002; van Praag and Ferrer-I-Carbonell 2004). Saving also has an inverse relationship with consumption (Wolff and Resnick 2012). As such, consumption is a countervailing force against saving.

The voluntaristic mechanism of utility optimization regards saving as resulting from its gain or value. Such gain is in terms of the interest rate of saving (Wolff and Resnick 2012). Meanwhile, having children in the family has lowered saving and family income (Chakrabarty et al. 2008; Vartanian 1999). This lowering would happen because of the need to consume for childcare. That is, consumption rather than saving is valuable for childcare.

The voluntaristic mechanism of norm conformity highlights learning from others as the cause of personal or family saving or income. Such learning has stemmed from socialization, particularly about finance (Webley and Nyhus 2006). Another source is the social network (Angelusz and Tardos 2008).

The voluntaristic mechanism of idea consistency maintains consistency between saving and various experiences, perceptions, dispositions, attitudes, and practices. This works through rationalizing, such as by finding saving as opposed to spending to be easy rather than difficult (Webley and Nyhus 2006). Similarly, conventionality or conservatism, conscientiousness, and planning have been consonant with saving (Webley and Nyhus 2006; Wolff and Resnick 2012). Conservatism has saving as its component (Yoos 2007). Conscientiousness champions conventionality and delaying gratification (Roberts et al. 2009). By contrast, spending has reduced saving (Chakrabarty et al. 2008; Wolff and Resnick 2012).

The direct deterministic mechanism works as the impact of collective saving on personal or family saving or income. Family income at the neighborhood level has indicated a positive impact on family income at the family level (Walder 2002). Conversely, poverty at the neighborhood level has eroded family income (Roscigno 1999). Similarly, the amounts of national income and savings have sustained the amount of personal savings (Obben and Waayer 2011; Zhang and Zhang 2004). Thus, sharing of experience or practice among people happens privately or vicariously.

The deterministic mechanism of empowerment works when contextual factors empower or disempower voluntaristic mechanisms in producing personal or family saving or income. Contextual empowering factors have been national export, economic growth, population size, and trade, which have sustained personal saving (Baharumshah 2003; Kazmi 1993). Conversely, national foreign aid received, import, population growth, and have impaired personal saving (Kazmi 1993). These national conditions reflect the lack or depletion of resources, thus disempowering saving. Moreover, foreign investment at the national level has diminished personal saving (Baharumshah 2003). This diminishment would happen as foreign investment takes profits away from the country, thus reducing people's savings within the country. In addition, employment, earnings, and wage at the neighborhood level have buttressed family income (Bellair and Roscigno 2000; Walder 2002). Employment at the national level has also lifted family income (Lin et al. 2015). These factors thus can empower personal saving and family income acquisition.

The deterministic mechanism of incentivizing indicates incentives available in the context boost personal and family saving or income through voluntaristic mechanisms. The national interest rate has been the chief incentive for raising saving (Kazmi 1993). Moreover, unemployment at the national level has lifted saving (Obben and Waayer 2011). Such unemployment would indicate the need for personal and family saving. What is more, neighborhood quality has encouraged earning and saving in the family (Vartanian 1999). Accordingly, neighborhood quality would raise the value of saving or investment in the neighborhood or its home. Conversely, national wealth and welfare or social security have discouraged personal saving (Obben and Waayer 2011; Salotti 2010). These national factors would diminish the value of saving.

Stress

Stress is a common factor derived from economic hardship, neighborhood nuisance, and victimization. Conversely, stress is the reverse of security and family saving. At the personal level, based on voluntaristic mechanisms, stress results from the failure to avoid, prevent, or protect against stress. By contrast, deterministic mechanisms maintain that collective or contextual factors create or share personal stress directly or indirectly through voluntaristic mechanisms.

The voluntaristic mechanism of power realization states that stress results from the lack of power or resources. Stress thus arises when depletion, disadvantage, or limitation is greater or social class is lower (Carr and Umberson 2013; Tokunaga 2016). Thus, age, earning reduction, having dependants, minority status, risk status, and underemployment have fomented stress (Aytac et al. 2015; Cepulic et al. 2022; Uddin 2011; Walen and Lachman 2016). Conversely, education and employment have relieved stress (Cepulic et al. 2022; Walen and Lachman 2016). In addition, emotional intelligence, such as in clarifying and repairing emotions, has prevented stress (Extremera et al. 2007). Power in terms of health or social capital has also dampened stress (Barrett 1999; Frank et al. 2014). Alternatively, stress results from power generated due to conflict or overload (Carr and Umberson 2013). As such, demand from work has generated stress (Fenwick and Tausig 1994). Conversely, coping has reduced stress (Aytac et al. 2015). As such, coping instills the power to alleviate stress.

The voluntaristic mechanism of utility optimization emphasizes exchange as a basis for stress. Accordingly, receiving positive affect prevents the experience of stress (Floyd 2019). This prevention maintains fairness in not generating a stressful response to positive affect received.

The voluntaristic mechanism of idea consistency indicates that stress resulting from maintaining consistency or rationalizing with various ideas related to experiences, dispositions, attitudes, feelings, and practices. Thus, the experiences of neighborliness and networking have dampened stress (Beaudoin 2009; Frank et al. 2014)). Meanwhile, the dispositions of optimism, positive reactivity, and self-differentiation have prevented stress (Boyes et al. 2017; Constantino et al. 2006; Extremera et al. 2007). Self-differentiation is a notably a way to separate oneself from stress. The attitude of trust has lessened stress (Cepulic et al. 2022). Conversely, the disposition of pessimism has sustained stress (Extremera et al. 2007). Communication about death and health or illness has increased stress (Cheng et al. 2017). Furthermore, obesity has raised stress (Beaudoin 2009). Death, illness, and obesity invoke ideas consonant with stress.

The deterministic mechanism of empowering identifies some disempowering collective factors raising personal stress. These factors have been unemployment and restriction stringency in the context (Cepulic et al. 2022; Fenwick and Tausig 1994). Their depletion or restriction of power and resources engenders stress.

Predictors of Social Experiences

The predictors of personal life quality include personal and national factors. Personal factors include various sociodemographic characteristics such as age and gender, whereas national factors include population, phone ownership, and land area per capita. Notably, the reverse of the effect of age squared indicates the effect of mid-age. Meanwhile, social experiences broadly comprise stressful and non-stressful or pleasant ones, with the former including economic hardship, neighborhood nuisance, and victimization, and the latter includes security and family saving.

Age

For the voluntaristic mechanism of power realization, age offers power or resources in adaptation, human capital, income, knowledge, resiliency, and skill (Charles and Carstensen 2009; Consedine 2011; Pena 2020; Von Krogh and Wallin 2011; Wagner and Lang 2011). Age also enables getting resources or support through marriage (Kuntla et al. 2013). Marriage has notably alleviated stress (Plagnol and Easterlin 2008). Hence, age has sustained affordability and knowledge (Hallerod 2006; Price et al. 2006). Affordability mainly means the absence of economic hardship. The other abilities or resources have also prevented stress (Zheng et al. 2020). Thus, stress has diminished with age (Beaudoin 2009; Cepulic et al. 2022).

Nevertheless, age also indicates a decline in power or resources, particularly in awareness, learning, relating, planning, and regulating (Charles and Carstensen 2009; Kliegel et al. 2007; Wagner and Lang 2011). Thus, the decline has happened in cognitive ability, friendship, memory, physical functioning, and social integration (Gerstorf et al. 2006; Goerres 2007; Herd et al. 2008; Stevens et al. 2001). The decline has also induced illness (Schaie 2013). Such a decline in personal and social resources has failed to prevent stress (Cepulic et al. 2022; Extremera et al. 2007). Hence, age increases stress (Frank et al. 2014; Barrett 1999; Walen and Lachman 2016).

For the voluntaristic mechanism of utility optimization, age has manifested declines in the need for achievement and valuation of material well-being (Yee 2006). These declines in demand or aspiration suggest greater experiences of finding something to be achievement and well-being. This suggestion lowers the utility of experiencing financial adequacy, security, and saving. Hence, the experiences of security and saving would decline with age, and the experiences of stress and hardship would increase with age.

For the voluntaristic mechanism of idea consistency, age has generated such dispositions as agreeableness, conservatism, materialism, religiosity, stability, and the values of order and trust (Cornelis et al. 2009; Fung and Ng 2006; Goerres 2007; Kurata 2015). Similarly, age has raised such attitudes as favor for accommodating, peace, and trust (Bonin-Scaon et al. 2009; Sneed et al. 2006). In addition, age has activated such practices as protection and self-regulating (Isaacowitz et al. 2003; Tam 2014). These have dampened the experience of stress, including hardship, insecurity, nuisance, victimization, and draining or inability to save (Cepulic et al. 2022; Zavala and Guadalupe-Diaz 2019). This dampening would maintain idea consistency based on rationalizing or wishful thinking. Conversely, age has weakened neuroticism (Stanley et al. 2014). This weakening has lowered the experience of stress, including economic hardship (Lincoln et al. 2003). However, age has diminished generosity, openness, tolerance, and community activity (Miner-Rubino et al. 2004). The diminishment has buttressed the experience of stress, including nuisance and insecurity (Extremera et al. 2007). Conversely, age has elevated emotional reactivity, concern for privacy, sensitivity to negativity, and the use of medical services (Fung et al. 2008; Kliegel et al. 2007; Schaie 2013). This elevation has raised the experience of stress, including nuisance and victimization (Beaudoin 2009).

Mid-age

For the voluntaristic mechanism of power realization, mid-age has generated more resources in terms of employment, homeownership, income, marriage, and cultural and social capital than have other age ranges (Benstock 2008; Keister 2003; Glaeser and Gottlieb 2006; Parrado 2005; Plagnol and Easterlin 2008). These resources have weakened the experience of stress, including hardship and insecurity (Barrett 1999; Cepulic et al. 2022). By contrast, mid-age has lowered resources regarding affordability, savings, wealth, and organizational membership (Anderson and Nevitte 2006; Apinunmahakul and Devlin 2008; Keister 2003). Such lowering has elevated the experience of stress, including hardship, insecurity, and victimization (Coffe and Geys 2007; Hallerod 2006; Reese et al. 2021).

For the voluntaristic mechanism of utility optimization, mid-age would affect the utility of stress avoidance to maintain security. Accordingly, mid-age has contributed to criminal involvement and reporting (Akers and Kaukinen 2009; Land et al. 1996). These have been causes of or responses to victimization (Wittebrood and Nieuwbeerta 2000). This relationship indicates reciprocity between perpetration and victimization, following the logic of exchange in the mechanism of utility optimization. That is, criminal involvement generates an expectation for victimization, thus culminating in the experience of victimization.

For the voluntaristic mechanism of idea consistency, mid-age has raised the experiences of gift receiving and social integration (Frei et al. 2009; Godoy et al. 2007). This raising has weakened the experience of stress, including hardship and nuisance (Treharne et al. 2001; Frank et al. 2014). Conversely, mid-age has diminished the practices of borrowing (Guiso et al. 2004). This diminishment reflects the absence of economic hardship (Guiso et al. 2004; Li 2010).

However, mid-age has reduced the experience of friendship (Prouteau and Wolff 2008). Mid-age has also weakened such attitudes as an orientation toward charity and political and social trust (Brown and Ferris 2007; Marien 2011; Traunmuller 2011). In addition, mid-age has impeded the practices of community participation (Richey 2007). Such impedance has raised the experience of stress, including neighborhood nuisance (Hunter et al. 2013). Conversely, mid-age has underlaid the experience of political alienation (Coffe and Geys 2007). Such alienation has raised the experience of stress (Treharne et al. 2001; Frank et al. 2014). Moreover, mid-age has upheld aspiration (Hallerod 2006; Plagnol and Easterlin 2008). Aspiration has elevated the experience of stress, notably economic hardship (Nickerson et al. 2007). That is, stress results from the inability to meet aspirations. Hence, mid-age has stimulated the experience of economic hardship (Hays and Seifert 2003).

Gender

Female gender is conducive to the experience of stress or threat, including victimization (Betz et al. 2013; de Coster 2005; Thapa et al. 2021). However, female gender has underlain the experience of security, thus eroding the experience of stress (Hraba et al. 2001).

For the voluntaristic mechanism of power realization, power and resources are crucial for the experience of stress. Due to discrimination, social construction, and other conditions, female gender has impeded power or resources in competence, knowledge, skill, and social status (Carli 2004; Irwin 2011; Rundman and Glick 2008; Kerrissey and Schofer 2013; Shin 2012; Valiente 2018). The impedance has fomented the experience of stress, including hardship and insecurity (Mutz 1998). This fomenting reflects the weakening of the ability to avoid or prevent stress. Moreover, female gender poses a risk of victimization such as raping (Kurz and Donaghue 2013). This posing indicates a positive effect of female gender on stress expereinced. However, female gender has less testosterone than does male gender (Lippa 2005). This fact means lower perpetration and thus victimization (Farrington 2007; Lilly et al. 2011). In practice, female gender has bolstered coping in various ways (Gattino et al. 2015; Tamres et al. 2002). Coping has relieved stress (Caplan and Schooler 2007). This relief supports the negative effect of female gender on stress experienced.

For the voluntaristic mechanism of utility optimization, personal demands, dependency, values, and social rewards are influential on the experience of stress. Accordingly, female gender receives less reward (Carli and Bukatko 2000; Franklin 2012). Female gender also maintains greater dependency on others (Rundman and Glick 2008). In addition, female gender has sustained the value of need, emphasizing need fulfillment (Gelissen 2002). Aspiration and dependency have sustained the experience of stress (Adams et al. 2009; Auerbach et al. 2011; Kachadourian et al. 2013).

Notably, the relationship between dependency and stress conforms to the logic of exchange. This logic bolsters a positive effect of female gender on stress experienced.

For the voluntaristic mechanism of idea consistency, ideas derived from dispositions, experiences, attitudes, and practices affect the experience of stress through rationalizing. Female gender maintains such dispositions as agreeableness, attachment, communality, controllability, deference, and endurance (Franklin 2012; Guimond et al. 2013; Fyall and Gazley 2015; Hopcroft 2016). Moreover, female gender has upheld such dispositions as religiosity and the value of conservation (Datler et al. 2013; Immerzeel and van Tubergen 2013). Female gender has also sustained such attitudes as tolerance for noise, support for security, and trust, notably in police (Anciaes et al. 2017; Feingold 1994; Mondak and Hurwitz 2012; Sun et al. 2013). These conditions indicate favorable social experiences. The conditions have prevented the experience of stress, including insecurity, nuisance, and victimization (Bardeen et al. 2016; Weinberg et al. 2021). Conversely, female gender has lower dispositions in aggressiveness, competitiveness, dominance, and violence than has male gender (Conway and Schaller 2002; Goldberg 1993; Hopcroft 2016; Rundman and Glick 2008). Female gender has also eroded the disposition of cynicism (Kirk and Papachristos 2011). Furthermore, female has dampened the experience of social rejection (Kaplan and Liu 2000). Practically, female gender has reduced aggression and criminal involvement (de Coster 2005; Lippa 2005). Female gender has also reduced such feelings as anger (Charles and Carstensen 2008). Such conditions have prevented the experience of stress, including nuisance and victimization (Kaukinen 2004; Zavala and Guadalupe-Diaz 2019). In addition, female gender is lower in aspiration, demandingness, or the pursuit of status than is male gender (Hopcroft 2016). Notably, female gender has dampened demand for safety (Anciaes et al. 2017). Such lower aspiration or demand has resulted in lower stress (Auerbach et al. 2011). This effect shows a negative effect of female gender on stress experienced. These conditions suggest that female gender is preventive of the experience of stress.

By contrast, female gender engenders dispositions of anxiety or fear, depression, jealousy, sensitivity (Guo et al. 2008; Hopcroft 2016; Rundman and Glick 2008). Female gender has also sustained the dispositions of morbidity, neuroticism, and the value of security (Caprara and Vecchione 2017; Walter-Ginzburg et al. 2005). Moreover, female gender has engendered perceptions about problem and risk (Lemyre et al. 2006; Wan 1999). Female gender has also buttressed the experiences of illness (Schaie 2013). In practice, female gender has sustained medication or the consultation with or use of medical services (Schaie 2013). Female gender has also bred such feelings as depression and distress (de Coster 2005). These conditions have underlain the experience of stress (Bellingtier et al. 2022; Constantino et al. 2006). Conversely, female gender diminishes self-esteem (Thapa et al. 2021). Female gender has also weakened the disposition of conservatism (Norris and Inglehart 2009). Moreover, female gender has dampened health (Gattino et al. 2015). Such weakening has led to the experience of stress, including a lack of savings (Barrett 1999; Hair et al. 2007). Saving is notably congenial to conservation (Ribeiro and Soares 2017). These influences suggest the positive effect of female gender on the experience of stress.

Immigration

Immigration, as indicated by parental immigration, has raised the experience of stress such as neighborhood nuisance and insecurity (Bask 2005; Lilly et al. 2011). However, immigration has lessened the experience of stress in terms of economic hardship (Fridberg and Kangas 2008). The influences of immigration work through the voluntaristic mechanisms of power realization, utility optimization, norm conformity, and idea consistency.

For the voluntaristic mechanism of power realization, immigration has engendered functional limitations (Herd et al. 2008). This engendering reflects the misfit of immigration with the host society. Furthermore, immigration has impeded employment, marriage, and social capital (Fanning et al. 2011; Ravanera et al. 2003; Thornton et al. 2007). The impedance would reduce the power or resources to avoid or prevent stress. These resources have been preventive of stress. Conversely, immigration has engendered poverty and unemployment (Posthumus et al. 2013; Kurz et al. 2005). These conditions have been conducive to the experience of stress. Hence, immigration would lead to the experience of stress sue to the lack of resources.

The voluntaristic mechanism of norm conformity emphasizes the social influence on the experience of stress through social interaction and learning. Such an influence arises from that of contact with criminals. Meanwhile, immigration has prevented such contact (Brayne 2014). Therefore, immigration would alleviate the experience of stress.

The voluntaristic mechanism of idea consistency indicates that the experience of stress results from ideas derived from other experiences, perceptions, dispositions, attitudes, feelings, and practices. Herein, immigration has weakened the experience of illness (Fridberg and Kangas 2008; Wen et al. 2010). Immigration has also raised feelings about health and social relationship quality (Fridberg and Kangas 2008; Wen et al. 2010). In practice, immigration has upheld social cohesion (Tolsma et al. 2009). Conversely, immigration has eroded depression and psychosis (Lofors and Sundquist 2007). In addition, Aspiration for egalitarianism has declined with immigration (Saunders and Wong 2012). The decline would lower the experience of stress. Thus, immigration would be preventive for the experience of stress.

However, immigration has delivered ideas consonant with the experience of stress. Herein, immigration has raised the experience of social exclusion and the lack of neighborhood social cohesion or control (Bask 2005; Lilly et al. 2011). Immigration has also weakened such attitudes as attachment to the community and social trust (Anton and Lawrence 2014). Furthermore, immigration has impeded such a feeling as life satisfaction (Ambrey and Fleming 2014). In practice, immigration has fomented suicide (Hassan 1995).

Education

Education has dampened the experience of stress in terms of hardship, hazards, insecurity, threat, and victimization (Cerin and Leslie 2008; Hraba et al. 2001; Kaukinen 2004; Raijman et al. 2003; Whyte and Gao 2009). Conversely, education has contributed to earnings and insurance (Knab et al. 2008; Schnittker and Behrman 2012). These conditions have enabled saving, particularly when married (Chakrabarty et al. 2008; Webley and Nyhus 2006). In marriage, income pooling for mutual support would add to family saving. Conversely, education has prevented poverty or economic hardship (Wang et al. 2013). The impacts of education work through the voluntaristic mechanisms of power realization, utility optimization, and idea consistency.

For the voluntaristic mechanism of power realization, education represents power or human resources for avoiding or preventing the experience of stress. Specifically, education registers human capital and resources for control based on learning (Dolton et al. 2004; Nordin 2011; Papastephanon 2015). Education also aims to enhance the ability of creativity (Yair 2003). Moreover, education has raised abilities based on health, intelligence, knowledge, memory, physical functioning, social competence, and verbal ability (Keightley et al. 2006; Kuppens et al. 2015; Pratt et al. 1996; Ross and Mirowsky 1995; Shin 2012; Straughn and Andriot 2011; Stevens et al. 2001). In addition, education has sustained employment, home resources, and social status (Cerin and Leslie 2008; Foster et al. 2001; Whyte and Gao 2009). Education has also elevated the practices of prevention and social distancing (Tsai 2006). This elevation would minimize the risk of nuisance and victimization. Such power or its exertion has diminished the experience of stress, including insecurity and victimization (Extremera et al. 2007). Conversely, education has impeded the practice of prostitution (Swader and Vorobeva 2015). Such impedance would prevent victimization. Hence, education would assure against the experience of stress.

For the voluntaristic mechanism of utility optimization, education champions the utility of avoiding or preventing the experience of stress. Accordingly, education has boosted the practices of civility, cohesion, cooperation, and volunteering (Chan 2014; Holbrook et al. 2003; Kerrissey and Schofer 2013; Letki 2006). According to the logic of exchange or fairness, this would indicate a demand for civility rather than victimization in return. This demand would raise the utility of stress or victimization avoidance. Such practices have thus prevented the experience of stress (Coffe and Geys 2007; Fernandes 2018). Conversely, education has prevented the practices of abusing others, deviance, discrimination, and violence (Atkinson et al. 2005; Backman and Nilsson 2011; Kwan and Law 1994; Michalski 2005). Such prevention has impeded the stress of stress, including victimization (Wittebrood and Nieuwbeerta 2000). This impedance would buttress the negative effect of education on the experience of stress.

However, education has reduced the utility of stress avoidance. Accordingly, education has weakened the demand or need for help and the practice of recourse (Lessler et al. 2000; Su and Feng 2013). The weakened need would lower the utility of stress avoidance, thus reducing stress avoidance and raising stress. This reduction suggests the positive effect of education on the experience of stress.

For the voluntaristic mechanism of idea consistency, education induces ideas congenial to avoiding or preventing the experience of stress, including draining and insecurity. Such ideas include the dispositions of conservatism and environmentalism, which have arisen from education (Norris and Inglehart 2009; Shen and Saijo 2008). In addition, education has raised the attitudes of concern for the environment, preference for insurance, support for environmental policy and social services, and tolerance for social experience (Franzen and Vogl 2013; Gibson 2013; Wong and Wan 2011; Seccombe 1996; Zumbrunnen and Gangl 2008). Education has also raised the practices of environmental protection and health maintenance (Welzel 2013). Furthermore, education has sustained the experiences of benefit, friendship, social networking, and social support (Cerin and Leslie 2008; Mau 2005a; Miyata et al. 2008; Prouteau and Wolff 2008). These ideas would be consonant with stress avoidance. The ideas have thus prevented the experience of stress, including hardship, insecurity, and victimization (Brisson 2009; Frank et al. 2014). Conversely, education has dampened the disposition of vulnerability (Langenderfer and Shimp 2001). Education has also weakened the attitudes of alienation and tolerance for violence (Weakliem and Borch 2006; Zumbrunnen and Gangl 2008). Furthermore, education has diminished perceptions about corruption, crime, and risk (Morris and Klesner 2010; Nabi and Sullivan 2001; Sjoberg 2003). Education has also dampened the experiences of arrest, crime, discrimination, and exclusion (Allwood and Widom 2013; Backman and Nilsson 2011; Cerin and Leslie 2008; Kessler et al. 1999). Such weakening would uphold stress avoidance, thus lowering the experience of stress. These weakening has eroded the experience of stress (Like 2011; Ross and Mirowsky 2009; Valera and Guardia 2014). Hence, education would attenuate the experience of stress.

However, education has maintained some ideas conducive to the experience of stress. Accordingly, education has eroded the attitudes of attachment to the community and country, social trust, and support for health spending, rehabilitation, public pension, security, and social welfare (Anton and Lawrence 2014; Gerxhani 2012; Lynch and Myrskyla 2009; Mondak and Hurwitz 2012; Rochelle 2015; Straughn and Andriot 2011; Taylor-Gooby et al. 2003). Education has also impeded perceptions about justice (Jasso 2015). These ideas would be incongruous with stress reduction to sustain security. Such weakening has reduced the experience of stress, including hardship, insecurity, and victimization (Cepulic et al. 2022; Ehrensuft et al. 2003). Conversely, education has increased perceptions about discrimination, inequality, problem, and violence (Brooks and Prysby 1999; Kluegal and Bobo 2001; Scharrer 2008; Whyte and Gao 2009). Education has also increased the experiences of demand or solicitation and mobilization (Foster et al. 2001; Kerrissey and Schofer 2013). These ideas have been conducive to the experience of stress, including insecurity, nuisance, and victimization (Fenwick and Tausig 1994; Patel et al. 2012; Reese et al. 2021). In addition, education has raised aspirations and protesting (Grasso 2014; Norris 2011). This raise would reduce the utility of stress avoidance, thus fomenting stress. Notably, aspiration has maintained the experience of stress (Auerbach et al. 2011). Hence, education would bolster the experience of stress.

Employment

Employment or social class has been conducive to stress avoidance, thus diminishing the experience of stress (Myer et al. 2008). Particularly, employment has impeded the experiences of hardship and victimization (DeMaris et al. 2003; Fan et al. 2004). Likewise, social class, which grades the quality of employment, has dampened stress, notably concerning economic hardship or poverty (Muhlau 2014; Stansfeld and Marmot 1992; Whelan and Maitre 2010). The grading of social class is from unemployment and the surplus class, including homemakers, retirees, and students, to the ownership class, including employers or capitalists, through the working class, middle class, service class or upper-middle class, and self-employed workers or the petty bourgeoisie. The service class includes professionals and managers, and the middle class includes clerks and technicians. Social class is associated with creative, intellectual, independent, and supervisory work. Conversely, unemployment has fomented the experience of stress, including hardship and victimization (Kaukinen 2004; Muhlau 2014; Schneider 2007). The impacts of employment on the experience of stress work through the voluntaristic mechanisms of power realization, utility optimization, and idea consistency.

The voluntaristic mechanism of power realization holds that employment or social class influences the experience of stress or its avoidance through power or resources. Employment or social class has raised abilities or power in terms of health, intelligence, self-efficacy, skill, and social capital (Chang 2009; Corcoran et al. 2011; Distante 2013; Kerrissey and Schofer 2013; Wink and Dillon 2003). In practice, employment has championed health maintenance (Lin et al. 2008). Likewise, social class has sustained power in terms of social capital (Wuthnow 2004). Such power or resources have prevented the experience of stress, including hardship and insecurity (Barrett 1999; Hansen-Nord et al. 2014; Valera and Guardia 2014). Conversely, unemployment has eroded power in terms of social capital (Manturuk et al. 2010; Webber and Huxley 2007). Such a lack of power has fueled the experience of stress, including hardship and insecurity (Hansen-Nord et al. 2014; Kachadourian et al. 2013). Meanwhile, employment has impeded functional disability and powerlessness (Li and Chung 2008; Ross and Mirowsky 2009). In practice, employment has reduced contact with criminals (Brayne 2014). Hence, employment would prevent the experience of stress through power and resources.

The voluntaristic mechanism of utility optimization stresses that employment or social class affects the experience of stress or its avoidance through the maintenance of utility. Employment and social class have diminished criminal behavior (Agnew and Brezina 2010; Savolainen 2009). This diminishment would reduce the risk of victimization according to the logic of exchange. Hence, employment would reduce the experience of victimization. Conversely, social class has induced prosocial behavior and volunteering (Wilson and Musick 1997). This would increase the expectation or desire for or the utility of reward rather than victimization, following the logic of exchange. This increase would heighten the utility of stress avoidance and the prevention of stress eventually. Alternatively, social class has dampened the demand for social welfare (Gelissen 2002). The dampening would lower the experience of economic hardship and insecurity. Conversely, unemployment has raised the demand for social welfare (Baslevent and Kirmanoglu 2011). This raising would sustain the experience of stress, including hardship and insecurity. Hence, employment would reduce the experience of stress.

However, unemployment has increased the value of need (Lewin-Epstein et al. 2003; Reeskens and van Oorschot 2013). The increase would thus boost the utility of stress reduction to reduce stress eventually. Hence, unemployment would prevent stress, and thus employment would raise the experience of stress.

The voluntarism mechanism of idea consistency holds that employment affects stress by generating related experiences, perceptions, attitudes, dispositions, and practices. Accordingly, employment or social class has sustained conservatism, disapproval of crime and strike, perception of justice, trust, and the experiences of friendship and social support (Evans 1993b; Elchardus and De Keere 2013; Gerteis and Savage 1998; Groot et al. 2007; Lennartsson 2010; Tsai 2006; Viewiebe and Wegener 2000; Wilson and Dunham 2001). Such ideas would be consonant with stress avoidance, including security maintenance as opposed to victimization. The ideas have been preventive of the experience of stress (Cepulic et al. 2022; Frank et al. 2014; Reese et al. 2021). Conversely, unemployment has eroded social trust (Reeskens and Vandecasteele 2017). The erosion would diminish the experience of security. Unemployment has also raised the experiences of homelessness and hospitalization (Anson 1988; Lelli 2008). Furthermore, employment or social class has prevented the experiences of arrest, deprivation, illness, insomnia, and social exclusion (Allwood and Widom 2013; Buck 2001; Green et al. 2014; Pettigrew 2002; Ross and Mirowsky 2009; Yamaoka 2008). Such prevention has weakened the experience of stress, including hardship, insecurity, and victimization (Peruzzi 2014; van der Bracht et al. 2017). Hence, employment would prevent the experience of stress.

However, employment or social class has impeded environmentalism (Davis and Davenport 1999). The impedance would reduce risk or stress avoidance. Moreover, employment has raised the experiences of violence and shaming (DeMaris et al. 2003). Conversely, social class has bred the perception about social problems (Andersen 1999). Hence, employment would sustain the experience of stress.

Creative Work

In general, creative work or creativity is germane to stress or its stress avoidance or prevention. Essentially, creative work fosters or realizes one's complexity in mind, defiance, human capital, and strengths, particularly for solving problems (Metzl and Morrell 2008; Runco 2014; Sternberg 2001). Creative work features or emphasizes adaptiveness, generation, ideation, implementation, innovation, novelty, problem-solving, research and development, self-efficacy, servicing, and technicality (Afsar and Masood 2018; Fontenot 1993; Gelade 1999; Harrison and Laberge 2002; Madrid and Patterson 2016; Kim et al. 2011; Puccio et al. 2000; Turnipseed and Turnipseed 2013). Such features are influential on the experience of stress or its avoidance through the voluntaristic mechanisms of power realization and idea consistency.

The voluntaristic mechanism of power realization highlights power or resources in creative work to activate the practice of stress avoidance to dampen the experience of stress. Accordingly, creative work is reflective or conducive to critical thinking and intelligence, particularly for diversification, mental ability, and technical skillfulness (Drus et al. 2014; Gadzella and Penland 1995; Shorthose and Maycroft 2017; Tacher and Readdick 2006). They are capacity or human capital features to enable stress avoidance or prevention. Hence, creative work would lessen the experience of stress.

The voluntaristic mechanism of idea consistency specifies ideas derived from creative work to rationalize stress avoidance to prevent the experience of stress. Herein, creative work generates the dispositions of adaptiveness, autonomy, carefreeness, flexibility, freedom, meaningfulness, openness, playfulness, uniqueness, and tolerance (Israelstam 2007; Joas 1996; Runco 2014; Taplin et al. 2013). Such dispositions have relieved the experience of stress (Extremera et al. 2007; Hong et al. 2018; Weinberg et al. 2021). Creative work also sustains the experience of acceptance by others (Leung and Koh 2018). Moreover, creative work has fostered the experience of achievement and accomplishment (Milgram and Hong 1994; Rindermann and Neubauer 2004). These experiences have cushioned the experience of stress (Beaudoin 2009; Treharne et al. 2001; Frank et al. 2014; Page and Jacobs 2011). Creativity work has furthermore raised the feelings of happiness, meaningfulness, resilience, pleasantness, satisfaction, self-esteem, and well-being generally (Chen et al. 2018; Diener et al. 2009; Gebbia and Honigsfeld 2012; Henderson 2004; Tavares 2016; Schneck 2014; Shimai et al. 2006; Turner 2013). These feelings have constrained the experience of stress (Gallie et al. 1998; Hair et al. 2007; Mak and Mueller 2000; Parent et al. 2016). Hence, creative work would forestall the experience of stress.

Independent Work

Independent work means autonomy, self-determination, or self-direction at work (Kelly and Kelly 1994). It involves taking charge at work (Morrison et al. 1999). The profession of social work is an example of independent work, characterized by discretion and street-level bureaucracy at work (Evans and Harris 2004).

The voluntaristic mechanism of power realization states that power or resources derived from independent work enable stress avoidance to dispel the experience of stress. Accordingly, independent work develops capitalists or leaders (Hammond et al. 2015; Steinberg 2003). Independent work also strengthens the worker's influence (Franzen and Hangartner 2006). Furthermore, independent work realizes autonomous and intrinsic motivation, capability, competence, competitiveness, creativity, and social skill (Gore 2014; Laruffa 2020; McLean 2015; Ntoumanis et al. 2009; Peng et al. 2019; Soenens and Vansteenkiste 2005; Vansteenkiste et al. 2008; Waterman et al. 2003; Yeh and Yang 2006). These power or resources have facilitated stress avoidance or prevention (McMahon et al. 2015; Wang 2013). They have eventually prevented the experience of stress (Acker and Lawrence 2009; Aloia and Solomon 2015; Bellingtier et al. 2022). In addition, independent work has generated higher earnings (Kalleberg and Marsden 1995; Ross and Mirowsky 1996). Earnings or income has lessened the experience of stress, including hardship, insecurity, and victimization (Hallerod 2006; Hraba et al. 2001; Kaukinen 2004; Schneider 2007). Furthermore, independent work has boosted social capital (Benton 2015). Hence, independent work would diminish the experience of stress.

The voluntaristic mechanism of idea consistency maintains that independent work derives ideas to constrain the experience of stress through rationalizing. Accordingly, independent work means satisfying one's own needs to heighten well-being (Reeve et al. 2004). Independent work has also strengthened well-being, including happiness, job, and life satisfaction, meaningfulness, pride, self-efficacy, self-esteem, and work quality (Anderson-Connolly 2002; De Moortel et al. 2015; Gahlawat et al. 2019; Hodson 1996; Martela and Riekki 2018; Schieman 2002; Schieman and Glavin 2017; Yeh and Yang 2006; Yoon 2001). The various forms of well-being have eroded the experience of stress (Gallie et al. 1998; Hair et al. 2007; Nahum-Shani et al. 2014; Parent et al. 2016). In addition, independent work has fostered the experiences of attaining goals, balance, justice, and organizational support (Haar et al. 2019; Pfeiffer and Pinquart 2012; Rhoades and Eisenberger 2002; Younts and Mueller 2001). These experiences have reduced the experience of stress (Bell et al. 1982; Page and Jacobs 2011). Independent work has also generated commitment to and desire for the career, organization, and work (Giffords 2009; Park and Searcy 2012; Soenens and Vansteenkiste 2005; Stiglbauer and Kovacs 2018). In practice, independent work has raised safe behavior (Parker et al. 2001). This raising has removed the experience of stress notably, including insecurity (Mak and Mueller 2000). Conversely, independent work has lessened the experiences of conflict and overload (Costigan et al. 2003; De Carlo et al. 2019). Reduction in such experiences has prevented the experience of stress (Lambert et al. 2017; Duxbury and Halinski 2018; Senjo 2011). In practice, independent work has diminished emotional labor and turnover (Kim and Stoner 2008; Smit et al. 2016). Reduction in these practices have dampened the experience of stress (Hong et al. 2018; Kane-Frieder et al. 2013). Thus, independent work would lessen the experience of stress.

Religiousness

Religiousness in terms of having religious faith is influential on the experience of stress. Such faith means the importance or value of god instead of the secular value (Diez-Nicolas 2002; Yuchtman-Yaar 2002). Essentially, religious faith represents the inculcation of ethics, social axioms, social practice, strictness, and supernaturality

(Gay and Lynxwiler 2009; Grayling 2013; Peifer 2010; Stavrova and Siegers 2014; Wuthnow 2011). The faith necessarily culminates in a community, fictive kinship, gathering, and solidarity among votaries (Peifer 2010; Saucier and Skrzypinska 2006). Moreover, the faith engenders conflict among votaries of different religions (Davidson 2008). Notably, religious faith has lessened the experience of economic hardship (Urbatsch 2014). Conversely, religious faith has sustained perception about security (Urbatsch 2014). Thus, religious faith would alleviate the experience of stress. The influence of religious faith on the experience of stress hinges on the voluntaristic mechanisms of power realization, utility optimization, norm conformity, and idea consistency.

The voluntaristic mechanism of power realization posits that personal and social power or resources accruing from religious faith affect the experience of stress. Such power emanates from the religious and non-religious community and institutions, sharing and providing power or resources (Haidt 2012; Norris 2002; Perks and Haan 2011; Turner 2009; von Stuckrad 2013). The sharing constitutes power due to solidarity (Marks 2004; Peifer 2010). Thus, religious faith has amounted to social capital (Chang 2009). Religious faith has also sustained marriage and thus its support in getting power or resources (Thornton et al. 2007; Uecher 2014). The power or resources also spring from education and privileges facilitated by religious faith (Muluk et al. 2013; Skerkat and Ellison 1999). Hence, religious faith has enhanced knowledge (Harris 1994). Religious faith is also compulsive to generate power for activism and assertion against oppression and racism (Forsyth 2003; Horell 2014; Maliepaard and Phalet 2012; Paterson 2018; Rip et al. 2012). All the power or resources have been conducive to stress avoidance to diminish the experience of stress, including hardship, insecurity, and victimization (Bellingtier et al. 2022; Chongatera 2013; Emery and Wu 2020; Hansen-Nord et al. 2014; Walen and Lachman 2016). Hence, religious faith would dispel the experience of stress.

However, religious faith deprives power and resources in some ways leading to the experience of stress. Herein, religious faith has diminished employment (Ravanera et al. 2003). Diminished employment has bolstered the experience of stress, including hardship, insecurity, nuisance, and victimization (Kaukinen 2004; Ravanera et al. 2003; Villarreal and Silva 2006). Thus, religious faith would maintain the experience of stress.

The voluntaristic mechanism of utility optimization finds utility or expectations from religious faith to avoid stress and thus dampen the experience of stress. Herein, religious faith maintains altruism, caring, compassion, ethics, forgiveness, humanitarianism, loving, and sacrificing (Ager and Ager 2011; Franks et al. 2013; Haustein 2021; Myers 2014; Peifer 2010; Rowatt et al. 2009; Simpson et al. 2008; Stavrova and Siegers 2014; Tenorio and Lo 2011). According to exchange logic, they would enhance expectations for others' altruism, ethics, humanitarianism, and sacrifice in return. The expectations have reduced expectations for nuisance and victimization from others. The reduction has, in turn, attenuated the experience of stress (Reese et al. 2021). Furthermore, religious faith has sustained the perception of harmony (Clemence 2001). In addition, religious faith has buttressed the disposition of civility (Keyes 2002). Religious faith has also raised preferences for benevolence, civility, and generativity or caring for younger generations (Devos et al. 2002; Letki 2006). In practice, religious faith has encouraged cohesion, donation, forgiving, prosocial behavior, and volunteering (Perks and Haan 2011; Ravanera et al. 2003; Wiepking and Maas 2009; Wuthnow 2004). All these have weakened the experience of stress, including hardship, insecurity, and victimization (Becker et al. 1997; Homant 2013). Conversely, religious faith has impeded criminal behavior and deviance (Skerkat and Ellison 1999). The impedance has prevented the experience of stress, notably including victimization (Kim et al. 2003). Consequently, religious faith would assuage the experience of stress.

However, the voluntaristic mechanism of utility optimization holds that religious faith generates utility in terms of expectations, needs, or values leading to practice and experience to avoid or reduce stress. Religious faith discounts materialism (Ager and Ager 2011; Dy-Liacco et al. 2009). Similarly, religious faith has weakened the disposition of hedonism and valuations of comfort and money-making (Devos et al. 2002; Wuthnow 2004). This weakening has discouraged the avoidance of economic hardship and insecurity (Kane-Frieder et al. 2013; Robinaugh et al. 2016; Sacks and Levi 2010). Conversely, religious faith maintains xenophobia (Werbner 2010). The faith has engendered prejudice and struggle (Hall et al. 2010; Werbner 2010). These would secure expectations for victimization in return, according to exchange logic. Furthermore, religious faith has fostered the dispositions of hawkishness or militancy, punitiveness, and racism (Hall et al. 2010; Pedahzur and Canetti-Nisim 2004; Saucier and Skrzypinska 2006). These raise expectations for stress, including nuisance and victimization from others, and thus have fomented the experience of stress (Grych and Kinsfogel 2010; Choi et al. 2011; Todd and Gesten 1999). Hence, religious faith would maintain the experience of stress.

The voluntaristic mechanism of norm conformity maintains that religious faith generates exposure to social norms to affect the experience of stress. A social norm is that for volunteering (Musick 2000). Exposure and conformity to this norm have prevented the experience of stress, including victimization. Hence, religious faith would relieve the experience of stress (Gallie et al. 1998; Gillath et al. 2005).

The voluntaristic mechanism of idea consistency hinges on the influences of ideas derived from various experiences, perceptions, dispositions, attitudes, and practices upheld by religious faith on the experience of stress. Ideas derived from religious faith to support stress avoidance to reduce the experience of stress include affiliation, attachment, certainty, coping, defensiveness, flourishing, holding an identity, leisure involvement, meaningfulness, optimism, recovery, relaxation, and trust (Forsyth 2003; Friedman 1992; Hoffman and Bagdanov 2020; Katz-Gerro and Shavit 1998; Levin and Chatters 1998; Malka and Soto 2011; Marks 2004; Furnham 1997; Peifer 2010; Shorey et al. 2018; Saroglou and Anciaux 2004; Tenorio and Lo 2011). Religious faith has also generated the experiences of friendship (Wuthnow 2002). In addition, religious faith has safeguarded the feeling of well-being, including adjustment, flourishing, health, mastery, pleasantness, relational quality, satisfaction, self-esteem, and socioemotional well-being (Chang 2009; Dy-Liacco et al. 2009; Flouri and Buchanan 2002; Helliwell and Putnam 2005; Moschis and Ong 2011; Ng and Fisher 2016; Schieman 2001; Skerkat and Ellison 1999; Wuthnow 2004). Moreover, religious faith has fostered the dispositions of conservatism and empathy (Jost 2020; Keyes 2002). Religious faith has also championed the attitudes of tolerance and trust (Gibson 2013; Zanin 2017). In practice, religious faith has raised coping, health maintenance, and protection (Myers 2008; Sherkat and Ellison 2007; Saroglou and Anciaux 2004). These raising has eroded the experience of stress, including hardship, insecurity, victimization, and draining of savings (Bardeen et al. 2016; Barrett 1999; Cepulic et al. 2022; Frank et al. 2014; Hair et al. 2007). Conversely, religious faith has reduced the experiences of illness and welfare reception (Muennig et al. 2013; Urbatsch 2014). Religious faith has also dampened the ill feelings of depression, fear, and loneliness (Ellison et al. 2001; Lauder et al. 2006). In practice, religious faith has prevented doping, gambling, protesting, and suicide (Andrews et al. 2015; Duberstein et al. 2004; Hatch 2007; van de Werfhorst and Kraaykamp 2001). The prevention has lessened the experience of stress, including insecurity and victimization (Constantino et al. 2006; Madlock and Westerman 2011; Zavala and Guadalupe-Diaz 2019). Thus, religious faith would erode the experience of stress.

However, the voluntaristic mechanism of idea consistency suggests enhancing the experience of stress by ideas generated by religious faith. Herein, ideas stemming from religious faith to sustain the experience of stress are dependency, discipline, harm, reliance, self-regulation, and threat (Grayling 2013; Koole et al. 2010; Rivera 2018). Religious faith has also engendered fear of death (Donahue 1985). In addition, religious faith has sustained the experience of marginalization (Wuthnow 2004). Religious faith has also sustained the disposition of restrictiveness (Woodrum 1992). Such enhancement has evolved the experience of stress, including insecurity, nuisance, and victimization (Kachadourian et al. 2013; Olthof and Grossens 2007; Schwartz et al. 2003). Conversely, religious faith downplays autonomy (Grayling 2013). Religious faith also has eroded acceptance of death (Donahue 1985). What is more, religious faith has dampened the dispositions of humor (Saraglou 2004). The dampening has lifted the experience of stress (Abel 2002). Therefore, religious faith would raise the experience of stress.

Marital Status

Marital status, comprising marriage, divorce, separation, widowhood, and nonmarriage, is influential on the experience of stress. Notably, marriage has raised the experience of stress through victimization (Pratt et al. 2010). This raising shows that marriage is not always helpful, as marriage can be greedy instead (Sarkisian 2006). Furthermore, marriage may not fulfill the integrative function to maintain social harmony (Ross 1995). Nevertheless, divorce as the obverse of marriage is stressful (Allemand et al. 2015). More generally, marital status influences the experience of stress through the voluntaristic mechanisms of power realization, utility optimization, and idea consistency.

The voluntaristic mechanism of power realization suggests that marriage raises power or resources to avoid stress and thus alleviate the experience of stress. The raising has appea4red in social capital, including affiliation, bonding, friendship, and social networking (Apinunmahakul and Devlin 2008; Chang 2009; Sampson 1991; Volker et al. 2007). In addition, marriage has sustained socioeconomic status, including homeownership as opposed to homelessness, poverty, studying, and welfare receipt (Chapman 1985; Pallas 2002; Vartanian 1999). These power or resources have prevented the experience of stress, including hardship and insecurity (Cepulic et al. 2022; Walen and Lachman 2016). Conversely, marriage has prevented functional disability or limitation (Lelli 2008; Li and Chung 2008). Such prevention has, in turn, prevented the experience of stress, such as insecurity (Kachadourian et al. 2013). Hence, marriage would facilitate power or resources for avoiding and thus lowering the experience of stress.

Conversely, divorce deprives power or resources in social capital (Demo and Buehler 2013). Meanwhile, divorce has engendered reliance (Cox and Paley 1997). Reliance has fueled the experience of stress (Kachadourian et al. 2013). Hence, divorce would raise the experience of stress.

The voluntaristic mechanism of utility optimization maintains that marriage raises the utility of avoiding and thus lowers the experience of stress. As such, marriage has raised such an attitude as charity orientation (Brown and Ferris 2007). Similarly, marriage has boosted the practice of donation, prosocial behavior, and social cohesion (Bednall et al. 2013; Mata and Pendakur 2014; Tolsma et al. 2009). According to exchange logic, the increases indicate the expectation for or utility of reward rather than stress such as victimization. Hence, the increases have reduced the experience of stress, including insecurity, nuisance, and victimization (Coffe and Geys 2007; Madlock and Westerman 2011). Conversely, marriage has impeded the practices of criminal behavior and violence (Savolainen 2009). Such impedance has prevented the experience of stress, notably victimization (Han and Connell 2020; Wittebrood and Nieuwbeerta 2000). Consequently, marriage would dampen the experience of stress.

The voluntaristic mechanism of idea consistency emphasizes marriage for generating ideas to weaken the experience of stress through rationalizing. At this juncture, ideas generated from marriage include gratitude and identity based on marriage (Hattery and Smith 2012; Su et al. 2015). Essentially, marriage has sustained the experiences of closeness and social integration (Cornwall 2009). Marriage has also boosted the feeling of well-being, including financial adequacy, health, quality of interaction and relationships, satisfaction, and self-esteem (Carrieri 2012; Lelli 2008; Marks 1996; McMullin and Cairney 2004; Molana and Adams 2019; Obucina 2013). Notably, satisfaction has included that with achievement, family, finance, friendship, health, life, and living standards (Koromeckyj-Cox et al. 2007; Louis and Zhao 2002; Mitrut and Wolff 2011; Rozer and Kraaykamp 2013; Yienprugsawan et al. 2010). In addition, marriage has elevated such attitudes as community attachment and evaluation, support for protection or relief, and trust (Okun et al. 1998; Prezza et al. 2001; Ross and Mirowsky 2009; Sampson and Raudenbush 2004). In practice, marriage has lifted community involvement, family functioning, and neighboring (McCabe 2014;

Smith and Hamon 2012; Swaroop and Morenoff 2006). Such increases have eroded the experience of stress, including hardship and insecurity (Barrett 1999; Beaudoin 2009; Hair et al. 2007). Conversely, marriage has impeded the experiences of discrimination and social exclusion (Carr and Friedman 2005; Wojcieszak and Mutz 2009). Marriage has also reduced the perception of social impact (Silbereisen et al. 2010). In addition, marriage has reduced ill feelings, including depression, fear, and loneliness (Koromeckyj-Cox et al. 2007; Michalski 2005). Furthermore, marriage has reduced community opposition (Takahashi and Gaber 1998). Such reduction has weakened the experience of stress, such as hardship, insecurity, nuisance, and victimization (Constantino et al. 2006; Frank et al. 2014; Parent et al. 2016). Hence, marriage would reduce the experience of stress.

However, the voluntaristic mechanism of idea consistency also indicates that marriage engenders ideas to raise the experience of stress. Herein, ideas stemming from marriage include obligation and the loss of freedom (Stanton and Maier 2004; Su et al. 2015). In practice, marriage has fueled protesting (Marsh 2005). In addition, marriage has lifted shaming experiences (Lu et al. 2002). These increases have bred the experience of stress (Duxbury and Halinski 2018; Fenwick and Tausig 1994). Conversely, marriage has impeded the attitudes of social acceptance and tolerance (Coffe and Geys 2007; Keyes and Shapiro 2004). Marriage has also weakened the feeling of satisfaction with security and spirituality (Yienprugsawan et al. 2010). Such weakening has raised the experience of stress (Gallie et al. 1998). Thus, marriage would escalate the experience of stress.

Conversely, divorce and widowhood or spousal bereavement have sustained ideas conducive to reducing the experience of stress. Such ideas have been about satisfaction with life and the country due to divorce, widowhood, or spousal bereavement (Tiliouine et al. 2006). Satisfaction has dampened the experience of stress, including hardship, insecurity, and victimization (Gallie et al. 1998; La Guardia et al. 2000; Madlock and Westerman 2011; Singer et al. 2019). Hence, divorce, widowhood, or widowerhood would alleviate the experience of stress.

Parenthood

Parenthood, having children, fertility, or the number of children has had mixed effects on stress. It has raised the experience of stress such as nuisance and victimization (Michalski 2005; Wilson and Hammer 2001; Wittebrood and Nieuwbeerta 2000); Meanwhile, it has impeded the experience of stress such as hardship and insecurity (Coffe and Geys 2007; Muhlau 2014). The impacts, anyhow, follow the voluntaristic mechanisms of power realization, utility optimization, and idea consistency.

The voluntaristic mechanism of power realization holds parenthood as a source of power or resources to facilitate stress avoidance and thus lower the experience of stress. As such, parenthood has raised power in knowledge, insurance, and social capital, notably that from bonding, neighbors, and neighborhood (Apinunmahakul and Devlin 2008; Kleinhans et al. 2007; Manturuk et al. 2010; Menahem 2001; Volker and Flap 2007). Such power has prevented the experience of stress, including hardship and insecurity (Narayan and Cassidy 2001; Walen and Lachman 2016). Hence, parenthood would facilitate stress avoidance to lower the experience of stress.

However, parenthood also weakens power or resources and their facilitation of stress avoidance. Herein, parenthood has impeded social capital in terms of friendship and networking (Groot et al. 2007; Sampson 1991; Tsai 2006). Similarly, parenthood has diminished friends' support regarding companionship and nurturance (Carbery and Buhrmester 1998). Furthermore, parenthood has impeded employment, home-ownership, personal and family income, savings, and wealth (Conley 2001; Kawabata 2014; Mulder and Wagner 1998; Pal 2000; Vartanian 1999). Such impedance would weaken power for preventing the experience of stress, including hardship and insecurity. The impedance has thus maintained the experience of stress (Barrett 1999; Cepulic et al. 2022; Frank et al. 2014). Conversely, parenthood has been conducive to poverty (Joassart-Marcelli 2005). Thus, parenthood would underlie the experience of stress.

The voluntaristic mechanism of utility optimization maintains that parenthood generates the utility of avoiding and thus weakening the experience of stress. Herein, parenthood means provisioning to offspring (Carbery and Buhrmester 1998). Parenthood thus has raised the disposition of generativity or caring for the younger generation (Peterson and Klohnen 1995). In practice, parenthood has boosted support for kin and volunteering (Oesterle et al. 2004; Wellman 1990). These would raise the expectation for or utility of social support to avoid and lower the experience of stress. The raising has attenuated the experience of stress, including victimization (Gillath et al. 2005; Pallante et al. 2018). Conversely, parenthood has reduced the practice of crime (Savolainen 2009). The reduction would lift the expectation for or utility of the avoidance of victimization to lower the experience of stress. Such reduction has prevented the experience of stress, notably victimization (Kim et al. 2003; Wittebrood and Nieuwbeerta 2000). Hence, parenthood would diminish the experience of stress.

The voluntaristic mechanism of idea consistency states that parenthood evolves ideas to rationalize stress avoidance to lower the experience of stress. Accordingly, parenthood has boosted the disposition of religiosity (Baker and Smith 2009). In practice, parenthood has reduced borrowing (Chou et al. 2006). Moreover, parenthood has upheld well-being, including health, satisfaction with health and neighborhood, and self-esteem (Bassani 2008; Schieman and Taylor 2001; van Praag and Ferrer-I-Carbonell 2004). Such increases would mean dispelling the idea of stress, including deficiency, hardship, and insecurity. The increases have weakened the experiences of stress, including deficiency and insecurity (Barrett 1999; Hair et al. 2007; Rader et al. 2012). Hence, parenthood would impede the experience of stress.

However, parenthood induces the experience of stress through some derived ideas based on the voluntaristic mechanism of idea consistency. Such ideas concentrate on childcare rather than contact with others. As such, parenthood has generated the experiences of disparity in housework and social exclusion (Bask 2005; A. Johnson et al. 2008). Parenthood has also raised risk perception (Dosman et al. 2001). In practice, parenthood has raised the practices of crime reporting and moving (Akers and Kaukinen 2009; Richmond 2003). Parenthood has also reduced well-being by raising depression (Anusic et al. 2014). Such raising would mean raising the idea of stress, including hardship, insecurity, and victimization. The raising has heightened the experience of stress, including hardship, insecurity, and victimization (Johnson et al. 2008; Kleiman and Riskind 2014). Conversely, parenthood has reduced the attitude of social acceptance (Lo and Jim 2012). Parenthood has also dampened well-being, including housing quality, neighborhood quality, pleasantness, satisfaction with finance, leisure, life, marriage, neighborhood, and social quality (Ambrey and Fleming 2014; Anusic et al. 2014; Brennan et al. 2001; Peiro 2006; Shapiro and Keyes 2008; van Praag and Ferrer-I-Carbonell 2004; Wilson and Hammer 2001; Woldoff and Ovadia 2009). Such reduction would indicate an increase in the idea of stress, including hardship, insecurity, and victimization. The reduction has been conducive to the experience of stress (Bardeen et al. 2016; Farrington 2018; Pulkkinen et al. 2009). Hence, parenthood would sustain the experience of stress.

Family Income

Family income represents power or resources to avoid stress for weakening the experience of stress. Notably, family income has lowered the experience of stress or threat, including economic hardship and victimization (Myer et al. 2008; Posthumus et al. 2013; Raijman et al. 2003; Zhang et al. 2007b). Conversely, family income has contributed to saving to lower the experience of stress (Chakrabarty et al. 2008). Such weakening manifests the voluntaristic mechanisms of power realization, utility optimization, and idea consistency.

The voluntaristic mechanism of power realization maintains that power or resources derived from family income facilitate stress avoidance to lower the experience of stress. As such, family income has strengthened education, knowledge, possession, organizational membership, social capital, including that from family and friends, social status, social support, and wealth (Andersson 2004; Apinunmahakul and Devlin 2008; Cerin and Leslie 2008; Keister 2003; Kleinhans et al. 2007; Lennartsson 2010; Shin 2012; Whyte and Gao 2009). Family income has also raised the environmental protection and use of health services (Cleary and Angel 1984). Hence, family income would generate power or resources and action for stress avoidance. Such generation has impeded the experience of stress, including hardship, insecurity, and victimization (Coffe and Geys 2007; Felson and Outlaw 2007; Sacks and Levi 2010; Walen and Lachman 2016). Conversely, family income has forestalled welfare reception, indicating poverty (Stenberg 2000). Hence, family income would dampen the experience of stress.

The voluntaristic mechanism of utility optimization emphasizes the utility of stress avoidance stemming from family income. Accordingly, family income has raised the dispositions of conservatism, environmentalism, and friendliness, the values of friendship and health, and support for gun control (Ishio 2010; La Grange and Yip 2001; Ludwig and Cook 2001; Norris and Inglehart 2009; Shen and Saijo 2008; Whynes and Sach 2007). In practice, family income has sustained civility, compliance, and donation (Alnsour and Meaton 2009; Shin 2012; Wiepking and Maas 2009).

According to exchange logic, such raising would manifest the utility of saving and stress avoidance to weaken the experience of stress, including insecurity, nuisance, and victimization. Such weakening has been evident (Huesmann 2018; Pulkkinen et al. 2009). Conversely, family income has reduced the practices of cheating and crime (Cerin and Leslie 2008; Ozbay 2008). Such reduction has lowered the experience of stress, including victimization (Wittebrood and Nieuwbeerta 2000). Hence, family income would prevent the experience of stress.

The voluntaristic mechanism of idea consistency states that family income engenders ideas to rationalize stress avoidance to dampen the experience of stress. As such, family income has bred the experiences of family cohesion and social integration (Crowder et al. 2006; van Oorschot and Arts 2005). Similarly, family income has sustained the perception of civility and fairness (Ferriss 2002; Viewiebe and Wegener 2000). Family income has also lifted well-being, including financial adequacy, living standards, mastery, neighborhood quality, physical and mental health, satisfaction with democracy, finance, friendship, housing, life, marriage, the neighborhood, and work, self-efficacy, and self-esteem (Ambrey and Fleming 2014; Cerin and Leslie 2008; Louis and Zhao 2002; Harris 2001; Kwok et al. 2015; Norris 2011; Oshio and Kobayashi 2010; Powdthavee 2009; Thoits and Hewitt 2001; van Praag et al. 2003; Whyte and Gao 2009; Woldoff and Ovadia 2009). Such raising has dispelled the experience of stress, including hardship, insecurity, nuisance, and victimization (Kanan and Pruitt 2002; Rader et al. 2012; Sacks and Levi 2010; Salehi 2012). Conversely, family income has impeded the experiences of badness, barriers, deprivation, discrimination, hazards, and social exclusion (Cerin and Leslie 2008; Moore and Aweiss 2003; Pettigrew 2002; Stanley et al. 2011; Whyte and Gao 2009). Likewise, family income has abated the perception of inequality, risk, and uncertainty (Castillo 2011; Noack et al. 2001; Oliver 2003). Such reduction has prevented the experience of stress, including hardship, insecurity, nuisance, and victimization (Peruzzi 2014; Gotzsche-Astrup 2020). Thus, family income would impede the experience of stress.

However, family income has also sustained ideas discouraging stress avoidance or chiming with the experience of stress. Accordingly, family income has bred the experiences of family conflict (Ruppanner 2010). Hence, family income would sustain the experience of stress, such as nuisance.

Population Size

National population size directly affects the personal experience of stress through the direct deterministic mechanism of sharing privately and/or publicly and the indirect deterministic mechanisms of empowering, incentivizing, standardizing, and framing. Population size has generated stress directly based on the population itself (Turner 2003). That is, population or people are the sources of stress.

The indirect deterministic mechanism of empowering maintains that population size generates resources personally and/or collectively for stress avoidance to diminish the experience of stress. Population size has raised the personal wage and collective resources, including levels of science and technology and government support (Florida 2005; Glaeser et al. 2009; Turner 2013; Pattie et al. 2004). These personal and collective resources have lessened the personal experience of stress, including hardship and insecurity (Barrett 1999; Schieman 2013). Hence, population size would weaken the personal experience of stress.

However, population size also deprives personal and/or collective resources for stress avoidance. Population size has impeded employment personally and collectively and education and physical and mental health collectively (Cotter et al. 1998; Liska et al. 1999; Queralt and Witte 1999; Sanders 1990). Hence, population size would sustain the personal experience of stress.

The indirect deterministic mechanism of incentivizing suggests that population size offers incentives for stress rather than its avoidance to raise the experience of stress. Herein, population size has generated a collective demand or incentive for productivity (Turner 1984). The demand would escalate personal demand for productivity through the voluntaristic mechanism of utility optimization to meet others' demand. Such demand would also raise stress through the voluntaristic mechanism of idea consistency, as the experience of demand is consonant with the experience of stress. Eventually, the demand has been stressful (Conard and Matthews 2008; Duxbury and Halinski 2018; Fenwick and Tausig 1994; Nahum-Shani et al. 2014; Senjo 2011). Thus, population size would raise the personal experience of stress.

The indirect deterministic mechanism of incentivizing suggests that population size offers incentives for stress rather than its avoidance to raise the experience of stress. Herein, population size has generated a collective demand or incentive for productivity (Turner 1984). The demand would escalate personal demand for productivity through the voluntaristic mechanism of utility optimization to meet others' demands. Such demand would also raise stress through the voluntaristic mechanism of idea consistency, as the experience of demand is consonant with the experience of stress. Eventually, the demand has been stressful (Conard and Matthews 2008; Duxbury and Halinski 2018; Fenwick and Tausig 1994; Nahum-Shani et al. 2014; Senjo 2011). Thus, population size would raise the personal experience of stress.

However, the indirect deterministic mechanism of framing also suggests that population size generates frames to raise the experience of stress. Herein, population size has raised protesting personally and conflict, crime, footprints, price or inflation, punishment, revolution, and terrorism collectively (Cho et al. 2013; Collier and Hoeffler 2004; Dodson 2016; Foster et al. 2013; Glaeser et al. 2009; Havinga 2002; Yagci 2017; York et al. 2003). Such raising has sustained the personal experience of stress, including hardship, insecurity, nuisance, and victimization (Gaitan-Rossi and Shen 2018; Lansford and Dodge 2008; Poveda 2011; Valera and Guardia 2014). Conversely, population size has reduced cohesion, development, quality, or well-being, liberty, and rights collectively (Abouharb and Cingranelli 2007; Coffe and Geys 2006; Kwan and Chiu 2018). Such reduction has bolstered the personal experience of stress, including hardship, insecurity, and nuisance (Gallie et al. 1998; Taylor-Gooby 2001; Salehi 2012; Schieman 2013). Thus, population size would sustain the personal experience of stress.

Population Density

National population density, as the reciprocal of the ratio of land size over population size, influences the personal experience of stress through deterministic mechanisms. Notably, population density has raised the personal experience of stress regarding illness (Pattie et al. 2004).

The direct deterministic mechanism suggests that population density influences personal experience through sharing contextual or collective experience privately or publicly. Accordingly, population density has raised the contextual experience of stress regarding pollution (Stretesky and Lynch 2009). Such experience would then escalate the personal experience of stress privately or vicariously.

The indirect deterministic mechanism of empowering maintains that population density reduces the personal experience of stress through empowering the avoidance or prevention of stress. Accordingly, population density has raised economic growth and government support for education and social services in the context (Obschonk et al. 2016; Pattie et al. 2004). Hence, population density would impede the personal experience of stress.

The indirect deterministic mechanism of incentivizing suggests that population density provides incentives for stress avoidance to dampen the personal experience of stress. Accordingly, population density has raised such attitudes as the personal preference for privacy, support for the environment, and the disposition of environmentalism (Ewing et al. 2016; Franzen and Vogl 2013). In practice, population density has induced the practices of donation, neighboring, and prosocial behavior (Graddy and Wang 2009; Swaroop and Morenoff 2006). These attitudes, dispositions, and practices would represent incentives for avoiding or preventing stress, notably including nuisance. Remarkably, the practices would be incentives to induce prosocial as opposed to stressful practices in return, following exchange logic. The attitudes, dispositions, practices, and their experiences have eroded the experience of stress, including nuisance and victimization (Beaudoin 2009; Page and Jacobs 2011). Hence, population density would impede the personal experience of stress.

The indirect deterministic mechanism of framing maintains that population density generates ideas for framing and rationalizing stress avoidance to lessen the personal experience of stress. Population density has sustained feelings of neighborhood quality and satisfaction with life and the neighborhood (Oliver 2003; Whitham 2012). These feelings would be incongruous with the experience of stress (Johnson et al. 2008; Salehi 2012; Villarreal and Silva 2006). The feelings thus have lowered the experience of stress, including nuisance and victimization. Hence, population density would lessen the personal experience of stress.

However, the indirect deterministic mechanism of framing also suggests that population density engenders ideas from framing the experience of stress. Herein, population size has reduced the practices of cohesion, giving, and volunteering (Andrews 2009; Glaeser and Gottlieb 2006; Phan et al. 2009). Failing to provide and receive such practices would be consistent with the experience of stress. Such a failure has bolstered the experience of stress, including insecurity (Beaudoin 2009; Carter and Wolfe 2021; Frank et al. 2014). Conversely, population density has invoked the feeling of depression (Oliver 2003). Depression has engendered the experience of stress (Kleiman and Riskind 2014). Thus, population density would sustain the personal experience of stress.

Talent

National talent or human capital comprises education and earnings (Dahlberg et al. 2018). It is influential on the personal experience of stress through direct and indirect deterministic mechanisms.

The indirect deterministic mechanism of empowering holds that national talent empowers the personal avoidance of stress to diminish the experience of stress. As such, national talent has contributed to personal income and leadership as opposed to illiteracy, poverty, and welfare reception (Carli and Eagly 2011; Florida 2005; Hostetler et al. 2007; Hyggen 2006; Muffels and Fouarge 2004). The contribution would represent the empowering of stress avoidance to dampen the experience of stress. Hence, national talent would erode the personal experience of stress.

The indirect deterministic mechanism of framing maintains that national talent frames ideas conducive to stress avoidance to weaken the personal experience of stress. Herein, national talent has raised the evaluation of the economy and diminished depression (Drope and Chowdhury 2014; Schieman et al. 2001). Such ideas would be incongruous with the experience of stress, including hardship and insecurity. Hence, national talent would diminish the personal experience of stress.

However, the indirect deterministic mechanism of framing also suggests that national talent frames ideas consistent with stress to sustain the personal experience of stress. Herein, national talent has fostered the feeling of aspiration and the practice of migration (Correll 2004; Gurak and Kritz 2000). Aspiration and migration would be stressful. They have fomented the experience of stress, including insecurity and victimization (Auerbach et al. 2011; Bask 2005). Hence, national talent would sustain the personal experience of stress.

Technology

National technology covers information and communication, infrastructure, education, biotechnology, and high or advanced forms (Florida 2005; Fukuyama 2003; Goetz et al. 2011; Schofer 2004). It influences the personal experience of stress through direct and indirect deterministic mechanisms.

The direct deterministic mechanism holds that national technology generates the collective experience of stress to determine the personal experience of stress through sharing privately or publicly. Herein, national technology evokes the collective experiences of dehumanization or the loss of humanity or being zombies, domination, risk, rivalry, and transformation (Fukuyama 2003; Roderick 2016). These experiences are integral to stress (Demertzis 2020; Fairris and Brenner 2001; Molz et al.

2013; Su et al. 2021; Walen and Lachman 2016). Thus, national technology would enhance the personal experience of stress.

The indirect deterministic mechanism of empowering emphasizes that national technology empowers collective and personal stress avoidance to reduce the personal experience of stress. Accordingly, national technology has generated employment, income, opportunities, productivity, prospects, and resources for goal attainment (Florida 2005; Goetz et al. 2011; Matthewman 2011; Roderick 2016; Welzel 2013). Hence, national technology would attenuate the personal experience of stress.

The indirect deterministic mechanism of framing suggests that national technology frames ideas for stress avoidance and relief reduce the personal experience of stress. As such, national technology has framed the ideas of agency, autonomy, convenience, emancipation, environmental quality, growth, independence, life-saving, progress, rationalization, self-expression, and solutions (Fukuyama 2003; Matthewman 2011; Roderick 2016; Schroeder and Swedberg 2002; Welzel and Inglehart 2010). These ideas would be consonant with stress avoidance. They have thereby erased the experience of stress, including hardship and insecurity (Schieman 2013). Hence, national technology would dispel the personal experience of stress.

However, the indirect deterministic mechanism of framing also suggests that national technology frames ideas consistent or promoting stress, thus increasing the personal experience of stress. Herein, national technology has framed the ideas of technological authority, coercion, hierarchy, negative externalities, and unsustainability (Fukuyama 2003; Matthewman 2011; Welzel 2013). These ideas would be consistent with the experience of stress. They have thereby raised the experience of stress, including hardship, nuisance, and victimization (Cepulic et al. 2022; Gallie et al. 1998; Schieman 2013; Valera and Guardia 2014). Hence, national technology would increase the personal experience of stress.

Financialization

National financialization, banking, or credit services, technology covers insurance, investment, securitization, shareholding, and speculation (Haiven 2014). It determines the personal experience of stress through direct and indirect deterministic mechanisms.

The indirect deterministic mechanism of empowering indicates that national financialization empowers stress avoidance to prevent the experience of stress. National financialization offers capital and liquidity or financial application (Haiven 2014). Such empowering has reduced the experience of stress, including hardship and insecurity (Reese et al. 2021; Sacks and Levi 2010). Thereby, national financialization would lessen the personal experience of stress.

The indirect deterministic mechanism of framing suggests that national financialization frames ideas conducive to stress reduction to weaken the experience of stress. Herein, national financialization raises the ideas of autonomy, creativity, freedom, and individuality (Harvey 2016). These ideas have dispelled the experience of stress, including nuisance (Schieman 2013; Starrs et al. 2017). Thus, national financialization would weaken the personal experience of stress.

However, the indirect deterministic mechanism of framing also holds that national financialization frames ideas consistent and thus conducive to the experience of stress. Accordingly, national financialization breeds the ideas of alienation, loneliness, disjuncture, and unmooring by liquidizing to erode social identity and obligation, indebtedness, and precarity in the face of financial institutions (Haiven 2014). These ideas have constituted the experience of stress, including hardship and insecurity (Cohen et al. 2013; Kachadourian et al. 2013). Hence, national financialization would secure the personal experience of stress.

Prosperity

National prosperity, economic development, income, product, or wealth covers industrialization, trade, and urbanization (Imbroscio 1997; Peet and Hatwick 2009; Schofer and Cranados 2006). Its reverses are national economic crisis and poverty (Wolff and Resnick 2012). It means a good economic life (Peet and Hatwick 2009). National prosperity determines the personal experience of stress through direct and indirect deterministic mechanisms.

The direct deterministic mechanism states that national prosperity creates the collective experience of stress to spread to the personal experience of stress through sharing privately or publicly. Herein, national prosperity has reduced the collective experiences of economic hardship, illness, and pain (Peet and Hatwick 2009; Fridberg and Kangas 2008). This reduction would weaken the personal experience of stress. Thus, national prosperity would dispel the personal experience of stress.

The indirect deterministic mechanism of empowering indicates that national prosperity empowers stress avoidance to lessen the experience of stress. Notably, national prosperity has raised people's education, knowledge, and social class (Baldacci et al. 2003; Norris 2011). Such raising has weakened the experience of stress, including hardship and insecurity (Beaudoin 2009; Schieman 2013). Thereby, national prosperity would lessen the personal experience of stress.

However, the indirect deterministic mechanism of empowering suggests that national prosperity disempowers stress avoidance, thus bolstering the experience of stress. National prosperity has reduced government support, notably for healthcare and welfare or social security (Finseraas 2010; Kittel 2006; Rudra and Haggard 2005). Moreover, national prosperity has lowered people's homeownership (Conley and Gifford 2006). Such reduction has sustained the experience of stress, including hardship and insecurity (Gaitan-Rossi and Shen 2018). National prosperity has also increased people's relative poverty (Moller et al. 2003). Thus, national prosperity would lift the personal experience of stress.

The indirect deterministic mechanism of incentivizing indicates that national prosperity fosters incentives for stress avoidance to relieve the experience of stress. Herein, national prosperity has lifted people's values of emancipation and independence (Fjellvang 2011; Welzel 2013). National prosperity has also elevated people's support for environmental protection and volunteering (Franzen and Vogl 2013; Salamon and Sokolowski 2003). The elevation would raise the incentive or utility for preventing stress, including nuisance and victimization. As such, the elevation has lowered the experience of stress (Like 2011; Salehi 2012; Schieman 2013). Hence, national prosperity would assuage the personal experience of stress.

The indirect deterministic mechanism of framing suggests that national prosperity frames ideas conducive to stress relief to erase the experience of stress. These ideas include emancipation, enjoyment of rights, happiness, health, the satisfaction of need and with consumption, and sustainability (Peet and Hatwick 2009; Wolff and Resnick 2012). Essentially, national prosperity has fostered the collective experiences of development, notably urban development, growth, notably economic growth, government effectiveness, justice, legal quality, and rights (Bjornskov 2005; Gani and Clemes 2006; Guisan 2009; Hunter 2016; Quinn and Woolley 2001; Rindermann 2008). In addition, national prosperity has raised people's attitudes of tolerance and trust, including that in institutions and people (Marien 2011; Tov and Diener 2008; Traunmuller 2011). Furthermore, national prosperity has upgraded people's well-being, including health, relational quality, satisfaction with democracy and life, and self-efficacy (Corcoran et al. 2011; Helliwell et al. 2010; Inglehart 2010; Norris 2011). Such framing would be incompatible with stress. Hence, the framed ideas have alleviated the experience of stress, including hardship and insecurity (Barrett 1999; Johnson et al. 2008). Conversely, national prosperity has eroded the ideas of indebtedness (Peet and Hatwick 2009). National prosperity has lessened imprisonment and segregation collectively (Liska et al. 1999; Moller and Li 2009). In addition, national prosperity has weakened people's perception of anomie, risk, and threat (Teymoori et al. 2016; Schneider 2007; Schwartz and Melech 2000). Such weakening has prevented the experience of stress, including insecurity and victimization (Valera and Guardia 2014; Viola et al. 2016). Thus, national prosperity would quell the personal experience of stress.

However, the indirect deterministic mechanism of framing also holds that national financialization frames ideas consistent and thus contributory to the experience of stress. National prosperity has raised the collective experiences of crime, notably theft, footprints, inequality, and terrorism (Cho et al. 2013; Ha 2012; Jorgenson et al. 2009; Neumayer and Plumper 2009; Sun et al. 2011; York et al. 2003). In addition, national prosperity has lifted people's perception of corruption (Uslaner 2008). Such framing would be compatible with stress. These framed ideas have elevated the experience of stress, including insecurity, nuisance, and victimization (Like 2011; Nepal et al. 2011; Wittebrood and Nieuwbeerta 2000). Hence, national prosperity would bolster the personal experience of stress.

Inequality

National income inequality has engendered the personal experience of stress in terms of disadvantage, illness, and social exclusion (Reardon and Bischoff 2011; Jones et al. 2015; Portes and Vickstrom 2011). Such engendering follows direct and indirect deterministic mechanisms, with the latter hinging on voluntaristic mechanisms. Notably, national inequality incentivizes doing something (Baldus 2017; Lui 2011).

The direct deterministic mechanism holds that national inequality raises collective stress to determine personal stress through sharing privately or publicly. As such, national inequality has fomented collective experiences about problems in health and social aspects and risk (Knack 2002; Wilkinson and Pickett 2017). Such collective experiences have translated into the personal experience of stress (Gaitan-Rossi and Shen 2018; Villarreal and Silva 2006). Hence, national inequality would breed the personal experience of stress, including insecurity and victimization.

The indirect deterministic mechanism of empowering emphasizes that national inequality is disempowering or depriving power or resources to avoid stress, thus sustaining the personal experience of stress. Accordingly, such disempowering engenders or manifests corruption, deprivation, disintegration, exploitation, poverty, segregation, and separation (Alesina and Angeletos 2005; Baldus 2017; Neckerman and Toche 2007; Pebley and Sastry 2004; Suchweh 2012). National inequality has bred functional disability (Kim and Kawachi 2007). Such disempowering has strengthened the experience of stress, including hardship, insecurity, nuisance, and victimization (Gallie et al. 1998; Valera and Guardia 2014). Conversely, national inequality thus has eroded social capital (Portes and Vickstrom 2011). Such erosion has sustained the experience of stress, including hardship and insecurity (Frank et al. 2014; Hansen-Nord et al. 2014; Valera and Guardia 2014). Hence, national inequality would spur the personal experience of stress.

The indirect deterministic mechanism of incentivizing suggests that national inequality diminishes the incentive for stress avoidance, thus sustaining stress. Conversely, national inequality reduces cooperation and solidarity (Baldus 2017; Collins 2000). Such reduction would invoke others' stressful reactions, according to exchange logic. In addition, national inequality has discouraged the disposition of environmentalism for environmental protection (Engel and Potschke 1998). In practice, national inequality has eroded cohesion and volunteering (Green et al. 2003; Lipford and Yandle 2009). Such erosion has bolstered the experience of stress, including nuisance and victimization (Olthof and Grossens 2007; Schwartz et al. 2009). Conversely, national inequality has boosted such practices as crime and violence (Ousey and Lee 2013; van Wilsem 2007). The boosting has raised the experience of stress, notably victimization (Han and Connell 2020; Wittebrood and Nieuwbeerta 2000). Hence, national inequality would raise the personal experience of stress.

However, the indirect deterministic mechanism of incentivizing maintains that national inequality provides incentives for stress avoidance to lessen the personal experience of stress. That is, inequality is incentivizing (Lui 2011). Accordingly, the incentivizing functions through individuating, self-creating, and responsibility-taking to promote autonomy and the realization of ability (Fein 2012; S. Smith 2011). Such work has diminished the experience of stress, including nuisance (Gallie et al. 1998; Schieman 2013). Hence, national inequality would erode the personal experience of stress.

The indirect deterministic mechanism of framing holds that national inequality frames ideas that are compatible and sustains the personal experience of stress. Such frame ideas are alienation, corruption, distancing, division, domination, exploitation, greed, unhappiness, injustice, marginalization, polarization, poverty, protest, struggle, unethicalness, unfairness, and wrongness (Alessio 2011; Baldus 2017; Bebbington et al. 2010; Collins 2000; Fein 2012; Gainsborough 2008; Godoy et al. 2004; Grover 2011; Jencks 2002; Jordahl 2009; Ryan 2002; Suchweh 2012). National inequality has also bred perceptions of anomie, corruption, injustice, and unfairness (Eriksson et al. 2015; Oishi et al. 2011; Uslaner 2008; Teymoori et al. 2016). Moreover, national inequality has raised the need for income (Winkelmann and Winkelmann 2010). National inequality has also bolstered the attitude of distrust (Oishi et al. 2011; van Oorschot and Arts 2005). Such bolstering has sustained the experience of stress, including hardship, insecurity, and victimization (Johnson et al. 2008; Parent et al. 2016; Peruzzi 2014). Hence, national inequality would foster the personal experience of stress.

Nevertheless, the indirect determinist mechanism of framing also maintains that national inequality generates frames for shaping ideas to prevent the personal experience of stress. Such frames include that highlight matching with personal talent (Baldus 2017). National inequality has also buttressed the experience of family cohesion (van Oorschot and Arts 2005). In addition, national inequality has fostered such attitudes as belief in the just world and tolerance (Castillo 2011; Malahy et al. 2009). Such fostering has weakened the experience of stress (Bardeen et al. 2016). Conversely, national inequality has impeded such practices as protesting (Dodson 2016; Solt 2015).

Liberty

National liberty is influential on the personal experience of stress through the direct and indirect deterministic mechanisms. Essentially, liberty means the absence of others' harm, interference, restriction, and government limitation (Bavetta et al. 2014; Sadurski 1999). The absence indicates the removal of stress (Barrett 1999; Carr and Umberson 2013). In addition, personal freedom has weakened the experience of stress (Gallie et al. 1998; Schieman 2013). This weakening can result from the direct deterministic mechanism through sharing liberty privately or publicly.

The indirect deterministic mechanism of empowering suggests that national liberty empowers stress avoidance to lessen the personal experience of stress. As such, national liberty represents capability (Bavetta et al. 2014). The capability has impeded the experience of stress, including hardship and insecurity (Acker and Lawrence 2009; Aloia and Solomon 2015; Valera and Guardia 2014). Hence, national liberty would dampen the personal experience of stress.

However, the indirect deterministic mechanism of empowering also maintains that national liberty disempowers stress protection, thus raising the personal experience of stress. In the first place, national liberty diminishes stress protection (Sadurski 1999). The diminishment has bred the experience of stress, notably insecurity, nuisance, and victimization (Ho 1998; Kanan and Pruitt 2002). Hence, national liberty would sustain the personal experience of stress.

The indirect deterministic mechanism of incentivizing suggests that national liberty disincentivizes stress prevention, thus sustaining the personal experience of stress. As such, national liberty has eroded people's support for security (Jenkins-Smith and Herron 2009). The erosion has bolstered the experience of stress, including hardship and insecurity (Carter and Wolfe 2021; Ho 1998). Conversely, national liberty has raised people's postmaterialism or the devaluation of security (Tov and Diener 2008). The disincentivizing has bolstered the experience of stress, notably insecurity (Oksanen et al. 2014). Hence, national liberty would sustain the personal experience of stress.

The indirect deterministic mechanism of framing holds that national liberty frames ideas that are incongruous with stress, thus lessening the personal experience of stress. These ideas include autonomy, individuality, insensitivity to harm, rights, self-expression, self-fulfillment, and self-realization (Bavetta et al. 2014; Moller and Skaaning 2014; Rasmussen and Den Uyl 2005; Sadurski 1999). Furthermore, national liberty has lifted people's trust in government (Wong et al. 2016). National liberty has also elevated people's well-being, including satisfaction with democracy and life (Abbott et al. 2011; Norris 2011). Such ideas have eroded the experience of stress, including hardship, insecurity, and nuisance (La Guardia et al. 2000; Schieman 2013). Conversely, national liberty has eroded deficit perception (Norris 2011). Hence, national liberty would impede the personal experience of stress.

However, the indirect deterministic mechanism of framing also maintains that national liberty frames ideas that raise stress. Such ideas include the neglect of flourishing, health, and justice (Rasmussen and Den Uyl 2005). Moreover, national liberty has raised corruption perception (Collier 2002). Such ideas have bolstered the personal experience of stress, including hardship and victimization (Oksanen et al. 2014; Rader et al. 2012). Therefore, national liberty would raise the personal experience of stress.

Democracy

National democracy, typically practiced in its electoral, liberal, and representative form, has induced people's stress in terms of collective unpredictability (Catley 2001). Such democracy distributes power to people to confront the authority. The induction works through direct and indirect deterministic mechanisms.

The direct deterministic mechanism maintains that democracy engenders collective stress to induce the personal experience of stress through sharing privately or publicly. Collective stress engendered by democracy includes antagonism, argument, conflict, confrontation, contention, contestation, dissensus, disharmony, instability, polarization, and rivalry among people and between the populace and authority (Brennan 2016; Dryzek and Dunleavy 2009; Fairfield 2008; Mukherjee 2000; Munck 2005; O'Dwyer 2003; O'Neill 2000; Peng et at. 2017; Pettit 2012; Shin 2012; Trainor

2008). Such collective stress corresponds to the stress of draining, hardship, insecurity, nuisance, and victimization. Notably, collective stress has induced the personal experience of stress. National democracy thus would sustain the personal experience of stress.

However, the direct deterministic mechanism also suggests that democracy reduces collective stress to dampen the personal experience of stress. Such reduction includes that in authoritarianism, coercion, domination, inequality, injustice, interference, moralizing, remonstrance; subjection, and unfairness by the authority (Brennan 2016; Dryzek 2006; Dryzek and Dunleavy 2009; Minogue 2010; Moller and Skaaning 2013; O'Neill 2000; F. Peter 2009; Pettit 2012; Shin 2012; Steiner 2012; Talisse 2009). Such experience is primarily conducive to the stress of nuisance and victimization. They have relieved the experience of stress, including nuisance and victimization (Aloia and Solomon 2015; Fenwick and Tausig 1994; Gallie et al. 1998; Johnson et al. 2008; Schieman 2013; Schmidt et al. 2015). Thus, national democracy would reduce the personal experience of stress.

The indirect deterministic mechanism of empowering holds that national democracy empowers stress alleviation to dampen the personal experience of stress. Such empowering applies to the raising or sharing capability, education, intelligence, welfare, and wisdom (Dryzek and Dunleavy 2009; Fairfield 2008; O'Dwyer 2003; Pettit 2012; Saward 1998). Essentially, empowerment and sharing are emphases in democracy (Abizadeh 2002; Munck 2005). Moreover, national democracy has raised people's knowledge and prosperity (Rindermann 2008; Shin 2012). Such raising has lessened the experience of stress, including draining, hardship, and insecurity (Aishwarya et al. 2019; Extremera et al. 2007; Gitto et al. 2020). Thus, national democracy would mitigate the personal experience of stress.

The indirect deterministic mechanism of incentivizing indicates that national democracy incentivizes stress prevention to alleviate the personal experience of stress. Such incentivizing applies to the promotion of people's adaptation, agency, assertiveness, autonomy, coping, emancipation, rationality, responsibility, self-determination, self-development, and self-regulation (Caprara and Vecchione 2017; Fairfield 2008; Levi 2003; Munck 2005; O'Neill 2000; Ringen 2007; Saward 1998; Warren 2011; Wood 2003). Essentially, incentivizing emphasizes democracy (Dryzek and Dunleavy 2009). Such incentivizing has alleviated the experience of stress (Furnham 1997; Hong et al. 2018; Mak and Mueller 2000; Schieman 2013). Hence, national democracy would minimize the personal experience of stress.

The indirect deterministic mechanism of framing states that national democracy frames ideas relieving people's experience of stress. Essentially, framing is notable in democracy (Brennan 2016). Framed ideas include civility, dignity, freedom, happiness, liberty, openness, respect, rights, and tolerance (Caprara and Vecchione 2017; Ceva and Zuolo 2013; Dryzek and Dunleavy 2009; Brennan 2016; Minogue 2010; Safford 2002; Saward 1998). Collectively, national democracy has raised the ideas of cooperation and peace (Hausermann 2006; Moller and Skaaning 2013). Moreover, national democracy has fostered perceptions about freedom (Moller and Skaaning 2013). These ideas have relieved the experience of stress, including insecurity, nuisance, and victimization (Antonukis and Dietz 2011; Bardeen et al. 2016; Oksanen et al. 2014). Conversely, national democracy alleviates such ideas as sentimentalism, rent-seeking, servitude, social obligation, and vigilance (Dryzek and Dunleavy 2009; Fairfield 2008; Minogue 2010; Pettit 2012). Furthermore, national democracy has dampened crime perception (Uslaner 2008). Such dampening has lessened the experience of stress, including nuisance and victimization (Fenwick and Tausig 1994; Schmidt et al. 2015; Wittebrood and Nieuwbeerta 2000). Hence, national democracy would weaken the personal experience of stress.

However, the indirect deterministic mechanism of framing also suggests that national democracy frames ideas conducive to people's experience of stress. Such ideas include hooliganism, licentiousness, protesting, and radicalism (Aytac and Stokes 2019; Brennan 2016; Hellinger 2008; Munck 2005; Ruggiero 2017). They have bolstered the experience of stress, including insecurity, nuisance, and victimization (Antonukis and Dietz 2011; Wittebrood and Nieuwbeerta 2000). Conversely, national democracy discourages such an idea as social cohesion (Dryzek and Dunleavy 2009). Such discouragement has boosted the experience of stress, including nuisance and victimization (Beaudoin 2009; Gaitan-Rossi and Shen 2018). Therefore, national democracy would sustain the personal experience of stress.

Government Effectiveness

National government effectiveness signifies the effectiveness of the whole country in national functioning or building, including fulfillment, adaptation, integration, and latency. The building is manifest in the development of the nation as a community and through a variety of physical or infrastructural construction (Loo 2020; Yogeeswaran and Dasgupta 2014). The building aims to cultivate people's voluntarism in national cohesion (Greenfield and Eastwood 2005). As such, national government effectiveness has raised experiences of the living standard and social harmony and diminished the experience of environmental problems (Mizrahi 2016; Wong and Shik 2011; Wong and Wan 2011). These experiences directly reflect stress, including hardship, insecurity, and nuisance, as opposed to saving or being well-off. The function of national government effectiveness works through direct and indirect deterministic mechanisms, including empowering, incentivizing, standardizing, and framing.

The direct deterministic mechanism holds that national government effectiveness creates the collective experience of stress to share with the person privately or publicly. National government effectiveness has established the living standard, social harmony, and prosperity and dampened environmental problems collectively (Guisan 2009; Mizrahi 2016; Wong and Shik 2011; Wong and Wan 2011). Essentially, national government effectiveness also applies to welfare and other social service provisions (Batta 2011). Such collective experiences have spread to the person to lower the personal experience of stress versus being well-off (Cepulic et al. 2022). Thus, national government effectiveness would weaken the personal experience of stress, including draining, hardship, insecurity, and nuisance.

The indirect deterministic mechanism of empowering relies on empowering stress avoidance or prevention to lessen the personal experience of stress. Such empowering transpires in national government effectiveness in co-creation, community, industrialization, rights protection, and social service provision (Altman and Wellman 2009; Batta 2011; Berger 2003; Loo 2020; Szondi 2010). These empowering measures have furnished power or resources, including income, possession, social class, social networking, social status, and wealth (Lin et al. 2015; Lipford and Yandle 2009; Walder 2002). Such power or resources have impeded the experience of stress, such as draining, hardship, insecurity, and nuisance (Cepulic et al. 2022; Schieman 2013). Hence, national government effectiveness would reduce the personal experience of stress.

The indirect deterministic mechanism of incentivizing proposes that national government effectiveness incentivizes stress avoidance or coping to impede the personal experience of stress. Such incentivizing transpires in national government effectiveness in promoting people's activeness, dutifulness, materialism, and rationality (Berger 2003; Loo 2020; Moore 2001). Hence, national government effectiveness has activated people to deal with problems and enjoy material life (Guisan 2009; Koch 2000). Such activation has dampened the experience of stress (Furnham 1997; Hong et al. 2018; Mak and Mueller 2000). Thus, national government effectiveness would prevent the personal experience of stress.

The indirect deterministic mechanism of standardizing states that national government effectiveness provides social standards for avoiding stress to dispel the personal experience of stress. Such standardizing is manifest in national advertising, campaigning, communication, culture, discussion, images, marketing, myths, and narratives to become social norms for sharing among people (Loo 2020; Moore 2001; Rivera 2008; Szondi 2010). Such social norms have dampened the experience of stress, including draining, hardship, and insecurity (Burns and Machin 2012). Hence, national government effectiveness would diminish the personal experience of stress.

The indirect deterministic mechanism of framing indicates that national government effectiveness frames ideas contradictory to stress for dispelling the personal experience of stress. These framed ideas involve community, identity, meaningfulness, recognition, and understanding or empathy (Hu 2015; Loo 2020; Szondi 2010; Sutherland 2005). Moreover, national government effectiveness has lifted people's well-being regarding life quality and satisfaction (Bohnke 2008; Helliwell 2006; Murphy 2009). These ideas have dissolved the experience of stress, including draining, hardship, insecurity, and victimization (Bardeen et al. 2016; Beaudoin 2009; Johnson et al. 2008; La Guardia et al. 2000; Salehi 2012). Hence, national government effectiveness would impede the personal experience of stress.

However, the indirect deterministic mechanism of framing also suggests that national government effectiveness frames ideas conducive to stress to shape people's experience of stress. These ideas are state demand, manipulation, rule, power, taxation, and war, warfare, national defense or security due to international rivalry (Altman and Wellman 2009; Barr 2012; Batta 2011; Loo 2020; Moore 2001). They have induced the experience of stress, including draining, hardship, and nuisance (Baba et al. 2013; Fenwick and Tausig 1994; Qouta et al. 2007; Schieman 2013;

Schmidt et al. 2015). Hence, national government effectiveness would raise the personal experience of stress.

Emission

National carbon dioxide (CO_2) emission, as an indicator of environmental degradation or demerit, is stressful. Accordingly, the emission is degrading, detrimental, hazardous, and risky, thus causing distress (Esaisason 2014; Riad and Norris 1992; Scafuto and La Barbera 2016). The stressful impact of national CO_2 emission on the personal experience of stress hinges on the direct and indirect mechanisms of empowering, incentivizing, and framing.

The direct mechanism maintains that national CO_2 emission is stressful collectively to induce the personal experience of stress privately or publicly. Such collective experience is about degradation, deterioration, hazard, poverty, and risk (Esaisason 2014; Riad and Norris 1992; Hengeveld 2012; Scafuto and La Barbera 2016; Swanson et al. 1992). They have spread and translated into the personal experience of stress, including draining, hardship, and insecurity (Like 2011; Taylor-Gooby 2001). Hence, national CO_2 emission would foment the personal experience of stress.

The indirect mechanism of empowering emphasizes that national CO_2 emission is disempowering in stress avoidance or prevention, thus breeding the personal experience of stress. Such disempowering figures in weakening social capital (Cummins et al. 2003). This weakening has engendered the experience of stress, including hardship, insecurity, nuisance, and victimization (Frank et al. 2014; Hansen-Nord et al. 2014). Therefore, national CO_2 emission would sustain the personal experience of stress.

The indirect mechanism of incentivizing accentuates that national CO_2 emission incentivizes stressful reactions to sustain the personal experience of stress. Such incentivizing has instigated detachment from community, migration, nimbyism or rejection of others, and protesting (Black et al. 2011; Esaisason 2014; Mesch and Manor 1998; Scafuto and La Barbera 2016). The instigation is socially agitating and harmful, according to exchange logic. It has thereby created the experience of stress, including nuisance and victimization (Emery and Wu 2020; Jonsson et al. 2003; Matthews et al. 2006). Consequently, national CO_2 emission would engender the personal experience of stress.

The indirect mechanism of framing holds that national CO_2 emission frames ideas consistent and conducive to stress, thus uplifting the personal experience of stress. Such ideas include crowding, dehumanization, dissatisfaction, uncleanliness, and vulnerability (Baum et al. 2002; Merrilees et al. 2009; Pujol 1999; Riad and Norris 1992; Sirgy 1998). These ideas are causative of the experience of stress, including insecurity and nuisance (Furnham 1997; La Guardia et al. 2000). Furthermore, national CO_2 emission has undermined well-being, including health and life satisfaction (Stafford et al. 2005; Tiliouine et al. 2006; Van Haaften et al. 2004). Such undermining has been the cause of the experience of stress, including hardship and insecurity (Gitto et al. 2020; La Guardia et al. 2000; Rader et al. 2012). Thus, national CO_2 emission would buttress the personal experience of stress.

Human Development

National human development, encompassing development in the economy, education, and life expectancy and reflecting talent or human capital, is likely to boost stress avoidance or prevention to relieve the personal experience of stress. The influence of national human development rests on the direct and indirect deterministic mechanisms, including empowering, incentivizing, standardizing, and framing.

The direct deterministic mechanism maintains that national human development diminishes collective stress and thus the personal experience of stress successively. Herein, national human development means national life quality or well-being and thus stress relief (Castles 2000). Such collective experience has carried over or translated into the personal experience of stress relief (Garfin et al. 2015; Page and Jacobs 2011; Ritchie 2012). This influence depends on private or public sharing, whereby the person appropriates collective experience vicariously (Garfin et al. 2015; Ritchie 2012). Hence, national human development would alleviate the personal experience of stress.

The indirect deterministic mechanism of empowering states that national human development empowers people's stress avoidance or prevention to reduce the personal experience of stress. Such empowering results in people's capability, earnings, education, entitlement to legal protection or support, motivation, and tenure (Dahlberg et al. 2018; Inglehart and Welzel 2005). Moreover, national human development has raised people's income, knowledge, and leadership as opposed to poverty and welfare dependency (Carli and Eagly 2011; Hyggen 2006; Muffels and Fouarge 2004; Norris 2011). Such raising of power or resources collectively or personally has weakened the experience of stress, including draining, hardship, and insecurity (Gaitan-Rossi and Shen 2018; Garfin et al. 2015; Gitto et al. 2020; Kanan and Pruitt 2002). Thus, national human development would impede the personal experience of stress.

The indirect deterministic mechanism of incentivizing holds that national human development incentivizes people's stress avoidance or prevention to lower the personal experience of stress. Such incentivizing has applied to people's practices of abidance or obedience, donation, and responsibility, opposed to extremism, lying, and protesting (Fridberg and Kangas 2008b; He et al. 2014; Jakobsen 2010; Norris 2002; van Hemert et al. 2002). These practices incentivize stress avoidance or prevention among people, according to exchange logic. As such, the practices have prevented the experience of stress, including nuisance and victimization (Han and Connell 2020; Jonsson et al. 2003; Wittebrood and Nieuwbeerta 2000). Hence, national human development would relieve the personal experience of stress.

The indirect deterministic mechanism of standardizing suggests that national human development de-standardizes social constraints alleviate the personal experience of stress. Such de-standardization applies to removing tradition and its constraint

(Quah 2003). Accordingly, tradition is constraining (Chu 2001). Such removal has diminished the experience of stress, including nuisance (Holman et al. 2011). Thus, national human development would reduce the personal experience of stress.

The indirect deterministic mechanism of framing maintains that national human development frames ideas inconsistent with and contradictory to stress to erode the personal experience of stress. Such framed ideas consist in life satisfaction (Basabe et al. 2002; Castles 2000). Moreover, national human development has raised acquiescence, the evaluation of the economy, social trust, and well-being, including health, as opposed to depression (Drope and Chowdhury 2014; Eikemo et al. 2008; Fridberg and Kangas 2008b; He et al. 2014; Meulemann 2010; Schieman et al. 2001). National human development has also boosted civility in society. (Bond and Lun 2014) These ideas have impeded the experience of stress, including draining, hardship, insecurity, nuisance, and victimization (Becker et al. 1997; Gitto et al. 2020; Johnson et al. 2008; Rader et al. 2012). Thereby, national human development would relieve the personal experience of stress.

However, the indirect deterministic mechanism of framing also suggests that national human development frames ideas consistent with and conducive to stress to raise the personal experience of stress. As such, national income development has increased the perception of corruption, the attitude of aspiration, and the practice of migration, (Correll 2004; Gurak and Kritz 2000; Uslaner 2008). These ideas have sustained the experience of stress, including hardship, nuisance, and victimization (Auerbach et al. 2011; Sacks and Levi 2010). Thus, national human development would bolster the personal experience of stress.

Time

Time, reflecting social change, is influential on the collective and personal experiences of stress. Such change includes denaturalization, globalization, individualization, modernization including industrialization and Westernization, postmodernization, secularization, and universalization or the diverse development of the public sphere (Adams 2007; de Graaf et al. 2001; Harper and Leicht 2011; Morody and Giza-Poleszczuk 2018). Notably, time has diminished the experience of threat (Sahar 2008). The influence works through direct and indirect deterministic mechanisms, including empowering, incentivizing, standardizing, and framing.

The direct deterministic mechanism states that time raises the collective experience of stress relief to induce the personal experience of stress relief through sharing privately or publicly. Such collective experiences have been a relief in conflict and increased social integration (Lange and Dawson 2009; Smith et al. 2001). These collective experiences have, in turn, weakened the personal experience of stress, including insecurity, nuisance, and victimization (Gaitan-Rossi and Shen 2018; Garfin et al. 2015; Kanan and Pruitt 2002; Kim and Lee 2020; Ritchie 2012). Hence, time would dampen the personal experience of stress.

The indirect deterministic mechanism of empowering maintains that time empowers stress avoidance or prevention to diminish the personal experience of stress. Such empowering has registered in employment, postindustrialization or knowledge-based production collectively, and prosperity collectively (Ladd 1995; Norris 2012; Shin 2013). Personally, empowering has also consolidated employment or social class, homeownership, income, knowledge, and reduction in poverty (Conley and Gifford 2006; Dekkers 2008; Francesconi and Golsch 2005; Lichter et al. 2002; Singer et al. 1999). In practice, time has raised exercising (Bianchi et al. 2004). Such empowering has alleviated the experience of stress, including hardship and insecurity (Cepulic et al. 2022; Gaitan-Rossi and Shen 2018; Garfin et al. 2015; Gitto et al. 2020; Schieman 2013). Hence, time would dwindle the personal experience of stress.

However, the indirect deterministic mechanism of empowering also suggests that time reduces power to avoid or prevent stress, thus sustaining the personal experience of stress. Such reduction has happened in social capital (Grenier and Wright 2006). Such reduction has bolstered the experience of stress, including nuisance and victimization (Brisson 2009; Frank et al. 2014; Hansen-Nord et al. 2014). Hence, time would lift the personal experience of stress.

The indirect deterministic mechanism of incentivizing holds that time escalates incentives for stress avoidance or prevention to dampen the personal experience of stress. Such incentives have figured in the dispositions of environmentalism, friendliness, and helpfulness (Scruggs 2003; Smith et al. 2001). In addition, time has raised the practices of cohesion, neighboring, sympathizing, and volunteering (de Beer and Kostere 2009; Sarracino 2010; Smith et al. 2001). These dispositions and practices would be incentives to induce favorable social returns. They have thereby reduced the experience of stress, including nuisance and victimization (Tom et al. 2010; Homant 2013). Conversely, time has reduced the practices of burrowing, protesting, resistance, and violence (Norris and Inglehart 2009; Pinker 2011). Such reduction would minimize unfavorable social returns, according to exchange logic. Thus, the reduction has eroded the experience of stress, including nuisance and victimization (Han and Connell 2020; Wittebrood and Nieuwbeerta 2000). Time would thereby attenuate the personal experience of stress.

The indirect deterministic mechanism of framing indicates that time creates frames providing ideas that are incongruous with stress to weaken the personal experience of stress. These framed ideas have included the collective experiences of development and the personal experiences of safety (Norris 2012; Smith et al. 2001). In addition, time has raised the attitudes of belief in a just world, tolerance, and trust (Malahy et al. 2009; Smith et al. 2001; Wang et al. 2004). Time has only lifted well-being in terms of relational quality, satisfaction with welfare, and survival (Beckfield 2004; Logan and Cobb 2013; Wong et al. 2010). These ideas have impeded the experience of stress, including hardship, insecurity, and nuisance (Bardeen et al. 2016; Cepulic et al. 2022; Furnham 1997; Johnson et al. 2008; Madlock and Westerman 2011). Conversely, time has reduced anomie or normlessness and smoking personally and inequality collectively (Bianchi et al. 2004; Bulmahn 2000; Diez-Nicolas 2002). Such reduction has lessened the experience of stress, including hardship and insecurity (Gitto et al. 2020; Lau et al. 2005). Hence, time would diminish the personal experience of stress.

However, the indirect deterministic mechanism of framing also suggests that time raises the personal experience of stress by framing ideas consistent with and conducive to stress. Time has buttressed narcissism or maladaptation, polarization, revolution, and suicide collectively (Chang et al. 2009; Egerton and Savage 2000; Lijphart 1997; Wilkinson and Pickett 2017). Notably, narcissism as a form of radicalism involves attacking, confusion, dependency, grandiosity, hedonism, lying, phantasy, pride, rage, solipsism, uncertainty, and violence (Jacoby 1990; Kilminster 2008; Lasch 1984; Tracy et al. 2009). Personally, time has bred the experiences of disconnection, exclusion, and generational gaps, and problem perception (McPherson et al. 2006; Smith 2005; Wong et al. 2010). Furthermore, time has raised the dispositions of pessimism and skepticism (Ladd 1995). These experiences, perceptions, and dispositions have fomented the experience of stress, hardship, insecurity, and nuisance (Han and Connell 2020; Ho 1998; Hodges and Perry 1999; Schwartz et al. 2003; Smith 2005). Conversely, time has attenuated the experiences of social integration and legitimacy perception (Inglehart 1999; McPherson et al. 2006). Time has also eroded well-being in terms of financial satisfaction, health, and marital quality and satisfaction (Hays and Seifert 2003; Islam et al. 2006; Murray et al. 2011; Umberson et al. 2005). Moreover, time has discounted the disposition of religiosity (Kaufmann et al. 2012). These reductions have sustained the experience of stress, including hardship and security (Gitto et al. 2020; Johnson et al. 2008; Khoo et al. 2021; Rader et al. 2012).

Summary

According to theory and research, the social experiences of economic hardship, neighborhood nuisance, victimization, security, and family saving are likely to be predictable by a host of personal and national factors in line with analytical functionalism. The main thread of prediction rests on the experience of stress to encompass hardship, insecurity, nuisance, victimization, and non-saving or draining. Based on voluntaristic mechanisms, the experience recedes due to the realization of power, optimization of utility, conformity to norms, and consistency with ideas for stress removal. Conversely, inadequate power, utility, norms, and ideas favorable to the removal lead to the maintenance or even raising of the experience of stress. These mechanisms operate with personal factors, including experiences, perceptions, dispositions, attitudes, feelings, practices, and sociodemographic characteristics. In addition, these voluntaristic mechanisms run with national factors through the indirect deterministic mechanisms of empowering, incentivizing, standardizing, and framing. The latter mechanisms furnish power, utility, norms, and ideas for voluntaristic mechanisms. In addition, the deterministic mechanism can work through a direct path

Table 5.1 Hypothesized functionalist effects on social experiences

Predictor	Hard	Nuisance	Victim	Secure	Saving
Wave	–	–	–	+	+
Personal					
Irreligious	+	+	+	–	–
Family income	–	–	–	+	+
Female	+	+	+	–	–
Age	–	+	–	+	+
Age squared	+	+	+	–	–
Married	–	–	–	+	+
Cohabited	–	–	–	+	+
Divorced	+	+	+	–	–
Separated	+	+	+	–	–
Widowed	+	+	+	–	–
Kid	+	+	+	–	–
Mother immigrant	+	+	+	–	–
Father immigrant	+	+	+	–	–
Education	–	–	–	+	+
Graduation age	–	–	–	+	+
Interest	–	–	–	+	+
Living with parents	+	+	–	+	–
Full-time employment	–	–	–	+	+
Part-time employment	–	–	–	+	+
Self-employment	–	–	–	+	+
Retired	+	+	+	–	–
Homemaking	+	+	+	–	–
Student	–	+	+	–	–
Unemployed	+	+	+	–	–
Public employment	–	–	–	+	+
Private business employment	–	–	–	+	+
Nonprofit organization employment	–	–	–	+	+
Intellectual work	–	–	–	+	+
Creative work	–	–	–	+	+
Independent work	–	–	–	+	+
Supervision	–	–	–	+	+
Earner	–	–	–	+	+
Earner employed	–	–	–	+	+
National					

(continued)

Table 5.1 (continued)

Predictor	Hard	Nuisance	Victim	Secure	Saving
Population	+	+	+	−	−
Phone	−	−	−	+	+
Land	+	−	−	+	−
Technology	−	−	−	+	+
Credit	−	−	−	+	+
Prosperity	−	−	−	+	+
Income inequality	+	+	+	−	−
Globalization	−	−	−	+	+
Government effectiveness	−	−	−	+	+
Democracy	−	−	−	+	+
Liberty	−	−	−	+	+
Human development	−	−	−	+	+
Human capital	−	−	−	+	+
CO_2	+	+	+	−	−

from collective factors to personal factors through sharing privately or publicly. Such sharing is to share collective experiences, power, utility, norms, ideas, and other factors to become personal experiences and other factors. The voluntaristic and deterministic mechanisms of the analytical-functionalist framework thereby sustain hypothesized effects on social experiences (Table 5.1).

Chapter 6
Life Experience Production: Findings

A series of regression analyses revealed significant influences of personal and national factors on the personal experiences of economic hardship, neighborhood nuisance, victimization, security, and family saving, based on the average person found in the world. The analyses also showed temporal differentials in personal and national influences. As such, regression analysis examined temporal and national variations first. Then, it scrutinized personal and national influences and their temporal differentials alternately. Notably, only a standardized effect stronger than the weak level of 0.10 was meaningful. A weaker effect was too slight to be notable.

Findings

In predicting personal social experiences about life quality, personal family income, education, student status, employment in a nonprofit organization, creative work and independent work, national population size, technology, bank credit, government effectiveness, democracy, liberty, human capital, and human development displayed some notable but sporadic effects. Some of these effects showed notable changes with time.

Economic Hardship

The first step of regression analysis revealed significant variations among the waves of surveys and nations. Time variation between the two waves indicated a moderate decrease in economic hardship experienced. National variations indicated that economic hardship was the highest in India, followed by Nigeria, Pakistan, and the Philippines, among the big countries. In addition, Russia, Mexico, Egypt, and Turkey had slightly higher economic hardship. By contrast, economic hardship was

C. Cheung, *Production Dynamics for Life Quality in the Incipient 21st Century*,
https://doi.org/10.1007/978-981-19-3827-6_6

the lowest in Germany among the big countries. The variation due to Germany, nevertheless, was slight.

The second step of regression analysis unraveled the significant effects of personal factors. Education indicated the strongest and negative effect on economic hardship among personal characteristics. Family income was the next strongest predictor, having a positive effect on economic hardship. Another weak effect emanated from nonprofit organization employment, which exhibited a negative effect on economic hardship. The other personal characteristics displayed weaker or negligible effects on economic hardship. Notably, the response characteristic of acquiescence showed a weak positive effect on economic hardship, indicating the need for control for acquiescence in the analysis.

The third step of regression analysis examined significant temporal variations in the effects of personal factors on economic hardship. Among the significant variations, the effect of student status was more positive in Wave 6 than in Wave 5. By contrast, the effects of family income became less positive, the effect of education became more negative, and the effect of full-time employment became less negative with time. The other temporal variations in effects were weaker and thus negligible (Table 6.1).

The first step of regression analysis of economic hardship on national factors screened significant national factors. Among the significant national factors, human development and credit evolved a weak negative effect, and democracy indicated a weak positive effect. In addition, income inequality displayed a slight negative effect on economic hardship.

The second step of regression analysis scrutinized the significant temporal variations in the effects of national factors on economic hardship and significant variations among nations in economic hardship. Among the temporal variations, the effects of human development, credit, and income inequality became more negative with time, and the effect of democracy became more positive with time. The temporal variation in the effect of income inequality was slight only. In addition, Germany showed the lowest economic hardship, followed by Japan, among the big countries. By contrast, Nigeria and the Philippines had the highest economic hardship after controlling national characteristics. Except Germany, other countries only manifested slight variations in economic hardship (Table 6.2).

Neighborhood Nuisance

The first step of regression analysis showed a significant but minimal reduction in neighborhood nuisance with time. Significant and notable national variations in neighborhood nuisance were lower nuisance in China, the United States, and Japan than in other countries. The other significant national variations were slight and not noteworthy.

The second step of regression analysis indicated that nonprofit organization employment had a significant negative effect on neighborhood nuisance, whereas

Table 6.1 Standardized effects on economic hardship

Predictor	(1)	(2)	(3)
Wave	−0.256***	−0.253***	−0.220***
India	0.229***	0.046***	−0.035***
Nigeria	0.225***	0.169***	0.139***
Pakistan	0.208***	0.144***	0.129***
Philippines	0.146***	0.109***	0.062***
Russia	0.093***	0.098***	0.089***
Mexico	0.090***	0.062***	0.028***
Egypt	0.059***	0.039***	0.042***
Germany	−0.058***	−0.069***	−0.081***
Turkey	0.034***	−0.005	0.000
Education		−0.243***	−0.167***
Acquiescence		0.162***	0.203***
Family income		0.155***	−0.166***
Nonprofit organization employment		−0.112***	−0.016*
Earner employed		−0.090***	−0.027***
Earner		0.088***	0.061***
Creative work		0.075***	0.081***
Full-time employment		−0.069***	−0.156***
Father immigrant		0.069***	0.057***
Self-employment		−0.061***	−0.093***
Age		−0.059***	−0.033***
Graduation age		0.057***	0.038***
Supervision		−0.052***	−0.011
Irreligious		−0.051***	−0.057***
Kid		0.050***	0.039***
Retired		0.045***	−0.016
Student		0.043***	0.047***
Age squared		−0.030***	−0.029***
Interest		0.028***	0.016***
Homemaking		−0.027***	−0.038***
Married		−0.026*	−0.011
Living with parents		0.024**	0.013
Separated		0.023**	0.016**
Public employment		−0.021**	0.029***
Private business employment		−0.020*	0.033***
Female		−0.017*	0.010

(continued)

Table 6.1 (continued)

Predictor	(1)	(2)	(3)
Divorced		0.016	0.008
Cohabited		0.015	0.024**
Independent work		−0.012	−0.052***
Part-time employment		0.009	−0.066***
Widowed		−0.006	−0.009
Wave × Acquiescence			0.228***
Wave × Student			0.174***
Wave × Family income			−0.164***
Wave × Education			−0.144***
Wave × Full-time employment			0.099***
Wave × Unemployed			0.095***
Wave × Homemaker			0.093***
Wave × Part-time employment			0.067***
Wave × Earner employed			−0.066***
Wave × Irreligious			−0.061***
Wave × Kid			0.056***
Wave × Retiree			0.051***
Wave × Father immigrant			0.047***
Wave × Self-employed			0.047***
Wave × Earner			0.038***
Wave × Private business employment			0.037***
Wave × Married			−0.032***
Wave × Age			−0.028***
Wave × Nonprofit organization employment			−0.025**
Wave × Separated			0.023***
Wave × Supervisor			−0.022***
Wave × Divorce			0.020**
Wave × Cohabited			0.019**
R^2	0.172	0.322	0.461

* $p < 0.05$, ** $p < 0.01$, *** $p < 0.001$

creative work had a significant positive effect on the nuisance. The other effects of background characteristics on neighborhood nuisance were slight.

The third step of regression analysis exhibited that being irreligious had a significant negative effect on neighborhood nuisance only in Wave 6. This differential effect and other differential effects were slight, even though many were statistically significant (Table 6.3).

Table 6.2 Standardized effects of national characteristics on economic hardship

Predictor	(1)	(2)
Wave	0.026^{***}	0.006
Human development	-0.136^{***}	-0.092^{***}
Democracy	0.110^{***}	0.136^{***}
Credit	-0.096^{***}	-0.112^{***}
Income inequality	-0.063^{***}	-0.124^{***}
Wave × Human development		-0.110^{***}
Wave × Democracy		0.102^{***}
Wave × Credit		-0.091^{***}
Wave × Income inequality		-0.046^{***}
Germany		-0.110^{***}
Nigeria		0.070^{***}
Philippines		0.061^{***}
Japan		-0.057^{***}
Egypt		0.036^{***}
R^2	0.047	0.109

$^{*}p < 0.05$, $^{**}p < 0.01$, $^{***}p < 0.001$

The first step of alternative regression analysis on national factors exhibited that national credit and national technology had significant negative effects on neighborhood nuisance, whereas national liberty and human capital indicated significant positive effects on the nuisance. These significant effects were weak.

The second step of alternative regression analysis showed some significant differentials in the effects of national factors due to time. As such, time strengthened the negative effect of national credit on neighborhood nuisance. By contrast, national democracy and income inequality had positive effects on neighborhood nuisance only in Wave 6. The other differentials were too slight to be noteworthy. The countries' control for national factors revealed only slight variations at best. Hence, China, the United States, and Japan no longer exhibited significant variations in neighborhood nuisance (Table 6.4).

Victimization

The first step of regression analysis showed that victimization did not significantly change with time. With the control for time, Mexico and Brazil showed significantly higher victimization than other countries. Other national variations were slight, even though statistically significant.

Table 6.3 Standardized effects on neighborhood nuisance

Predictor	(1)	(2)	(3)
Wave	−0.020***	−0.002	0.036***
China	−0.330***	−0.231***	−0.207***
US	−0.109***	−0.071***	−0.058***
Japan	−0.104***	−0.059***	−0.065***
Germany	−0.082***	−0.055***	−0.053***
Turkey	−0.080***	−0.075***	−0.066***
Indonesia	−0.052***	−0.046***	−0.013***
Brazil	0.046***	0.042***	0.068***
Philippines	0.041***	0.038***	0.022***
Vietnam	−0.032***	−0.023***	−0.019***
Ethiopia	−0.031***	−0.019***	0.015**
Mexico	0.031***	0.044***	0.055***
Iran	−0.030***	−0.030***	−0.011***
Nigeria	−0.022***	−0.040***	−0.052***
Egypt	0.018***	0.038***	0.046***
Russia	0.013**	0.047***	0.074***
Acquiescence		0.150***	0.162***
Nonprofit organization employment		−0.105***	−0.021***
Creative work		0.099***	0.085***
Earner employed		−0.072***	−0.048***
Age		−0.066***	−0.045***
Graduation age		0.066***	0.028***
Education		−0.062***	−0.022***
Father immigrant		0.054***	0.048***
Part-time employment		0.052***	0.022***
Public employment		−0.050***	−0.008
Private business employment		−0.046***	0.010
Retired		0.040***	0.034***
Family income		−0.038***	−0.045***
Full-time employment		0.036***	0.018**
Married		−0.029***	−0.033***
Earner		0.027***	0.012**
Homemaking		0.020***	0.000
Independent work		−0.020**	−0.052***
Kid		0.018**	0.007
Living with parents		0.013**	0.009*

(continued)

Table 6.3 (continued)

Predictor	(1)	(2)	(3)
Supervision		-0.011^{**}	0.009*
Female		-0.011^{*}	−0.006
Cohabited		0.011^{*}	0.011^{*}
Separated		0.010^{*}	0.009
Interest		0.010	−0.001
Self-employment		-0.008^{***}	0.005
Age squared		−0.008	−0.007
Widowed		−0.007	−0.009
Student		0.007	0.009
Divorced		0.001	0.000
Wave × Acquiescence			0.155^{***}
Wave × Irreligious			-0.091^{***}
Wave × Earner employed			-0.061^{***}
Wave × Orthodox			0.054^{***}
Wave × Age			-0.053^{***}
Wave × Catholic			0.049^{***}
Wave × Mother immigrant			0.044^{***}
Wave × Nonmanual work			0.044^{***}
Wave × Graduation age			0.042^{***}
Wave × Married			-0.040^{***}
Wave × Family income			-0.037^{***}
Wave × Kid			0.036^{***}
Wave × Hindu			0.032^{***}
Wave × Cohabited			0.027^{***}
Wave × Private business employment			0.026^{***}
Wave × Idle			0.023^{***}
Wave × Student			0.019^{***}
Wave × Buddhist			-0.018^{***}
Wave × Separated			0.018^{***}
Wave × Female			-0.017^{***}
Wave × Earner			0.010^{*}
R^2	0.181	0.213	0.245

* $p < 0.05$, ** $p < 0.01$, *** $p < 0.001$

Table 6.4 Standardized effects of national characteristics on neighborhood nuisance

Predictor	(1)	(2)
Wave	0.007	0.002
Credit	-0.220^{***}	-0.280^{***}
Liberty	0.185^{***}	0.171^{***}
Technology	-0.184^{***}	-0.169^{***}
Human capital	0.129^{***}	0.154^{***}
Wave × Credit		-0.149^{***}
Wave × Democracy		0.139^{***}
Wave × Income inequality		0.118^{***}
Wave × Land		0.063^{***}
Wave × Population		-0.025^{***}
Turkey		-0.092^{***}
Indonesia		-0.042^{***}
R^2	0.108	0.220

* $p < 0.05$, ** $p < 0.01$, *** $p < 0.001$

The second step of regression analysis indicated that personal background effects on victimization were slight, even if statistically significant. Even the strongest effect of graduation age was negligibly weak.

The third step of regression analysis showed significant differentials in background effects due to time. Such differentials were slight. At most, being Catholic displayed a slight positive effect on victimization only in Wave 6 (Table 6.5).

The first step of alternative regression analysis of victimization on national factors showed four significant national factors. Only national population size displayed a notable significant weak negative effect on victimization among these factors.

The second step of alternative regression analysis showed two notable significant time variations in the effects of national factors. Accordingly, the effect of national population size on victimization was more negative with time. Meanwhile, the effect of national income inequality on victimization was more positive with time. With the control for national factors, no more national variation was notable (Tabel 6.6).

Security

The first step of regression analysis of security exhibited that security reduced significantly with time. Given this reduction, Egypt, Brazil, and Mexico displayed significantly lower security than other countries. By contrast, Germany fared significantly higher security than did other countries.

The second step of regression analysis revealed significant personal background influences on security. Among the influences, independent work indicated a positive

Table 6.5 Standardized effects on victimization

Predictor	(1)	(2)	(3)
Wave	−0.006	0.001	0.008
Mexico	0.116***	0.115***	0.142***
Brazil	0.094***	0.082***	0.115***
US	0.039***	0.042***	0.061***
Nigeria	0.025***	0.018***	0.012*
China	−0.024***	0.011	0.035***
Pakistan	0.015**	0.015**	0.012*
Turkey	−0.015**	−0.013**	−0.018***
Japan	−0.012**	−0.005	−0.002
Egypt	−0.011*	−0.007	−0.006
Acquiescence		0.041***	0.046***
Graduation age		0.031***	0.004
Supervision		0.030***	0.031***
Age		−0.028***	−0.018**
Family income		−0.026***	−0.021***
Kid		0.026***	0.020***
Creative work		0.024***	0.029***
Public employment		0.022***	0.024***
Earner		−0.020***	−0.018**
Student		0.019***	0.014**
Nonprofit organization employment		−0.016**	−0.009
Independent work		−0.016*	−0.025**
Cohabited		0.014**	0.013*
Widowed		0.012*	0.012*
Full-time employment		0.012*	0.013*
Married		−0.012	−0.015*
Divorced		0.009	0.009
Part-time employment		0.009	0.003
Retired		0.009	0.006
Irreligious		−0.008	−0.027***
Living with parents		−0.006	−0.010
Self-employment		−0.005	−0.005
Father immigrant		0.005	0.004
Homemaking		−0.004	−0.009
Education		0.004	0.015**
Separated		0.003	0.001

(continued)

Table 6.5 (continued)

Predictor	(1)	(2)	(3)
Age squared		−0.001	−0.004
Private business employment		−0.001	0.011**
Female		0.001	0.003
Earner employed		0.001	0.001
Interest		0.000	−0.002
Wave × Catholic			0.079***
Wave × Married			−0.063***
Wave × Acquiescence			0.046***
Wave × Age			−0.034***
Wave × Supervision			0.032***
Wave × Kid			0.031***
Wave × Unmarried			−0.027***
Wave × Nonprofit organization employment			−0.024***
Wave × Graduation age			0.023***
Wave × Earner			−0.019***
Wave × Islam			−0.017**
Wave × Living with parents			−0.016**
Wave × Protestant			0.014**
Wave × Full-time employment			0.012*
R^2	0.026	0.033	0.046

* $p < 0.05$, ** $p < 0.01$, *** $p < 0.001$

effect on security, whereas student status and nonprofit organization employment displayed negative effects on security.

The third step of regression analysis served to reveal significant differentials in personal background effects due to time. None of these significant effects, however, was notably strong enough. Thus, the differentials across time were only slight (Table 6.7).

The first step of alternative regression analysis of security on national factors found that national government effectiveness and population size generated significant positive effects on security, whereas national credit indicated a significant negative effect on security. These effects, though statistically significant, were weak.

The second step of alternative regression analysis showed significant temporal differentials in the effects of national factors on personal security. Accordingly, national population size was more positively influential on security with time. Meanwhile, national democracy and land per capita showed positive effects on security only in Wave 6. By contrast, national income inequality exhibited a negative effect on security only in Wave 6. With the control for national factors, Egypt and

Table 6.6 Standardized effects of national characteristics on victimization

Predictor	(1)	(2)
Wave	−0.002	0.003
Population	-0.103^{***}	-0.131^{***}
Income inequality	0.080^{***}	0.091^{***}
Credit	0.029^{***}	0.044^{***}
Liberty	0.023^{***}	0.004
Wave × Population		-0.139^{***}
Wave × Income inequality		0.120^{***}
Wave × Credit		0.040^{***}
Wave × Technology		0.018^{*}
Wave × Land		-0.020^{***}
Mexico		0.075^{***}
Philippines		-0.048^{***}
Turkey		-0.037^{***}
Russia		-0.037^{***}
Japan		-0.023^{***}
R^2	0.010	0.032

$^{*}p < 0.05$, $^{**}p < 0.01$, $^{***}p < 0.001$

Brazil displayed significantly lower security than other countries. The other national differences were slight (Table 6.8).

Family Saving

The first step of regression analysis of family saving showed that the saving increased significantly with time. Given this increase, China was significantly higher in family saving than was the other country. The other national variations were slight.

The second step of regression analysis of family saving revealed significant personal background influences on the experience. Among the influences, those of family income were notably positive. The other influences were slight.

The third step of regression analysis detected significant temporal differentials in the background influences on family saving. None of the differentials was notably strong (Table 6.9).

The first step of alternative regression analysis of family saving on national factors showed some significant effects of national factors. However, none of them was notably strong.

The second step of alternative regression analysis of family saving on national factors showed that the effect of national democracy on family saving significantly

Table 6.7 Standardized effects on security

Predictor	(1)	(2)	(3)
Wave	−0.064***	−0.194***	−0.232***
Egypt	−0.227***	−0.206***	−0.204***
Brazil	−0.131***	−0.096***	−0.086***
Mexico	−0.094***	−0.077***	−0.064***
Germany	0.092***	0.091***	0.097***
Nigeria	−0.083***	−0.051***	−0.026**
India	0.050***	0.126***	0.135***
Pakistan	−0.047***	−0.025**	−0.007
Philippines	0.022**	0.033***	0.050***
Independent work		0.205***	0.257***
Creative work		−0.123***	−0.145***
Student		−0.104***	−0.110***
Nonprofit organization employment		−0.103***	−0.135***
Acquiescence		−0.091***	−0.102***
Private business employment		−0.086***	−0.115***
Full-time employment		−0.079***	−0.058***
Graduation age		−0.070***	−0.017
Family income		0.065***	0.064***
Age		0.065***	0.043***
Retired		−0.063***	−0.029**
Part-time employment		−0.049***	−0.032***
Education		0.045***	0.011
Earner employed		0.045***	0.036***
Public employment		−0.044***	−0.049***
Father immigrant		−0.040***	−0.035***
Homemaking		−0.039***	−0.038***
Kid		−0.032**	−0.031**
Separated		−0.027***	−0.029***
Cohabited		−0.027**	−0.036***
Irreligious		−0.020*	0.004
Supervision		−0.017*	−0.031***
Interest		0.015*	0.021**
Married		0.015	0.014
Earner		−0.014	−0.013
Age squared		0.014	0.014
Widowed		−0.012	−0.013

(continued)

Table 6.7 (continued)

Predictor	(1)	(2)	(3)
Self-employment		−0.011	−0.029**
Female		0.011	0.007
Divorced		−0.010	−0.010
Living with parents		−0.009	−0.001
Wave × Acquiescence			−0.086***
Wave × Age			0.082***
Wave × Creative work			0.078***
Wave × Private business employment			−0.072***
Wave × Graduation age			−0.069***
Wave × Public employment			−0.045***
Wave × Family income			0.045***
Wave × Earner employed			0.044***
Wave × Married			0.043***
Wave × Kid			−0.041***
Wave × Retiree			−0.039***
Wave × Homemaker			−0.039***
Wave × Education			0.039***
Wave × Nonprofit organization employment			−0.036***
Wave × Student			−0.034***
Wave × Earner			−0.033***
Wave × Supervisor			−0.030***
Wave × Separated			−0.029***
Wave × Living with parents			0.029***
Wave × Irreligious			0.027**
Wave × Age squared			0.026**
Wave × Cohabited			−0.023**
R^2	0.106	0.163	0.197

* $p < 0.05$, ** $p < 0.01$, *** $p < 0.001$

increased with time. Given the control for national factors, no national variation was notable (Tabel 6.10).

Discussion

At the personal level, education was the most influential factor in lowering economic hardship and sustaining family saving. By contrast, family income sustained

Table 6.8 Standardized effects of national characteristics on security

Predictor	(1)	(2)
Wave	−0.009*	−0.019***
Government effectiveness	0.201***	0.154***
Population	0.174***	0.067***
Credit	−0.099***	−0.091***
Land	0.031***	0.013*
Wave × Population		0.307***
Wave × Democracy		0.188***
Wave × Income inequality		−0.176***
Wave × Land		0.097***
Wave × Technology		0.017*
Egypt		−0.153***
Brazil		−0.106***
Mexico		−0.072***
Philippines		0.067***
Iran		−0.049***
Vietnam		−0.049***
Japan		−0.015**
R^2	0.028	0.094

* $p < 0.05$, ** $p < 0.01$, *** $p < 0.001$

economic hardship as well as family saving. Besides education and family income, student status, nonprofit organization employment, creative work, and independent work were personal factors showing notable effects on some life experiences. Meanwhile, national factors impacting some of the personal experiences were population size, technology, liberty, democracy, bank credit, government effectiveness, human capital, and human development. Additional national variations were notable due to Germany, Egypt, and Brazil. Specifically, economic hardship decreased with education, nonprofit organization employment, national bank credit, national democracy, national human development, and increased, and time with family income and student status. Moreover, the reduction in economic hardship through education and national development increased with time. By contrast, the reduction of economic hardship by full-time employment, national democracy, and national human development shrank with time. The increase in economic hardship by family income reduced with time. The increase in economic hardship by student status and unemployment increased with time. Neighborhood nuisance decreased with nonprofit organization employment, national technology, national bank credit, and national human capital and increased with creative work, national liberty. Moreover, the reduction in neighborhood nuisance by national bank credit decreased with time. By contrast, the reduction in neighborhood nuisance by national democracy shrank with time. The increase in

Table 6.9 Standardized effects on family saving

Predictor	(1)	(2)	(3)
Wave	0.089***	0.077***	0.076***
China	0.099***	0.125***	0.111***
Germany	0.065***	0.054***	0.055***
US	0.054***	0.025***	0.024***
Ethiopia	0.035***	0.029***	0.019***
India	−0.034***	0.020**	0.033***
Philippines	−0.034***	−0.028***	−0.015***
Vietnam	0.033***	0.022***	0.021***
Mexico	−0.028***	−0.016***	−0.018***
Indo	0.027***	0.007	−0.002
Russia	0.016**	−0.002	−0.006
Pakistan	0.012*	0.009*	0.021***
Family income		0.216***	0.215***
Education		0.103***	0.085***
Earner employed		0.057***	0.045***
Public employment		0.046***	0.022***
Supervision		0.045***	0.035***
Private business employment		0.042***	0.019**
Kid		−0.038***	−0.031***
Earner		−0.037***	−0.039***
Nonprofit organization employment		0.034***	−0.007
Self-employment		0.030***	0.057***
Independent work		−0.027***	−0.016**
Age squared		0.026***	0.027***
Age		0.025***	0.014*
Female		−0.019***	−0.024***
Part-time employment		−0.017***	0.025***
Acquiescence		0.011*	0.011*
Interest		0.011*	0.016***
Divorced		−0.010*	−0.010*
Father immigrant		−0.010*	−0.009*
Widowed		0.009	0.006
Cohabited		−0.008	−0.010*
Separated		−0.008	−0.008
Student		−0.008	−0.001
Creative work		0.008	0.015**

(continued)

Table 6.9 (continued)

Predictor	(1)	(2)	(3)
Full-time employment		−0.007	0.043***
Graduation age		0.005	0.009
Homemaking		0.005	0.022***
Retired		0.003	0.041***
Married		−0.001	−0.009
Living with parents		0.000	0.003
Wave × Irreligious			0.073***
Wave × Full-time employment			−0.067***
Wave × Acquiescence			−0.066***
Wave × Student			−0.064***
Wave × Retired			−0.064***
Wave × Homemaking			−0.053***
Wave × Part-time employment			−0.046***
Wave × Self-employed			−0.045***
Wave × Idle			−0.043***
Wave × Unmarried			−0.024***
Wave × Islam			0.020***
Wave × Public employment			−0.018***
Wave × Nonprofit organization employment			0.018***
Wave × Living with parents			0.018***
Wave × Divorced			−0.017***
Wave × Education			0.016**
Wave × Interest			0.013**
Wave × Supervision			−0.012**
Wave × Earner employed			0.012*
Wave × Protestant			0.011*
R^2			0.011*

* $p < 0.05$, ** $p < 0.01$, *** $p < 0.001$

neighborhood nuisance by national income inequality increased with time. Victimization decreased with population size and more with time. The increase in victimization by national inequality grew with time. Security increased with independent work, national population size, and national government effectiveness, and decreased with student status, nonprofit organization employment, creative work, and national bank credit. The increase in security by National population size and democracy increased with time. Moreover, the reduction in security by national inequality increased with time. Family saving increased with education and family income. The decrease in family saving by national democracy grew with time (Tabel 6.11).

Table 6.10 Standardized effects of national characteristics on family saving

Predictor	(1)	(2)
Wave	0.075^{***}	0.081^{***}
Democracy	-0.082^{***}	-0.074^{***}
Income inequality	-0.048^{***}	-0.065^{***}
CO_2	0.047^{***}	0.034^{***}
Technology	0.041^{***}	0.025^{**}
Population	0.019^{**}	0.015^{*}
Wave × Democracy		-0.110^{***}
Wave × Technology		0.029^{***}
Wave × Credit		0.025^{***}
Wave × Population		0.013^{*}
Vietnam		0.026^{***}
Philippines		-0.021^{***}
Iran		-0.010^{*}
R^2	0.025	0.042

$^{*}p < 0.05$, $^{**}p < 0.01$, $^{***}p < 0.001$

Education Effects

Education showed notable effects in preventing economic hardship and sustaining family saving. Likewise, education has reduced economic hardship and facilitated saving (Fridberg and Kangas 2008b; Lusardi and Beeler 2007). These effects register the voluntaristic mechanisms of power realization, utility optimization, norm conformity, and idea consistency.

Activating the voluntaristic mechanism of power realization, education embodies or constitutes power in terms of capability, creativity, expertise, human capital, including cultural capital, learning, personal control, rationalization, self-efficacy, and social status (Corcoran et al. 2011; Dolton et al. 2004; Fiske et al. 1990; Horowitz 2018; Nordin 2011; Papastephanon 2015; Yair 2003). Moreover, education has secured health, knowledge, social status, and verbal ability (Kuppens et al. 2015; Shin 2012; Straughn and Andriot 2011; Whyte and Gao 2009). Social status and other resources raised by education have weakened economic hardship (Whelan et al. 2016). Health and other resources have bolstered saving (Chakrabarty et al. 2008; Lum and Lightfoot 2003).

Relevant to the voluntaristic mechanism of utility optimization, education has reduced the value of hardship (Bullock 2021). Education thus increased the disutility of hardship. Conversely, education has boosted the values of achievement, independence, and work (Fjellvang 2011; James and Luo 1999; Lu, Lum, and Chen 2001). These values indicate the utility of saving as opposed to hardship.

Table 6.11 Substantiation of hypothesized effects on social experiences

Predictor	Hard	Nuisance	Victim	Secure	Saving
Wave	⊖	-	-	+	+
Personal					
Irreligious	+	+	+	-	-
Family income	◇−↓	-	-	+	⊕
Female	+	+	+	-	-
Age	-	+	-	+	+
Age squared	+	+	+	-	-
Married	-	-	-	+	+
Cohabited	-	-	-	+	+
Divorced	+	+	+	-	-
Separated	+	+	+	-	-
Widowed	+	+	+	-	-
Kid	+	+	+	-	-
Mother immigrant	+	+	+	-	-
Father immigrant	+	+	+	-	-
Education	⊖↓	-	-	+	⊕
Graduation age	-	-	-	+	+
Interest	-	-	-	+	+
Living with parents	+	+	-	+	-
Full-time employment	-↑	-	-	+	+
Part-time employment	-	-	-	+	+
Self-employment	-	-	-	+	+
Retired	+	+	+	-	-
Homemaking	+	+	+	-	-
Student	(+)↑	+	+	⊖	-
Unemployed	+↑	+	+	-	-
Public employment	-	-	-	+	+
Private business employment	-	-	-	+	+
Nonprofit organization employment	⊖	⊖	-	◇−	+
Intellectual work	-	-	-	+	+
Creative work	-	◇+	-	◇−	+
Independent work	-	-	-	⊕	+
Supervision	-	-	-	+	+
Earner	-	-	-	+	+
Earner employed	-	-	-	+	+
National					
Population	+	+	◇−↓	◇+↑	-
Phone	-	-	-	+	+
Land	+	-	-	+	-

(continued)

Table 6.11 (continued)

Technology	-	⊖	-	+	+
Credit	⊖	⊖↓	-	◇(-)	+
Prosperity	-	-	-	+	+
Income inequality	+	+↑	+↑	-↓	-
Globalization	-	-	-	+	+
Government effectiveness	-	-	-	⊕	+
Democracy	◇(-)↑	-↑	-	+↑	(-)↓
Liberty	-	◇(+)	-	+	+
Human development	⊖↓	-	-	+	+
Human capital	-	◇(-)	-	+	+
CO_2	+	+	+	-	-
Germany	-				
Egypt				-	
Brazil				-	

Note. Circle: notable and agreeing with the hypothesis; Diamond: notable but contrary to the hypothesis; Bracket: contrary to hypothesis; upward arrow: notably more positive with time; downward arrow: notably more negative with time

In sustaining the voluntaristic mechanism of norm conformity, education registers conformity to social norms through norm acquisition, role modeling or exemplification, and social control (O'Dwyer 2003; Papastephanon 2015; Vanderstraeten 2003). The social norms justify endurance and order as opposed to hardship. Such social norms, socialization, or social control have been conducive to saving as opposed to the experience of hardship (Webley and Nyhus 2006).

In triggering the voluntaristic mechanism of idea consistency, education conveys such ideas of choice, entertainment or enjoyment, excitation, and progress (Teodoro 2003; Yair 2003). Moreover, education has raised well-being including life satisfaction, including satisfaction with safety and security, living standards, self-esteem, and youthfulness (Cerin and Leslie 2008; James and Amato 2013; Kuppens et al. 2015; van Praag and Frijters 1999; Yienprugsawan et al. 2010; Whyte and Gao 2009). Education has buttressed the experiences of benefit, opportunity, security, and support (Hraba et al. 2001; Mau 2005a; Emler and Frazer 1999). Education has also generated willingness to pay, perception about equal opportunity, and justice (Barker and Tinnick 2006; Bullock 2021; Fasakin 2000). In practice, education has facilitated choice, musical involvement, and purchase (Pratt et al. 2010; Stone and Buttice 2010; Van Eijck 2001). These ideas indicate comfort and ease as opposed to hardship. Eventually, education has raised earnings, home possession, and insurance coverage (Cerin and Leslie 2008; Schnittker and Behrman 2012). Earnings, satisfaction, and other ideas have been compatible with the experience of saving as opposed to the experience of hardship (Whelan et al. 2016). Conversely, education has reduced distress, including depression, paranoia, psychoticism, and somatization (Al-krenawi et al. 2011; Snyder et al. 2020). Education has dampened the experiences of arrest, badness, constraint, crime, discrimination, hazards, social exclusion, threat, and victimization (Allwood and Widom 2013; Backman and Nilsson 2011; Cerin and Leslie 2008; Kaukinen 2004; Kessler et al. 1999; Raijman et al. 2003; Stavrova and Ehlebracht 2018; Whyte and Gao 2009). Education has also reduced perception about crime, problems including environmental and unemployment ones, and risk (Nabi and Sullivan 2001; Sjoberg 2003; Staples et al. 1999; Treno and Holder 1997; Wan 1999). In practice, education has diminished deviance, protesting, recourse, and resistance (Backman and Nilsson 2011; Behr et al. 2014; Lubbers et al. 2006; Su and Feng 2013). Education has weakened such dispositions as a need for help (Lessler et al. 2000). These ideas represent hardship. Hence, the weakening of social exclusion and others has sustained the experience of saving as opposed to the experience of hardship (Robila 2006).

Family Income Effects

Family income strengthened the experience of family saving but raised the experience of economic hardship. Likewise, family income has sustained saving (Chakrabarty et al. 2008; Webley and Nyhus 2006). The effects of family income hinge on the voluntaristic mechanisms of power realization, utility optimization, norm conformity, and idea consistency.

Using the voluntaristic mechanism of power realization, family income provides economic resources for saving, and thus family saving. Accordingly, family income has secured family resources, home possession, and homeownership (Cerin and Leslie 2008; Henretta 1987; Yeung et al. 2002). Family resources thus afford family saving.

Through the voluntaristic mechanism of utility optimization, family income sustains saving by raising the utility of saving, and thus family saving. As such, family income has favored saving as opposed to reliance on the public pension and support (Hudson and Jones 2005; Yang and Barrett 2006). The favor or utility of saving or self-reliance thus buttresses saving.

In applying the voluntaristic mechanism of idea consistency, family income generates ideas consistent with and thus propelling family saving. Herein, family income has sustained the feeling of financial adequacy (Powdthavee 2009). Adequacy is consonant with saving (Ribeiro and Soares 2017). Conversely, family income has impeded risk and uncertainty perceptions and the experience of hazards (Cerin and Leslie 2008; Noack et al. 2001; Oliver 2003). Such impedance is consonant with saving (Ribeiro and Soares 2017).

However, based on the voluntaristic mechanism of idea consistency, family income raises economic hardship by boosting aspiration for luxurious living. Herein, hardship and aspiration mean insufficiency and are consonant (Chulef et al. 2001;

Robinaugh et al. 2016). Hence, family income has heightened aspiration (Stutzer 2004; Norris 2011). In turn, aspiration has raised the experience of hardship (Ferssizidis et al. 2010). Moreover, family income has engendered dissatisfaction, protesting, and violence (Farrington 2007; Norris 2011; Norris and Inglehart 2009; Oliver 2003). Dissatisfaction, protesting, and violence are compatible with hardship. Hence, dissatisfaction, protesting, and violence have bred hardship (Ahnquist et al. 2012; Cramer 2000; Zalewski et al. 2017).

With the voluntaristic mechanism of norm conformity, family income provides a social norm about conflict and dysfunction to raise the experience of hardship. Family income has bred the social experience of conflict and dysfunction (Ma et al. 2009; Ruppanner 2010). Such social experiences or norms have sustained the experience of hardship (Walen and Lachman 2016).

Student Status Effects

Student status weakened the experience of security and raised the experience of economic hardship. These effects result from the voluntaristic mechanisms of power realization and idea consistency.

According to the voluntaristic mechanism of power realization, student status impedes the acquisition of power or resources to maintain the experience of security and prevent the experience of economic hardship. Such power or resources include knowledge, social capital, and wealth (Growiec and Growiec 2010; Webber and Huxley 2007; Winterdyk and Thompson 2008). Knowledge, social capital, and wealth have buttressed the experience of security and dispelled the experience of hardship (Brisson 2009; Frank et al. 2014; Sacks and Levi 2010; Scholz and Pinney 1995; Whelan et al. 2016). Thus, student status breeds the experiences of hardship and insecurity.

Applying the voluntaristic mechanism of idea consistency, student status sustains ideas compatible with and thus conducive to the experience of hardship and insecurity. These ideas have transpired in the experiences of stress and victimization (Arsandaux et al. 2021; Hansen-Nord et al. 2014). Student status has also raised the perception of theft (Winterdyk and Thompson 2008). Moreover, student status has engendered feelings of anxiety, depression, dissatisfaction with life, and stagnation (Arsandaux et al. 2021; Rampichini and D'Andrea 1998). In practice, student status has evoked evasion of payment and purchase, protesting, reliance on government and its welfare, and suicidal ideation (Arsandaux et al. 2021; Bosma et al. 2016; Matheson and Wearing 1999; Olcese et al. 2014; Winterdyk and Thompson 2008). Stress and the others are idealistically consistent with hardship and insecurity. The former thus have sustained the experiences of hardship and insecurity (Fernandes 2018; La Guardia et al. 2000; Suldo 2004; Yu and Gamble 2008).

Nonprofit Organization Effects

Nonprofit organization employment, meaning work engagement without gaining profit from work, relieved the experiences of economic hardship and neighborhood nuisance and diminished the experience of security. The latter echoes the existing finding that nonprofit organization employment has raised the experience of stress, notably job security (Brolis and Nyssens 2020; Hamann and Foster 2014). These employment or organizational effects embody the voluntaristic mechanisms of power realization, utility optimization, norm conformity, and idea consistency.

Through the voluntaristic mechanism of power realization, nonprofit organization employment enhances power or resources to prevent economic hardship and nuisance. Such power or resources have appeared in seniority, training, wage, and earning efficacy (Ben-Ner and Ren 2015; Brolis and Nyssens 2020; Noe and Forgione 2014). These resources have lessened the experiences of hardship and nuisance (Tenorio and Lo 2011; Whelan et al. 2016).

Working with the voluntaristic mechanism of utility optimization, nonprofit organization employment buttresses the utility of avoiding economic hardship and neighborhood nuisance. Accordingly, such employment has raised the values of community and freedom as opposed to hardship and nuisance (Robichau and Sandberg 2022). The values, in turn, have eroded the experiences of hardship and nuisance (Frantz 2013).

Relying on the voluntaristic mechanism of norm conformity, nonprofit organization employment induces the norms of preventing economic hardship and neighborhood nuisance. Such norms, inherent in the nonprofit organization, advocate autonomy, commonwealth, desirability, development, freedom, helpfulness, opportunity, philanthropy, problem-solving, safety, and self-determination (Harkema 2022; Hatcher and Hammond 2018; Heinrich 2000; LeRoux 2007; Polson 2017; Wo 2018; Salamon and Sokolowski 2016; Zatepilina-Monacell 2012). In addition, the nonprofit organization breeds the norms of charity, religion, and welfare (Hasenfeld and Powell 2004; Kovic and Hänsli 2018; Miller-Stevens et al. 2018). The nonprofit organization has also maintained the norms of altruism, flexibility, quality, and service as opposed to debt (Brolis and Nyssens 2020; Miller-Stevens et al. 2018; Noe and Forgione 2014). As such, the norms emphasize helpfulness and wellness as opposed to hardship and nuisance. These emphases have mitigated the experiences of hardship and nuisance (Amiot et al. 2017; Brisson 2009; Sampson and Raudenbush 2004).

Applying the voluntaristic mechanistic mechanism of idea consistency, nonprofit organization employment upholds ideas contradicting and thus dismissing economic hardship and neighborhood nuisance. Such ideas have transpired in the experiences of autonomy as opposed to monotony (Ariza-Montes and Lucia-Casademunt 2016). In addition, nonprofit organization employment has boosted satisfaction with salary and emotional involvement (Ariza-Montes and Lucia-Casademunt 2016). These ideas have prevented the experiences of economic hardship and nuisance (Reeskens and Vandecasteele 2017; Moen et al. 2013).

Creative Work Effects

Creative work increased the experience of neighborhood nuisance and diminished the experience of security. This increase and diminishment work through the voluntaristic mechanisms of power realization, utility optimization, norm conformity, and idea consistency.

With the voluntaristic mechanism of power realization, creative work deprives power or resources to prevent the experiences of insecurity and nuisance. Such deprivation happens in difficulty, persistence, and social isolation in creative work (Prabhu et al. 2008; Runco 2014; Sternberg 2001; Whitton 2018). Resource deprivation has fomented the experience of insecurity and nuisance (Ostberg 2003; Peruzzi 2014; Sacks and Levi 2010).

Applying the voluntaristic mechanism of utility optimization, creative work downplays the utility or values of comfort and security, thus substantiating the experiences of insecurity and nuisance. Such downplaying transpires in the values of insecurity and nuisance in terms of complexity, detachment, normlessness, obsession, radicalism, self-control, self-effacement, and unpredictability in creative work as opposed to conservatism (Joas 1996; Lan and Kaufman 2012; Niu and Kaufman 2013; Rubenstein 2000; Runco 2014; Shorthose and Maycroft 2017; Sundararajan and Raina 2016; Simonton 2003; Zhang and Sternberg 2012). These values have maintained the experiences of insecurity and nuisance (Brown and Symons 2016; Hocking et al. 2016; Muris et al. 2003; Weinberg et al. 2021).

Using the voluntaristic mechanism of norm conformity, creative work reflects the norms of the creative organization to breed the experiences of insecurity and nuisance. Such organizational norms advocate change and protesting (Mosca and della Porta 2009; Wang and Soule 2016). These norms have been conducive to the experiences of insecurity and nuisance (Kanan and Pruitt 2002; Peltonen et al. 2010).

Working with the voluntaristic mechanism of idea consistency, creative work engenders ideas consonant and thus underlies the experiences of insecurity and nuisance. Such ideas highlight aggression, contradiction, flexibility, redirection, and transformation (Israelstam 2007; Runco 2014; Sternberg 2003; Van Leeuwen and Baas 2017; Zittoun and Gillespie 2016). These ideas have sustained the experiences of insecurity and nuisance (Carter and Wolfe 2021; Valera and Guardia 2014).

Independent Work Effects

Independent work raised the experience of security. Notably, the experience of independence has contributed to the experience of security (Valera and Guardia 2014). The contribution of independence or its setting hinges on the voluntaristic mechanisms of power realization, utility optimization, norm conformity, and idea consistency.

Based on the voluntaristic mechanism of power realization, independent work affords power or resources to sustain the experience of security. Essentially, independence reflects capability including employability, competitiveness, and resourcefulness (Laruffa 2020; McLean 2015; Ryan and Deci 2017; Stavrova and Ehlebracht 2018). Specifically, power or resources generated by independent work include influence and productivity (Franzen and Hangartner 2006; Wells et al. 2003). Independent work has also fostered competence, creativity, earnings, knowledgeability, and skill (Bekker et al. 2011; de Witte et al. 2007; Peng et al. 2019; Ross and Mirowsky 1996; Soenens and Vansteenkiste 2005; Yeh and Yang 2006). These power or resources have enabled the experience of security (Gaitan-Rossi and Shen 2018; Knight and Song 2005; Valera and Guardia 2014).

Through the voluntaristic mechanism of utility optimization, independent work boosts the utility or value of security to sustain the experience of security. Such utility embraces commitment and predictability (Giffords 2009; Reeve et al. 2004; Xanthopoulou et al. 2009). These values underlie the experience of security (La Guardia et al. 2000; Probst 2000).

Applying he voluntaristic mechanism of norm conformity, independent work registers the workplace norm to raise the experience of security. Such a norm has contributed to job satisfaction (Tsai and Huang 2007). Job satisfaction, in turn, has buttressed the experience of security (La Guardia et al. 2000).

Through the voluntaristic mechanism of idea consistency, independent work generates ideas consistent and thus conducive to the experience of security. Such ideas signify achievement, consistency, identity, satisfaction well-being, as opposed to problems (Christopher et al. 2012; Franzese 2013; Laruffa 2020; Pfeiffer and Pinquart 2012; Reeve et al. 2004; Yeh and Yang 2006). Thus, independent work has raised effectiveness, performance, well-being, including financial adequacy, mastery, quality of work, satisfaction with the job and life, and self-esteem (Anderson-Connolly 2002; De Moortel et al. 2015; Delhey 2010; Gagne and Deci 2005; Gahlawat et al. 2019; Kam et al. 2012; Roy and Chaudhuri 2008; Ryan and Deci 2017; Schieman 2002; Schieman and Narisada 2014; Visser et al. 2016; Weinstein and Ryan 2010). These ideas have been conducive to the experience of security (Gaitan-Rossi and Shen 2018; La Guardia et al. 2000; Salehi 2012).

National Population Effects

National population size reduced the personal experience of victimization and raised the personal security experience. The effects work through direct and indirect deterministic mechanisms, emphasizing empowering, incentivizing, and framing.

With the direct deterministic mechanism, national population size diminishes the experiences of insecurity and victimization and share them among people privately or publicly. Herein, national population size has reduced insecurity and victimization (Browning et al. 2004; Hughes et al. 2015). Collective insecurity and victimization have induced the personal experiences of insecurity and victimization (Gaitan-Rossi and Shen 2018; Kanan and Pruitt 2002; Schutte 2015).

Through the indirect deterministic mechanism of empowering, national population size enhances power or resources for prevention to undercut the experiences of insecurity and victimization. Such power or resources are evident in wages and others (Glaeser et al. 2009; J. Turner 2013). National population size also reflects the power of talent and technology (J. Turner 2010). The power or resources have prevented the experience of insecurity and victimization (Emery and Wu 2020; Hansen-Nord et al. 2014; Reese et al. 2021; Valera and Guardia 2014).

Leveraging the indirect deterministic mechanism of incentivizing, national population size generates incentives for preventing insecurity and victimization to dampen the personal experiences of insecurity and victimization. Such incentives have stemmed from demand for productivity and punishment, notably capital punishment (Havinga 2002; Turner 1984). The incentive and sanctioning have discouraged the practices of risk and violence (Berger 2005; Van Knippenberg et al. 2007). The practices experienced in society have eventually lessened the experiences of insecurity and victimization (Valera and Guardia 2014; Viola et al. 2016).

Equipped with the indirect deterministic mechanism of framing, national population size frames ideas for preventing insecurity and victimization to lessen the corresponding personal experiences. Such ideas have highlighted development, quality of life, or well-being and discouraged conflict, migration, and rebellion (Abouharb and Cingranelli 2007; Frey et al. 1997; Morenoff and Sampson 1997; Ryckman 2019). The highlighting and discouragement have impeded the experiences of insecurity and victimization (Graham et al. 2010; Schwartz et al. 2003; Valera and Guardia 2014; Vitoroulis and Georgiades 2017).

National Bank Credit Effects

National bank credit offered by banks weakened the experiences of economic hardship and neighborhood nuisance, and the experience of security. The effects work through direct and indirect deterministic mechanisms, emphasizing empowering and framing.

Through the direct deterministic mechanism, national bank credit substitutes immaterial credit for physical security (Haiven 2014). This substitution thereby diminishes the experience of security collectively and personally. Moreover, national bank credit facilitates liquidity to raise alienation, disjuncture, deregulation, precarity, uncertainty, and unmooring (Haiven 2014). National bank credit also creates debts (Haiven 2014). These are experiences of insecurity. Conversely, national bank credit or its induced investment weakens national stability and people's social identity and obligation (Haiven 2014; Hollyer et al. 2018). This weakening translates into the erosion of the personal experience of security.

Using the indirect deterministic mechanism of empowering, national bank credit strengthens power or resources to prevent personal experiences of economic hardship and nuisance. Such power has consisted in creativity, economic growth, and prosperity (Chang et al. 2008; Haiven 2014). The national power has eroded the personal experiences of economic hardship and nuisance (Fridberg and Kangas 2008; Grasso and Giugni 2016), creativity has notably facilitated stress management (Gebbia and Honigsfeld 2012). Furthermore, national bank credit facilitates investment and production and thus shareholding (Haiven 2014). National investment, in turn, has fostered economic development and growth, employment, export, and urbanization (Farla 2015; Schofer and Cranados 2006). Moreover, national investment has raised personal income (Lei and Yao 2008). These contributions of national investment have eroded economic hardship and nuisance (Fridberg and Kangas 2008; Olson et al. 2016; Tenorio and Lo 2011; Whelan et al. 2016).

Meanwhile, in using the indirect deterministic mechanism of empowering, national bank credit also introduces disempowering to erode the experience of security. National bank credit or its facilitated investment has diminished national environmental sustainability and elevated national inequality (Chatterjee and Turnovsky 2012; Frey et al. 1997). These impacts have impaired the experience of security (Ho 1998; Salehi 2012).

Applying the indirect deterministic mechanism of framing, national bank credit induces the frames to lessen the personal experiences of hardship and nuisance. The framed ideas are autonomy, freedom, imagination, individuality, and possibility (Haiven 2014). Moreover, national investment facilitated by national bank credit has boosted national and personal quality of life or well-being, notably life satisfaction (Frey et al. 1997; Gehring 2013; Ram 2009). These framed ideas have eroded the experience of hardship and nuisance (Cramer 2000; Greenberg 1999; Suldo 2004).

National Technology Effects

In terms of the number of scientific and technical journal articles apiece, national technology diminished the personal experience of neighborhood nuisance. The diminishment realizes through the indirect deterministic mechanisms of empowering, standardizing, and framing.

Applying the indirect deterministic mechanism of empowering, national technology endows power or resource to prevent the personal experience of nuisance. Such power enhances people's autonomy, communication, cooperation, and learning (Chen 2008; Fukuyama 2003; Welzel and Inglehart 2010). National technology has also raised people's employment, environmental quality, income, knowledge, and resources for action (Chen 2008; Florida 2005; Goetz et al. 2011; Welsch 2002; Welzel 2013). These power or resources have been bases for boosting neighborhood quality and alleviating neighborhood nuisance (Olson et al. 2016; Sampson and Raudenbush 2004; Whitham 2012).

With the indirect deterministic mechanism of standardizing, national technology disseminates social norms to prevent the practice and experience of nuisance. Such norms evolve from schooling facilitated by national technology (Dahlberg et al.

2018). Specifically, school norms emphasize citizenship, civic-mindedness, collaboration, compliance, cultivating, humanizing, pacifying, and serving, as opposed to risk (Brown 2001; Elmore 2009; George et al. 1998; Lawrence 2000; Sung and Yang 2009). Such norms have minimized nuisance practice (Dahlberg 2007; Foshee et al. 2013; Heyman and Slep 2007; Lee and Song 2012; Walters 2020). These norms and practices in the neighborhood have eroded the personal experience of neighborhood nuisance (Olson et al. 2016; Whitham 2012).

With the indirect deterministic mechanism of framing, national technology frames ideas conducive to preventing the practice and thus experience of nuisance. These ideas highlight ease, education, lifesaving, opportunity, possibility, or prospect, pleasure, rationality, resolution, and satisfaction (Goetz et al. 2011; Matthewman 2011; Roderick 2016; Zhu 1995). Such ideas have discouraged people's practice of nuisance (Felson and Outlaw 2007; Gotzsche-Astrup 2020; Pulkkinen et al. 2009; Pauwels and De Waele 2014; Santoro and Broidy 2014). The ideas have thus lessened the personal experience of others' nuisance (Arnett 2018; Cramer 2000; Palker-Corell and Marcus 2004; Suldo 2004).

National Talent Effects

National talent or human capital, which includes earnings and education, diminished the personal experience of neighborhood nuisance. Hence, national talent has reduced people's practice nuisance (Poveda 2011). This reduction thus leads to the diminishment of the personal experience of nuisance. The diminishment hinges on the indirect deterministic mechanisms of empowering, standardizing, and framing.

Using the indirect deterministic mechanism of empowering, national talent empowers people to prevent nuisance, thus lessening the personal experience of nuisance. National talent embodies capability, knowledge, and skill (Kelly 2020; Olssen et al. 2004). Furthermore, national talent boosts productivity to generate resources and afford accomplishment (Corrigan et al. 2013; Olssen et al. 2004). National talent also enables coping, deliberation, dialogue, self-reflection, and self-regulation or self-control (Bowker 2016; Corrigan et al. 2013; Olssen et al. 2004; Stevenson 2011). Hence, national talent has lifted people's health, income, intelligence, and social capital (Herian et al. 2014; Lipford and Yandle 2009; Portes and Vickstrom 2011; Schaie 2013). Such power or resources have prevented people's practice of nuisance (Ishoy 2017; Stogner et al. 2014). The prevention, in turn, has reduced the personal experience of nuisance (Greenberg 1999). Conversely, national talent has reduced people's illness, obesity, and poverty (Goetz et al. 2011; Herian et al. 2014; Jones et al. 2015). The reduction has lessened the experience of nuisance (Sampson and Raudenbush 2004).

By the indirect deterministic mechanism of standardizing, national talent generates social norms to prevent the practice and experience of nuisance. Such norms evolve from schooling sustained by national talent (Hostetler et al. 2007). Schooling upholds norms treasuring citizenship, civic-mindedness, collaboration, compliance, cultivating, humanizing, pacifying, and serving, as opposed to risk (Brown 2001;

Elmore 2009; George et al. 1998; Lawrence 2000; Sung and Yang 2009). Such norms have forestalled the practice of nuisance (Dahlberg 2007; Foshee et al. 2013; Heyman and Slep 2007; Lee and Song 2012; Walters 2020). These norms and practices in the neighborhood have mitigated the personal experience of neighborhood nuisance (Olson et al. 2016; Whitham 2012).

Applying the indirect deterministic mechanism of framing, national talent fosters ideas resisting the practice and experience of nuisance. Such framed ideas are caring, compassion, or sympathy, citizenship, cohesion, commonwealth, community, empathy, moderation, prosociality, rationality, respect, and virtue (Corrigan et al. 2013; Olssen et al. 2004; Shan 2017; Stevenson 2011). These ideas have prevented people's practice of nuisance (Pauwels and De Waele 2014; Pulkkinen et al. 2009; Su et al. 2010). The prevention, in turn, has diminished the experience of nuisance (Greenberg 1999; Olson et al. 2016). Conversely, national talent frames ideas against blackmailing, domination, interference, and subversion (Lee and Song 2012; Olssen et al. 2004; Stevenson 2011). National talent has also reduced people's perception of corruption, practice of smoking, and disposition of extremity, racism, and violence (Collier 2002; Herian et al. 2014; Meisenberg and Williams 2008; Oliver and Mendelberg 2000; Poveda 2011). The reduction has diminished the nuisance experience (Olson et al. 2016).

National Human Development Effects

National human development, comprising that in economic, educational, and health aspects, alleviated the personal experience of economic hardship. The alleviation rests on the direct deterministic mechanism and indirect deterministic mechanisms of empowering and framing.

With the direct deterministic mechanism, national human development successfully reduces the collective and personal experiences of hardship. The reduced collective experience involves those of cost, hunger, loss, poverty, and welfare dependence (Harkhess 2007; Johnson 2009; Rabbani 2011).

Through the indirect mechanism of empowering, national human development strengthens power or resources for preventing economic hardship and thus its personal experience. Such power or resources are capabilities, education, employment, income, motivation, social capital, and wealth (Booysen 2002; Charles 2011; Inglehart and Welzel 2005; Nederveen Pieterse 2010). They enable capacitation, production, and productivity (C. Johnson 2009; Nederveen Pieterse 2010). National human development has also raised people's health and knowledge (Eikemo et al. 2008; Hadden et al. 2003; Norris 2011).

Working with the indirect mechanism of framing, national human development generates ideas contradictory to and thus preventing the personal experience of economic hardship. These framed ideas foreground well-being, notably happiness and life satisfaction (Castles 2000; Diener and Tov 2012). Well-being has lessened the experience of economic hardship (Caputo 2003; Julkunen 2002; Redmond and Skattebol 2019).

National Liberty Effects

National liberty raised the personal experience of neighborhood nuisance. The raising works through the indirect deterministic mechanisms of incentivizing and framing.

With the indirect deterministic mechanism of incentivizing, national liberty incentivizes nuisance and thus its experience. Accordingly, national liberty lessens the values of character, commonwealth, community, duty, morality, non-harm, protection for other people, regulation, responsibility, and virtue (Bavetta et al. 2014; Pevnick 2015; Rasmussen and Den Uyl 2005; Sadurski 1999). Such lessening has bred the practice of nuisance (Belanger et al. 2019; Farrington 2018; Piquero and Hickman 2002; Pulkkinen et al. 2009). The practice has constituted the experience of neighborhood nuisance (Olson et al. 2016; Sampson and Raudenbush 2004).

Through the indirect deterministic mechanism of framing, national liberty frames ideas conducive to the personal experience of neighborhood nuisance. These ideas involve immorality, incivility, interference, protesting, and uncooperativeness (Hamilton 2008; Kekes 1997; Zhang 2022). National liberty has also lifted perception about corruption (Collier 2002). These ideas have sustained the experience of neighborhood nuisance (Greenberg 1999; Olson et al. 2016).

National Democracy Effects

National democracy lowered the personal experience of economic hardship. The lowering works through the direct deterministic mechanism and indirect deterministic mechanisms of empowering, incentivizing, standardizing, and framing.

Using the direct deterministic mechanism, national democracy sustains collective experience to erode the personal experience of economic hardship. This collective experience has been national prosperity (Rindermann 2008). National prosperity, in turn, has diminished the personal experience of economic hardship (Fridberg and Kangas 2008).

Activating the indirect deterministic mechanism of empowering, national democracy affords power or resources to prevent the personal experience of economic hardship. Such power or resources are people's capability, education, information, motivation, and welfare or subsidies (Abizadeh 2002; Mukherjee 2000; O'Dwyer 2003; O'Neill 2000; Peter 2009; Pettit 2012; Tilly 2009). The power or resources have prevented the experience of economic hardship (Fridberg and Kangas 2008; Ireland and Kim 2001).

By the indirect deterministic mechanism of incentivizing, national democracy incentivizes practices to avoid the personal experiences of economic hardship. Such incentivizing applies to the practices of cooperation, entrepreneurship, sharing, and work (Abizadeh 2002; Christians et al. 2009; Peng et al. 2017). These practices or their experiences have prevented the personal experience of economic hardship (Robila 2006; Saunders et al. 2014).

Using the indirect deterministic mechanism of standardizing, national democracy cultivates social norms against the personal experience of economic hardship. Such norms, which constitute the democratic culture, emphasize people's education, efficacy, and powerfulness (Tan 2003). These norms have induced the prevention of economic hardship to lower the corresponding experience (Clain 2007; Goetz et al. 2011).

Applying the indirect deterministic mechanism of framing, national democracy frames ideas contradicting and thus mitigating the personal experience of economic hardship. Such ideas include people's abundance, access, autonomy, dignity, emancipation, empowerment, entitlement, freedom, happiness, justice, life quality, peace, protection, security, self-determination, self-development, stability, and tolerance (Blokker 2018; Brennan 2016; Caprara and Vecchione 2017; Ceva and Zuolo 2013; Femia 1993; Glasson 2015; Levi 2003; Munck 2005; Ney and Molenaars 1999; O'Neill 2000; Peng et al. 2017; Ringen 2007; Safford 2002; Saward 1998; Tilly 2009; Warren 2011). Furthermore, national democracy has raised the person's perception of freedom and feeling of life satisfaction and self-efficacy (Corcoran et al. 2011; Frey and Stutzer 2000; Moller and Skaaning 2013). National democracy has also sustained trust in the institution and law (Norris 1999a, 1999b). In addition, national democracy has buttressed national peace (Moller and Skaaning 2013). These ideas have dispelled the experience of economic hardship (Caputo 2003; Dekkers 2008). Conversely, national democracy demeans such ideas as alienation, coercion, domination, exploitation, interference, oppression, manipulation, and violence (Brennan 2016; Fairfield 2008; Femia 1993; Mukherjee 2000; O'Neill 2000; Pettit 2012). Moreover, national democracy has diminished the person's protesting (Solt 2015). Such diminishment has weakened the experience of economic hardship (Dekkers 2008; Julkunen 2002; Robila 2006; Whelan and Maitre 2013).

National Government Effectiveness Effects

National government effectiveness lifted the personal experience of security. This lifting accords with reducing the personal experience of problems by the effectiveness (Wong and Wan 2011). The lifting applies the indirect deterministic mechanisms of empowering, incentivizing, and framing.

Using the indirect deterministic mechanism of empowering, national government effectiveness raises people's power or capability to maintain security. As such, national government effectiveness has sustained economic resources or prosperity in the country. (Guisan 2009). These resources have sustained the experience of security (Gaitan-Rossi and Shen 2018; Kanan and Pruitt 2002).

By the indirect deterministic mechanism of incentivizing, national government effectiveness incentivizes the provision of social security to boost the personal experience of security. National government effectiveness has raised the desire for or utility of social security (Wong et al. 2005). The provision of social security has evolved from people's desire for social security (Brooks and Manza 2006). This provision, in turn, has contributed to health or living (Coburn 2004). Such contribution has eventually buttressed the experience of security (Rader et al. 2012; Sacks and Levi 2010).

Through the indirect deterministic mechanism of framing, national government effectiveness frames ideas conducive to the experience of security. These ideas have been well-being, notably satisfaction with democracy and police, perceptions of government legitimacy, justice, living standards, and social harmony, and trust in government, other institutions, people, and policy (Bohnke 2008; Bratton and Mattes 2001; Grimes 2006; Guisan 2009; Heatherington and Globetti 2002; Mizrahi 2016; Nunkoo and Smith 2013; Tankebe 2009; Wolfe et al. 2016; Wong and Shik 2011). These ideas have contributed to the experience of security (La Guardia et al. 2000). Conversely, national government effectiveness has reduced suicidal attempts (Carter and Wolfe 2021; Helliwell 2006; Sacks and Levi 2010). The reduction sustains productivity, income, and thus the experience of security as opposed to suffering (Cosculluela 1995; Feldman 2006).

Time Effects

Time or the survey wave diminished the personal experience of economic hardship and its susceptibility to education, family income, and national human development. By contrast, time raised the susceptibility of the experience of economic hardship to full-time employment, student status, unemployment, and national democracy. Time also escalated the influences of national population size on the experience of security, the influences of national income inequality on the experiences of neighborhood nuisance and victimization, and the influences of national democracy on neighborhood nuisance and security. Meanwhile, time shrank the influences of national population size on the experience of victimization, the influence of national bank credit on the experience of neighborhood nuisance, the influence of national inequality on the experience of security, and the influence of national democracy on family saving. These time effects apply the direct and indirect deterministic mechanisms of empowering and framing.

With the direct deterministic mechanism, time reduces national or collective economic hardship and the personal experience of economic hardship successively. Notably, time has escalated national or collective prosperity (Norris 2012). The sharing of collective prosperity privately or publicly has reduced the experience of economic hardship (Fridberg and Kangas 2008).

Using the indirect deterministic mechanism of empowering, time raises people's power or resources for preventing the personal experience of economic hardship. Such power or resources include employment or working, homeownership, knowledge, wage, and family income (Campbell and Pearlman 2013; Conley and Gifford 2006; Francesconi and Golsch 2005; Gershuny 2000; Singer et al. 1999; van Praag and Ferrer-I-Carbonell 2004). These resources have mitigated the experience of economic hardship (Muhlau 2014; Robinaugh et al. 2016; Whelan et al. 2016).

With the indirect deterministic mechanism of framing, time increases the frames of ideas diminishing the personal experience of economic hardship. These ideas register in the experience of safety and satisfaction with finance and welfare (Hsieh 2002; Smith et al. 2001; Wong et al. 2010). These ideas have weakened the experience of economic hardship (Hallerod 2006; Ireland and Kim 2001). Conversely, time has reduced people's borrowing (Brown et al. 2005). Borrowing has been indicative of economic hardship (Li 2010).

Time increased employment status influences, including full-time employment, student status, unemployment, national income inequality, and national democracy. The increased influences of employment or work, inequality, and democracy reflect modernization (Andreeva et al. 2017; Han and Shim 2010; Inglehart and Welzel 2005; Sanchez 2007; Scaff 2000). Notably, the influence of employment means a difference due to employment or social class, and the difference signifies inequality. The influences apply the direct deterministic mechanism to sharing ideas for employment, inequality, and democracy. With the indirect deterministic mechanism of framing, modernization additionally raises the frames of ideas for choice, earning, economic activity, and professionalization (Andreeva et al. 2017; Heaphy 2007; Inglehart and Welzel 2005; Martinelli 2005). These ideas have strengthened the values of democracy, employment, and inequality (Castillo 2011; Chen and Zhong 1998; Sing 2004; Sing and Lee 1999).

Time eroded the influences of education, family income, national bank credit, and national human development. As such, the influences of resources declined with time. According to the indirect deterministic mechanism of incentivizing, this decline follows the increased abundance of resources. Herein, resources including education, employment, homeownership, knowledge, skill, wage, wealth, family income, and national prosperity have grown with time (Campbell and Pearlman 2013; Conley and Gifford 2006; Francesconi and Golsch 2005; Greenfield 2009; Norris 2012; Singer et al. 1999; van Praag and Ferrer-I-Carbonell 2004).

Summary

The stressful social experiences of economic hardship, neighborhood nuisance, victimization, insecurity, and family non-saving were somehow consistently predictable by education, nonprofit organization employment, creative work, national population size, and national bank credit. These experiences were also sporadically predictable by time, family income, student status, independent work, national technology, national government effectiveness, national liberty, national democracy, national talent, and national human development. The predictions follow the voluntaristic and deterministic mechanisms of analytical functionalism.

The voluntaristic mechanism of power realization emphasizes the availability of power or resources to prevent stressful experiences. Such power stems from education and independent work, which lowered the stressful experience. In addition, family income can provide resources to sustain family saving specifically.

The voluntaristic mechanism of utility optimization accentuates the utility of stress reduction as a contributor to stress reduction. This utility can grow with education, which turned out to be an essential contributor to stress reduction.

The voluntaristic mechanism of norm conformity highlights social norms for stress reduction as a contributor to stress reduction. Such norms can originate from nonprofit organization employment, which dampens the stressful experience.

The voluntaristic mechanism of idea consistency focuses on ideas for rationalizing the experience of stress or its reduction. Ideas conducive to stress reduction can emanate from independent work, which lessened the stressful experience. By contrast, ideas sustaining stress can derive from creative work, which raised the stressful experience.

The direct deterministic mechanism maintains that private or public sharing of collective experience determines personal experience. Such collective experience is national human development, which weakened the personal experience of stress.

The indirect deterministic mechanism of empowering holds that national empowering enables the reduction of stressful personal experiences. Such empowering can evolve from national population size, talent, technology, bank credit, government effectiveness, and democracy, which dampened the experiences.

The indirect deterministic mechanism of incentivizing posits that the nation provides incentives for boosting stress reduction, thus lowering stressful personal experiences. Such incentives can increase with national government effectiveness, which diminished the stressful personal experience. Notably, the mechanism underlies the dwindled influence of resources with time because of the increase in resources. That is, the deterministic incentivizing mechanism constrains the voluntaristic power realization mechanism.

The indirect deterministic mechanism of standardizing rests on the collective provision of norms for or against the personal practice and experience of stress. Such provision can arise from national democracy and government effectiveness, which are institutional factors promulgating norms to weaken stressful personal experiences.

The indirect deterministic mechanism of framing postulates that national frames of ideas shape the personal practice and experience of stress. Such frames can be widely available from all national factors. Notably, national liberty can frame ideas raising stressful practices and experiences.

Chapter 7
Life Practice Production: Theory

Personal practices relevant to life quality are public engagement and informational activity. Public engagement comprises appealing, strike participation, organizational participation, green demonstration, spiritual activity, green donation, and informational activity comprises e-activity and learning. Appealing, in turn, encompasses joining boycotts, attending peaceful demonstrations, and signing a petition. Organizational participation includes that in an environmental, consumer, humanitarian, professional, art, music, or education, labor, political, sport or recreational, self-help, and religious organization. E-activity comprises using the Internet, personal computer, and email. Learning comprises reading printed magazines, reading daily newspapers, listening to radio news, using the mobile phone, talking with friends or colleagues, and watching TV news. Among the practices, risk aversion raised worry, while weapon carrying diminished it (see Table 4.8). Generally, the practices indicated negative effects on life quality, including health, life satisfaction, delight, and non-worry. Thus, while weapon carrying represents defending or safeguarding and other practices manifest fidgeting worsening life quality. This worsening indicates that inaction or tranquility is typically salutary.

Functionalist Explanation for Practices

Analytical-functionalist theory specifies voluntaristic and deterministic mechanisms to explain practice with personal and collective factors. Voluntaristic mechanisms embody power realization to achieve the function of fulfilling or goal attainment, utility optimization to achieve the function of adaptation, norm conformity to achieve the function of integration, and idea consistency to achieve the function of latency. Deterministic mechanisms work directly or indirectly through empowering to achieve the function of fulfilling, incentivizing to achieve the function of adaptation, standardizing to achieve the function of integration, and framing to achieve the function of latency.

C. Cheung, *Production Dynamics for Life Quality in the Incipient 21st Century*,
https://doi.org/10.1007/978-981-19-3827-6_7

The voluntaristic mechanism of realization emphasizes using power for driving practice to attain goals. Such power arises from personal activation or arousal due to emotion, mood, or needs and mobilization received (Donohew et al. 1987; Matthewman 2011; Silver 2011). Such emotions as anxiety and passion are influential accordingly (Silver 2011). Needs rest on psychic or emotional forces toward autonomy, cognitive closure, cognitive consonance, cognitive equilibrium, egocentrism, justice, meaning, novelty, reason, security, and self-love (Elster 2011, 2015; Turner 2013). Similarly, practice happens to attain goals (Eccles and Wigfield 2002). Such attainment involves the force of motivation, notably the intrinsic kind (Eccles and Wigfield 2002; Turner 2013). Motivation, in turn, builds on the consciousness of others' discourses and practices (Turner 2013). Power also rests on competence and self-efficacy (Eccles and Wigfield 2002). Conversely, power can constrain practice with self-control or self-regulation (Eccles and Wigfield 2002; Hofmann et al. 2012). More socially grounded, power can derive from education, income, organizational membership, and social class, characterized by the ownership of cultural, economic, social, and symbolic or status capital (Donohew et al. 1987; Michael 2017; Stolle 2001; Turner 2013). Hence, education and income have facilitated practice (Bonke and Fallesen 2010; Donohew et al. 1987).

The voluntaristic mechanism of optimization highlights the weighing of expected or received gain from practice for gravitating toward the practice. Such gain can be affective such as affective attachment and the feelings of attainment, enjoyment, equity, flow, functionality, instrumentality, justice, meaning, saving, self-worth, success, utility, and the demonstration of values (Bunge 1996; Gears and Lassiter 2002; Cook et al. 2013; Eccles and Wigfield 2002; Elster 2000; Scaff 2014; Tyler 2012). The feeling of flow upholds awareness, control, focus, and immersion as opposed to self-consciousness (Eccles and Wigfield 2002). Conversely, practice arises to avoid effort, futility, loss, risk, and shame or shamefulness (Bunge 1996; de Jonge 2012; Elster 2015; Michael 2017). Meanwhile, the feeling of self-worth rises with the sense of improvement, mastery, or perseverance and declines with competition, evaluation, or social comparison (Eccles and Wigfield 2002). Expected gain means the attribution, expectancy for, hope for, and understanding of the gain and its feasibility from the practice or similar ones, as under dependence and deprivation (Cook et al. 2013; de Jonge 2012; Eccles and Wigfield 2002; Ginev 2018; Snyder 2000). The expected gain can rest on the gain from similar practices (Mallard 2020). Gain from personal practice, and thus the practice diminishes with companionship or marriage through shared or vicarious gain (Donohew et al. 1987). Expectation also concerns the availability of resources for practice (Watts 2014). The expectation, in turn, hinges on the realization of opportunity or vacancy to gain from practice (Hedstrom 2005). Such realization evolves from learning about gain (Donohew et al. 1987). More generally, in fulfilling the function of adaptation, practice is a response to a stimulus (Cook et al. 2013; Jones 2001). Notably, personal practice has declined with marriage and companionship because of spousal sharing and thus reducing the utility of personal practice (Donohew et al. 1987). By contrast, personal practice has increased with parenthood or the number of children because of the responsibility and thus utility of the practice, such as parenting (Bonke and Fallesen 2010). Personal practice has also increased with residency, which raises the utility of practice for living places (Stolle 2001).

The voluntaristic mechanism of conformity regards social norms to guide practice as assimilating. Conformity can take the forms of affinity, contagion, imitation, and learning about norms (Donohew et al. 1987; Hedstrom 2005; Tharp 2012). The social domain identifies a field covering atmosphere, ecology, life space, self-category, and teamwork (Ellemers and Haslam 2012; Martin 2011). Social norms are manifest in acceptance, custom, expert judgment, injunction, popularity, and tradition (Cialdini 2012; Elster 2000, 2015; Scaff 2014).

The voluntaristic mechanism of consistency cherishes rationalizing to maintain consistency among practices, attitudes, and dispositions. Accordingly, practice arises from the personal consciousness about deflection or the discrepancy between expectation and experience in affect in terms of activeness, evaluation, and potency in the definition of a situation (Heise 1999; Owens et al. 2010). More generally, practice results from dissonance among practices, attitudes, and dispositions (Westermann 1989). Social dominance orientation is a crucial disposition or orientation orienting practice to dominate others (Sidanius and Pratto 2012). Another vital disposition is identity, including social one, which entails monitoring and verification (Burke and Stets 2009; Ellemers and Haslam 2012; Owens et al. 2010). Similarly, the perceived role, rule, and self-category are other criteria for maintaining consistency with practice (Eagly and Wood 2012; Ellemers and Haslam 2012; Jost and van der Toom 2012; Miller 2001). Other influential dispositions are altruism, authoritarianism, belief in fairness, creativity, fatalism, gambling, magical thinking, perfectionism, and reactance or demand for freedom (Elster 2015; Hofmann et al. 2012; Martin 2011; Silver 2011). Similarly, practice ensues from agreement to the practice, desire for the practice, intent on the practice, interest in the practice, justification for the practice, and stability attributed to the practice (Eccles and Wigfield 2002; Fishbein and Ajzen 2010; Gross 2009; Hedstrom 2005; Jost and van der Toom 2012; Manstead 2011; Mantet and Serra 2003; Miller 2001). The latter indicates the continuity, habituality, and stability of practice, resting on concern for sunk costs (Elster 2015; Silver 2011). Consistency among practices happens between practice and its learning and testing, which prepare the practice (Raab 2019). Such practice results from self-fulfilling prophecy or wishful thinking involving face-saving, impression management, and self-presentation (Hedstrom 2005; Raab 2019). Moreover, practice can respond socially to advertising and frames (Raab 2019). Most evidently, practice has increased with favor for and intent on the practice to maintain consistency between attitude and behavior (Cooke and Sheeran 2004; Jenkins and Dragojevic 2011).

The direct deterministic mechanism maintains that collective practice induces personal practice through private or public sharing. Private sharing works through collaboration or joint practice, whereas public sharing allows free riding to claim practice without practicing.

The indirect deterministic mechanism of empowering states that collective power empowers or disempowers personal practice through the voluntaristic mechanism of realization. Collective power means an opportunity structure for empowering or disempowering with authorization, capital, coercion, conflict, control, domination, regulation, resistance, and the provision of resources (Eagly and Wood 2012; Hofmann et al. 2012; Michael 2017; Munch 1987; Swartz 2013; Townley 2014). They involve power in a credential, cultural, economic, ideological, informational, military, political, social, or symbolic form, strengthened by bureaucratization and professionalization (Swartz 2013).

The indirect deterministic mechanism of incentivizing asserts that social structure provides incentives for practice to attract personal practice through the voluntaristic mechanism of optimization. A unique form of social structure is the hierarchy, which provides rewards according to hierarchical position (Sidanius and Pratto 2012). Hierarchical position thereby incentivizes practice, such as dominance, to sustain the gain from the position.

The indirect deterministic mechanism of standardizing specifies the maintenance of social norms as a determinant of personal practice through the voluntaristic mechanism of conformity. Such norms are social constructions setting habitus and rituals embedded and promulgated by institutions (Elder-Vass 2010; Swartz 2013; Townley 2014). The constructions flow as feeding, instruction, and structuring (Tharp 2012).

The indirect deterministic mechanism of framing posits that collective ideas serve as frames for rationalizing personal practice through the voluntaristic mechanism of idea consistency. Framing can happen as agenda-setting, meaning-making, legitimizing, questioning, signifying, and the enactment of roles and rules to exert influences through anchoring, availability, ordering, and representativeness (Eagly and Wood 2012; Elster 2015; Michael 2017; Miller 2001; Swartz 2013; Tharp 2012).

Explaining Practices

Analytical-functionalist theory explains the private practices of e-activity, learning, spiritual activity, risk aversion, and weapon carrying, and the public practices of organizational participation, appeal, strike participation, voting, green demonstrating, and green donation. Among them, appealing, strike participation, organizational participation, green demonstrating, green donation, and spiritual activity identify public engagement, whereas e-activity and learning reflect informational engagement. In addition, these practices, except weapon carrying, register fidgeting, considering their detrimental effects on life quality. Thus, the practices imply life inadequacy or poor life quality.

E-activity

E-activity, comprising using the Internet, personal computer, and email, represents engagement in a private or individualized but connected and globalized world for communication, consumption, and interaction (Dutton 2013; Fuchs 2008; Kellerman

2014). The characteristics of e-activity include anonymity, connection, immediacy, interactivity, and multiplexity or multidimensional connection (Caldwell 2020; Fuchs 2008; Fullwood 2019; Kellerman 2014). As such, e-activity thrives with the deterministic forces of globalization, individualization, postindustrialization, and time-space compression or distanciation among netizens (Caldwell 2020; Fuchs 2008; Kellerman 2014; Wallace 2016). Meanwhile, e-activity grows with personal entitlement, freedom, information, knowledge, and networking (Fuchs 2008; Katz and Rice 2002; Mesch and Coleman 2007; Norris 2001; Wong et al. 2010). These bases for e-activity are illustrative of the deterministic and voluntaristic mechanisms of analytical-functionalism. Relevant to functionalism, e-activity fulfills the goals of dating, entertainment, gaming, informing, networking, and publicizing (Caldwell 2020; Gunter 2013; Ho and Ng 2022; Livingstone et al. 2007; Settle 2018).

The voluntaristic mechanism of power realization specifies personal power or resources for activating e-activity. Such power or resources arise from or consist in access, affordability, arousal, capability, curiosity, interest, and pleasantness (Cheng et al. 2019; Fang et al. 2019; Griffiths 2000; Khang et al. 2014). Specifically, capability encompasses that for self-reflection, self-regulation, symbolization or use of symbols, and vicarious learning or learning from others' experiences and practice (Khang et al. 2014). Pleasantness is influential in broadening and building thinking or a cognitive repertoire, and thus capability (Cheng et al. 2019). The contribution of curiosity stems from need for information (Fang et al. 2019). Power, such as expertise, knowledge, and skill about e-activity, has enabled e-activity (Katz and Rice 2002; Loader 2007). More fundamentally, socioeconomic status, including class, education, homeownership, and personal, the household head's and family income, has facilitated e-activity (Livingstone et al. 2007; Norris 2001; Pratt et al. 2010). Notably, the student has higher e-activity than has the other, such as the unemployed person (Chak and Leung 2004; Zhu and He 2002). In addition, friendship and social capital have boosted e-activity (Katz and Rice 2002; Miyata and Kubayashi 2008). The impetus for e-activity to help achievement, advancement, escapism, and social interaction has been the key to e-activity (Khang et al. 2014; Sun et al. 2008; Yee 2006).

The voluntaristic mechanism of utility optimization highlights expected or perceived utility, including gain and other values, as the cause of e-activity. Such utility consists in anonymity, convenience, and escape (ACE) (Griffiths 2000; Meerkerke et al. 2006). Utility can arise from using e-activity to compensate for social anxiety, social connection difficulty, and self-depreciation (Peter and Valkenburg 2007; Wallace 2016; Zsido et al. 2021). Social compensation works when e-activity is personally controllable and focused (Peter and Valkenburg 2007). As such, e-activity is a hyperpersonal activity compensating for anxiety and loneliness (Cheng et al. 2019). Similarly, e-activity generates the utility of building social identity to lessen stigmatization (Bargh and McKenna 2004). Furthermore, e-activity provides usefulness in self-extension (Suler 2016). The utility of e-activity also transpires in recreation and gathering information to reduce uncertainty (Peter and Valkenburg 2007; Tsiotsou 2015). Beliefs that e-activity is advantageous, compatible rather than interfering with other activities, convenient, easy, and valuable have contributed to e-activity (Johnson and Kaye 2002; Zhu and He 2002). Moreover, e-activity has resulted from neuroticism, social anxiety, and fear of missing out (Blackwell et al. 2017; Zsido et al. 2021). In addition, e-activity has grown with its reliance and valuation and privacy concern (Livingstone et al. 2007; Vitak 2017). Conversely, e-activity has diminished with self-esteem (Brandenberg et al. 2019; Vitak 2017). This susceptibility of e-activity reveals its utility in tackling personal problems.

The voluntaristic mechanism of norm conformity treasures social norms to influence e-activity through assimilating. Such norms are evident in the belief about the popularity of e-activity (Zhu and He 2002).

The voluntaristic mechanism of idea consistency regards e-activity as arising with other factors, practices, attitudes, dispositions, experiences, and feelings consonant with e-activity. These other factors include extraversion, narcissism, particularly its component of self-extension, recreational orientation, and sensation seeking (Cheng et al. 2019; Suler 2016; Peter and Valkenburg 2007). Such factors generally boost activity and outside contact. Similarly, e-activity has risen with innovativeness, interest in politics, particularly elections, permissiveness, and trust in politics (Katz and Rice 2002; Johnson and Kaye 2002; Livingstone et al. 2007; Loader 2007; Peter and Valkenburg 2007). In practice, e-activity has risen with addiction, deception, involvement in politics, and the use of various media conveying news or others (Chak and Leung 2004; Hardy et al. 2009; Johnson and Kaye 2002; Wheatley and Buglass 2019). Conversely, e-activity has diminished with conservatism and reliance on traditional media (Hardy et al. 2009; Johnson and Kaye 2002).

The direct deterministic mechanism maintains that personal e-activity results from sharing privately or publicly through collective e-activity. Thus, personal e-activity arises with connection with others in the cyberworld, such that the former is essential for the latter and vice versa (Settle 2018). This sharing indicates that personal e-activity can be passive, as engaged with others' e-activity.

The indirect deterministic mechanism of empowering applies collective power to empower personal e-activity through the voluntaristic mechanism of power realization. Such power hinges on national technology development, mobilization, networking, postindustrialization, and social or community capital to compress time and space to allow distance communication (Fuchs 2008; Kellerman 2014; Livingstone et al. 2007; Mesch and Coleman 2007). Postindustrialization emphasizes applying and sharing information and knowledge (Fuchs 2008). Collective power has included national economic development and spending on research and development (Norris 2001). This power has raised collective e-activity (Norris 2001). Collective e-activity, in turn, engages personal e-activity as an integral part.

The indirect deterministic mechanism of incentivizing raises the utility of e-activity to boost e-activity through the voluntaristic mechanism of utility optimization. Such incentivizing happens in the societal promotion of e-democracy, e-politics, e-rights, globalization, and networking to heighten the utility of e-activity in various life domains (Livingstone et al. 2007; Norris 2001; Wallace 2016; Wong et al. 2010).

The indirect deterministic mechanism of standardizing or normalizing imposes social norms to boost personal e-activity through the voluntaristic mechanism of norm conformity or assimilating. Such norms for e-activity, including information and knowledge sharing, reside in peer groups and the larger society (Fuchs 2008; Livingstone et al. 2007; Norris 2001). Moreover, the norms emanate from post-Fordist culture emphasizing automation, decentralization, and globalization, and self-culture notably treasuring e-activity and narcissism (Beck and Beck-Gernsheim 2002; Burgess 2018; Fuchs 2008).

The indirect deterministic mechanism of framing relies on social discourses to rationalize and thus induce personal e-activity through the voluntaristic mechanism of idea consistency. Such discourses prize the ideas of communality, engagement, expression, freedom or liberty, individualization, immediacy, information, multiplexity, networking, self-determination, and romanticism (Allmer 2015; Dahlberg 2007; Fuchs 2008; Ingrams 2017; Kellerman 2014; Norris 2001; Toews 2018). Among these ideas, individualization favors agency, autonomy, choice, emancipation, heterogeneity, immediacy, knowledge, liberty, narcissism, sensation seeking, singleness, and notably, e-activity (Beck and Beck-Gernsheim 2002; Burgess 2018; Krys et al. 2019; Bauman 2001). Meanwhile, romanticism hails expression, freedom, self-fulfillment, and self-realization (TenHouten 2017). All these ideas are consonant with and rationalize e-activity.

Learning

Learning, comprising reading, listening, watching through various media, and talking with friends or colleagues, is vital in this runaway world fraught with irrationality and uncertainty attributed to globalization (Robert and Bukodi 2005). With globalization, conventional local knowledge lapses and requires perennial supplanting with rapidly changing global knowledge. Such requirement registers functionalist deterministic and voluntaristic mechanisms for the functioning of society and its members. Hence, learning represents empowerment (Clark and Inglehart 1998). Precisely, learning attains the goals of adaptation, capacitation, entertainment, health maintenance, impulse-control, and problem-solving (Brannstrom and Lindblad 1994; Gadsden 2008; Maltseva 2016; Mesirow 2003; Rigby and Ryan 2017).

The voluntaristic mechanism of power realization capitalizes on personal power to drive learning. Such power rests on motivation or need for accuracy, curiosity, defense, self-enhancement, and self-efficacy in learning (Knobloch-Westerwick 2015). More fundamentally, education, employment experience, homeownership, insurance coverage, knowledge, savings, skill, social class, and family incomes have been resources affording to learn (Chou 2003; Kerrissey and Schofer 2013; Lavrijsen and Nicaise 2017; Pallas 2002; Verba et al. 1995; Wink and Dillon 2003). In addition, one's popularity or acceptance by others has been a necessary condition for others to provide information for one's learning (Pei and Pan 2018).

The voluntaristic mechanism of utility optimization upholds the utility of learning to attract learning. This utility, expectancy, or value arises from adjustment, improvement, management, and optimization of mood or self, cooperation, and comparison with others through learning (Chilton 2004; Knobloch-Westerwick 2015). Hence, learning has risen with negative moods (Robinson and Knobloch-Westerwick 2017).

The voluntaristic mechanism of idea consistency rationalizes and induces learning with other factors conveying ideas consonant with learning. These factors include such attitudes as identification with or establishing a social identity with the source of learning, liking for and satisfaction with learning, or its attractiveness (Knobloch-Westerwick 2015; Rigby and Ryan 2017). In addition, the factors encompass impulsivity and sensitivity to information or messages (Exelmans and Van den Bulck 2021). Political interest, discussion, and study have also raised learning (Howe 2010; Verba et al. 1995).

The indirect deterministic mechanism of empowering brings collective power or resources to facilitate personal learning such as through continuing and further education. Essentially, national technology in hardware and software empowers learning (Wood 2010). Moreover, information for learning and media disseminating the information increase with globalization (Wood 2010). Propaganda in society and other manipulation causes also disseminate information for learning (Carmines and Kuklinski 1990; Miller 1991).

The indirect deterministic mechanism of incentivizing provides societal incentives to boost personal learning. Such incentivizing stems from the belief that learning is productive, profitable, and thus worth investment (Joeckel and Dogruel 2017).

The indirect deterministic mechanism of framing or agenda setting applies social discourses to rationalize and encourage personal learning (Iyengar 1987; Lopez-Escobar et al. 1998). Such discourses emphasize individualization, life planning, normalization or establishing normalcy, self-work, socialization, and trendiness (Herda-Rapp 2003; Mutz 1998; Sidanius 1988; Wood 2010). Individualization accentuates competition, life planning, self-help, self-work, and selfhood (Wood 2010).

Spiritual Activity

Spiritual activity, comprising praying, religious attendance, and thinking about the meaning and purpose of life. Essentially, spiritual activity features internality or soul work, nonconformity, religiosity, sacredness, and transcendence (Dalby 2006; Kalkstein and Tower 2009; Pargament and Mahoney 2009; Schwartz 2012). Among these spiritual features, religiosity, in turn, features altruism, authoritarianism, community, ethicalness, fraternity, ritualism, sacredness, solidarity, strictness, and supernaturalism (Franks et al. 2013; Kalkstein and Tower 2009; Peifer 2010; Stavrova and Siegers 2014). While subsuming religious activity, spiritual activity does not explicitly emphasize those religious features, except sacredness. Spiritual activity stems from humanity, particularly the awakened form (Lerner et al. 2006). The activity is functional to thus humanity with diverse goals to achieve asceticism, calmness, compassion, comprehension, collaboration, enjoyment, enlightenment, forbearance, forgiveness, fullness, gratitude, harmony, hope, humility, integrity, justice, love, meaningfulness, mindfulness, peace, power, reasoning, sacredness, self-satisfaction, serenity, and transcendence variously (Connors et al. 1999; Gorsuch and Miller 1999; Kelly 2012; MacDonald and Friedman 2002; Patch 2012; Richards 2012; Sandeerson and Linehan 1999; Shek 2010; Yahne and Miller 1999). Conversely, spiritual activity has diverse goals to dispel egocentrism, craving, delusion, hatred, and vice (Kelly 2012; Richards 2012; Semple and Hott 2012). Spiritual activity follows voluntaristic and deterministic functionalist mechanisms as functional to humanity.

The voluntaristic mechanism of power realization capitalizes on personal power to energize spiritual activity. Such power consists in the production processes of goal setting, self-monitoring (Martin and Booth 1999). These processes rely on such power as autonomy (Eliason et al. 2010). Power or drive also arises from motivation or the need to compensate for or heal alienation, conflict, guilt, helplessness, ignorance, insecurity, meaninglessness, neuroticism, nihilism, nothingness, purposelessness, or trauma (Browning and Cooper 2004; Day 2011; Forsyth 2003; Immerzeel and van Tubergen 2013; Rose and Exline 2012). Such need has resulted from divorce, illness, minority status, underemployment, and unemployment (De Vaus and McAllister 1987; Immerzeel and van Tubergen 2013; Medvedovski and Allison 2017; Wuthnow 1992). Additionally, drive emanates from needs for affiliation, beauty, belonging, conscience, goodness, integration, justice, meaning, relaxation, truth (Day 2011; Forsyth 2003). Need for justice, in turn, rests on income inequality perceived (Jasso 2002). Furthermore, power or drive springs from hostility, rebelliousness, and the instinct of death (Forsyth 2003). Power or energy also evolves from ritualistic activity to prop spiritual activity (Wollschleger 2012). In addition, spiritual activity has risen with social capital (Rivera 2018).

The voluntaristic mechanism of utility optimization consolidates the utility of spiritual activity to attract engagement in the activity. Such utility consolidates from contracting, effectiveness, reward, or positive reinforcement received as opposed to cost from spiritual activity (De Graaf 2013; Forsyth 2003; Martin and Booth 1999). The utility also concerns harmony, liberation, love, self-awareness, and transcendence (Forsyth 2003). Furthermore, the utility of spiritual activity rises with education and other forms of human capital (Medvedovski and Allison 2017; Skerkat and Ellison 1999).

The voluntaristic mechanism of norm conformity applies social norms to assimilate spiritual activity (Gorsuch 1994). Such norms spread from modeling, religious education, and social construction (Day 2011; Martin and Booth 1999).

The voluntaristic mechanism of idea consistency leverages ideas to rationalize and encourage spiritual activity. Such ideas favor generosity, morality, self-determination, and tolerance (Day 2010). In addition, ideas derived from agreeableness, authoritarianism, conscientiousness, exhibitionism, extraversion, and openness have lifted spiritual activity (Hall and Edwards 2002; MacDonald 2000; Saucier and Skrzypinska 2006). Spiritual activity ensues to please others (Skerkat and Ellison 1999). Secure attachment has also facilitated spiritual activity (Hall and Edwards 2002). Conversely, egocentricity and neuroticism have dampened spiritual activity (Hall and Edwards 2002; MacDonald 2000).

The direct deterministic mechanism operates with collective spiritual activity determining personal spiritual activity through private or public sharing. As such, collective or contextual spiritual activity has determined personal spiritual activity (Stavrova and Siegers 2014). Herein, one is either involved in others' spiritual activity privately or takes the activity as one's activity vicariously in a public way.

The indirect deterministic mechanism of empowering draws on collective power to enable personal spiritual activity through the voluntaristic mechanism of power realization. Such collective power includes the accessibility of religion and individualization (Land and Deane 1992; Lane 1991). Herein, individualization is overloading, thus boosting one's need for coping through spiritual activity. Similarly, spiritual activity has risen with contextual disaster (Rivera 2018). Conversely, contextual plurality and regulation are a disempowering force diluting or opposing power to drive spiritual activity (De Graaf 2013). Likewise, contextual diversity has weakened personal spiritual activity (Land and Deane 1992). Contextual civilization or social development also reduces the drive for spiritual activity (Browning and Cooper 2004). Similarly, contextual economic development and education have dampened spiritual activity. (Fjellvang 2011; Land and Deane 1992).

The indirect deterministic mechanism of incentivizing mobilizes incentives collectively to enhance the utility and thus practice of spiritual activity through the voluntaristic mechanism of utility optimization. As such, contextual conditions affect personal spiritual activity through the logic of competition (De Graaf 2013). When alternatives to spiritual activity are numerous, the activity diminishes.

The indirect deterministic mechanism of standardizing promulgates social norms to assimilate personal spiritual activity through the voluntaristic mechanism of norm conformity. The social norms have been more influential with increased popularity and strictness (Wollschleger 2012).

The indirect deterministic mechanism of framing popularizes ideas to rationalize and boost personal spiritual activity through the voluntaristic mechanism of idea consistency. As such, conservatism and expressivity in the context have sustained spiritual activity (Wollschleger 2012). Conversely, cosmopolitanism or disfavor for traditional culture in the context has weakened spiritual activity (Norris and Inglehart 2009).

Risk Aversion

Risk aversion, comprising not going out at night and carrying much money, typically represents a reaction to a perceived or expected threat (Makhanova and Shepherd 2020). Furthermore, risk aversion manifests disgust, infectibility perceived, prejudice, and sensitivity, as opposed to openness (Tybur et al. 2014). In addition, risk aversion registers as a dysfunction detrimental to one and one's social integration (Alonso-Arbiol et al. 2007; Barber et al. 2010; Makhanova and Shepherd 2020; Van Haaften et al. 2004). Meanwhile, risk aversion rests on the voluntaristic and deterministic mechanisms of analytical functionalism.

The voluntaristic mechanism of power realization hinges on personal power to parry risk aversion. Such power included collective efficacy perceived to maintain social order (Brown and Zoorob 2022). In addition, education and homeownership have generated power to dampen risk aversion (Brown and Zoorob 2022). Similarly, social support received has reduced risk aversion. Conversely, power also arises from the need to avoid risks. Hence, the experiences of broken windows, criminality, disorder, non-benevolence, pathogen, and threat have increased risk aversion (Bock et al. 2016; Brayne 2014; Brown and Zoorob 2022; Ruiter et al. 2003; Lee-Baggley et al. 2004; Tybur et al. 2014). In addition, indebtedness, indicative of insufficient economic power, has raised risk aversion (Bock et al. 2016).

The voluntaristic mechanism of utility optimization adduces the utility of risk aversion as a cause of the aversion. Such utility has been evident in support for independence and dislikes for coping and endurance (Hsu et al. 2019; Ruiter et al. 2003). Moreover, the utility of risk aversion or expectation for risk would rise with criminal involvement and wishful thinking. Such practices have raised risk aversion (Brayne 2014; Lee-Baggley et al. 2004).

The voluntaristic mechanism of idea consistency applies alternative ideas consonant with risk aversion to rationalize and encourage the aversion. Thus, anxiety has raised risk aversion (Brayne 2014). Conversely, authoritarianism, empathy, and social dominance orientation have diminished risk aversion (Lee-Baggley et al. 2004).

Organizational Participation

Organizational participation, comprising that in environmental, consumer, humanitarian, professional art, music, education, labor, political, sport, recreational, self-help, and religious organizations, serves the goals of belonging, bonding, empowering, recreating (Delgado and Staples 2008; Jacobs et al. 2009; Larson 1994; Wetterbeng 2007). Specifically, such empowerment enhances choice, collaboration, consultation, help, information, partnership, resiliency, success, support, therapy, and other resources (Delgado and Staples 2008). It is a form of civic engagement and social capital for the function of integration or networking and adaptation through learning from the organization (Cotterell 2007; Palmer et al. 2011; Quinn 1995; Wang and Graddy 2008). The participation also rests on the voluntaristic and deterministic mechanisms of analytical functionalism.

The voluntaristic mechanism of power realization leverages power or resources to enable organizational participation. Such power has stemmed from education and organizational membership, which secures the condition or opportunity for organizational participation (Guillen et al. 2011; Nussio 2019). The latter illustrates organizational participation as realizing the power of organization membership. Furthermore, power or energy evolves from positive beliefs and feelings. Belief in agency or voluntariness and satisfaction have boosted organizational participation (Bagherior et al. 2009).

The voluntaristic mechanism of utility optimization emphasizes the contribution of the utility or organizational participation expected or realized to the participation. This utility indicates the function of organizational participation to tackle problems (Delgado and Staples 2008). Hence, problems such as conflict, crime, and victimization have raised organizational participation (Nussio 2019). Conversely, security perception has dampened organizational participation (Nussio 2019). More generally, organization participation results from the utility or gain in self-interest and fulfilling reciprocity in exchange (Bagherior et al. 2009).

The voluntaristic mechanism of norm conformity maintains that the social norm for organizational participation assimilates the participation. Such a norm evolves from social integration, including contact with and learning from others and their encouragement, mores, and values (Larson 1994).

The voluntaristic mechanism of idea consistency highlights practices and other factors to provide ideas rationalizing and inducing organizational participation. Thereby, civic practice has contributed to organizational participation (Bowman et al. 2015).

Appealing

Appealing, comprising joining boycotts, peaceful demonstrations, and petitions, represents collective action and identity, confidence, contention, democracy, grouping, idealism, mobilization, polarization, politicization, and voicing (Armony and Armony 2005; Barker et al. 2021; Kutlaca et al. 2020; Morgan and Chan 2016; Sexton and Benson 2006; Pfaff and Kim 2003; Rucht 2007; Shriver et al. 2003; Stewart et al. 2012; Wulff et al. 2015). By contrast, appealing contradicts civility, institutionalization, and production (Jasper 2005; Opp 2009; Stewart et al. 2012). The appealing goals include democracy, counter-hegemony, justice, and liberalization (Bosi and Della Porta 2012; de Costa 2006; Youngs 2019). More specifically, the goals cover anti-austerity, anti-capitalism, anti-corporation, anti-globalization, anti-neoliberalism, anti-market, or anti-commodification, anti-nuclear technology, anti-refugees, anti-violence, equality, identity, ideology including localism, militarism, nativism, nimbyism, populism, and radicalism, peace, rights for children, humans, minority, or women, and religion (Belanger et al. 2019; Chesters and Welsh 2005; Crossley 2012; Drury 2002; Esaiasson 2014; Fumagalli 2007; Lopez et al. 2019; McCright and Dunlap 2008; Morselli and Passini 2018; Moskolenko and McCauley 2009; McVeigh and Sikkink 2001; Rice 2013; Rudig and Karyotis 2014; Selvanathan and Lickel 2019; Wulff et al. 2015; Youngs 2019). Appealing draws on the voluntaristic and deterministic mechanisms of analytical functionalism with these properties and goals.

The voluntaristic mechanism of power realization specifies power to achieve appealing goals as the basis for appealing. Such power can emanate from affect for appealing, alliances, anger, compassion, connection, education, emboldening, empowerment, effervescence, energy in the emotion form, fellowship, intellectual status, need, networking, opportunity, resources, social capital, space, and feelings about invulnerability, prowess, outrage, self-efficacy, shock, strain, support received, tension, and youthfulness (Aytac and Stokes 2019; Benford and Snow 2000; Brusting and Postmes 2002; Buechler 2011; Coley et al. 2020; Cronin et al. 2012; Crossley 2012; Flam 2015; Hoffman et al. 2016; Jost et al. 2017; Karatzogianni and Robinson 2010; McPhail and Tucker 2003; Moss and Snow 2016; Olcese et al. 2014; Oliver and Marwell 2002; Opp 2009; Ostrom and Ahn 2009; Pearlman 2013; Ryan 2015; Sing 2020; Summers-Effler 2002; Turner 2015; Van Ness and Summers-Effler 2016; Zhuang 2020). Anger, compassion, outrage, shock, strain, and tension, in turn, arise from consciousness, experiences, or feelings about adversity, breakdown, clash, collusion, competition, conflict, conspiracy, deprivation, deterioration, devaluation, disadvantage, disruption, downgrading, frustration, grievances, injustice, insecurity, instability, isolation, loss, marginality, nuisance, precarity, problems, repression, struggle, threat, turmoil, under-reward, unemployment, unfairness, victimization, and violation (Aytac and Stokes 2019; Bassoli and Monticelli 2018; Braun and Vliegenthart 2008; Buechler 2011; Choi and Kim 2019; Dalton et al. 2010; Esaiasson 2014; Hart 2008; Hirsch 1993; Hoffman et al. 2016; Klandermans and van Stekelenburg 2013; Koopmans 2007; Kowalchuk 2005; Jenkins and Form 2005; Passini 2019; Passini and Morselli 2011; Rydgren 2007; Snow and Owens 2014; Somma et al. 2020; Su and Feng 2013; Thomas and Louis 2013; Van Ness and Summers-Effler 2016; Van Zomeren 2009). Need or motivation concerns cohesion, efficacy, facticity, identity or self, payoff, and trust (Turner 2013; Van Ness and Summers-Effler 2016). Payoff, in turn, incorporates fairness and justice (Turner 2013). Specifically, breakdown comprises social change, crisis, disintegration, and uncontrol (Buechler 2011; Khoshneviss and Benford 2018; Somma et al. 2020; Stewart et al. 2012; Van Ness and Summers-Effler 2016). Disruption includes that in control, community, demand, expectation, privacy, resources, safety, subsistence, and survival, as in crisis (Moss and Snow 2016; Van Ness and Summers-Effler 2016). Resources cover labor, material, money, skill, technology, and time (Choi and Kim 2019; Opp 2009). Such resources accrue with the new class, including the knowledge worker and one working in the public sector in the wake of postindustrialization (Jenkins and Wallace 1996). Eventually, power fueling appealing has been economic or financial capability, political knowledge, particularly on democracy (Bassoli and Monticelli 2018; Child and Nikolova 2020; Menahem 2001; Norris 2011). Such power has stemmed from employment, health, organizational membership, self-efficacy, social capital, and socioeconomic status, notably in occupation (Bassoli and Monticelli 2018; Child and Nikolova 2020; Pattie et al. 2004; Somma et al. 2020; Su and Feng 2013; Thyen and Gerschewski 2018). By contrast, incapacity in terms of irrationality and simple-mindedness has propelled appealing (Li and Song 1992). Moreover, power has risen from discontent provoked by perceptions about corruption, crisis, harm, inequality, risk, and threat (Cho and Hwang 2021; Cronin et al. 2012; Renger et al. 2020; Scafuto and La Barbera 2016; Swart et al. 2020). Similarly, appealing has risen with experiences of deprivation, deterioration in living, discrimination, failure, grievance, injustice, marginalization, provocation, rejection, repression, and threat (Aytac and Stokes 2019; Charrad and Reith 2019;

Esaiasson 2014; Grasso and Giugni 2016; Just and Anderson 2014; Kaplan and Liu 2000; Mannarini et al. 2015; Sabucedo et al. 2018; Shriver et al. 2003; Wahlstrom 2011). Furthermore, appealing has resulted from the feelings of anger, dissatisfaction, excitement, frustration, outrage, strain, and worry (Akinboade et al. 2014; Giugni and Grasso 2019; Selvanathan and Lickel 2019; Weeber and Rodenheaver 2003). Conversely, power for appealing diminishes with experiences of control, dependency, regulation, repression, and injustice (Crossley 2012; Kowalchuk 2005). Such control can arise from social connection, integration, and overlapping networking (Fillieule 2015; Jasper 2005). With lowered motivation, appealing has reduced with experience about advantage, government, rights, and social support (Borbath and Gessler 2020; Christensen 2016; Pradel-Miquel 2017; Jost et al. 2017). Meanwhile, the experience of difficulty in finance has also diminished appealing (Bassoli and Monticelli 2018). The feelings of depression and hopelessness have deactivated appealing (Adnanes 2004; Omoto et al. 2010).

The voluntaristic mechanism of utility optimization highlights the utility of appealing as the influence on appealing (Pearlman 2013). Such utility, including demand, effectiveness, efficacy, expectancy, hope, instrumentality, interest, preference, urgency, and value, stems from comparison, evaluation, and perception of incentives (Aytac and Stokes 2019; Benford and Snow 2000; Gillham et al. 2019; Klandermans 2015, 2015a; Kowalchuk 2005; Ibrahim 2011; Opp 2009; Passy and Giugni 2000; Sa'di 2015; Summers-Effler 2002; Van Zomeren 2009; Wenzel 2000; Wilkinson 2009). The utility covers achievement, dignity, expression, fairness, gain, identity, joy, pride, security, and success, as opposed to sadness, shame, and stigma expected or received (Klandermans and van Stekelenburg 2013; Mizen 2015; Opp 2009; Pearlman 2013; Sturmer and Simon 2009; Tsai 2019; Turner 2013; Van Stekelenburg et al. 2009; van Troost et al. 2018; Wilkinson 2009). Appealing has thus risen with expectancy for effectiveness, opportunity, or success, valuation of emancipation, freedom, politics, and self-transcendence (Cho and Hwang 2021; Corcoran et al. 2011; Datler et al. 2013; Jones and Brewster 2017; Rudig and Karyotis 2014; Zhuang 2020), Conversely, the utility reduces with constraint, free ridership, responsibility, and sanctions expected (Opp 2009; Snow and Owens 2014; Turner 2013; Zurbriggen 2013). Appealing has diminished with the expected cost, dependence on government, and risk valuation (Ayanian and Tausch 2016; Scafuto and La Barbera 2016). Similarly, appealing has receded with the perception of violence (Sing 2020).

The voluntaristic mechanism of norm conformity foregrounds social norms for appealing to assimilate appealing (Brusting and Postmes 2002; Thomas and Louis 2013; Van Ness and Summers-Effler 2016). These norms inherent in social entities promulgate antagonism, competition, and threat (Lopez et al. 2019). Such social norms evolve from social connection, construction, contagion, diffusion, identification, learning, media exposure, modeling, recruitment, ritual, rumor, sharing, and validating to heighten consensus and normativity (Bennett et al. 2014; Buechler 2011; Braun and Vliegenthart 2008; Eder 2015; Giugni and Grasso 2019; McPhail and Tucker 2003; Mizen 2015; Sing 2020; Taylor et al. 2009; Van Ness and Summers-Effler 2016; Wahlstrom 2011; Wulff et al. 2015). Notably, social connection with brokers, comrades, leaders, or mobilizers is influential (Buechler 2011; Opp 2009).

Appealing has risen with experience with the norm, campaigning, or mobilization emanating from organizations or social networks for justice, protest and its support (Berman and Wittig 2004; Brusting and Postmes 2002; Giugni and Grasso 2019; Hwang and Kim 2015; Li and Song 1992; Monfortia and McGlynn 2015).

The voluntaristic mechanism of idea consistency applies ideas consistent with appealing to rationalize and lift appealing. Such ideas highlight anarchism, anomie, aspiration, autonomy, blaming, challenging, childishness, collective identity, contentiousness, criminality, crowd mentality, cynicism, decivilization, dehumanization, delusion or madness, deviance, discontent, disorganization, dissatisfaction, entitlement, environmentalism, expressivity, extremity, fellowship, feminism, heroism, homosexuality, individualism, justification, leadership, masculinity, meaningfulness, narcissism, opposition, partisanship, politicization, postmaterialism, rightfulness in appealing, sharing, social dominance orientation, tolerance for appealing, and valuation of anti-hegemony, justice, and liberalism (Braun and Vliegenthart 2008; Bassoli and Monticelli 2018; Buechler 2011; Choi and Kim 2019; Grasso and Giugni 2016; Hewitt 1991; Hirsch 1993; Ibrahim 2011; Jasper 2005; Jenkins and Wallace 1996; Kaufman 2003; Khoshneviss and Benford 2018; Klandermans and van Stekelenburg 2013; Kowalchuk 2005; Koopmans 2007; McVeigh and Sikkink 2001; Reese et al. 2019; Reznek 2010; Snow and Owens 2014; Su and Feng 2013; Summers-Effler 2002; Taylor et al. 2009; Thomas and Louis 2013; Torfing 1999; Van Ness and Summers-Effler 2016; Verkuyten and Martinovic 2015; Zhuang 2020; Zurbriggen 2013). Specifically, crowd mentality comprises anonymity, barbarism, delirium, hypnosis, ignorance, impulsivity, invincibility, suggestibility, unconsciousness, and unity (Borch 2013; Koopmans 2007; McPhail and Tucker 2003). Delusion includes confirmation bias, fundamentalism, illusory correlation, and irrationality (Reznek 2010). Notably, justification or legitimization derives from beliefs about enemies, hierarchy, morality, opposition, and conspiracy theories (Buechler 2011; Stewart et al. 2012; Van Zomeren 2009; Zurbriggen 2013). These ideas also originate from working-class and youth cultures (Braun and Vliegenthart 2008). In practice, civic, organizational, or political participation, community or organizational involvement, political discussion, social networking, and voting have translated into appealing (Achilov 2016; Christensen 2016; Klandermans and de Weerd 2000; Mannarini et al. 2009; Slavina and Brym 2020; Somma et al. 2020; van der Meer and van Ingen 2009; Van Vugt et al. 2003). More fundamentally, the dispositions of altruism, anti-traditionalism, assertiveness, careerism, fanaticism, feminism, humanitarianism, idealism, individualism, innovativeness, leftism, libertarianism, openness, oversensitivity, postmaterialism, progressivism, and radicalism (Adnanes 2004; Braithwaite 1997; Cho and Hwang 2021; Curtin et al. 2010; Duncan 1999; Grasso 2014; Giugni and Grasso 2019; Li and Song 1992; McVeigh and Sikkink 2001; Neilson 2010; Rudig and Karyotis 2014; Somma et al. 2020). Attitudinally, aspiration, attachment to the party, belief in others' sinfulness, concern for the economy, commitment to democracy, consciousness about politics, conviction about morality, identification with the party or protest, interest in politics, motivation for defense, expressing, ideology, morality, or raising public awareness, support for democracy, sympathy, have raised appealing (Bassoli and Monticelli 2018; Borbath and Gessler 2020; Cho and Hwang 2021; Curtin et al. 2010; Fernandes-Jesus et al. 2020; Giugni and Grasso 2019; Lee and Chan 2011; McVeigh and Sikkink 2001; Norris 2011; Saab et al. 2015; Skitka and Morgan 2014). Conversely, ideas based on authoritarianism, guilt, morality, social contact, and social harmony erode appealing (Borch 2013; Hassler et al. 2021; Turiel 2014; Yuchtman-Yaar and Hermann 1998; Zhuang 2020). The dispositions of authoritarianism, nationalism, rightism, and social responsibility have prevented appealing (Flanagan and Lee 2000; Grasso and Giugni 2016; Lahusen 2021). Similarly, appealing has weakened with orientation to the economic or legal aspect and trust in government or politics (Lee and Chan 2011; Nikolayenko 2008; Tang 2009; Zhuang 2020).

The direct deterministic mechanism holds that collective appealing in the contest generates personal appealing through private or public sharing. Such contextual influence has prevailed (Andrews et al. 2015; Choi and Kim 2019; Gillham et al. 2019; Jenkins et al. 2003). In private sharing, personal appealing is part of collective appealing. Meanwhile, public sharing happens in free ridership in others' appealing.

The indirect deterministic mechanism of empowering works with the collective provision of power to facilitate personal appealing through the voluntaristic mechanism of power realization. Such empowering derives from leadership, mobilization, modernization, openness, opportunity, prosperity, sponsoring, social capital, support, and technology externally in the context (Aytac and Stokes 2019; Braun and Vliegenthart 2008; Buechler 2011; Gillham et al. 2019; Grasso 2014; Jenkins and Form 2005; Klandermans and van Stekelenburg 2013; Opp 2009; Slavina and Brym 2020). Furthermore, power springs from the alienation, dehumanization, and exploitation of capitalism and its resultant inequality, clash in civilization, colonization, conflict, crisis, damage, loss, and threat to the political economy (Buechler 2011; Crossley 2012; McCammon and Moon 2015; Mesch 1996; Olcese et al. 2014; Rydgren 2007; Stewart et al. 2012). Such springing is attributable to globalization (Rydgren 2007). Thereby, physical and mental power raised by autonomy, bureaucracy, capital, casualties in war, civil society strength, communism, conflict, crowding, division in government, education, empowerment in women, heterogeneity, income, inequality, inflation, issues, media coverage, organization, population size, risk, social networking, telephone connectivity, transparency in government, unemployment, unionization in labor, urbanization, and youthfulness in the context have energized appealing (Bahry and Lipsmeyer 2001; Bates and Yackovkev 2002; Braun and Vliegenthart 2008; Child and Nikolova 2020; Cho and Hwang 2021; Choi and Kim 2019; Corcoran et al. 2011; Cornell and Grimes 2015; Gillham et al. 2019; Grasso and Giugni 2016; Hollyer et al. 2018; Jenkins et al. 2003; Mesch 1996; Quaranta 2016; Sampson et al. 2005; Schatzman 2005; Sexton and Benson 2006; Suh et al. 2017; Uslaner and Brown 2005). Contextual issues have involved change, crime, housing, noise, and unwanted business (Burningham 1998; Mesch 1996). Conversely, disempowering arises from control, countering, hegemony, opposition, regulation, repression, surveillance, and threat in the context (Andrews et al. 2016; Buechler 2011; Crossley 2012; Kowalchuk 2005; Jenkins et al. 2003; Moss and Snow 2016; Opp 2009). Such control declines with breakdown, crisis, or disintegration in the context (Van Ness and Summers-Effler 2016). In addition, power agitated from discontent declines with democracy (Tilly 2005). Hence, appealing has diminished with contextual freedom, military power held by government, policing, repression, and rights (Choi and Kim 2019; Sexton and Benson 2006; Slavina and Brym 2020; Welzel 2013).

The indirect deterministic mechanism of incentivizing issues incentives collectively to attract personal appeal through the voluntaristic mechanism of utility optimization (Opp 2009). Such incentives reward solidarity (Buechler 2011). Conversely, disincentives for appealing evolve from law enforcement, punishment, and sanctions against appealing (Varga 2008). Disincentives for appealing have also risen from contextual investment in non-appealing (Mesch 1996).

The indirect deterministic mechanism of standardizing imposes social norms to assimilate personal appealing through the voluntaristic mechanism of norm conformity. Such norms as consensuses prevail in classes, cultures, ghettos, groups, institutions, organizations, parties, and polities (Buechler 2011; Choi and Kim 2019; Hechter 2004; Opp 2009; Schofer and Fourcade-Gourinchas 2001; Su and Feng 2013). They advocate claiming, contest, democracy, and solidarity (Buechler 2011; Choi and Kim 2019; Taylor et al. 2009). Meanwhile, social dissensus is also conducive to appealing (Thomas and Louis 2013). Eventually, social norms for polarization have induced appealing (Kleiner 2018). Conversely, social norms against appealing diminish with social isolation (Koopmans 2007).

The indirect deterministic mechanism of framing provides frames of ideas in the context to popularize ideas for justifying and invoking appealing (Buechler 2011; Khoshneviss and Benford 2018; Klandermans and van Stekelenburg 2013; Schwirian et al. 2001). These contextual ideas comprise anarchism, antagonism, assertion, cosmopolitanism, competition, criminalization, demoralization, expressivity, humanitarianism, justice, liberation, neoliberalism, politicization, populism, radicalism, revolution, rights, uprising, and we-ness (Buechler 2011; Chaitin et al. 2017; Kaufman 2003; Kowalchuk 2005; Opp 2009; Parson 2015; Rojo 2014; Stewart et al. 2012; Torfing 1999; Turiel 2014). Anarchism notably emphasizes autonomy as opposed to consent, duty, fairness, gratitude, and obligation (Gans 1992). Antagonism highlights a disparity between the ingroup and outgroup in representing fundamentalism (Coley et al. 2020). Cosmopolitanism favors equality and denounces disparity, exclusion, and hegemony with globalization and neoliberalism (Rojo 2014). Nevertheless, neoliberalism also braces anarchism (Roberts 2012). Humanitarianism detests disease, exile, hunger, instability, and violence (Lo 2021). Justice cherishes coalition, community, cooperation, and dialogue as opposed to violence (Chaitin et al. 2017). Liberation popularizes struggles, notably among classes, and opposes conservatism (Drury 2002; Mantena 2012). Moreover, the frames attribute problems to collusion, conspiracy, injustice, misrule, and victimization (Benford and Snow 2000; Kowalchuk 2005; Moss and Snow 2016). Such contextual ideas originate from social disorganization (Hirsch 1993). Hence, appealing has risen from contextual cohesion, democratization, pluralism, and valuation of emancipation (Norris 2002; Sexton and Benson 2006; Solt 2015; Welzel 2013). Conversely, appealing has subsided with contextual religiousness, support for government, and statism (DeLeon and Naff 2004; Mesch 1996; Schofer and Fourcade-Gourinchas

2001). Herein, framing in the context evolves conservatism, familialism, pathologizing of the mob, realism, security or securitization, and sovereigntism or statism to denounce appealing (Drury 2002; Jusufi 2018; Mantena 2012). Conservativism treasures traditional morality (Mantena 2012; Stewart et al. 2012). Familialism values the family (Drury 2002). Mob pathology highlights atavism, contagion, hysteria, irrationality, opportunism, regression, and incivility as opposed to peace and normativity in appealing (Drury 2002). Realism, instrumentalism, or Machiavellianism, premised on consequentialism, dispels idealism, morality, utopianism, and violence (Mantena 2012).

Strike participation

Strike participation or joining strikes dealing with work or employment is a negotiation typically fulfilling the function of the labor union (Litor 2019). The function of strike participation, in turn, rests on the functionalist mechanisms of voluntarism and determinism.

The voluntaristic mechanism of power realization activates power to drive strike participation to achieve its goals. Such power emanates from unionization (Roscigno and Hodson 2004). Moreover, power for strike participation has evolved from seniority, work skill, and union membership (Dixon and Roscigno 2003). Conversely, power to strike diminishes with self-control and imposed control over or constraint on the power (Roscigno and Hodson 2004).

The voluntaristic mechanism of utility optimization raises the utility of strike participation to attract strike participation. Such utility includes gain or benefit over cost from strike participation over alternatives (Rhomberg 2010). The utility of strike participation has been lower with higher come (Dixon and Roscigno 2003).

The voluntaristic mechanism of norm conformity foregrounds social norms for strike participation to assimilate strike participation. Such norms transpire in the group culture (Healy and Kirton 2013).

The voluntaristic mechanism of idea consistency highlight ideas consonant with strike participation to rationalize and induce strike participation. Such ideas consist in bargaining, conflict, consciousness about the class disparity, disagreement, disconnection, dissatisfaction, frustration, and misunderstanding concerning employment or its issues (Healy and Kirton 2013; Kramer and Hyclak 2002; Roscigno and Hodson 2004). Hence, the feeling of job dissatisfaction and experience of conflict have boosted strike participation (Dixon et al. 2004; Roscigno and Hodson 2004).

The direct deterministic mechanism reflects the influence of strike participation in the context on personal strike participation through private or public sharing. Personal strike participation is simply part of collective strike participation in private sharing. Alternatively, the claim of strike participation happens due to free ridership in public sharing. The direct contextual influence on strike participation has been evident (Dixon and Roscigno 2003).

The indirect deterministic mechanism of empowering imposes power to drive strike participation through the voluntaristic mechanism of power realization. Such empowering springs from the labor union and its pressure (Rhomberg 2010). Hence, labor and union strength have boosted strike participation (Isaac and Christiansen 2002; Kim and Gandhi 2010). Conversely, disempowering for strike participation stems from administrative control and regulation (Roscigno and Hodson 2004). Similarly, strike participation has subsided with national dictatorship (Kim and Gandhi 2010).

The indirect deterministic mechanism of incentivizing offers incentives to raise the utility of appealing and thus appealing through the voluntaristic mechanism of utility optimization. Such utility rises with strike participation to meet inflation in the context (Litor 2019). Hence, national inflation has raised strike participation (Kim and Gandhi 2010). Furthermore, national income is the reference for demand and thus gain through strike participation. Therefore, national income has been conducive to strike participation (Kim and Gandhi 2010). Conversely, the utility of strike participation declines with unemployment in the context (Litor 2019). Thereby, national unemployment has discouraged strike participation (Isaac and Christiansen 2002).

The indirect deterministic mechanism of standardizing consolidates social norms for strike participation to enable normative influence on strike participation through the voluntaristic mechanism of norm conformity. Such norms flow from mobilization (Healy and Kirton 2013).

The indirect deterministic mechanism of framing popularizes frames to invoke ideas to rationalize and induce strike participation through the voluntaristic mechanism of idea consistency. Such frames in the context highlight autonomy, deprivation, deregulation, and rights concerning employment (Litor 2019). As such, strike participation has risen with national civil rights movements, democrat strength, and deprivation (Isaac and Christiansen 2002; Kim and Gandhi 2010). Notably, deprivation particularly applies to minority labor (Coleman et al. 2008; Semyonov et al. 2002). Thus, minority labor in the context has induced strike participation (Roscigno and Hodson 2004). Conversely, contextual frames discouraging strike participation laud bureaucracy, efficiency, flexibility, hierarchy, institutionalism, managerialism, and neoliberalism in employment as opposed to labor rights (Greenberg 2004; Litor 2019).

Voting

Voting is a conventional political practice under political competition (Chaney 2014). This practice realizes and sustains the function of democracy to safeguard political accountability, empowerment, fulfillment, legitimacy, and sovereignty (Aldrich and Simon 1986; Bennett and Resnick 1990; Joslyn and Cigler 2001). Voting also demonstrates the function of good citizenship (Abelson et al. 1992). Essentially, voting serves the goal for individual instead of collective political participation (Aldrich

1993). To fulfill the function and goal, voting builds on analytical functionalism's voluntaristic and deterministic mechanisms.

The voluntaristic mechanism of power realization applies power to attain the goal of voting to activate voting. Such power encompasses competence, information, knowledge, and various resources for voting (Carreras 2018; de Zuniga et al. 2016; Lassen 2005; Norris 2002). As such, voting has risen from cognitive and verbal or vocabulary abilities, political information or knowledge, leadership, self-efficacy, social capital, and civic, job, organizational, and political competence or skill (Anderson 2009; Ayala 2000; de Zuniga et al. 2016; Glanville 1999; Schlozman et al. 1994; Straughn and Andriot 2011; Verba et al. 1995; Weinschenk and Dawes 2022). Furthermore, voting has increased with education, employment, health, homeownership, income, social class, time availability, parental education and income, and family income or socioeconomic status, as opposed welfare dependence (Aytac and Stokes 2019; Bruch et al. 2010; Child and Nikolova 2020; Goerres 2007; Hansen and Tyner 2019; Heath et al. 1991; McCabe 2014; Norris 2002; Verba et al. 1995; Weinschenk and Dawes 2022; Zaff et al. 2003), In addition, voting has escalated with experience or feeling about anger, pride, satisfaction with the job or life, and shame, which would energize action (Aytac and Stokes 2019; Delli Carpini 1986; Panagopoulos 2010; Flavin and Keane 2011). Conversely, voting declines with emotionality, fatigue, and belief about the complexity of politics (Anderson 2009; Lijphart 1997; Shockley and Fairdosi 2015).

The voluntaristic mechanism of utility optimization highlights the utility of voting to attract voting. Such utility arises from the gain or benefit over cost from voting, fulfilling duty or rules, self-expression or signaling, and perceived election competitiveness (Aytac and Stokes 2019; Gallego 2009). Conversely, the disutility of not voting or abstention emanates from social pressure (Aytac and Stokes 2019). Belief in, support for, and the valuation of voting or election has raised voting (Aytac and Stokes 2019; Echabe et al. 1988; Hennessy et al. 2015). Similarly, attachment to community and belief in government responsiveness have buttressed voting (Echabe et al. 1988; Finkel 1995; Petrocik 1991). Voting has risen with experience of blame, ease in voting or its preparation, incentive, prosperity, and social connection, which would buttress the utility of voting (Aytac and Stokes 2019; Chan and Lee 2007; Hansen and Tyner 2019; Shockley and Fairdosi 2015; Wilking and Zhang 2013). Meanwhile, the utility of voting declines with the perceived uncontrollability of politics or electoral outcomes and consensus or certainty of the outcomes (Clark and Inglehart 1998; Shockley and Fairdosi 2015). By reducing the utility of voting, the dispositions of nationalism, patriotism, and submissiveness to government have discouraged voting (Goel 1980; Huddy and Khatib 2007). Moreover, voting has diminished with liberty perceived, which would dampen the utility of voting (Schwartz et al. 2010).

The voluntaristic mechanism of norm conformity builds on social norms for voting to assimilate voting. Such norms arise from the culture, institution, mobilization, and party normalizing choice and rights rather than independence and skepticism (Carreras 2018; Chaney 2014; Gallego 2009; Goldstein and Holleque 2010; Lister 2007; Norris 2002; Schecter 2009). Moreover, voting has risen with the experience of media, mobilization, promotion, recruitment, social norms and pressure, and others' partisanship perceived (Anderson 2009; Green et al. 2009; Hennessy et al. 2015; Kennamer 1990; McGregor 2018; Sobieraj and White 2004).

The voluntaristic mechanism of idea consistency gathers ideas compatible with voting to rationalize and encourage voting (Fife and Breakwell 1990). Such ideas favoring voting cover or consist in agency, alternative participation connections concerning voting, and social desirability generally (Aytac and Stokes 2019; Belli et al. 1999; Lijphart 1997; Hennessy et al. 2015; Norris 2002). In practice, voting has risen with compliance, extracurricular activity, mobility, organizational or union involvement, parasocial interaction, political activism and discussion, public engagement, radio listening, and religious attendance (Delli Carpini 1986; Frenk et al. 2013; Kruikemeier et al. 2014; Lassen 2005; Lee 2012; Marsh 2005; McGregor 2018; Rhodes 2011; Straughn and Andriot 2011; Zaff et al. 2003). The dispositions of attentiveness to politics, internal control, partisanship, and religiosity have also buttressed voting (Claassen and Povtak 2010; Pasek et al. 2008; Weinschenk and Dawes 2022). Furthermore, voting has risen with such attitudes as belief in civic duty, concern for politics, favor for politicians, identification with a party or the country, interest in politics, orientation toward equality, sensitivity to government, support for the regime, trust in politics or others (Aldrich and Simon 1986; Aytac and Stokes 2019; Carreras 2018; Chen and Zhong 2002; Goerres 2007; Hansen and Tyner 2019; Huddy and Khatib 2007; Hutcheson and Prather 1981; Lelieveldt 2004; Mattes and Southall 2004; Schwartz et al. 2010; Verba et al. 1995). Conversely, belief in tradition and egocentric orientation have discouraged voting (Papadakis 2000; Schwartz et al. 2010).

The indirect deterministic mechanism of empowering generates power for voting collectively to facilitate voting through the voluntaristic mechanism of power realization. Such empowering derives from the requirement of compulsory voting in the context (Lijphart 1997). Thus, voting has increased with compulsory voting, electoral permissiveness, and human development in the country (Norris 2002; Singh 2011). Conversely, disempowering for voting results from frequent voting (Lijphart 1997). Moreover, voting has diminished with inflation and poverty in the country, which would be disempowering (Bruch et al. 2010; Finegold and Swigt 2001).

The indirect deterministic mechanism of incentivizing raises the utility of voting collectively to attract voting through the voluntaristic mechanism of utility optimization. Such incentives evolve from the competition and competitiveness, choices, and proportional representation of election (Gallego 2009; Lijphart 1997; Norris 2002). Hence, voting has risen with bicameralism, candidates' policy agreement, economic problems, government expenditure, notably on welfare, income inequality, party competition, proportional representation in the country, tax revenues, and voting on Sunday, which would escalate the utility of voting (Bahry and Lipsmeyer 2001; Bruch et al. 2010; Franklin 1996; Hobolt and Klemmensen 2005; Lister 2007; Lockerbie 1999; Schecter 2009). Indicative of electoral competitiveness, population size per elected seat has also raised voting (Norris 2002). Similarly, unemployment in the context has encouraged voting (Bruch et al. 2010). Furthermore, the electoral administration has sustained voting by safeguarding its utility (Freeman 2004). Conversely, incentives reduce with the consensus or certainty of the electoral result and wastage of votes (Clark and Inglehart 1998; Lijphart 1997). Hence, voting has declined with ethnic diversity and associational activity in the context, which would reduce the utility of voting (Pattie et al. 2004; Schecter 2009).

The indirect deterministic mechanism of standardizing popularizes social norms for voting to assimilate voting through the voluntaristic mechanism of norm conformity. As such, voting has risen with labor unionization and electorate size in the country, which would mobilize voting (Uslaner and Brown 2005; Norris 2002). Similarly, population size in the context has boosted voting (Gilberbloom and Markham 1995).

The indirect deterministic mechanism of framing provides frames for voting collectively to rationalize and induce voting through the voluntaristic mechanism of idea consistency. Such ideas uphold agency, altruism, beneficence, bonding, collaboration, commonwealth, democracy, equality, freedom, instrumentality, justice, populism, responsibility, rights, self-interest, virtue, and welfare provision as opposed to domination and free ridership to justify voting (Brennan 2011; Nyenhuis 2020). Based on framing, voting has risen with democratization and its history in the country (Norris 2002). In addition, social trust in the context has escalated voting (Pattie et al. 2004). Conversely, voting has declined with repression in the country, which discourages political participation (Booth and Richard 1998). In addition, religiosity in the context has dampened voting (DeLeon and Naff 2004).

Green Demonstrating and Donation

Green demonstration and donation reflect environmentalist practice (Zhang et al. 2007; Vesalon and Creţan 2015). The practice displays political and social-movement properties (Anderson 2010; Lee and Norris 2000). This movement holds goals to achieve balance in the nature or ecosystems, biodiversity, biophilia, cleanliness, compassion, connectedness to nature, conservation, greening, health, postmaterialism, preservation, protection, recycling, renewability, safety, sustainability, and transcendentalism (Bostrom et al. 2012; Cantzler 2007; Combes et al. 2018; Dayton 2000; Domina and Koch 2002; Foss 2009; Gonzalez et al. 2021; Hultgren 2018; McGrail 2011; O'Connor et al. 2002; O'Neill et al. 2008; Richards 2001; Taylor 2000). Conversely, the goals are to resist danger, degradation, economism, exploitation, extinction, growth, marketing, militarization, pollution, risk, savagery, and wastage (Cantzler 2007; Eugene and Holland 2000; Gatersleben et al. 2002; Glasson 2015; Korfiatis et al. 2004; McGrail 2011; Scruton 2014; Sinn and Hayes 2017; Taylor 2000; Tonglet et al. 2004). To attain these goals, environmentalist practice builds on the voluntaristic and deterministic mechanisms of analytical functionalism.

The voluntaristic mechanism of power realization mobilizes power to drive environmentalist practice to attain its goals. Such power consists in availability, cognition or knowledge for environmentalist practice, consciousness, efficacy personally and collectively, income, intelligence, resourcefulness, and wealth for environmentalist goals or practice (Briscoe et al. 2019; Brulle 2000; Franzen and Vogl 2013; Lubell

2002; O'Connor et al. 2002; Reese et al. 2019; Yates et al. 2015). The availability rises with homemaking, usually associated with female gender (Yates et al. 2015). Power also springs from drive provoked by terror, such as mortality (Fritsche et al. 2010). In addition, environmentalist practice benefits capability or competence enabled by knowledge, social capital, and motivation based on self-determination (Chow et al. 2019; Corral-Vergugo 2002; Geerts et al. 2020; Lubell 2002). Hence, environmentalist practice has benefited from education, health, and self-efficacy (Adeola 2000; Heath and Gifford 2006; Kanji and Nevitte 1997). Conversely, environmentalist practice has diminished with full-time employment and children in the family, which reduces availability for the practice (Shen and Saijo 2008; Yates et al. 2015).

The voluntaristic mechanism of utility optimization emphasizes the utility of environmentalist practice to attract the practice. Such utility or value inheres in gain or benefit over cost, reward from environmentalist practice, controllability of the practice, and the risk, severity, threat, and vulnerability of environmental issues (Carmeli et al. 2017; Poortinga et al. 2014; Lubell 2002; Truelove et al. 2019). Therefore, environmentalist practice has risen with beliefs in controllability over risk, effectiveness, moral responsibility, and fragility and harm due to environmental issues (Bostrom et al. 2012). Perception of the problems of climate change, corruption, dysfunction, and harm and their seriousness would also raise environmentalist practice and government efficacy, empowerment, and transparency, possibly through enhancing the utility of the practice, as supported by government (Curtis and Lockwood 2000; Harring 2014; Heath and Gifford 2006; Lubell 2002; O'Connor et al. 2002; Sherkat and Ellison 2007). Similarly, the experience of benefit from environmentalist practice and danger and threat from environmental issues has boosted environmentalist practice (Domina and Koch 2002; Hafner et al. 2019; Lubell 2002; Yates et al. 2015). Conversely, the utility reduces with the discounting of the future (Hantula 2012). Similarly, environmentalist practice has diminished with resilience, which would reduce the utility of the practice (Plutzer et al. 1998).

The voluntaristic mechanism of norm conformity highlights social norms for environmentalist practice to assimilate the practice. Such norms evolve from culture, consensus, dialogue, institutions, roles, and socialization concerning environmentalist practice (Briscoe et al. 2019; Brulle 2000; Truelove et al. 2019; Yates et al. 2015). Environmentalist practice has risen from discussion and information, mobilization, and norms observed or received concerning the practice (Clark et al. 2003; Fujii et al. 2004; Kanji and Nevitte 1997; Kempton et al. 1995; Siu and Xiao 2015; Steel 1999).

The voluntaristic mechanism of idea consistency champions ideas consonant with environmentalist practice to rationalize and safeguard the practice. This mechanism sustains the generalization or spillover of ideas and their connection and organization to minimize dissonance (Ghazali et al. 2018; Poortinga et al. 2014). These ideas concern morality, partisanship, safety, transcendence concerning environmentalist identity, intention, liking, obligation, or practice (Briscoe et al. 2019; Brulle 2000; O'Connor et al. 2002; Truelove et al. 2019; Yates et al. 2015). As such, environmental practice has evolved from the dispositions of acquiescence, agreeableness, altruism, conscientiousness, cynicism, democratic partisanship, egalitarianism, empathy, environmentalism, extraversion, future orientation, inclusiveness, independence, leftism, liberalism, libertarianism, morality, openness, postmaterialism, progressivism, republican partisanship, and universalism (Barker and Tinnick 2006; Briscoe et al. 2019; Clark et al. 2003; Combes et al. 2018; Franzen and Vogl 2013; Gonzalez et al. 2021; Harring 2014; Kanji and Nevitte 1997; Jones 2011; Lee and Norris 2000; Lubell 2002; Sinn and Hayes 2017; Tam 2013; Thomas et al. 1998). Moreover, environmentalist practice has grown with the values of benevolence and self-transcendence (Bain et al. 2013). Environmentalist practice has also increased with membership in environmentalist organizations (Combes et al. 2018; Kanji and Nevitte 1997). The practices of cohesion, political discussion and involvement, and visiting parks have sustained environmentalist practice (Guardia and Pol 2002; Lee and Norris 2000). Such attitudes as concern for morality and the world, identification with the place, interest in politics, liking for sustainability, and support for sacrificing have underlain environmentalist practice (Carmeli et al. 2017; Guardia and Pol 2002; Kanji and Nevitte 1997; Korfiatis et al. 2004; Sherkat and Ellison 2007; Tonglet et al. 2004). Conversely, ideas discounting environmental practice reside in careerism, individualism, and possessiveness (Brulle 2000). Furthermore, environmentalist practice has declined with the dispositions of conservatism, Darwinism, fatalism, individualism, materialism, neuroticism, and religiosity (Briscoe et al. 2019; Combes et al. 2018; Engel and Potschke 1998; Gonzalez et al. 2021; Jones 2011; Sherkat and Ellison 2007). In addition, environmentalist practice has diminished with the value of binding, including authority, loyalty, and purity (Rossen et al. 2015). The practices of purchasing and traveling have weakened environmentalist practice (Schiebel et al. 2015). Support for development, government, and the market has eroded environmentalist practice (Barker and Tinnick 2006; Heath and Gifford 2006; Papadakis 2000). Environmentalist practice has also evolved from identity and satisfaction concerning the practice (Adeola 2000; Heinen 2016; Siu and Xiao 2015).

The direct deterministic mechanism operates with collective environmentalist practice raising personal environmentalist practice through private or public sharing (Sell et al. 2002). In private sharing, personal practice is part of collective practice, whereas in public sharing, free ridership in the practice works.

The direct deterministic mechanism operates with collective environmentalist practice raising personal environmentalist practice through private or public sharing (Sell et al. 2002). In private sharing, personal practice is part of collective practice, whereas, in public sharing, free ridership in the practice works.

The indirect deterministic mechanism of incentivizing boosts the utility of environmentalist practice to attract the practice through the voluntaristic mechanism of utility optimization. Such incentivizing works through funding and professionalization for environmentalist practice (Brulle 2000). In addition, incentivizing highlights environmental problems in the context due to colonialism, disaster, shortage, and unsustainability (Erickson 2020; Goldblatt 1996; Heath and Gifford 2006; Milbrath 1986). Hence, corruption, economic inequality, and population density in the country, indicating ineffectiveness in tackling environmental problems, have raised environmental practice (Franzen and Vogl 2013; Harring 2014). Similarly, environmental hazards, hazardous waste, and population size in the context have urged the citizen's environmentalist practice (Adeola 2000; Engels and Jacobson 2007). Attractiveness in the context has also attracted environmentalist practice, possibly to sustain the attractiveness (Adeola 2000). Charging plastic bags and environmental indicator programming in the context have also boosted citizens' environmentalist practice (Blair 2005; Poortinga et al. 2014). Conversely, government democracy and spending, possibly tackling environmental problems, have discouraged the citizen's environmentalist practice (Combes et al. 2018).

The indirect deterministic mechanism of empowering imposes power to lift environmentalist practice through the voluntaristic mechanism of power realization. National prosperity and its growth have empowered environmentalist practice (Franzen and Vogl 2013; Scruggs 2003). Similarly, income in the context has facilitated the citizen's environmentalist practice (Engel and Potschke 1998). Conversely, disempowering against environmentalist practice stems from control, domination, and exploitation in the context (Briscoe et al. 2019).

The indirect deterministic mechanism of framing propagates ideas for environmentalist practice to rationalize and sustain the practice through the voluntaristic mechanism of idea consistency. Framing involves amplifying and constructing ideas (McGrail 2011; Taylor 2000). Frames or discourses for environmentalist practice highlights adversaries, conservation, cosmopolitanism, ecology, destiny, individualization and thus personal responsibility, intellectualism, postmaterialism, preservation, reflexivity, responsibility, survival, sustainability, utilitarianism, and the future (Anderson 2010; Brulle 2000; Cantzler 2007; Dryzek 1997; Glasson 2015; Guneratne 2008; Humphrey 2010; Inglehart 1990). Intellectualism treasures science and technology and their administration (Glasson 2015). Reflexivity emphasizes personal knowledge and rationality to deal with global issues (Borne 2009). Notably, postmaterialism in the country has encouraged environmentalist practice. Conversely, frames countering environmentalist practice signify anthropocentrism, conservatism, consumerism, heroism or Prometheanism, modernization, nationalism, neoliberalism, and pragmatism (Anderson 2010; Dryzek 1997; Glasson 2015; Maxton-Lee 2020; Scruton 2014). Consumerism treasures advertising or marketing, commodification, fetishism, and romanticism (Glasson 2015). Neoliberalism advocates deregulation, marketization, liberalization, and privatization (Hultgren 2018; Maxton-Lee 2020; Vesalon and Creţan 2015). Hence, conservatism in the context has discouraged environmentalist practice (de Oliver 1999).

Predictors of Practices

The predictors of personal private and public practices or activeness include personal and national factors. Personal factors consist of various sociodemographic characteristics such as age and gender, whereas national factors include population size, phone ownership, and land area per capita. Meanwhile, practices encompass e-activity, learning, spiritual activity, risk aversion, weapon carrying, organizational participation, appealing, strike participation, voting, green demonstrating, and green donation.

Age

Age, representing experience and the life course and stage, is influential (Hess et al. 2005; O'Rand 1996; Riley and Riley 1999). Essentially, age as an individual variable is a typical antecedent because of its insusceptibility and uncontrollability (Frazier et al. 2007). Instead, age assimilates and controls other factors, including practices. In practice, age has escalated activity generally, including attention to news and problems, compensation or recovering losses, discussion about politics, eating, engagement, exercising, influencing others, investment, leisure activity, negotiation, protecting the environment, religious activity, self-regulation, spending on medicine, using medical services, visiting hospitals, volunteering, and working in the household (Charles and Carstensen 2009; Datler et al. 2013; Freund 2006; Fung et al. 2008; Howe 2013; Inglehart 2003; Isaacowitz et al. 2003; Marcum 2013; Schaie 2013; Shindler et al. 2006; Tam 2014). These practices are mostly private. By contrast, age has diminished attention to politics, caring, choosing, communication, cultural practice, educating, exploring, gardening, optimizing, participation, political activity, search for meaning, seeking varieties, self-disclosure, sleeping, and traveling (Anciaes et al. 2017; Freund 2006; Guillen et al. 2011; Howe 2010; Isaacowitz et al. 2003; Marcum 2013; Novak and Mather 2007; Scherger 2009; Steger et al. 2009; Van den Broeck et al. 2015). These practices are primarily public or interactive. The influence of age would undergo the voluntaristic mechanisms of analytical functionalism.

The voluntaristic mechanism of power realization works with power for practice rooted in age or aging. Power for practice grows with age through adaptability, learning, and talent or human capital learned and developed (Consedine 2011; Von Krogh and Wallin 2011; Wagner and Lang 2011). Hence, age has increased affordability, identification with a party, knowledge, reactivity, and vocabulary, underpinning power for practice (Goerres 2007; Hallerod 2006; Kliegel et al. 2007; Price et al. 2006; Stanley et al. 2014). Age has also escalated organizational membership and social class, thus strengthening power for practice (Inglehart 2003; Parrado 2005). Such power has been activating (Stolle 2001). Conversely, age has lessened depression and thus power loss (Stanley et al. 2014). By contrast, power weakens with age because of decline or deterioration in strength and even time for use, disengagement, isolation from social connection, and thus its resources and support, and incapability (Charles and Carstensen 2009; Marcum 2013; Morgan and Robinson 2013). Age has reduced extrinsic motivation, health, intelligence and thinking, memory, need for achievement, physical functioning, and self-efficacy, which would constitute power for practice (Ferssizidis et al. 2010; Gerstorf et al. 2006; Goerres 2007; Li and Chung

2008; Stevens et al. 2001). Moreover, education and income have been lower in the older person (Goerres 2007). Age has also diminished experience about friendship, social integration, and thus power or opportunities for practice (Goerres 2007). Age has dampened anger regarding the feeling as power to activate practice (Charles and Carstensen 2008). These declines have been deactivating (Bonke and Fallesen 2010). Conversely, age has escalated the experience of illness, thus weakening power for practice (Schaie 2013).

The voluntaristic mechanism of utility optimization operates with the utility of practice changed by age. Age has increased the preference for creativity, the values of voting and work, and thus the utility of practice (Kiecolt 2003). By contrast, the utility of practice declining with age stems from a decline in future orientation and materialism (Morgan and Robinson 2013; Wagner and Lang 2011). The utility of personal practice also declines with age due to marriage or spousal sharing (Kuntla et al. 2013). Age has also increased authoritarianism and conservatism, which would dampen the utility of practice (Cornelis et al. 2009). Authoritarianism and conservatism uphold passivity and inaction by favoring the government and custom (Braun 2011; Scruton 2014). Conversely, age has diminished leftism and the value of independence, thus the utility of practice (Fjellvang 2011; Tilley 2002).

The voluntaristic mechanism of norm conformity hinges on social norms for practice evolving with age. Social norms affecting practice arise from enculturation, parenthood, or grandparenthood (Holstein and Gubrium 2000; Wagner and Lang 2011).

The voluntaristic mechanism of idea consistency functions with ideas for practice growing with age. Ideas for practice increasing with age include generativity, parenting, and grandparenting (Wagner and Lang 2011; Morgan and Robinson 2013). Age has also raised the duty for voting, extraversion, political interest, and self-reliance (Fung and Ng 2006). By contrast, ideas discouraging practice arises with age due to disengagement, detachment, compensation, limitation in time and the horizon, optimization, selectivity, self-regulation, short-termism, stress, and its sensitivity (Charles and Carstensen 2009; Chow et al. 2007; Consedine 2011; Marcum 2013; Morgan and Robinson 2013; Wagner and Lang 2011). Age has also increased agreeableness and neuroticism (Fung and Ng 2006; Stanley et al. 2014). Conversely, ideas for practice decline with age, including acquisition, searching, and self-presentation (Morgan and Robinson 2013; Wagner and Lang 2011). Age has also diminished integrity and support for social movements (Sneed et al. 2006; Tilley 2002).

Mid-Age

Mid-age shows an effect to indicate that the age effect is not straightly linear. Accordingly, mid-age has raised civic engagement, criminal activity, and its reporting, giving, prosocial behavior, religious activity, volunteering, and voting (Akers and Kaukinen 2009; Apinunmahakul and Devlin 2008; Bellemare and Kroger 2007;

Flavin and Keane 2011; Land et al. 1996; Phan et al. 2009; Sarracino 2010; Taniguichi and Thomas 2011). These effects would transmit through the voluntaristic mechanisms of analytical functionalism.

The voluntaristic mechanism of power realization envisions the contribution of power stemming from mid-age to activate practice. Power enabling practice stemming from mid-age has included cultural and social capital, education, employment, financial adequacy, homeownership, income, and social class (Benstock 2008; Glaeser and Gottlieb 2006; Keister 2003; Parrado 2005; Plagnol and Easterlin 2008). Mid-age has also raised social integration to engage practice (Frei et al. 2009). Furthermore, mid-age has sustained the feeling about mastery or self-efficacy to activate practice (Schieman 2001). By contrast, mid-age has weakened power based on affordability, health, wealth, and family income (Hallerod 2006; Jorgensen et al. 2010; Keister 2003; van Praag and Ferrer-I-Carbonell 2004).

The voluntaristic mechanism of utility optimization attracts practice by its utility evolving from mid-age. Mid-age has sustained belief about collective efficacy and thus the utility of practice (Grasso 2014). Furthermore, mid-age has increased experience with gifts received to enhance the utility of reciprocating practice (Godoy et al. 2007). By contrast, mid-age has reduced belief about government responsiveness and thus the utility of practice (Shi 2000).

The voluntaristic mechanism of norm conformity accentuates the impacts of social norms concerning mid-age on practice. Social norms stemming from mid-age conducive to practice derive from organizational membership and parenthood (Apinunmahakul and Devlin 2008; Parrado 2005).

The voluntaristic mechanism of idea consistency relies on ideas generated from mid-age to rationalize and sustain practice. Ideas rationalizing practice arising from mid-age include aspiration, orientation toward practice, and partisanship (Grasso 2014; Plagnol and Easterlin 2008; Sheldon and Kasser 2001). By contrast, mid-age has generated experience of political alienation to weaken practice (Coffe and Geys 2007).

Gender

Gender is crucial as an easily recognizable and prominently socialized status characteristic (Carli and Bukatko 2000; Franklin 2012). Female gender has sustained commitment, coping, kin visiting, medical service use, medication, modeling, political awareness, tax-paying, teacher interaction, and traveling (Ferssizidis et al. 2010; Lippa 2005; Lockwood 2006; Schaie 2013; Tamres et al. 2002; Tang 2011; Young and Willmont 1957). By contrast, female gender has impeded environmentalist participation, exercising, Internet use, political discussion, sacrificing, tax evasion, volunteering, and voting (Fyall and Gazley 2015; Gerxhani and Schram 2006; Kerrissey and Schofer 2013; Roy 2009; Sherkat and Ellison 2007; Walter-Ginzburg et al. 2005; Welzel 2013). These effects would work through the voluntaristic mechanisms of analytical functionalism.

The voluntaristic mechanism of power realization refers to power differential due to gender in driving practice. Female gender has generated power for practice based on cognitive complexity, intelligence, intrinsic motivation, mastery, and verbal ability (Ferssizidis et al. 2010; Hansen et al. 2012; Sternberg 2006; Straughn and Andriot 2011). By contrast, female gender has reduced health, information, knowledge, and time free to furnish power for practice (Gattino et al. 2015; Shin 2012). Female gender has also lessened anger and extrinsic motivation, thus generating power for practice (Charles and Carstensen 2008; Ferssizidis et al. 2010; Verba et al. 1995). Conversely, female gender has raised depression and illness to dampen power for practice (Schaie 2013).

The voluntaristic mechanism of utility optimization emphasizes the gender differential in the utility of practice for gravitating to the practice. Accordingly, female gender has championed the values of benevolence, conservation, emancipation, family, friendship, material, power, security, stimulation, tradition, voting, work, and thus their related practices (Bonin-Scaon et al. 2009; Caprara and Vecchione 2017; Datler et al. 2013; Gross 1995; Kiecolt 2003; Straughn and Andriot 2011; Welzel 2013; Wuthnow 2004). Conversely, female gender has diminished authoritarianism, conservatism, and thus the utility of personal practice (Hooghe 2003; Norris and Inglehart 2009). Similarly, female gender has weakened the values of conformity, independence, marriage, responsibility, wealth, and thus related practices (Guo et al. 2008; Nie and Hillygus 2001; Ulbig 2002).

The voluntaristic mechanism of norm conformity highlights social norms arising from gender for assimilating practice. Female gender has sustained experience with mobilization to realize the norm for practice (Olcese et al. 2014). By contrast, female gender has weakened the perception of the norm for violence and thus related practices (Scharrer 2008).

The voluntaristic mechanism of idea consistency hinges on idealistic differences due to gender for rationalizing and sustaining practice. Female gender has sustained ideas concerning caring and extraversion to uphold practice (Feingold 1994; Lippa 2005). Accordingly, female gender has sustained altruism, familism, hedonism, liberalism, and meritocratism. Multiculturalism, patriotism, progressivism, radicalism, religiosity, and universalism for raising justifications for relevant practices (Caprara and Vecchione 2017; Dietz et al. 2002; Evans et al. 2010; Hagan et al. 1999; Hughes 2001; Immerzeel and van Tubergen 2013; Norris and Inglehart 2009; Pehrson et al. 2011; Kunovich 2009; McCright and Dunlop 2008). By contrast, female gender has bred ideas concerning agreeableness to discourage practice (Caprara and Vecchione 2017). Furthermore, female gender has discounted environmentalism, individualism, leftism, nationalism, neoliberalism, postmaterialism, racism, rightism, socialism, and thus justifications for related practices (Curry and O'Connell 2000; Datler et al. 2013; Finseraas 2010; Gilberbloom and Markham 1995; Norris and Inglehart 2009; Paterson 2008; Shen and Saijo 2008; Welzel 2013). Conversely, female gender had dampened ideas upholding assertiveness, civic duty, helpfulness, and interest in politics to reduce practice (Datler et al. 2013; Feingold 1994; Lippa 2005; Weimann and Brosius 1994).

Immigration

Immigration, as indicated by parental immigration, has withheld such practices as cohesion, contact, civic engagement, migration, political participation, volunteering, and voting (Brayne 2014; Hui and Yu 2009; Lien 1994; Ravanera et al. 2003; Sonderskov 2011; Stromblad and Myrberg 2013). Such deactivating effects would hinge on the voluntaristic mechanisms of analytical functionalism.

The voluntaristic mechanism of power realization employs power to activate practices to attain its goal. However, the immigrant has lessened power in health, functional ability, and social capital (Fanning et al. 2011; Herd et al. 2008; Islam et al. 2006). Moreover, power has diminished with immigration through illness, poverty, and unemployment as opposed to employment (Kurz et al. 2005; Posthumus et al. 2013; Ravanera et al. 2003; Wen et al. 2010).

The voluntaristic mechanism of utility optimization hinges on the utility of practice experienced or expected to attract practice. Such utility has declined with immigration through social exclusion, which has impeded reasoning and practice (Bask 2005; Guillen et al. 2011).

The voluntaristic mechanism of norm conformity highlights social norms to assimilate practice. Meanwhile, immigration has encountered social norms suggesting incapability (Lilly et al. 2011). These norms, in turn, discourage practice (Zurcher 2017).

The voluntaristic mechanism of idea consistency rests on ideas compatible with practice to rationalize and encourage the practice. Such ideas or practices have diminished with depression and life dissatisfaction (Flavin and Keane 2011; Moran et al. 2012). The latter, in turn, has arisen from immigration (Ambrey and Fleming 2014; Lofors and Sundquist 2007).

Education

Education has been activating in raising a full range of practice, including choosing, civic engagement, civility, collective action, cultural activity, environmentalist participation, exercising, formal and informal participation, health behavior, media use, persistence, political awareness, discussion, and participation, prevention, social activity, studying, traveling, using, such as services and skills, visiting, and voting (Chan 2014; Corcoran et al. 2011; Djupe and Lewis 2015; Guillen et al. 2011; Horowitz 2018; Lelli 2008; Lewis 2003; McCabe 2014; McClelland 1982; Mirowsky and Ross 2001; Morenoff et al. 2008; Norris 2011; Pallas 2002; Norris and Inglehart 2009; Papadakis 2000; Singer et al. 1999; Stone and Buttice 2010; Tang 2011; Welzel 2013; Yang et al. 2012). Hence, education has driven practice (Bonke and Fallesen 2010; Soderberg and Wester 2012). By contrast, education has been deactivating in withholding birthing, deviance, discriminating, housework, intergenerational association, personal care, prostitution, resistance, returning from migration, and violence (Backman and Nilsson 2011; Gershuny 2000; Huang 2002; Korinek et al. 2005; Lee et al. 2004; Lubbers et al. 2006; Michalski 2005; Swader and Vorobeva 2015; Torche 2011). These influences fulfill the goals of education as deliberation, entertainment, knowledge acquisition, learning, normalizing, rationalization, responsibilizing, social control, integration, positioning, and working (Horowitz 2018; Izquierdo and Minguez 2003; Nordin 2011; O'Dwyer 2003; Papastephanon 2015; Teodoro 2003; Vanderstraeten 2003). The fulfillment would thereby build on the voluntaristic mechanism of analytical functionalism.

The voluntaristic mechanism of power realization hinges on power generated by education to drive practice for attaining its goals. Education is power, known as talent or human capital, and cultural capital for accumulating various forms of capital (Dolton et al. 2004; Horowitz 2018; Nordin 2011). Precisely, power evolving from education has consisted in eloquence, expertise, functioning, health, intelligence, knowledge, memory, and skill, as opposed to vulnerability (Cerin and Leslie 2008; Fiske et al. 1990; Langenderfer and Shimp 2001; Pratt et al. 1996; Ross and Mirowsky 1995; Shin 2012; Stevens et al. 2001; Straughn and Andriot 2011; Verba et al. 1995). Education has also nurtured feelings about mastery and self-efficacy, such as exercising and politics (Cerin and Leslie 2008; Corcoran et al. 2011; Rasmussen et al. 2018; Stavrova and Ehlebracht 2018). Furthermore, education has generated power located in earnings, employment, insurance coverage, possession, social class, and status, as opposed to poverty (Cerin and Leslie 2008; Knab et al. 2008; Pettigrew 2002; Schnittker and Behrman 2012; Vartanian 1999; Wang et al. 2013; Whyte and Gao 2009). In addition, education has fostered social support experiences such as from family (Cerin and Leslie 2008). Such power has been activating (Donohew et al. 1987; Flint and Luloff 2007). Conversely, education has lessened the experience of arrest, constraint, discrimination, exclusion, and threat, which impede practice (Allwood and Widom 2013; Backman and Nilsson 2011; Kessler et al. 1999; Emler and Frazer 1999; Raijman et al. 2003; Stavrova and Ehlebracht 2018).

The voluntaristic mechanism of utility optimization works with utility raised by education for practice to attract the practice (Fiske et al. 1990). Such utility raised by education has consisted in the values of autonomy, childbearing, independence, voting, and work (Fjellvang 2011; James and Luo 1999; Weimann and Brosius 1994; Wu and MacNeill 2003; Xiao 2000). Education has also raised experience about the benefit of exercising and opportunity instead of hazards (Cerin and Leslie 2008; Emler and Frazer 1999).

The voluntaristic mechanism of norm conformity leverage social norms drawn from education to assimilate practice. Such norms emanate from instruction to nourish authenticity, challenging, choosing, competition, creativity, discovering, and peaking (Yair 2003). Norms for practices induced by education have also arisen from mobilization (Kerrissey and Schofer 2013).

The voluntaristic mechanism of idea consistency highlights ideas gleaned from education to rationalize and induce practices. Ideas nurtured from education to activate practice has consisted in the dispositions of conscientiousness, expressivism, humanism, individualism, meritocratism, and progressivism (Evans et al. 2010; McCright and Dunlop 2008; Rossi 2001; Sotirovic 2000; Yuchtman-Yaar 2002; Welzel 2013). Herein, conscientiousness upholds work (Bogg 2008). Humanism champions agency, construction, cooperation, creativity, vitality, and work (Browning and Cooper 2004; Doane 2017; Selznick 2008; Visher 1997; Waterman 2013). Individualism accentuates achievement, choosing, competing, contribution, responsibility, and restlessness (Braun 2011; Davis and Robinson 1999; Oyserman et al. 2002; Sullivan et al. 2015). Meritocratism treasures performance (Evans et al. 2010). Progressivism favors collective action, cooperation, employment, and labor (Box 2008; Fukuyama 2018b; Mahoney 2004; Wilson 2001). Education has also fostered attitudes such as aspiration, consciousness about rights, endorsement for duty, and interest in politics, as opposed to alienation (Coffe and Geys 2007; Kerrissey and Schofer 2013; Norris 2011; Straughn and Andriot 2011; Weimann and Brosius 1994). Furthermore, education has lifted feeling about youthfulness (van Praag and Frijters 1999). Conversely, education has diminished ideas impeding practice, as consisting in the dispositions of authoritarianism, Buddhism, conservatism, and traditionalism (Achterberg and Houtman 2009; Coffe and Geys 2007; Datler et al. 2013; Tang 2001).

Employment

Employment has activated practices including civic engagement, collective action, community involvement, donation, health behavior, political discussion, and participation, protesting, role-taking, social interaction, and voting (Corcoran et al. 2011; Fridberg and Kangas 2008b; Kerrissey and Schofer 2013; Lin et al. 2008; Lu et al. 2002; McCabe 2014; Stalker 2008; Tsai 2006). Meanwhile, employment has deactivated caring, criminal activity, exercising, moving, and volunteering (Bianchi et al. 2004; Kleinhans 2009; Savolainen 2009; Sarasa 2008; Taniguchi 2013). Such diverse influences reflect the goal of employment for career development (Hakim 2006). To attain the goal, employment would activate the voluntaristic mechanisms of analytical functionalism.

The voluntaristic mechanism of power realization hinges on power generated from employment to drive practice. Power has evolved from functional ability, health, skill, social capital, and social support received enhanced by employment (Distante 2013; Groot et al. 2007; Kerrissey and Schofer 2013; Li and Chung 2008). In addition, employment has sustained feelings about mastery and self-efficacy as opposed to depression, dysfunction, and powerlessness (Corcoran et al. 2011; Hansen et al. 2012; Keyes 2002; Ross and Mirowsky 2009). Moreover, employment has generated power in terms of income and insurance as opposed to poverty (Growiec and Growiec 2010; Fan et al. 2004). Conversely, employment has reduced experience of arrest, exclusion, and stress (Allwood and Widom 2013; Myer et al. 2008; Ross and Mirowsky 2009).

The voluntaristic mechanism of utility optimization refers to the utility of practice raised by employment to attract the practice. Such utility has consisted in the value of work sustained by employment (Moen et al. 1997).

The voluntaristic mechanism of norm conformity foregrounds social norms surrounding employment to assimilate practice. Such norms have evolved from shaming encourage abstinence from crime (Lu et al. 2002).

The voluntaristic mechanism of idea consistency engages ideas arising from employment to rationalize and induce practice. Ideas rationalizing practice stemming from employment have included growth and purposefulness (Ryff et al. 2004). Notably, purposefulness registers acting, motivation, and planning (George and Park 2013). Conversely, employment has reduced anomie, deterring practice (Zhao and Cao 2010).

Creative Work

More generally, creative work or creativity has fomented abusing substances, leisure activity, managing stress, vigorous activity as opposed to sleeping and volunteering (Gebbia and Honigsfeld 2012; Milgram and Hong 1994; Plucker and Dana 1998; Montgomery et al. 2004; Runco 2010). Hence, creative work is activating, likely in an unconventional way. Such work fulfills goals for adaptation, amorality, art, authoring, autonomy, carefreeness, complexity, drama, expression, flexibility, individualism, liberation, meaning, music, openness, playfulness, problem finding and solving, romanticism, self-enhancement, sensitivity as opposed to technocratism (Israelstam 2007; Joas 1996; Kozbelt et al. 2010; Leung and Koh 2018; Runco 2014; Shorthose and Maycroft 2017; Silvia et al. 2012). To attain these goals, creative work would draw on the voluntaristic mechanisms of analytical functionalism.

The voluntaristic mechanism of power realization applies creative work to generate power for practice. Such power has consisted in health and intelligence as opposed to feeling about despondence (Drus et al. 2014; Montgomery et al. 2004; Richards 2010).

The voluntaristic mechanism of utility optimization emphasizes the utility of practice evolving from creative work to buttress the practice. Such utility has emanated from experience or feeling about accomplishment, achievement, and meaningfulness and rested on creative work (Milgram and Hong 1994; Rindermann and Neubauer 2004; Turner 2013).

Independent Work

Independent work or autonomy at work has activated such practices as cohesion, involvement in the organization, productivity, safe work, use of family care policy, and the Internet (Kelly and Kelly 1994; Man and Lam 2003; Mortimer and Lorence 1989; Parker et al. 2001). Meanwhile, independent work has deactivated such practices as control over the spouse, emotional labor such as hiding agitation, and turnover (Erickson and Ritter 2001; Kim and Stoner 2008; Smit et al. 2016; Stets 1995). These effects reflect the goals of independent work for influence, responsibility, and taking charge (Franzen and Hangartner 2006; Morrison et al. 1999). The goal attainment would benefit from the voluntaristic mechanisms of analytical functionalism.

The voluntaristic mechanism of power realization harnesses power through independent work to drive practice to achieve its goals. Such power has consisted in creativity, health, leadership, skill, social capital, and support from the organization (Au and Cheung 2004; Benton 2015; de Witte et al. 2007; Garcia et al. 2017; Ng et al. 2008; Peng et al. 2019; Rhoades and Eisenberger 2002). This power depends on earnings raised by independent work (Ross and Mirowsky 1996). The power has also arisen from feeling about energy, mastery, and self-efficacy (Garcia et al. 2017; Schieman and Narisada 2014; Yoon 2001). Such power or its bases enable practice (Caprara and Vecchione 2013; Eccles and Wigfield 2002; Skyttner 2005; Silver 2011).

The voluntaristic mechanism of utility optimization highlights the utility of practice affected by independent work to influence the practice. Herein, independent work has diminished the experience of conflict, overload, and stress from work (Costigan et al. 2003; De Carlo et al. 2019; Garcia et al. 2017; Schieman and Glavin 2017). Such diminishment encourages practice (Hofmann et al. 2012). Conversely, independent work has lifted experience about balance and distributive justice regarding work to sustain work (Haar et al. 2019; Younts and Mueller 2001). Such experience sustained practice (Tyler 2012). However, diminishment would raise the utility of work. Herein, independent work has reduced the value of extrinsic work or work to obtain rewards (Haivas et al. 2012). Such reduction discourages extrinsic work (Eccles and Wigfield 2002; Cook et al. 2013).

The voluntaristic mechanism of idea consistency foregrounds ideas generated by independent work to rationalize and sustain practice. Such ideas have transpired in attitude or feelings about commitment, desire, and quality of work or work evaluation (Giffords 2009; Stiglbauer and Kovacs 2018). Such attitude or feeling is conducive to practice (de Jonge 2012; Owens et al. 2010; Silver 2011).

Religiousness

Religiousness or having religious faith has activated such practices as civic activism and engagement, cohesion, particularly religiously, compliance, coping, donation, emotional expression, environmental protection, forgiving, health behavior, helping, political participation, religious activity, role-taking, volunteering, and voting (Claassen and Povtak 2010; Finke et al. 2006; Fridberg and Kangas 2008b; Marien and Hooghe 2011; Myers 2008; Norris 2002; Perks and Haan 2011; Phalet et al. 2010; Ravanera et al. 2003; Saroglou and Anciaux 2004; Sherkat and Ellison 2007; Stalker 2008; Wiepking and Maas 2009; Wuthnow 2004). Meanwhile, religiousness has deactivated such practices as collective action, consumption, crime or deviance, doping, gambling, social interaction, suicide, and using (Ayalon et al. 1993; Corcoran et al. 2011; Duberstein et al. 2004; Hatch 2007; Skerkat and Ellison

1999; Singer et al. 1999; van de Werfhorst and Kraaykamp 2001). These influences reflect the goals of religiousness for the affiliation, altruism, attachment, belongingness, character, community, discipline, forgiveness, hospitality, humanity, love, meaning, morality, recovery, relaxation, sacredness, sacrifice, solidarity, as opposed to free ridership, individualization, opposition, and oppression (Ager and Ager 2011; Franks et al. 2013; Friedman 1992; Grayling 2013; Haddorff 2000; Horell 2014; Marks 2004; Medvedovski and Allison 2017; Myers 2014; Peifer 2010; Rowatt et al. 2009; Shorey et al. 2018; Tenorio and Lo 2011; Turner 2009; von Stuckrad 2013). The attainment of such goals would hinge on the voluntaristic mechanisms of analytical functionalism.

The voluntaristic mechanism of power realization drives practice with power generated by religiousness. This driving reflects the compulsion of religiousness (Forsyth 2003). The compulsion has rested on power in health, knowledge, and social capital furnished by religiousness (Harris 1994; Helliwell and Putnam 2005; Chang 2009). Religiousness has also sustained a feeling of mastery (Schieman 2001). Such power, in turn, has stemmed from organizational membership as opposed to poverty and welfare dependency, as facilitated by religiousness (Perks and Haan 2011; Urbatsch 2014). The power energizes practice (Eccles and Wigfield 2002; Ellemers and Haslam 2012).

The voluntaristic mechanism of utility optimization attracts practice with the utility of the practice raised by religiousness. Such utility has consisted of the values of bettering the world, conformity, and helping, as opposed to comfort, freedom, money-making, and survival (Devos et al. 2002; Shmueli 1999; Wuthnow 2004). The values underlie practice (Eccles and Wigfield 2002).

The voluntaristic mechanism of norm conformity assimilates practice with social norms associated with religiousness. Such norms arise from social inclusion, manifested in the invitation, as facilitated by religiousness (Pfeifer 2019; Schwadel 2012). For instance, the norms have emanated from recruitment to volunteering (Musick 2000). Such experience is conducive to practice (Matthewman 2011; Zurcher 2017).

The voluntaristic mechanism of idea consistency rationalizes and thus induces practice with ideas derived from religiousness. Such ideas conducive to practice are responsibility, self-actualization, and self-regulation (Forsyth 2003; Koole et al. 2010). These ideas have emerged from the dispositions of civility, empathy, familism, patriotism, progressivism, radicalism, and responsibility sustained by religiousness (Ishio 2010; Kim and Wilcox 2013; Keyes 2002; Killian and Ganong 2002; McCright and Dunlop 2008; Pedahzur and Canetti-Nisim 2004). Furthermore, religiousness has raised such attitudes as identification with a party and race and support for abortion, charity, a party, and social movements (Barker and Tinnick 2006; Brown and Ferris 2007; Ellison 1991; Marx 2014; Nie et al. 1979; Schafer and Fourcade-Gourinchas 2001). These dispositions and attitudes activate practice (Burke and Stets 2009; Cook et al. 2013; Silver 2011). Religiousness has also reduced a feeling of depression (Ellison et al. 2001). By contrast, ideas discouraging practice have sprung from the dispositions of authoritarianism, conservatism, restrictiveness, and traditionalism

(Diez-Nicolas 2002; Hooghe 2003; Jost 2020; Woodrum 1992). Conversely, religiousness has reduced the dispositions of individualism and leftism (Coffe and Geys 2007; Jou 2011). Such reduction deactivates practice (Glaeser 2016).

Marital Status

Marriage is beneficial to the couple through spousal sharing and support (Solomon 2006). For conventional practice, marriage has sustained civic engagement, involvement, consumption, donation, family functioning, investment, neighboring, political participation, reciprocating, religious activity, social cohesion and interaction, taxpaying, and voting (Apinunmahakul and Devlin 2008; Cornwall 2009; Degenne et al. 2004; Dressler 1991; Flavin and Keane 2011; Frye 2007; Molana and Adams 2019; McCabe 2014; Smith and Hamon 2012; Swaroop and Morenoff 2006). By contrast, marriage has diminished such unconventional practices as collective action, criminal activity, cyber involvement, self-help group attendance, and violence (Bjerk 2009; Corcoran et al. 2011; Kessler and Michelson 1997; Tolsma et al. 2009; Zhu and He 2002). However, marriage has raised protesting, sexual activity, and smoking (Bianchi et al. 2004; Guo et al. 2008; Marsh 2005). Anyhow, marriage seeks to attain its goals of fulfilling needs, intimacy, problem-solving, provisioning, and supporting (Carbery and Buhrmester 1998; Lichter et al. 2002). The goals also expand to achieve childrearing, companionship, conventionality, and partnership (Agha 2016; Noguera et al. 2005; Turner 2005a). To attain the goals through practice, marriage would draw on the voluntaristic mechanisms of analytical functionalism.

The voluntaristic mechanism of power realization drives practice with power enhanced by marriage. Such power rests on functional ability, health, social capital, and social support received (Chang 2009; Hou et al. 2015; Li and Chung 2008; Mata and Pendakur 2014). Marriage has also secured the power bases of socioeconomic status, including homeownership as opposed to poverty and welfare dependency (Chapman 1985; Manturuk et al. 2010; Vartanian 1999). Such power or its bases activates practice (Eccles and Wigfield 2002; Molana and Adams 2019; Walker et al. 2010).

The voluntaristic mechanism of utility optimization attracts practice with its utility sustained by marriage. Such utility has included the value of work (James and Luo 1999). The value underlies practice (Yukl et al. 1999).

The voluntaristic mechanism of idea consistency rationalizes and lifts practice with ideas evolving from marriage. Such ideas consistent with and thus conducive to practice have consisted in such attitudes as an orientation toward or support for the charity, community attachment, police, relief, and protection (Brown and Ferris 2007; Prezza et al. 2001; Okun et al. 1998; Thompson and Lee 2004). Such attitudes underlie practice (Flint and Luloff 2007; Jenkins and Dragojevic 2011; Sidanius and Pratto 2012). Conversely, marriage has diminished depression (Wright et al. 2015). This diminishment has activated practice (Holzel et al. 2011).

Parenthood

Parenthood. Has activates such conventional practices as civic engagement, commuting, crime reporting, supporting kin, and voting (Akers and Kaukinen 2009; Kim and Wilcox 2013; Lau 2010; Schlozman et al. 1994; Wellman 1990). By contrast, parenthood has retarded such unconventional activities as borrowing, criminal activity, and moving (Chou et al. 2006; Richmond 2003; Savolainen 2009). However, parenthood has also diminished volunteering (Oesterle et al. 2004). These influences reflect the goals of parenthood for fulfilling needs and provisioning for offspring (Carbery and Buhrmester 1998). To activate practice to attain these goals and deactivate practice deviating from the goals, parenthood would display its influences through the voluntaristic mechanisms of analytical functionalism.

The voluntaristic mechanism of power realization activates or deactivates practice with power generated by parenthood to attain its goals. Such power has rested on health and homeownership (Bassani 2008; Keister 2003).

The voluntaristic mechanism of norm conformity assimilates practice through social norms facing parenthood. Such norms have arisen from others' invitations (Schwadel 2012).

The voluntaristic mechanism of idea consistency rationalizes and induces practice through ideas consistent and thus conducive to the practice, as raised by parenthood. Such ideas have consisted in the dispositions of generativity, religiousness, and moral traditionalism (Baker and Smith 2009; Peterson and Klohnen 1995; Weisberg 2005). These dispositions are conducive to practice to attain the goals of parenthood (Alexander 1998; Scaff 2014). Conversely, parenthood has weakened depression (Anusic et al. 2014). Such weakening activates practice (Holzel et al. 2011).

Family Income

Family income reflects the goals for effort, legitimacy, opportunity, and wealth as opposed to poverty (Wolff and Resnick 2012; Zhang and Eriksson 2010). It has afforded such legitimate practice as civic engagement, civility, collective action, community involvement, compliance, consumption, cultural activity, decision-making, donation, environmentalist participation, migration, moving, political participation, protesting, popular lifestyle, social interaction, using automobiles and health services, violence, and voting (Alnsour and Meaton 2009; Clark et al. 2003; Cleary and Angel 1984; Doff and Kleinhans 2011; Farrington 2007; Frank et al. 2007; Hanser 2010; Katz-Gerro 1999; Kleinhans 2009; Norris 2002, 2011; Norris and Inglehart 2009; Oliver 2003; Shin 2012; van Eijck and Knulst 2005; Xu and Lai 2002; Wiepking and Maas 2009; Xu et al. 2010; Yip et al. 2007). By contrast, family income has deactivated such illegitimate or alternative practices as cheating, criminal activity, and rural life (Cerin and Leslie 2008; Katz-Gerro 1999; Ozbay 2008).

These family income effects would rest on the voluntaristic mechanisms of analytical functionalism.

The voluntaristic mechanism of power realization drives practice along the path of power generated by family income. Such power has rested on health, language capability, knowledge, social capital, particularly from family and friends, social integration, social status, and social support received, particularly from family (Crowder et al. 2006; Lee et al. 2012; Kleinhans et al. 2007; Lennartsson 2010; Oshio and Kobayashi 2010; Shin 2012; Whyte and Gao 2009). Family income has also raised feelings about financial adequacy, mastery, and self-efficacy (Cerin and Leslie 2008 Powdthavee 2009; Thoits and Hewitt 2001). Moreover, family income has raised power based on education, possession, savings, wealth, and family resources as opposed to welfare dependency (Cerin and Leslie 2008; Belzil and Hansen 2020; Chakrabarty et al. 2008; Keister 2003; Stenberg 2000; Yeung et al. 2002). Such power underlies practice (Caprara and Vecchione 2013; Cook et al. 2013; Eccles and Wigfield 2002; Soderberg and Wester 2012; Swartz 2013; Watts 2014). Conversely, family income has diminished the experience of barriers, deprivation, discrimination, hardship, hazards, social exclusion, stress, and threat to weaken power (Cerin and Leslie 2008; Pettigrew 2002; Posthumus et al. 2013; Myer et al. 2008; Raijman et al. 2003; Stanley et al. 2011; Zhang et al. 2007). Such diminishment has enabled practice (Flint and Luloff 2007).

The voluntaristic mechanism of utility optimization attracts practice with its utility fostered by family income. Such utility has rested on the values of friendship and health to boost corresponding practices (Ishio 2010; Whynes and Sach 2007). The values champion practice (Cook et al. 2013; Eccles and Wigfield 2002; Fishbein and Ajzen 2010; Schwinn 1998).

The voluntaristic mechanism of norm conformity assimilates practice through social norms buttressed by family income. Such norms have originated from the family, organizational membership, and urbanity (Apinunmahakul and Devlin 2008; Bramley and Morgan 2003; van Oorschot and Arts 2005). Notably, family income has sustained experience in family cohesion (van Oorschot and Arts 2005). Meanwhile, urbanity champions capacitation, citizenship, competition, economic activity, entrepreneurship, independence, innovation, networking, reciprocating, and self-help (Cochrane 2007; Kelly and Becker 2000). Family income has also mainly raised the perceived social norm of civility (Ferriss 2002). The norms activate practice (Elster 2015; Fishbein and Ajzen 2010; Swartz 2013; Turner and Reynolds 2012; Zurcher 2017). Mainly, civility practice has grown with the norm of civility (Pattie et al. 2004).

The voluntaristic mechanism of idea consistency rationalizes and thus induces practice with its consistent ideas fostered by family income. Such ideas conducive to practice have emanated from the dispositions of environmentalism, familism, friendliness, individualism, nationalism, and neoliberalism (Hughes 2001; La Grange and Yip 2001; Norris and Inglehart 2009; Shen and Saijo 2008). Family income has also boosted such attitudes as aspiration, notably for democracy, commitment, interest in politics, and willingness to pay (Norris 2011; Schur et al. 2004; Shin 2012; Stutzer 2004). In addition, family income has sustained job satisfaction (van Praag et al. 2003). These ideas activate practice (Burke and Stets 2009; Eccles and Wigfield 2002; Fishbein and Ajzen 2010; Jones 2001; Manstead 2011; Mantet and Serra 2003; Schwinn 1998; Silver 2011; Swartz 2013; Watts 2014). Conversely, family income has dampened the dispositions of authoritarianism (Diez-Nicolas 2002). This dampening activates practice (Diez-Nicolas 2002; Stone 1993).

Population Size

National population size has raised the person's practices of lying and protesting (Dodson 2016; van Hemert et al. 2002). By contrast, national population size has impeded the person's practices of civic engagement and migration (Beinc et al. 2001; Fridberg and Kangas 2008b). These influences would rely on the direct and indirect deterministic mechanism of analytical functionalism.

With the direct deterministic mechanism, national population size activates practice collectively, raising personal practice through private or public sharing. The activation has applied to conflict, crime, footprinting or using environmental resources, revolution, social interaction, and terrorism (Cho et al. 2013; Collier and Hoeffler 2004; Foster et al. 2013; Turner 2003; Yagci 2017; York et al. 2003). These collective practices have been conducive to personal practice such as protesting (Gillham et al. 2019; Jenkins et al. 2003; Smidt 2020). Conversely, national population size has reduced people's cohesion and employment (Coffe and Geys 2006; Cotter et al. 1998). This reduction has dampened such personal practice as civic engagement (Bruch et al. 2010; Sampson et al. 2005; Swaroop and Morenoff 2006).

Running the indirect deterministic mechanism of empowering, national population size empowers or disempowers people's practice through the voluntaristic mechanism of power realization. Such disempowering has appeared in reducing personal employment (Sanders 1990). The reduction has impeded such practice as civic engagement, collective action, community involvement, donation, health behavior, political discussion and participation, protesting, role-taking, social functioning and interaction, and voting (Corcoran et al. 2011; Fridberg and Kangas 2008b; Kerrissey and Schofer 2013; Lin et al. 2008; Lu et al. 2002; McCabe 2014; Stalker 2008; Tsai 2006).

Employing the indirect deterministic mechanism of framing, national population size frames or provides ideas to rationalize and activate people's practice through the voluntaristic mechanism of idea consistency. Such frames advocate internationalization and neoliberalism (Dean 2015). The frames have also fostered people's belief in capitalism, support for environmentalism, and tolerance for violence (Bjornskov and Paldam 2012; Franzen and Vogl 2013; Tadjoeddin 2013). These framed ideas have underlain practice (Elster 2000; Gross 2009; Swartz 2013).

Population Density

National population density has raised the person's civic activity, donation, exercising, neighboring, political activity, and prosocial behavior (Graddy and Wang 2009; Morenoff et al. 2008; Nai et al. 2018; Pattie et al. 2004; Swaroop and Morenoff 2006). This raising would hinge on the deterministic mechanism of analytical functionalism.

With the direct deterministic mechanism, national population density raises personal practice through increasing practice collectively and sharing it privately or publicly. Herein, national population density has raised pollution collectively (Stretesky and Lynch 2009). Such raising boosts practice correspondingly (Flint and Luloff 2007).

Leveraging the indirect mechanism of standardizing, national population density engendered social norms to assimilate personal practice through the voluntaristic mechanism of norm conformity. Such norms have consisted in corruption and risk perceived in the context (Uslaner 2008; Oliver 2003). The norms activate practice correspondingly (Cialdini 2012; Swartz 2013).

Using the indirect mechanism of framing, national population size frames ideas to rationalize and induce personal practice through the voluntaristic mechanism of idea consistency. Such frames have foregrounded ideas concerning collectivism, entrepreneurship, environmentalism and its support, and privacy preference (Ewing et al. 2016; Franzen and Vogl 2013; Pattie et al. 2004; Triandis 1995). These ideas contribute to practice correspondingly (Elster 2000; Swartz 2013).

Talent

National talent or human capital comprises earnings, education, and working experience (Dahlberg et al. 2018). It can boost people's migration (Gurak and Kritz 2000). The boosting would hinge on the deterministic mechanism of analytical functionalism.

Leveraging the indirect deterministic mechanism of empowering, national talent empowers and thus drive personal practice through the voluntaristic mechanism of power realization. Such empowering has applied to personal power based on income and leadership as opposed to poverty and welfare dependency (Carli and Eagly 2011; Florida 2005; Hyggen 2006; Muffels and Fouarge 2004). The power has afforded migration (Brown and Connell 2004; Hu 2005). Moreover, the power activates practice generally (Bryce 2009; Donohew et al. 1987).

Using the indirect deterministic mechanism of framing, national talent frames ideas to rationalize and thus induce personal practice through the voluntaristic mechanism of idea consistency. Such ideas can consist in aspiration (Correll 2004). Aspiration is conducive to practice (Jones 2001).

Technology

National technology maintains goals for facilitating communication, education, information, and infrastructure for people's betterment and independence (Chen 2008; Florida and Gates 2004; Goetz et al. 2011; Matthewman 2011; Schofer 2004). Hence, national technology has facilitated persona; self-expression (Welzel and Inglehart 2010). The facilitation would unfold through the deterministic mechanisms of analytical functionalism.

With the direct deterministic mechanism, national technology raises practice collectively to uplift personal practice through private or public sharing. Private and public sharing means own and vicarious or taking others' practice, respectively. Such practice has included employment, footprinting or using environmental resources, and online involvement (Goetz et al. 2011; Norris 2001; Welzel 2013). The practice in the context has upheld personal practice correspondingly, such as through collaboration and networking (Sanchez 2007; Miyata and Kubayashi 2008; Wheatley and Buglass 2019).

Activating the indirect deterministic mechanism of empowering, national technology empowers people to drive their practice through the voluntaristic mechanism of power realization. Such power has consisted in income and resources (Florida 2005; Welzel 2013). This power has driven practice (Donohew et al. 1987; Watts 2014).

Hinging on the indirect deterministic mechanism of incentivizing, national technology raises the utility of practice to attract personal practice through the voluntaristic mechanism of idea consistency. Such utility has concerned the value of emancipation (Welzel 2013). This value can attract practice (Elder-Vass 2010).

Financialization

National financialization means raising financial capital through banking or similar enterprises (Haiven 2014). It holds goals for achieving people's autonomy, creativity, freedom, individuality, insurance, investment, prosperity, and speculation (Haiven 2014). Eventually, national financialization has boosted national economic growth. Such growth can activate personal practice through the indirect deterministic mechanism of empowering and voluntaristic mechanism of power realization successively. Accordingly, the growth can generate power to empower personal practice (Swartz 2013; Turner 2013). More specifically, the growth has raised personal protesting and voting (Finegold and Swigt 2001; Welzel 2013). Meanwhile, the empowering has materialized in such power as personal employment as opposed to poverty (Brady 2006; Sanders 1990).

Prosperity

National prosperity signifies economic efficiency and modernity (Deller and Maher 2009; Peet and Hatwick 2009). The goals of national prosperity are for achieving better living, emancipation, happiness, rights, satisfaction, science, technology, and urbanization, as opposed to crises and poverty (Hunt 1989; Imbroscio 1997; Peet and Hatwick 2009; Schofer and Cranados 2006; Wolff and Resnick 2012). National prosperity has raised such practices as collective activity, cyber involvement, political activity, protesting, and volunteering (Corcoran et al. 2011; Dodson 2016; Norris 2001; Salamon and Sokolowski 2003; van Oorschot and Arts 2005). By contrast, national prosperity has dwindled such practices as birthing and cohesion (Adsera 2003; de Beer and Kostere 2009). The effects of national prosperity would unfold with the deterministic mechanisms of analytical functionalism.

With the direct deterministic mechanism, national prosperity boosts people's practice collectively to induce personal practice through private or public sharing. Such practice has included criminal activity, notably theft, terrorism, and trading (Cho et al. 2013; Neumayer and Plumper 2009; Oneal et al. 2003; Sun et al. 2011). The practice can be sharable to become one's own or vicarious practice (Cook et al. 2013). Notably, trading involves the practice of one and one's partner.

Activating the indirect deterministic mechanism of empowering, national prosperity empowers personal practice through the voluntaristic mechanism of power realization. Such empowering has transpired in reducing people's imprisonment (Liska et al. 1999; Meier 1994). Moreover, national prosperity has boosted personal health, knowledge, and self-efficacy and their bases on education (Corcoran et al. 2011; Baldacci et al. 2003; Norris 2011). Such empowering has activated practice (Soderberg and Wester 2012; Swartz 2013). Conversely, national prosperity has lessened economic hardship and illness (Fridberg and Kangas 2008). Such lessening has activated practice. (Mirowsky and Ross 2001; Wuthnow 2004)

Through the indirect deterministic mechanism of incentivizing, national prosperity raises the utility of practice to attract the practice with the voluntaristic mechanism of utility optimization. Such utility has involved the values of emancipation and independence (Fjellvang 2011; Welzel 2013). These values have activated practice (Church 2010; Elder-Vass 2010).

Based on the indirect deterministic mechanism of standardizing, national prosperity standardizes social norms to assimilate personal practice through the voluntaristic mechanism of norm conformity. Such norms concern corruption as opposed to risking and threatening (Schneider 2007; Schwartz and Melech 2000; Uslaner 2008). These norms have activated personal practices correspondingly (de Jonge 2012; Flint and Luloff 2007; Stephan 1989).

Applying the indirect deterministic mechanism of framing, national prosperity frames ideas to rationalize and sustain personal practice through the voluntaristic mechanism of idea consistency. Such ideas have consisted in the dispositions of cosmopolitanism, environmentalism, individualism, liberalism, postmaterialism, rights, and universalism (Hunter 2016; Minkov 2011; Pichler 2009; Franzen and

Vogl 2013; Tov and Diener 2008; Yuchtman-Yaar and Alkalay 2007). These dispositions have justified and sustained corresponding practices (Glaeser 2016; Michael 2017; Swartz 2013). By contrast, national prosperity has weakened the dispositions of industry, materialism, patriotism, racism, and religiousness. National prosperity has also dampened the attitudes of support for democracy and law (Magalhaes 2014; Norris 1999b). Such dampening has discouraged corresponding practices, including cohesion (Granzin and Olsen 1998; Kasser 2016; Lane 2000; Ravanera et al. 2003).

Inequality

National income inequality has activated such practices as collective action, criminal activity, smoking, and violence (Corcoran et al. 2011; Siahpush et al. 2006; Ousey and Lee 2013; van Wilsem 2007). By contrast, national income inequality has diminished such practices as cohesion, cooperation, protesting, solidarity, volunteering, and voting (Baldus 2017; Dodson 2016; Green et al. 2003; Lipford and Yandle 2009; Lister 2007). The influences of national income inequality would hinge on the indirect deterministic mechanisms of analytical functionalism.

By the direct deterministic mechanism, national income inequality has raised practice collectively to induce personal practice through private or public sharing. Such practice has included criminal activity, gambling, risking, self-enhancement, and violence collectively (Hipp et al. 2009; Hughes et al. 2015; Knack 2002; Wilkinson and Pickett 2017). By contrast, national income inequality has reduced civic engagement collectively (Wilkinson and Pickett 2017). These practices have translated from the collective to the personal level (Silverman and Miller 2011; Tanner-Smith et al. 2013).

Activating the indirect deterministic mechanism of empowering, national income inequality empowers or disempowers personal practice through the voluntaristic mechanism of power realization. Such empowering has happened to personal self-efficacy and income and its needs and thus impetus (Gundersen and Ziliak 2004; Markowski 2006; Winkelmann and Winkelmann 2010). Furthermore, collective power can emanate from conflict and struggle (Alessio 2011). This power has driven practice (Caprara and Vecchione 2013; Donohew et al. 1987; Eccles and Wigfield 2002; Elster 2011, 2015). By contrast, national income inequality has diminished personal education, functional ability, health, homeownership, and social capital (Kim and Kawachi 2007; Martin 2000; Maurer 2011; Portes and Vickstrom 2011). Such diminishment has deactivated practice, including volunteering and voting (Brown and Ferris 2007; Goerres 2007; Soderberg and Wester 2012; Son and Wilson 2012).

With the indirect deterministic mechanism of incentivizing, national income inequality raises the utility of practice for attracting personal practice. Such utility has consisted in reciprocating others' practice experienced, notably disadvantaging and exclusion (Portes and Vickstrom 2011; Reardon and Bischoff 2011). These experiences have activated corresponding practices (Williams et al. 2000).

Using the indirect deterministic mechanism of standardizing, national income inequality standardizes social norms for assimilating practice through the voluntaristic mechanism of norm conformity. Such norms have popularized anomie, corruption, injustice, and unfairness (Eriksson et al. 2015; Oishi et al. 2011; Uslaner 2008; Teymoori et al. 2016). These norms have assimilated corresponding practices (van Prooijen et al. 2008).

Leveraging the indirect deterministic mechanism of framing, national income inequality frame ideas to rationalize and sustain personal practice (Alessio 2011). Such ideas for activating practice consist in frames highlighting autonomy, capitalism, competition, efficiency, fairness or justice, individuality, inequality, particularism, and responsibility, as opposed to universalism (Alessio 2011; Fein 2012; Smith 2011; Sun 2011). As such, national income inequality has championed the disposition of rightism (Pontusson and Rueda 2010). These ideas have justified and raised corresponding practices (Elster 2011, 2015; Cook et al. 2013; Fishbein and Ajzen 2010; Glaeser 2016).

Liberty

National liberty cherished goals for autonomy, democracy, individuality, rights, satisfaction, and self-realization (Bavetta et al. 2014; Moller and Skaaning 2014). In practice, national liberty has diminished personal voting (Schwartz et al. 2010). The diminishment would rest on the deterministic mechanisms of analytical functionalism.

With the indirect deterministic mechanism of empowering, national liberty has sustained power to activate personal practice through the voluntaristic mechanism of power realization. Such power has rested on national prosperity (Rindermann 2008). Such power has deactivated personal voting (Bahry and Lipsmeyer 2001). This deactivation indicated the activation of personal voluntary practice instead of complying with and relying on government, as indicated by voting (Dodson 2016; Salamon and Sokolowski 2003).

Using the indirect deterministic mechanism of incentivizing, national liberty reduces the utility of practice and thus the personal practice. Such reduction has stemmed from perception about corruption in government (Collier 2002). This perception has impeded voting (Aldrich and Simon 1986; Flavin and Keane 2011; Travers 1982).

Applying the indirect deterministic mechanism of framing, national liberty frames ideas rationalizing and sustaining personal practice. Such ideas have consisted in postmaterialism and trust in government (Tov and Diener 2008; Wong et al. 2016). Trust in government has remarkably diminished voting (Fife and Breakwell 1990). Postmaterialism has also embraced ideas departing from voting (Norris 2011; Passini and Morselli 2011).

Democracy

National democracy represents national development, equality, liberty, and citizens' agency, dignity, rationality, and self-determination (Caprara and Vecchione 2017; Rindermann 2008). The goals of national democracy concern facilitating accountability, agreement, autonomy, balance, belonging, capability, checking, choice, civility, commonwealth, community, competition, compromise, cooperation, cultivation, deliberation, dialogue, diversity, education, efficacy, election, emancipation, equality, flourishing, freedom, friendship, harmony, identity, inclusion, information, justice, justification, lawfulness, legitimacy, modernization, negotiation, neutrality, openness, participation, peacefulness, plurality, reconciliation, rationality, redistribution, reflexivity, representation, respect, responsibility, rights, security, sharing, solidarity, tolerance, transparency, and truthfulness, as opposed to coercion, conflict, corruption, domination, interference, manipulation, oppression, radicalism, sentimentalism, unity, utopia, vigilance, and war (Abizadeh 2002; Blokker 2018; Brennan 2016; Ceva and Zuolo 2013; Chakrabarti 2016; Christians et al. 2009; Dryzek 2006; Dryzek and Dunleavy 2009; Fairfield 2008; Fukuyama 1992; Haskell 2001; Kim 2018; Levi 2003; Lo 2015; Minogue 2010; Moller and Skaaning 2013; Mukherjee 2000; O'Dwyer 2003; O'Neill 2000; Peng et at. 2017; Pettit 2012; Ringen 2007; Safford 2002; Saward 1998; Shin 2012; Steiner 2012; Talisse 2009; Tan 2003; Thomson 2005; Tilly 2009; Yack 2012; Wiklund 2005; Wood 2003). Thus, national democracy aims to raise personal agency, choice, compromise, deliberation, and social integration (Aucoin 1990; Fairfield 2008; Saward 1998). In practice, national democracy has activated personal collective action, political activity, protesting, and voting (Corcoran et al. 2011; Norris 2002, 2011). By contrast, national democracy has reduced lying and volunteering (Ruiter and De Graaf 2006; van Hemert et al. 2002). Such influences would engage the deterministic mechanisms of analytical functionalism.

With the direct deterministic mechanism, national democracy lifts practice collectively to boost personal practice successively. Such practice has stood as alliance and peacemaking and trading, as opposed to conflicting (Hausermann 2006; Hegre et al. 2010; Moller and Skaaning 2013). Correspondingly, the practice has sustained personal practice (Sexton and Benson 2006; Sorens 2011).

Activating the indirect mechanism of empowering, national democracy empowers personal practice according to democratic goals through the voluntaristic mechanism of power realization. Power empowered has consisted in people's knowledge, prosperity, and self-efficacy (Corcoran et al. 2011; Rindermann 2008; Shin 2012). The power has facilitated practice (Caprara and Vecchione 2013; Donohew et al. 1987; Eccles and Wigfield 2002; Flint and Luloff 2007; Soderberg and Wester 2012; Swartz 2013).

Using the indirect deterministic mechanism of incentivizing, national democracy raises the utility of practice to attract personal practice through the voluntaristic mechanism of utility optimization. Such utility has consisted in the value of obedience as opposed to independence (Fjellvang 2011). The value of obedience has attracted personal organizational practice (Finegan 2000; Stride and Higgs 2014).

Relying on the indirect deterministic mechanism of standardizing, national democracy upholds social norms assimilating personal practice through the voluntaristic mechanism of norm conformity. Such norms have highlighted freedom and legitimacy as opposed to crime (Gilley 2009; Moller and Skaaning 2013; Uslaner 2008). These norms have assimilated corresponding practices (Costello 2013; Crandall and Beasley 2001; Lilly et al. 2011; Van Knippenberg et al. 2007).

Applying the indirect deterministic mechanism of framing, national democracy frames ideas influencing personal practice through the voluntaristic mechanism of idea consistency. Such frames imply ideas for agency, checking, choosing, consent, expression, inclusion, individualism, lawfulness, liberty, protest, and respect (Brennan 2016; Munck 2005; Ringen 2007; Warren 2011). National democracy has also fostered the personal dispositions of individualism, leftism, and religiousness as opposed to patriotism. Furthermore, national democracy has induced the attitudes of commitment to the association (Shin 2012). These ideas have justified and sustained corresponding practices (de Jonge 2012; Matthewman 2011). Notably, the reduction in personal patriotism by national democracy would diminish cohesion and volunteering practices (Granzin and Olsen 1998).

Government Effectiveness

National government effectiveness functions to achieve goals for citizens' belongingness, civility, commonwealth, cooperation, education, happiness, harmony, health, justice, legality, livelihood, modernization, peacefulness, problem-solving, prosperity, rationality, responsibility, safety, security, solidarity, as opposed to pain, poverty, resistance, revolution, risk, and violence (Bluhm and Heineman 2007; Bozeman 2007; Brooks 2013; Dillon 2019; Grcic 2000; Hagopian 2000; Knittila and Kubik 2000; Lessnoff 1999; Luthar 2009; O'Mahony 2013; Roazen 2003; Rothstein 2005; Scourfield and Welsh 2003; Sorell 2013; Spicker 2013; Weber 2011; Wenz 2009; Yanagisawa 2011). The effectiveness has raised such practices as choosing and voicing as opposed to suicide (Helliwell 2006; Guisan 2009; Koch 2000). Hence, national government effectiveness is activating and livening rather than debilitating. Such contribution would benefit from the deterministic mechanisms of analytical functionalism.

Using the indirect deterministic mechanism of empowering, national government effectiveness empowers personal practice through the voluntaristic mechanism of power realization. Power has arisen from national prosperity enabled by national government effectiveness (Guisan 2009). National prosperity has activated the personal practices of collective action, cyber involvement, political participation, and protesting (Corcoran et al. 2011; Dodson 2016; Norris 2001; van Oorschot and Arts 2005). By contrast, national government effectiveness has diminished personal power derived from personal employment (Jonasson 2012). This diminishment has reduced such personal practices as civic engagement, collective action, community involvement, donation, health behavior, political discussion and participation, protesting, role-taking, social functioning and interaction, and voting (Corcoran et al. 2011; Fridberg and Kangas 2008b; Kerrissey and Schofer 2013; Lin et al. 2008; Lu et al. 2002; Magdol and Bessel 2003; McCabe 2014; Stalker 2008). By contrast, the diminishment has raised the personal practices of caring, criminal activity, exercising, moving, and volunteering (Bianchi et al. 2004; Kleinhans 2009; Savolainen 2009; Sarasa 2008; Taniguchi 2013). Hence, national government effectiveness has empowered and disempowered personal practice in various ways.

Based on the indirect deterministic mechanism of standardizing, national government effectiveness sustains social norms to assimilate personal practice through the voluntaristic mechanism of norm conformity. Such norms have concerned harmony, justice, and living standards (Mizrahi 2016; Wong and Shik 2011). These norms have guided corresponding personal practices, including cooperation and political participation, as opposed to protesting (Lawrence and Daniels 1997; van Prooijen et al. 2008; Wenzel 2000).

Applying the indirect deterministic mechanism of framing, national government effectiveness frames ideas for rationalizing and lifting personal practice through the voluntaristic mechanism of idea consistency. Such framed ideas champion citizens' agency, autonomy, civility, diligence, entitlement, fellowship, legality, participation, rationality, sympathy, and solidarity (Atkins 2008; Friedman 2011; Gandjour and Lauterbach 2003; Khatchadourian 1999; Newey 2001; Selznick 2002). Moreover, national government effectiveness has boosted personal willingness to pay (Wong et al. 2005). These ideas have guided personal practice (Boudon 2011; Eccles and Wigfield 2002; Fishbein and Ajzen 2010; Heise 1999; Scaff 2014). Notably, agency or autonomy has buttressed exercising and performance (Gagne and Deci 2005; Levesque et al. 2007).

Emission

National carbon dioxide (CO_2) emission concerns climate change and degradation in the environment (Black et al. 2011). The emission has urged the personal practice of migration, which has reduced contact with relatives (Black et al. 2011; Young and Willmont 1957). This urging works through the deterministic mechanisms of analytical functionalism.

Activating the indirect deterministic mechanism of empowering, national carbon dioxide emission empowers personal practice through the voluntaristic mechanism of power realization. Such power has emanated from contextual temperature and its stress, as generated by national carbon dioxide emission (Giridharan et al. 2007). The temperature has activated the practices of competition, consumption, lying, and violence as opposed to civic engagement, compliance, and volunteering (Cai et al. 2021; Cohn et al. 2004; Craig and Douglas 2012; Glaeser and Gottlieb 2006; van de Vliert et al. 2000; van Hemert et al. 2002).

Through the indirect deterministic mechanism of standardizing, national carbon dioxide emission has raised the social norm for legitimacy in government (Gilley 2009). This norm legitimizes coercion, conflict, criticalness, and resistance (Zelditch 2001). Eventually, the norm has boosted migration, protesting, and violence (Mummendey et al. 1999; Van Knippenberg et al. 2007). By contrast, the norm has diminished criminal activity and discrimination (Crandall and Beasley 2001; Lilly et al. 2011).

Human Development

National human development features people's capability, entitlement, motivation, and satisfaction with life (Castles 2000; Inglehart and Welzel 2005). Such development has buttressed such personal practices as donation, obedience, law-abiding, and voting as opposed to lying (Fridberg and Kangas 2008b; Norris 2002; van Hemert et al. 2002). The buttressing would hinge on the deterministic mechanisms of analytical functionalism.

With the direct deterministic mechanism, national human development sustains people's practice collectively to raise personal practice through private or public sharing, which upholds one's own or vicarious practice, respectively. Such practice has been civility and self-direction (Bond and Lun 2014).

Activating the indirect deterministic mechanism of empowering, national human development empowers personal practice through the voluntaristic mechanism of power realization. Such empowering has applied to personal health and knowledge, as raised by national human development (Eikemo et al. 2008; Norris 2011). The power has activated personal practice (Soderberg and Wester 2012; Swartz 2013). Notably, health has enabled such practices as activism, cohesion, coping, cultural activity, religious activity, role-taking, search for meaning, self-enhancement, social activity, volunteering, and voting (Adeola 2000; Ben-Zur 2002; Goerres 2007; Immerzeel and van Kazarian and Tubergen 2013; Scherger 2009; Son and Wilson 2012; Stalker 2008; Tolsma et al. 2009; Tomich and Helgeson 2002). Knowledge has similarly facilitated the practices of choosing, cohesion, civic engagement, community participation, complaining, cooperation, cyber involvement, environmentalist participation, health behavior, political participation, prevention, protection, protesting, volunteering, and voting (Anderson 2009; Bish and Michie 2010; Blalock 2007; Hunter et al. 2013; Cheng and Ng 2006; Kosecik and Sagbas 2004; Lepkowski and Couper 2002; Loader 2007; Lubell 2002; McClurg 2006; Miller 2010; Norris 2011; Simon-Bemd and Steffens 2000; Volker et al. 2007; Wernet et al. 2005).

Applying the indirect deterministic mechanism of standardizing, national human development secures social norms to assimilate personal practice through the voluntaristic mechanism of norm conformity. A social norm has concerned corruption (Uslaner 2008). This norm has assimilated bribing and lying (Cabelkova and Honousek 2004; van Hemert et al. 2002). Moreover, national human development has reduced party membership (Norris 2002). Such reduction has impeded choosing, civic engagement, donation, political awareness, attention, and discussion, and voting (Claassen and Povtak 2010; Djupe and Lewis 2015; Echabe et al. 1988; Huber et al. 2022; Hutchings 2003; Marcus et al. 2000; McClurg 2006).

By the indirect deterministic mechanism of framing, national human development frames ideas to influence personal practice through the voluntaristic mechanism of idea consistency. Such framing has discouraged the personal disposition of communitarianism (Davis and Robinson 2006) Hence, this discouragement reduces such communitarian practices as caring, dependence, reciprocating, settling, social activity, and volunteering (Frazer 1999).

Time

Time prominently proceeds with individualization and secularization (de Graaf et al. 2001). In practice, time has raised cohesion, exercising, immigration, neighboring, visiting physicians, volunteering, and working (Bianchi et al. 2004; de Beer and Kostere 2009; Gershuny 2000; Helliwell 2003; Sarracino 2010; Smith et al. 2001). By contrast, time has reduced the practices of borrowing, consumption, cooperation, fertility, protesting, recreation, religious activity, resistance, smoking, social interaction, violence, and voting (Bianchi et al. 2004; Brown et al. 2005; Claassen and Povtak 2010; de Ruijter 2004; Foster et al. 2001; Garcia et al. 2015; Glaeser and Gottlieb 2006; Norris and Inglehart 2009; Pinker 2011; Requena and Stanek 2014; Zhu 1996). These changes would rest on the deterministic mechanisms of analytical functionalism.

With the direct deterministic mechanism, time has influenced people's practice collectively to affect personal practice by private or public sharing. Practices thus raised collectively have been employment, revolution, social integration, and suicide (Chang et al. 2009; Lijphart 1997; Shin 2013; Smith et al. 2001). Notably, social integration collectively has sustained personal civic engagement, financial support, political participation, and recourse as opposed to violence (Lee 2012; Mitrut and Wolff 2011; Palmer et al. 2011; Su and Feng 2013).

Activating the indirect deterministic mechanism of empowering, time empowers or disempowers personal practice through the voluntaristic mechanism of power mechanism. Power has evolved from personal affluence, employment, homeownership, income from marriage, and wage raised with time (Campbell and Pearlman 2013; Dekkers 2008; Francesconi and Golsch 2005; Lichter et al. 2002). Such power has driven associational life, civic engagement, civility, collective action, community involvement, cultural activity, cyber involvement, donation, health behavior, leisure activity, media use, paying taxes, planning, political activism, discussion, and participation, prosocial behavior, protesting, purchase, role-taking, social functioning, and interaction, using health services, and voting (Bjornberg and Ekbrand 2008; Corcoran et al. 2011; Fridberg and Kangas 2008b; Glaeser and Gottlieb 2006; Janoski and Wilson 1995; Kerrissey and Schofer 2013; Chen et al. 2004; Letki 2006; Lin et al. 2008; Lu et al. 2002; McCabe 2014; Norris and Inglehart 2009; Pratt et al. 2010; Ross and Mirowsky 1989; Scherger 2009; Stalker 2008; Straughn and Andriot 2011; Treiman and Gartner 2006; Treno and Holder 1997; Tsai 2006). By contrast, such power has deactivated birthing, borrowing, caring, cohesion, compliance, criminal activity, exercising, gardening, migration, moving, neighboring, social comparison, suicide, violence, and volunteering (Anciaes et al. 2017; Bianchi et al. 2004; Broom et al. 2013; Fischer et al. 1996; Guiso et al. 2004; Joseph and Chaskin 2010; Kleinhans 2009; Rahe and Stegman 1994; Sarasa 2008; Sarkheyli et al. 2012; Savolainen 2009; Swanson et al. 1992; Taniguchi 2013; Wang et al. 2010; Varady and Raffel 1995). In addition, time has eroded power based on personal health and social integration (Islam et al. 2006; McPherson et al. 2006). Conversely, time has diminished power by raising social disconnection and exclusion, and illness (Smith 2005; McPherson et al. 2006; Ruta and Cernescu 2008). These time effects have reduced personal practice, including activism, cohesion, cultural activity, reasoning, religious activity, role-taking, self-enhancement, social activity, volunteering, and voting (Adeola 2000; Goerres 2007; Guillen et al. 2011; Immerzeel and van Tubergen 2013; Kazarian and Martin 2006; Son and Wilson 2012; Scherger 2009; Stalker 2008; Tolsma et al. 2009; Wuthnow 2004).

Leveraging the indirect deterministic mechanism of incentivizing, time changes the utility of practice to affect the personal practice through the voluntaristic mechanism of utility optimization. Such utility has consisted in the value of tradition rising with time (Brynin et al. 2009). This value has buttressed voting for the conservative and diminished donation, protesting, and theft (Blackwell and Eschholz 2002; Datler et al. 2013; Yeung et al. 2000).

By the indirect deterministic mechanism of standardizing, time evolves social norms assimilating personal practice through the voluntaristic mechanism of norm conformity. Such norms have popularized illegitimacy and problems (Inglehart 1999; Wong et al. 2010). These norms have assimilated personal practices, including criminal activity, deviance, discriminating, paying, religious activity, sacrificing, and surrendering, as opposed to migration, political participation, and protesting (Backman and Nilsson 2011; Cole and Pargament 1999; Crandall and Beasley 2001; Fahmy 2006; Lilly et al. 2011; Macias 2015; McCullough and Larson 1999; Mummendey et al. 1999; Van Zomeren 2009).

Applying the indirect deterministic mechanism of framing, time frames ideas influencing personal practice through the voluntaristic mechanism of idea consistency. Framed ideas originate from empiricism emphasizing empirical evidence, humanism emphasizing humanity, materialism emphasizing material such as money, postmodernism emphasizing liquidity, playfulness, and plurality, and rationalism emphasizing reasoning (Atkinson 2008; Lemon 2003). Essentially, time has escalated such personal dispositions as environmentalism, friendliness, helpfulness, multiculturalism, pessimism, prosociality, rightism, and skepticism (Haller 2002; Ladd 1995; Persell 1997; Ramarajan et al. 2017; Scruggs 2003; Smith et al. 2001; Smith 2005). Time has also elevated such personal attitudes as support for hooking or the one-night stand, and tolerance (Wang et al. 2004; Watt and Elliot 2017). These personal dispositions and attitudes have generated ideas rationalizing and conducive to corresponding personal practices (Cooke and Sheeran 2004; Fishbein and Ajzen 2010; Jenkins and

Dragojevic 2011; Swartz 2013). For instance, pessimism has raised practice or effort generally but discouraged comparison with others with better position, coping, and detection (Charke et al. 2000; Nes and Segerstrom 2006; Oettingen and Cachia 2016; Wood and VanderZee 1997). Tolerance has boosted such practices as cohesion, civic engagement, protesting, and voting (Ayob 2019; Houtman 2000; Lodewijkx et al. 2008; DiRenzo 1990).

Summary

Personal practice, in general, has been positively predictable by the personal characteristics of age, education, female gender, immigrant background, income, non-marriage, parenthood, social class, and family income (Bonke and Fallesen 2010; Donohew et al. 1987; Heller 2020; Soderberg and Wester 2012). According to the voluntaristic mechanism of analytical functionalism, among the predictors, age, education, income, family income, and social class provide power to drive practice. Moreover, according to the voluntaristic mechanism of utility optimization, marriage reduces the utility of personal practice and thus the practice because of spousal sharing. Conversely, parenthood raises the utility of personal practice for the parent and his or her offspring, according to the mechanism of utility optimization. Social class, particularly as opposed to unemployment, rationalizes practice such as working and similarly productive practices according to the mechanism of idea consistency. Similarly, education, immigration, and parenthood rest on and thus rationalize practice according to the mechanism of idea consistency.

As a private practice, e-activity has been positively predictable by the personal characteristics of education, homeownership, income, and family income (Chen 2015; Dan et al. 2011). These characteristics generate power to drive e-activity, considering the mechanism of power realization.

E-activity has been inversely predictable by such personal characteristics as age, mid-age, marriage, and self-employment. These characteristics diminish power for e-activity by alternative engagement, considering the mechanism of power realization. Marriage reduces the utility of personal e-activity and thus the activity by spousal sharing or vicarious practice, considering the mechanism of utility optimization.

E-activity has risen with national prosperity and technology (Norris 2001). These effects reflect the indirect deterministic mechanism of empowering, which raises personal power for e-activity.

As a private practice, learning has increased with such personal characteristics as education, employment, female gender, homeownership, and family income (Chou 2003; Pallas 2002 Wink and Dillon 2003). According to the mechanism of power realization, education, employment, homeownership, and family income provide power to drive learning. The female characteristics of caring and thus carefulness are conducive to learning, according to the mechanism of idea consistency (Fyall and Gazley 2015; Lippa 2005).

As a private practice, spiritual activity has depended on the personal characteristics of age and female gender (Dalby 2006; Kalkstein and Tower 2009). More specifically, religious activity as a spiritual activity has risen with age, parenthood, and religious faith (Baker and Smith 2009; Copen and Silverstein 2008; Fjellvang 2011; Stavrova and Siegers 2014). These influences reflect consistency between the characteristics and spiritual activity, based on the mechanism of idea consistency. Meanwhile, religious activity has diminished with employment or social class (Fjellvang 2011; Immerzeel and van Tubergen 2013). Such activity is inconsistent with employment, which demonstrat4s personal agency instead of religious predestination, considering the mechanism of idea consistency (Laruffa 2020).

As a private practice, risk aversion has risen with such personal characteristics as age and female gender and declined with education and homeownership (Brown and Zoorob 2022). Education, homeownership, male gender, and young age have sustained power to face risk (Aral and Walker 2012; Manturuk et al. 2010; Ross and Mirowsky 2009). They thus lessened risk aversion through the mechanism of power realization.

As a private practice, weapon carrying has increased with such personal characteristics as education, parenthood, and family income and diminished with marriage (Cassino and Besen-Cassino 2020; Ludwig and Cook 2001). Education, parenthood, and family income raise the utility of weapon carrying and thus weapon carrying, with the mechanism of utility optimization. Conversely, marriage lessens the utility of weapon carrying due to sharing the weapon by the spouse or vicarious weapon carrying.

As a public practice, organizational participation has increased with such a personal characteristic as age. Age has elevated the utility of organizational participation and thus support (Lu and Kao 2002). This elevation boosts organizational participation through the mechanism of utility optimization.

Appealing, as a public practice, has risen with such personal characteristics as majority status, socioeconomic status, family income, and urbanity, and declined with parenthood and religious affiliation (Bassoli and Monticelli 2018; Corcoran et al. 2011; Kolczyuska 2020; Somma et al. 2020; Swank and Fahs 2016). Majority status, socioeconomic status, urbanity, and family income have increased power (Flores and Telles 2012; Keltener et al. 2008; Kleinhans et al. 2007; Shin 2012; Verschuur et al. 2010; Zhang and Eriksson 2010). They thus raise appealing, according to the power realization mechanism. Meanwhile, parenthood and religious affiliation have generated such ideas as authoritarianism, conservatism, empathy, optimism, responsibility, and traditionalism (Barker and Tinnick 2006; Diez-Nicolas 2002; Hooghe 2003; Keyes 2002; Killian and Ganong 2002; Weisberg 2005). These ideas have discouraged appealing (Akkus et al. 2020; Bahry and Lipsmeyer 2001; Datler et al. 2013; Furnham 1997; Jones and Brewster 2017; Li and Song 1992). Such ideas discourage appealing according to the mechanism of idea consistency.

Appealing has also risen with national democracy and prosperity and reduced with national liberty (Norris 2011; Quaranta 2016; Slavina and Brym 2020). National democracy advocates appealing, agonism, competition, confrontation, expression, and emancipation to eliminate injustice and oppression (Dryzek and Dunleavy 2009;

Moller and Skaaning 2013; O'Neill 2000; Z. Peng et al. 2017; Tracy and Hughes 2014). Thus, national democracy raises appealing according to the indirect deterministic mechanism of framing. National prosperity has boosted personal postmaterialism and the value of emancipation (Tov and Diener 2008; Welzel 2013). The ideology and value have underlain appealing (Rudig and Karyotis 2014; Welzel 2013; Zhuang 2020). Thus, national prosperity has sustained personal appealing through the indirect deterministic mechanisms of framing and incentivizing. By contrast, national liberty has raised personal satisfaction with democracy and life (Abbott et al. 2011; Norris 2011). Such satisfaction has been an idea incongruous with and thus dampening appealing (Akinboade et al. 2014; Giugni and Grasso 2019). Hence, according to the indirect deterministic mechanism of framing, national liberty reduces appealing.

As a public practice, strike participation has increased with such personal characteristics as age and minority status and diminished with female gender, income, and social class (Dixon and Roscigno 2003; Gerteis and Savage 1998). Age and minority status have elevated the utility of strike participation for self-interest (An and Winship 2017; Fjellvang 2011). The elevation raises strike participation, according to the mechanism of utility optimization. Conversely, income and social class have reduced the utility of strike participation (Thompson et al. 1999; Ulbig 2002). Such reduction discourages strike participation, according to the mechanism of utility optimization. Meanwhile, female gender has generated such ideas as agreeableness and tender-mindedness (Caprara and Vecchione 2017). These ideas have been antithetical to strike participation (Houndkpatin et al. 2015). Thus, female gender reduces strike participation, according to the mechanism of idea consistency.

Strike participation has increased with national democracy and prosperity (Isaac and Christiansen 2002; Kim and Gandhi 2010). National democracy and prosperity have activated the personal practices of collective action, political participation, and protesting (Corcoran et al. 2011; Dodson 2016; Norris 2002, 2011; van Oorschot and Arts 2005). The activation of such practices congruous and conducive to strike participation raises strike participation, according to the indirect deterministic mechanism of framing. Moreover, national prosperity has raised the values of disobedience and emancipation (Fjellvang 2011; Welzel 2013). According to the indirect deterministic mechanism of incentivizing, the influence of national prosperity on personal strike participation hinges on these values.

Voting, as a public practice, has risen with such personal characteristics as parenthood, education, employment, homeownership, income, religious affiliation, residency, social class, and family income (Aytac and Stokes 2019; Child and Nikolova 2020; Franklin 1996; Heath et al. 1991; McCabe 2014; Norris 2002; Schlozman et al. 1994; Weinschenk and Dawes 2022). Education, employment, homeownership, income, residency, social class, and family income have contributed to power (Hofstetter et al. 1999; Ross and Mirowsky 2009). The power drives voting, according to the mechanism of power realization. Parenthood, education, homeownership, residency, social class, and family income have sustained citizenship or civic obligation (Gilberbloom and Markham 1995; Jukes et al. 2018; Kim and Wilcox 2013; Norris 2011; Shin 2012). Citizenship has underlain voting (Aytac and Stokes 2019). These characteristics thus buttress voting according to the mechanism of idea consistency. In addition, religious affiliation has engaged the social norm for voting (Claassen and Povtak 2010). The affiliation thus assimilated voting, according to the mechanism of norm conformity.

Voting has also risen with national democracy and human development and receded with national prosperity (Bahry and Lipsmeyer 2001; Norris 2002). According to the direct deterministic mechanism, national democracy is the basis for voting. Meanwhile, national human development has strengthened personal knowledge, notably on voting (Norris 2011). The development thus activates personal voting, according to the indirect deterministic mechanism of empowering. National prosperity has diminished personal support for democracy. The support has been conducive to voting (Echabe et al. 1988; Hennessy et al. 2015). Thus, according to the indirect deterministic framing mechanism, national prosperity dampens personal voting. Furthermore, national prosperity has raised the personal perception of corruption (Collier 2002; Uslaner 2008). Corruption indicates the disutility of voting (O'Connor and Fischer 2012). Hence, the prosperity hindered personal voting, according to the indirect mechanism of incentivizing.

Donation, as a public activity, has built on such personal characteristics as education, employment, homeownership, income, majority status, marriage, religious affiliation, rural residence, savings, social class, and family income (Bekkers 2008; Fridberg and Kangas 2008b; Rhodes 2011; Van de Vyver and Abrams 2018; Wang and Graddy 2008; Wiepking and Maas 2009; Yeung et al. 2000). Education, employment, homeownership, income, majority status, marriage, savings, social class, and family income have contributed to power (Hofstetter et al. 1999; Keltener et al. 2008; Manturuk et al. 2010; Ross and Mirowsky 2009; Shin 2012). Thus, according to the mechanism of power realization, these characteristics drive donation. Religious affiliation and rural residence have brought such ideas as civility, collectivism, and egalitarianism (Keyes 2002; Saunders and Wong 2012; Triandis and Gelfand 2012). These ideas have contributed to donation (Jones 2006; Rossi 2001). Hence, according to the mechanism of idea consistency, the characteristics boost donation. In addition, religious affiliation has foregrounded the social norm for donation (Ager and Ager 2011; Peifer 2010). Hence, the affiliation raises donation, according to the mechanism of norm conformity.

Table 7.1 Hypothesized functionalist effects on practices

Predictor	E-act	Learn	Spirit	Avert	Weapon	Organ	Appeal	Strike	Vote	Donate
Wave	+	+	+	+	–	–	+	+	–	–
Personal										
Irreligious	+	–	–	+	+	–	–	–	–	–
Family income	+	+	+	–	–	+	–	–	+	+
Female	–	–	–	+	–	–	–	–	–	–
Age	–	–	+	+	–	+	–	–	+	+
Age squared	+	–	+	+	+	+	+	+	–	–
Married	–	–	–	+	–	–	–	–	+	+
Cohabited	–	–	–	+	–	–	–	–	+	+
Divorced	+	+	+	–	+	+	+	+	–	–
Separated	+	+	+	–	+	+	+	+	–	–
Widowed	+	+	+	–	+	+	+	+	–	–
Kid	–	–	–	+	–	–	–	–	–	–
Mother immigrant	–	–	–	+	+	–	–	–	–	–
Father immigrant	–	–	–	+	+	–	–	–	–	–
Education	+	+	+	+	–	+	–	–	+	+
Graduation age	+	+	+	+	–	+	–	–	+	+
Interest	+	+	+	–	–	+	+	+	+	+
Living with parents	–	–	–	+	–	–	–	–	–	–
Full-time employment	+	–	–	–	–	–	–	+	+	+
Part-time employment	+	–	–	–	–	–	–	+	+	+

(continued)

Table 7.1 (continued)

Predictor	E-act	Learn	Spirit	Avert	Weapon	Organ	Appeal	Strike	Vote	Donate
Self-employment	+	–	–	–	–	–	–	–	+	+
Retired	–	–	+	+	–	+	–	–	–	–
Homemaking	–	–	–	+	–	–	–	–	–	–
Student	+	+	–	–	+	–	+	–	–	–
Unemployed	–	–	–	+	+	–	+	–	–	–
Public employment	+	–	–	–	–	–	–	+	+	+
Private business employment	+	–	–	–	–	–	–	+	+	+
Nonprofit organization employment	+	–	–	–	–	–	–	+	+	+
Intellectual work	+	–	–	–	–	–	–	+	+	+
Creative work	+	–	–	–	–	–	–	+	+	+
Independent work	+	–	–	–	–	–	–	+	+	+
Supervision	+	–	–	–	–	–	–	+	+	+
Earner	+	–	–	–	–	–	–	+	+	+
Earner employed	+	–	–	–	–	–	–	+	+	+
National										
Population	–	–	–	+	+	–	–	–	–	–
Phone	+	+	+	–	+	+	+	+	–	–
Land	–	–	–	–	+	–	–	–	–	–
Technology	+	+	–	–	–	–	+	+	–	–
Credit	+	+	–	+	+	–	+	+	–	–
Prosperity	+	+	+	–	–	+	–	–	–	–

(continued)

Table 7.1 (continued)

Predictor	E-act	Learn	Spirit	Avert	Weapon	Organ	Appeal	Strike	Vote	Donate
Income inequality	–	–	+	–	+	–	+	+	–	–
Globalization	+	+	–	–	–	–	+	+	–	+
Government effectiveness	–	–	–	–	–	–	–	–	–	–
Democracy	+	+	–	–	–	+	+	+	+	+
Liberty	+	+	–	–	–	–	+	+	–	–
Human development	+	+	–	–	–	–	–	–	+	+
Human capital	+	+	–	–	–	–	–	–	+	+
CO_2	–	–	–	+	+	–	+	+	–	–

Donation has also risen with national human development (Fridberg and Kangas 2008b). Such development has sustained such personal power as health and knowledge (Eikemo et al. 2008; Norris 2011). The development thus boosts donation, according to the indirect deterministic mechanism of empowering. Moreover, the development has secured personal social trust (Fridberg and Kangas 2008b). The development thereby elevates personal donation through the indirect deterministic mechanism of incentivizing to raise donation utility.

Overall, analytical-functionalist theory sustains the following expectations for the effects of personal and national characteristics on personal practices (Table 7.1).

Chapter 8
Life Practice Production: Findings

Production dynamics for personal life practices evolve from regression analyses of the practices on personal and national characteristics. The practices comprise private and public ones. Private practices comprise e-activity, learning, spiritual activity, risk aversion, and weapon carrying, whereas public practices comprise organizational participation, appealing, strike participation, voting, and green demonstrating and donation. The series of regression analyses had the first step examining the effects of time and countries on each practice. Additionally, the second step examined the effects of personal characteristics on the practice. Afterward, the third step estimated significant time differentials in the effects of personal characteristics. Alternatively, the analysis first scrutinized the significant effects of national characteristics on the practice and the time effect. The next step added the significant interaction effects involving time and national characteristics to estimate time differentials in the effects of national characteristics. In addition, this step introduced the remaining significant effects due to countries. In all the analyses, when an effect of a personal or national characteristic on the practice was statistically significant and stronger than 0.1, the effect was noteworthy.

Findings

Personal e-activity increased significantly with time in the person. This time effect remained significant after controlling for personal characteristics. The activity was significantly higher in the United States and Germany and significantly lower in India. In addition, e-activity rose significantly with creative work, family income, and supervisory work (Table 8.1).

Alternatively, personal e-activity increased significantly and substantially with national prosperity. By contrast, the activity significantly declined with national democracy. The decline significantly strengthened with time. In addition, time

C. Cheung, *Production Dynamics for Life Quality in the Incipient 21st Century*,
https://doi.org/10.1007/978-981-19-3827-6_8

Table 8.1 Standardized effects on e-activity

Predictor	(1)	(2)	(3)
Wave	0.146***	0.144***	0.144***
US	0.287***	0.282***	0.281***
India	−0.194***	−0.219***	−0.219***
Germany	0.108***	0.102***	0.101***
Japan	0.090***	0.084***	0.083***
Pakistan	−0.074***	−0.091***	−0.091***
China	−0.073***	−0.054***	−0.054***
Brazil	0.051***	0.071***	0.070***
Nigeria	−0.049***	−0.060***	−0.061***
Egypt	−0.046***	−0.037***	−0.037***
Vietnam	−0.030***	−0.034***	−0.033***
Philippines	−0.022***	−0.024***	−0.025***
Russia	0.018***	0.024***	0.025***
Creative work		0.134***	0.134***
Family income		0.115***	0.115***
Supervision		0.102***	0.102***
Earner employed		0.088***	0.087***
Living with parents		0.084***	0.083***
Self-employment		−0.062***	−0.061***
Student		0.057***	0.057***
Earner		−0.056***	−0.056***
Widowed		−0.047***	−0.048***
Female		−0.046***	−0.045***
Homemaking		0.040***	0.040***
Part-time employment		−0.039***	−0.040***
Age squared		−0.038***	−0.037***
Interest		0.037***	0.037***
Separated		−0.018***	−0.018***
Father immigrant		0.016***	0.016***
Nonprofit organization employment		0.009***	0.009***
Divorced		−0.006***	−0.006
Wave × widowed			−0.010**
Wave × public employment			0.009*
R^2	0.195	0.288	0.288

*$p < 0.05$, **$p < 0.01$, ***$p < 0.001$

Table 8.2 Standardized effects of national characteristics on e-activity

Predictor	(1)	(2)
Wave	0.100^{***}	0.096^{***}
Prosperity	0.422^{***}	0.441^{***}
Democracy	-0.092^{***}	-0.109^{***}
Land	0.063^{***}	0.053^{***}
Population	-0.052^{***}	-0.075^{***}
Income inequality	0.036^{***}	0.061^{***}
Wave × democracy		-0.087^{***}
Wave × technology		0.086^{***}
Wave × income inequality		0.079^{***}
Wave × land		0.044^{***}
Wave × CO_2		-0.016^{*}
Vietnam		-0.023^{***}
Turkey		0.012^{**}
R^2	0.185	0.193

$^{*}p < 0.05$, $^{**}p < 0.01$, $^{***}p < 0.001$

displayed a significant positive effect on e-activity, even after controlling for national characteristics (Table 8.2).

Personal learning significantly but weakly increased time, even after controlling for personal characteristics. In addition, learning was significantly lower in China, India, and Egypt than in other countries. After controlling for time and countries, education exhibited a significant positive effect on learning. The education effect did not significantly change with time (Table 8.3).

Alternatively, national liberty and land size per capita displayed significantly positive effects on personal learning, whereas national income inequality indicated a significant negative effect. Furthermore, the negative effect of national inequality significantly weakened with time. In addition, national globalization delivered a significant but weaker negative effect on personal learning. Meanwhile, the significant negative effect of national population size on personal learning was very weak (Table 8.4).

Personal spiritual activity significantly diminished with time, even after controlling for countries and personal characteristics. The activity was significantly lower in China, Russia, Japan, Germany, and the United States and significantly higher in Nigeria than in other countries. In addition, the activity was significantly lower with nonprofit organization employment. The other effects of personal characteristics were weaker (Table 8.5).

Alternatively, personal spiritual activity rose with national democracy and waned with national government effectiveness, population size, and land size per capita. The positive effect of national democracy significantly increased with time, and the negative effects of government effectiveness, population size, and land per capita

Table 8.3 Standardized effects on learning

Predictor	(1)	(2)	(3)
Wave	0.119***	0.125***	0.122***
China	−0.348***	−0.187***	−0.187***
India	−0.198***	−0.123***	−0.114***
Egypt	−0.109***	−0.078***	−0.080***
Pakistan	−0.093***	−0.064***	−0.055***
Germany	0.071***	0.095***	0.097***
Mexico	−0.059***	−0.029***	−0.021***
Turkey	−0.047***	−0.033***	−0.034***
Vietnam	−0.041***	−0.034***	−0.034***
Japan	0.028***	0.042***	0.052***
Brazil	−0.024***	0.020***	0.025***
Iran	0.017***	0.017***	0.010***
Nigeria	−0.012**	−0.015***	−0.008*
Acquiescence		0.294***	0.301***
Education		0.286***	0.267***
Public employment		0.088***	0.082***
Private business employment		0.069***	0.041***
Kid		−0.059***	−0.052***
Supervision		0.050***	0.044***
Married		−0.041***	−0.039***
Family income		0.040***	0.039***
Age		0.040***	0.029***
Full-time employment		−0.038***	−0.018**
Cohabited		−0.037***	−0.032***
Creative work		0.032***	0.038***
Nonprofit organization employment		0.029***	0.008
Interest		0.028***	0.032***
Father immigrant		0.026***	0.029***
Graduation age		0.025***	0.025***
Part-time employment		−0.024***	−0.003
Female		−0.022***	−0.020***
Age squared		−0.017***	−0.024***
Earner		0.012**	0.011*
Earner employed		0.012**	0.010*
Widowed		−0.011**	−0.013**
Living with parents		0.011**	0.011**

(continued)

Table 8.3 (continued)

Predictor	(1)	(2)	(3)
Student		−0.009*	−0.002
Homemaking		0.008	0.024***
Self-employment		−0.005	0.015**
Retired		0.005	0.020***
Independent work		0.005	0.002
Divorced		−0.003	−0.001
Separated		0.001	0.002
Wave × retired			−0.055***
Wave × irreligious			0.052***
Wave × public employment			−0.045***
Wave × unmarried			−0.036***
Wave × idle			−0.036***
Wave × private business employment			−0.031***
Wave × father immigrant			−0.030***
Wave × full-time employment			−0.025***
Wave × student			−0.023***
Wave × part-time employment			−0.021***
Wave × creative work			−0.020***
Wave × separated			−0.019***
Wave × age squared			−0.018***
Wave × Buddhist			0.018***
Wave × Catholic			0.017***
Wave × supervision			−0.015***
Wave × homemaking			−0.015**
Wave × divorced			−0.014***
Wave × cohabited			0.014***
Wave × living with parents			0.012**
Wave × earner employed			0.010**
R^2	0.114	0.374	0.384

*$p < 0.05$, **$p < 0.01$, ***$p < 0.001$

significantly strengthened with time. However, such strengthening of the negative effects with time was very weak. With the control of national characteristics, personal spiritual activity was significantly higher in the United States than in others (Table 8.6).

Personal risk aversion significantly but negligibly rose with time only after controlling for personal characteristics. The aversion was significantly lower in the United States than in other countries. Apart from acquiescence, personal characteristics only

Table 8.4 Standardized effects of national characteristics on learning

Predictor	(1)	(2)
Wave	0.123***	0.125***
Liberty	0.227***	0.222***
Income inequality	−0.156***	−0.138***
Land	0.116***	0.115***
Globalization	−0.094***	−0.086***
Population	−0.058***	−0.048***
Wave × democracy		−0.073***
Wave × technology		0.058***
Wave × income inequality		0.058***
Wave × CO_2		−0.030***
Wave × population		0.008
Iran		0.052***
Germany		0.049***
Brazil		0.019***
R^2	0.102	0.114

$^{*}p < 0.05$, $^{**}p < 0.01$, $^{***}p < 0.001$

slightly influenced risk aversion. The effects of personal characteristics also did not substantially change with time (Table 8.7).

Alternatively, personal risk aversion significantly reduced with national prosperity. The aversion also significantly but slightly rose with national credit provision and subsided with national globalization and income inequality. These effects did not significantly change with time (Table 8.8).

Personal weapon carrying did not significantly change with time. The carrying was significantly but slightly higher in India than in other countries. Furthermore, the carrying was at best only significantly and slightly predictable by creative work. The predictability was significantly but negligibly rose with time (Table 8.9).

Alternatively, personal weapon carrying significantly but slightly increased with national democracy. The increase significantly strengthened with time. Personal weapon carrying also significantly declined with national technology and rose with national government effectiveness and population size, but only slightly (Table 8.10).

Personal organizational participation declined significantly with time, even after controlling for personal characteristics. The participation was significantly higher in India, the United States, Nigeria, Mexico, and the Philippines than in the other countries. Furthermore, the participation significantly rose with nonprofit organization employment. The participation also significantly and slightly declined with independent work (Table 8.11).

Alternatively, personal organizational participation significantly rose with national democracy and bank credit and declined with national human development. The positive effect of national democracy, however, significantly weakened

Table 8.5 Standardized effects on spiritual activity

Predictor	(1)	(2)	(3)
Wave	−0.220***	−0.273***	−0.274***
China	−0.521***	−0.506***	−0.506***
Russia	−0.159***	−0.170***	−0.169***
Japan	−0.123***	−0.122***	−0.121***
Nigeria	0.114***	0.099***	0.103***
Germany	−0.106***	−0.115***	−0.115***
US	−0.104***	−0.117***	−0.115***
India	−0.095***	−0.084***	−0.081***
Vietnam	−0.079***	−0.092***	−0.091***
Philippines	0.067***	0.057***	0.058***
Pakistan	0.037***	0.036***	0.039***
Iran	−0.035***	−0.038***	−0.040***
Turkey	−0.026***	−0.031***	−0.031***
Ethiopia	0.022***	0.029***	0.027***
Egypt	−0.018***	−0.007	−0.007
Nonprofit organization employment		−0.109***	−0.108***
Private business employment		−0.083***	−0.085***
Interest		0.080***	0.080***
Creative work		0.071***	0.072***
Part-time employment		0.043***	0.041***
Female		0.034***	0.032***
Supervision		0.027***	0.027***
Homemaking		−0.026***	−0.021***
Education		0.024***	0.021***
Earner employed		−0.023***	−0.023***
Family income		0.020***	0.020***
Student		−0.016***	−0.019***
Age squared		0.016***	0.015***
Cohabited		−0.013***	−0.012**
Living with parents		0.009*	0.008*
Separated		0.006	0.006
Divorced		−0.001	−0.001
Father immigrant		−0.001	−0.001
Widowed		0.001	0.002
Self-employment		0.000	−0.009*
Wave × age			0.040***

(continued)

Table 8.5 (continued)

Predictor	(1)	(2)	(3)
R^2	0.283	0.317	0.318

$^{*}p < 0.05$, $^{**}p < 0.01$, $^{***}p < 0.001$

Table 8.6 Standardized effects of national characteristics on spiritual activity

Predictor	(1)	(2)
Wave	−0.174***	−0.178***
Democracy	0.352***	0.322***
Government effectiveness	−0.268***	−0.364***
Population	−0.248***	−0.245***
Land	−0.148***	−0.186***
Income inequality	0.054***	0.055***
Wave × democracy		0.258***
Wave × income inequality		0.072***
Wave × government effectiveness		−0.066***
Wave × population		−0.045***
Wave × land		−0.014**
US		0.164***
Vietnam		−0.076***
Brazil		0.032***
R^2	0.264	0.360

$^{*}p < 0.05$, $^{**}p < 0.01$, $^{***}p < 0.001$

with time. Meanwhile, the effect of national globalization became more positive with time, and the effect of national population size became more negative with time (Table 8.12).

Personal appealing reduced significantly but slightly with time, even after controlling for personal characteristics. The appealing was significantly higher in the United States, Indica, Brazil, and Germany than in the other countries. In addition, personal appealing at most significantly but slightly rose with supervisory work (Table 8.13).

Alternatively, personal appealing rose significantly with national time and national bank credit. The effects of these national characteristics did not significantly change with time (Table 8.14).

Personal strike participation significantly but negligibly declined with time. The time effect, nonetheless, become nonsignificant after controlling for personal characteristics. The participation was significantly higher in Nigeria and India than in other countries. Creative work significantly but only slightly increased strike participation. Other personal characteristics yielded only weaker effects on the participation. After controlling for national characteristics, strike participation was significantly higher in Nigeria than in other countries (Table 8.15).

Table 8.7 Standardized effects on risk aversion

Predictor	(1)	(2)	(3)
Wave	−0.002	0.031***	0.025***
US	−0.102***	−0.086***	−0.075***
Turkey	−0.076***	−0.074***	−0.075***
Germany	−0.068***	−0.051***	−0.042***
Philippines	−0.044***	−0.048***	−0.056***
Pakistan	0.046***	0.041***	0.040***
Japan	0.035***	0.057***	0.056***
China	0.035***	0.077***	0.092***
Russia	−0.013**	0.007	0.004
Acquiescence		0.115***	0.145***
Female		0.079***	0.085***
Creative work		−0.056***	−0.060***
Full-time employment		0.042***	0.034***
Self-employment		0.038***	0.036***
Family income		−0.030***	−0.033***
Public employment		−0.030***	−0.032***
Retired		0.030***	0.006
Age squared		0.019***	0.018**
Part-time employment		0.018***	0.024***
Independent work		0.017*	0.003
Father immigrant		0.015***	0.013**
Private business employment		−0.014*	−0.077***
Age		0.013	0.022**
Education		0.012*	0.018**
Irreligious		−0.012	−0.009
Married		0.012	0.022**
Nonprofit organization employment		−0.011*	−0.011
Interest		−0.010*	−0.008
Separated		0.009*	0.009*
Cohabited		0.008	0.011*
Earner employed		0.007	0.008
Student		0.006	0.017**
Kid		−0.004	−0.006
Living with parents		−0.004	−0.003
Homemaking		−0.002	0.009
Graduation age		0.002	0.007

(continued)

Table 8.7 (continued)

Predictor	(1)	(2)	(3)
Widowed		0.001	0.003
Supervision		0.001	0.007
Divorced		0.000	0.004
Earner		0.000	−0.003
Wave × acquiescence			0.148***
Wave × irreligious			0.078***
Wave × female			0.077***
Wave × private business employment			−0.066***
Wave × nonmanual work			−0.061***
Wave × unmarried			−0.036***
Wave × family income			−0.030***
Wave × interest			−0.028***
Wave × retired			−0.022***
Wave × divorced			−0.019***
Wave × living with parents			0.015**
R^2	0.029	0.050	0.079

*$p < 0.05$, **$p < 0.01$, ***$p < 0.001$

Table 8.8 Standardized effects of national characteristics on risk aversion

Predictor	(1)	(2)
Wave	0.016***	0.017***
Prosperity	−0.125***	−0.116***
Credit	0.075***	0.077***
Globalization	−0.068***	−0.082***
Income inequality	−0.045***	−0.044***
Wave × liberty		−0.079***
Wave × technology		−0.034***
Wave × population		0.016**
R^2	0.016	0.027

*$p < 0.05$, **$p < 0.01$, ***$p < 0.001$

Alternatively, personal strike participation significantly declined with national human development and rose with national liberty. The decline and rise significantly strengthened with time (Table 8.16).

Personal voting increased significantly but negligibly with time. The increase was no longer significant after controlling for personal characteristics. Furthermore, the voting significantly decreased with nonprofit organization employment (Table 8.17).

Table 8.9 Standardized effects on weapon carrying

Predictor	(1)	(2)	(3)
Wave	0.003	0.011	0.023***
India	0.098***	0.038***	0.000
US	0.049***	0.053***	0.050***
Nigeria	−0.018***	−0.038***	−0.046***
Germany	−0.016***	−0.015***	−0.018***
Philippines	0.015***	0.005	−0.006
Russia	−0.013**	−0.010*	−0.012*
Japan	0.013**	0.024***	0.016**
Egypt	−0.012**	−0.014**	−0.017***
Indonesia	0.012**	0.004	0.001
Pakistan	−0.011*	−0.035***	−0.050***
Acquiescence		0.098***	0.114***
Creative work		0.075***	0.057***
Education		−0.054***	−0.031***
Nonprofit organization employment		−0.047***	−0.017**
Age		−0.035***	−0.023**
Father immigrant		0.035***	0.029***
Earner employed		−0.034***	−0.025***
Living with parents		0.034***	0.035***
Independent work		−0.030***	−0.035***
Female		−0.028***	−0.027***
Private business employment		−0.025***	−0.008
Earner		0.022***	0.015**
Family income		0.021***	0.013**
Retired		0.021***	0.020**
Self-employment		−0.016**	−0.010
Divorced		0.014**	0.013**
Widowed		0.013**	0.011**
Kid		0.013**	0.006
Cohabited		0.013*	0.009
Married		0.013	0.009
Full-time employment		−0.012*	−0.012***
Public employment		−0.008	0.008
Separated		0.008	0.006
Supervision		−0.007	0.003
Irreligious		0.007	0.010

(continued)

Table 8.9 (continued)

Predictor	(1)	(2)	(3)
Student		0.007	0.004
Graduation age		−0.004	−0.003
Interest		0.004	−0.001
Homemaking		0.004	−0.011**
Age squared		−0.003	0.002
Part-time employment		0.000	−0.009
Wave × acquiescence			0.110***
Wave × living with parents			0.032***
Wave × father immigrant			0.031***
Wave × idle			0.031***
Wave × retired			0.027***
Wave × creative work			0.026***
Wave × female			−0.022***
Wave × education			−0.022***
Wave × earner employed			−0.021***
Wave × earner			0.021***
Wave × divorced			0.015**
Wave × student			0.015**
Wave × nonprofit organization employment			−0.014**
Wave × family income			0.014**
Wave × irreligious			0.013*
Wave × protestant			0.012**
R^2	0.013	0.035	0.052

*$p < 0.05$, **$p < 0.01$, ***$p < 0.001$

Alternatively, personal voting increased significantly with national inequality, democracy, and technology. The increase by national inequality and technology strengthened with time. In addition, the effect of national liberty became more positive with time (Table 8.18).

Personal participation in environmental demonstrations significantly but negligibly declined with time. However, with the control for personal characteristics, the participation significantly but negligible rose with time. Participation was significantly higher in India than in other countries. In addition, participation significantly increased with creative work (Table 8.19).

Alternatively, personal participation in environmental demonstrations significantly increased with national democracy and declined with national human development. Both the increase and decline strengthened significantly with time (Table 8.20).

Table 8.10 Standardized effects of national characteristics on weapon carrying

Predictor	(1)	(2)
Wave	−0.005	−0.008
Democracy	0.086***	0.094***
Technology	−0.078***	−0.053***
Government effectiveness	0.064***	0.040***
Population	0.061***	0.070***
Wave × democracy		0.115***
Wave × population		0.060***
Wave × technology		−0.051***
Wave × credit		0.041***
Wave × land		−0.009**
Philippines		0.025***
Brazil		−0.019***
R^2	0.012	0.023

*$p < 0.05$, **$p < 0.01$, ***$p < 0.001$

Personal green donation significantly but negligibly shrank with time. However, the shrinking was no longer significant with the control for personal characteristics. The donation was significantly but only slightly lower in China than in other countries. In addition, the donation significantly but only slightly rose with creative work (Table 8.21).

Alternatively, personal green donation significantly rose with national liberty. This rise did not significantly change with time. Instead, the effect of national democracy became more positive with time (Table 8.22).

Discussion

Notable effects on personal practices sprang from some personal characteristics, national characteristics, and time. These personal characteristics were nonprofit organization employment, creative work, supervisory work, education, and family income. The national characteristics were democracy, human development, prosperity, bank credit, income inequality, land share, population size, and technology.

Personal Influences

Nonprofit organization employment significantly reduced spiritual activity and voting and raised organizational participation. Such reduction or raising builds on the

Table 8.11 Standardized effects on organizational participation

Predictor	(1)	(2)	(3)
Wave	-0.257^{***}	-0.172^{***}	-0.187^{***}
India	0.418^{***}	0.231^{***}	0.242^{***}
US	0.187^{***}	0.122^{***}	0.137^{***}
Nigeria	0.157^{***}	0.095^{***}	0.110^{***}
Mexico	0.103^{***}	0.066^{***}	0.091^{***}
Philippines	0.100^{***}	0.044^{***}	0.065^{***}
Brazil	0.089^{***}	0.035^{***}	0.059^{***}
Indonesia	0.076^{***}	0.001	-0.013^{**}
Ethiopia	0.062^{***}	0.044^{***}	0.039^{***}
Germany	0.034^{***}	0.017^{***}	0.024^{***}
Egypt	-0.029^{***}	-0.063^{***}	-0.064^{***}
Pakistan	0.028^{***}	-0.020^{***}	−0.004
Turkey	-0.024^{***}	-0.063^{***}	-0.064^{***}
Japan	0.018^{***}	−0.002	0.009^{*}
Russia	-0.016^{***}	-0.041^{***}	-0.037^{***}
Acquiescence		0.361^{***}	0.354^{***}
Nonprofit organization employment		0.102^{***}	0.047^{***}
Independent work		-0.094^{***}	-0.071^{***}
Public employment		0.094^{***}	0.078^{***}
Education		0.091^{***}	0.069^{***}
Supervision		0.062^{***}	0.045^{***}
Creative work		0.055^{***}	0.066^{***}
Father immigrant		0.054^{***}	0.055^{***}
Age		0.053^{***}	0.046^{***}
Private business employment		0.051^{***}	0.049^{***}
Irreligious		-0.050^{***}	-0.051^{***}
Married		-0.043^{***}	-0.041^{***}
Graduation age		0.038^{***}	0.032^{***}
Student		0.037^{***}	0.025^{***}
Widowed		-0.026^{***}	-0.025^{***}
Self-employment		0.025^{***}	0.023^{***}
Kid		-0.022^{***}	-0.018^{***}
Part-time employment		-0.021^{***}	0.000^{**}
Retired		-0.019^{***}	-0.010^{*}
Homemaking		-0.014^{**}	−0.002
Female		0.014^{**}	0.006

(continued)

Table 8.11 (continued)

Predictor	(1)	(2)	(3)
Divorced		-0.012^{**}	-0.012^{**}
Interest		-0.012^{**}	−0.007
Living with parents		0.012^{**}	0.018^{***}
Full-time employment		−0.008	0.013
Age squared		0.007	0.002
Cohabited		−0.003	−0.003
Separated		−0.003	−0.003
Family income		0.003	0.008^{*}
Earner		0.003	0.012^{**}
Earner employed		0.000	-0.015^{***}
Wave × acquiescence			-0.095^{***}
Wave × irreligious			0.078^{***}
Wave × student			-0.049^{***}
Wave × Catholic			0.046^{***}
Wave × family income			0.034^{***}
Wave × public employment			-0.032^{***}
Wave × living with parents			-0.025^{***}
Wave × idle			-0.019^{***}
Wave × divorced			0.019^{***}
Wave × earner			0.018^{***}
Wave × kid			-0.017^{***}
Wave × private business employment			0.012
Wave × female			0.010^{*}
Wave × widowed			0.009^{*}
R^2	0.237	0.398	0.422

$^{*}p < 0.05$, $^{**}p < 0.01$, $^{***}p < 0.001$

voluntaristic mechanisms of power realization, idea consistency, and norm conformity. Considering the mechanism of power realization, the employment is deactivating because it has weakened power by raising experience about complexity, stress, workload, inadequacy in salary and support from the labor union, and insecurity in employment (Ariza-Montes and Lucia-Casademunt 2016; Comartin et al. 2020; Hamann and Foster 2014). The experience has reduced power (Hofstetter et al. 1999; Meng and Abrokwah 2021). Such reduction has eroded spiritual activity and voting (Aytac and Stokes 2019; Hall and Edwards 2002; Shockley and Fairdosi 2015). Meanwhile, organizational participation and nonprofit organization employment share the idea of organization, and thus their relationship follows the mechanism of idea consistency. As such, nonprofit organization employment would represent

Table 8.12 Standardized effects of national characteristics on organizational participation

Predictor	(1)	(2)
Wave	-0.218^{***}	-0.245^{***}
Democracy	0.400^{***}	0.414^{***}
Human development	-0.292^{***}	-0.224^{***}
Credit	0.167^{***}	0.194^{***}
Income inequality	0.055^{***}	0.096^{***}
Wave × globalization		0.192^{***}
Wave × democracy		-0.159^{***}
Wave × population		-0.115^{***}
Wave × income inequality		0.064^{***}
Wave × land		-0.040^{***}
Nigeria		0.085^{***}
Japan		-0.083^{***}
Turkey		-0.075^{***}
Philippines		0.043^{***}
Egypt		-0.038^{***}
Iran		0.026^{***}
R^2	0.211	0.276

$^{*}p < 0.05$, $^{**}p < 0.01$, $^{***}p < 0.001$

a form of organizational participation. The nonprofit organization spreads norms about civil society and government failure (Fric 2008; Sanyal 2006). These norms have assimilated organizational participation as opposed to voting in support of government (Hennessy et al. 2015; O'Mahony 2013).

Creative work raised e-activity and green donation. The raising works through the voluntaristic mechanism of idea consistency. Accordingly, creative work fosters ideas concerning contribution, curiosity, environmentalism, exploration, gaming, playfulness, and searching (Gelade 1999; Joas 1996; Kozbelt et al. 2010; Paletz and Peng 2009; Qian et al. 2010; Rudowicz and Hui 1997; Runco 2014; Silvia and Kimbrel 2010). These ideas contribute to e-activity and donation (Ho and Ng 2022; Mesch 2009; Renger and Reese 2017; Wang and Chiou 2006).

Supervisory work boosted e-activity, possibly through the voluntaristic mechanism of utility optimization. Accordingly, supervisory work raises the utility of supervising, including monitoring and networking (Wuthnow 2002). Meanwhile, such utility is inherent in e-activity (Settle 2018; Wheatley and Buglass 2019). Supervisory work thus attracts e-activity to achieve its utility.

Education activated the practice of learning, possibly through the voluntaristic mechanisms of power realization, utility optimization, and idea consistency. Regarding the mechanism of power realization, education has raised such power as expertise, functionality, health, intelligence, knowledge, mastery, memory, self-efficacy, skill, and verbal ability (Cerin and Leslie 2008; Corcoran et al. 2011; Fiske

Table 8.13 Standardized effects on appealing

Predictor	(1)	(2)	(3)
Wave	−0.054***	−0.063***	−0.063***
US	0.244***	0.237***	0.233***
India	0.190***	0.201***	0.203***
Brazil	0.136***	0.147***	0.157***
Germany	0.107***	0.103***	0.103***
Japan	0.095***	0.087***	0.088***
China	−0.072***	−0.047***	−0.047***
Pakis	0.039***	0.037***	0.036***
Ethiopia	0.032***	0.034***	0.032***
Nigeria	0.030***	0.027***	0.028***
Vietnam	−0.029***	−0.030***	−0.029***
Egypt	−0.026***	−0.014	−0.014**
Mexico	0.022***	0.029***	0.029***
Iran	0.021***	0.018***	0.018***
Supervision		0.088***	0.089***
Independent work		0.054***	0.054***
Family income		0.051***	0.050***
Female		−0.047***	−0.047***
Living with parents		0.035***	0.035***
Earner		0.034***	0.033***
Homemaking		0.031***	0.033***
Self-employment		0.029***	0.030***
Divorced		0.022***	0.022***
Part-time employment		0.021***	0.022***
Father immigrant		0.016***	0.017***
Earner employed		0.013**	0.014**
Creative work		−0.011*	−0.011*
Widowed		−0.008	−0.008
Separated		−0.007	−0.007
Cohabited		−0.004	−0.004
Nonprofit organization employment		−0.004	−0.005
Age squared		−0.002	−0.003
Wave × graduation age			−0.030***
Wave × protestant			−0.016***
R^2	0.125	0.156	0.157

*$p < 0.05$, **$p < 0.01$, ***$p < 0.001$

Table 8.14 Standardized effects of national characteristics on appealing

Predictor	(1)	(2)
Wave	−0.050***	−0.056***
Liberty	0.350***	0.362***
Credit	0.085***	0.102***
Human development	−0.066***	−0.070***
Wave × government effectiveness		−0.031***
Wave × population		0.030***
Wave × globalization		0.021**
Brazil		0.048***
Pakis		0.046***
Turkey		−0.043***
Iran		0.039***
Indo		−0.030***
Philippines		−0.029***
Japan		−0.023***
R^2	0.110	0.121

$^{*}p < 0.05$, $^{**}p < 0.01$, $^{***}p < 0.001$

et al. 1990; Pratt et al. 1996; Shin 2012; Straughn and Andriot 2011; Stavrova and Ehlebracht 2018; Stevens et al. 2001; Verba et al. 1995), such power has driven learning (Lavrijsen and Nicaise 2017). Regarding the mechanism of utility optimization, education has fostered the values of learning and reasoning (Armon and Dawson 2003; Ulbig 2002). Such values attract learning (Hagger and Hamilton 2018). Regarding the mechanism of idea consistency, education has cultivated ideas embedded in or related to awareness, conscientiousness, meritocratism or support for meritocracy, including rewarding according to education, media use, and openness (Evans et al. 2010; Norris and Inglehart 2009; Rossi 2001; Tang 2011). Such ideas are consonant and conducive to learning (Kanar and Bouckenooghe 2022; Katz-Schiavone et al. 2008; Roberts et al. 2009).

Family income facilitated personal e-activity, possibly through the voluntaristic mechanism of power realization. Personal power enhanced by family income has consisted in health, knowledge, self-efficacy, social capital, social integration, and social support received (Cerin and Leslie 2008; Crowder et al. 2006; Kleinhans et al. 2007; Lennartsson 2010; Oshio and Kobayashi 2010; Shin 2012). Moreover, family income has secured such power bases as education, home equipment, resources, savings, urbanity, and wealth as opposed to barriers, discrimination, hardship, social exclusion, stress, threat experienced, and welfare dependence (Raijman et al. 2003; Belzil and Hansen 2020; Bramley and Morgan 2003; Cerin and Leslie 2008; Chakrabarty et al. 2008; Keister 2003; Moore and Aweiss 2003; Myer et al. 2008; Posthumus et al. 2013; Stanley et al. 2011; Stenberg 2000; Yeung et al. 2002). Such power or bases have sustained e-activity (Chen 2015; Katz and Rice 2002;

Table 8.15 Standardized effects on strike participation

Predictor	(1)	(2)	(3)
Wave	−0.037***	−0.006	0.019***
Nigeria	0.232***	0.210***	0.197***
India	0.095***	0.065***	0.054***
China	−0.063***	−0.048***	−0.034***
Pakistan	0.047***	0.040***	0.029***
Brazil	0.035***	0.043***	0.044***
Philippines	−0.026***	−0.040***	−0.058***
Egypt	−0.021***	−0.017***	−0.022***
Russia	−0.020***	−0.011*	−0.024***
Germany	0.018***	0.025***	0.022***
Turkey	−0.012**	−0.018***	−0.025***
Acquiescence		0.151***	0.183***
Creative work		0.070***	0.062***
Nonprofit organization employment		−0.068***	−0.013*
Retired		−0.048***	−0.015*
Independent work		−0.037***	−0.063***
Part-time employment		0.034***	0.015**
Private business employment		−0.032***	0.000
Earner		0.030***	0.021***
Female		−0.029***	−0.027***
Age		0.026***	0.028***
Living with parents		0.026***	0.023***
Homemaking		0.025***	0.011*
Father immigrant		0.018***	0.015***
Irreligious		0.017**	0.033***
Public employment		−0.016**	0.010
Family income		0.015**	0.003
Divorced		0.009	0.009
Cohabited		−0.006	−0.007
Interest		0.005	0.005
Full-time employment		0.005	0.020**
Married		0.004	0.000
Education		0.004	0.025***
Separated		−0.003	−0.004
Supervision		0.003	0.018***
Earner employed		−0.003	0.005

(continued)

Table 8.15 (continued)

Predictor	(1)	(2)	(3)
Graduation age		−0.002	0.001
Age squared		0.002	−0.007
Widowed		−0.001	−0.006
Kid		−0.001	−0.006
Self-employment		−0.001	0.019***
Student		0.000	−0.003
Wave × acquiescence			0.181***
Wave × Islam			−0.030***
Wave × irreligious			−0.029***
Wave × female			−0.026***
Wave × education			0.025***
Wave × earner			0.024***
Wave × living with parents			0.024***
Wave × age			0.022***
Wave × orthodox			−0.020***
Wave × supervision			0.020***
Wave × self-employed			0.019***
Wave × retired			−0.019**
Wave × nonmanual work			0.017***
Wave × mother immigrant			0.017***
Wave × protestant			−0.014**
Wave × part-time employment			0.013**
Wave × full-time employment			0.012*
Wave × Buddhist			−0.011**
Wave × divorced			0.009*
R^2	0.075	0.114	0.155

*$p < 0.05$, **$p < 0.01$, ***$p < 0.001$

Loader 2007; Vitak 2017). Conversely, family income has reduced personal employment and work (Lau et al. 2006; Stier and Lewin-Epstein 2003). Such reduction has buttressed e-activity (Wheatley and Buglass 2019).

National Influences

National democracy sustained personal e-activity, spiritual activity, voting, and green donation, possibility through the direct and indirect deterministic mechanisms of

Table 8.16 Standardized effects of national characteristics on strike participation

Predictor	(1)	(2)
Wave	0.032***	0.000
Human development	−0.227***	−0.153***
Liberty	0.140***	0.141***
Income inequality	−0.075***	−0.044***
Population	−0.037***	0.023**
Land	0.027***	0.022***
Wave × human development		−0.148***
Wave × liberty		0.132***
Wave × income inequality		−0.036***
Wave × land		0.014**
Nigeria		0.160***
Philippines		−0.043***
Turkey		−0.016***
Brazil		0.014**
Germany		0.012*
R^2	0.038	0.094

*$p < 0.05$, **$p < 0.01$, ***$p < 0.001$

analytical functionalism. The mechanisms are feasible because of the function of national democracy to achieve such goals as people's agency, capacitation, dignity, equality, liberty, rationality, self-determination, and self-development (Caprara and Vecchione 2017; Hyland 1995; Rindermann 2008; Warren 2011). These goals are also common for e-activity and voting (Brennan 2011; Fuchs 2008; Jackman 1993; Norris 2002; Schecter 2009; Toews 2018).

Activating the indirect deterministic mechanism of empowering, national democracy empowered personal power to drive personal practice through the voluntaristic mechanism of power realization. Personal power raised by national democracy has consisted in knowledge, prosperity, and self-efficacy (Corcoran et al. 2011; Rindermann 2008; Shin 2012). Such power has driven e-activity, voting, and donation (Anderson 2009; Bednall et al. 2013; Chen 2015; de Zuniga et al. 2016; Hansen and Tyner 2019; Kerrissey and Schofer 2013; Khang et al. 2014; Loader 2007).

Leveraging the indirect deterministic mechanism of incentivizing, national democracy raises the personal utility of practice to attract the practice through the voluntaristic mechanism of utility optimization. The utility raised has consisted in the value of obedience and the experience of unpredictability (Catley 2001; Fjellvang 2011). This value has underlain voting, which means obedience to the corresponding government requirement or regulation (Aytac and Stokes 2019). Meanwhile, the experience of unpredictability bolsters the value and thus the practice of spiritual activity to tackle unpredictability (van den Bos et al. 2001). In addition, national democracy establishes the mechanism for election and voting (Kiser and Powers

Table 8.17 Standardized effects on voting

Predictor	(1)	(2)	(3)
Wave	0.022***	−0.005	0.003
Nigeria	−0.125***	−0.133***	−0.138***
India	0.115***	0.116***	0.106***
China	−0.101***	−0.093***	−0.089***
Pakistan	−0.087***	−0.090***	−0.096***
Russia	−0.078***	−0.075***	−0.080***
US	−0.060***	−0.066***	−0.066***
Brazil	0.055***	0.042***	0.039***
Philippines	0.049***	0.044***	0.035***
Japan	−0.034***	−0.029***	−0.034***
Egypt	−0.034***	−0.027***	−0.030***
Turkey	0.017***	0.014**	0.012***
Nonprofit organization employment		−0.101***	−0.077***
Independent work		0.075***	0.059***
Public employment		−0.058***	−0.048***
Interest		0.044***	0.046***
Earner		0.040***	0.036***
Age squared		0.038***	0.044***
Part-time employment		0.038***	0.031***
Private business employment		−0.035***	−0.026***
Student		−0.029***	−0.023***
Education		−0.028***	−0.013*
Creative work		−0.028***	−0.030***
Graduation age		0.025***	0.028***
Full-time employment		0.024***	0.026***
Earner employed		−0.021***	−0.016**
Widowed		−0.018***	−0.020***
Homemaking		−0.013**	−0.032***
Kid		0.013**	0.006
Living with parents		0.013**	0.016***
Female		0.011*	0.006
Divorced		−0.008	−0.007
Separated		−0.008	−0.009*
Retired		0.006	0.009
Cohabited		−0.005	−0.005
Family income		0.004	0.002

(continued)

Table 8.17 (continued)

Predictor	(1)	(2)	(3)
Self-employment		−0.002	−0.002
Father immigrant		0.001	0.000
Supervision		0.001	0.008
Wave × acquiescence			0.106***
Wave × homemaking			−0.043***
Wave × age squared			0.036***
Wave × widowed			−0.015**
R^2	0.073	0.094	0.016

*$p < 0.05$, **$p < 0.01$, ***$p < 0.001$

Table 8.18 Standardized effects of national characteristics on voting

Predictor	(1)	(2)
Wave	−0.013**	−0.019***
Income inequality	0.189***	0.247***
Democracy	0.118***	0.102***
Technology	0.097***	0.139***
CO_2	−0.075***	−0.051***
Land	−0.030***	−0.035***
Wave × income inequality		0.196***
Wave × liberty		0.126***
Wave × technology		0.097***
Wave × CO_2		−0.074***
Wave × land		−0.023***
Egypt		−0.044***
Mexico		−0.037***
Turkey		0.031***
Japan		0.013**
Philippines		0.012**
R^2	0.079	0.110

*$p < 0.05$, **$p < 0.01$, ***$p < 0.001$

2013). The contribution of national democracy to personal voting has been evident (Norris 2002).

Based on the indirect deterministic mechanism of standardizing, national democracy propagates social norms to boost personal practice through the voluntaristic mechanism of norm conformity. Such norms have favored freedom and legitimacy as opposed to criminality (Gilley 2009; Moller and Skaaning 2013; Uslaner 2008). The norm for freedom has assimilated e-activity (Khang et al. 2014; Peter and Valkenburg

Table 8.19 Standardized effects on participation in environmental demonstration

Predictor	(1)	(2)	(3)
Wave	−0.020***	0.019**	0.045***
India	0.095***	0.068***	0.045***
Nigeria	0.082***	0.057***	0.040***
China	−0.076***	−0.028***	−0.012
Pakistan	0.050***	0.033***	0.017***
Mexico	0.038***	0.043***	0.040***
Japan	−0.028***	−0.009	−0.010*
Russia	−0.024***	−0.010*	−0.013**
Egypt	−0.022***	−0.017***	−0.022***
Germany	−0.012**	−0.004	−0.007
Turkey	−0.011*	−0.018***	−0.026***
Acquiescence		0.157***	0.190***
Creative work		0.115***	0.104***
Independent work		−0.063***	−0.081***
Nonprofit organization employment		−0.053***	0.001
Homemaking		0.049***	0.040***
Family income		0.047***	0.036***
Earner		0.047***	0.039***
Father immigrant		0.041***	0.034***
Living with parents		0.034***	0.031***
Private business employment		−0.027***	0.005
Full-time employment		0.026***	0.050***
Part-time employment		0.024***	0.006
Public employment		−0.017**	0.013*
Student		0.014**	0.015**
Earner employed		−0.013**	−0.007
Interest		0.013**	0.012**
Married		−0.013	−0.012
Graduation age		0.010*	0.013**
Self-employment		−0.008	0.011*
Education		−0.007	0.015**
Cohabited		0.007	0.012*
Retired		0.007	0.024***
Supervision		−0.006	0.009*
Age		−0.005	0.006
Divorced		−0.005	−0.004

(continued)

Table 8.19 (continued)

Predictor	(1)	(2)	(3)
Widowed		−0.003	−0.006
Age squared		−0.002	−0.007
Separated		−0.002	−0.002
Kid		−0.002	−0.012*
Female		0.002	0.009
Wave × acquiescence			0.192***
Wave × mother immigrant			0.039***
Wave × full-time employment			0.038***
Wave × living with parents			0.037***
Wave × family income			0.034***
Wave × earner			0.034***
Wave × nonmanual work			0.031***
Wave × homemaking			0.031***
Wave × cohabited			0.022***
Wave × education			0.020***
Wave × student			0.020***
Wave × Islam			−0.016**
Wave × supervision			0.013**
Wave × irreligious			−0.013*
Wave × nonprofit organization employment			0.012*
Wave × Catholic			0.011*
Wave × self-employed			0.010**
Wave × interest			0.009**
R^2	0.083	0.126	0.136

*$p < 0.05$, **$p < 0.01$, ***$p < 0.001$

2007). Meanwhile, the norm for legitimacy as opposed to criminality has assimilated voting as a legitimate practice (Bednall et al. 2013).

Relying on the indirect deterministic mechanism of framing, national democracy frames personal ideas to rationalize and induce personal practice through the voluntaristic mechanism of idea consistency. Such framed ideas have consisted in personal favor for politicians, individualism, political participation, and religiousness (Fjellvang 2011; Norris 2002; Remmer 2012; Shin 2012). Favor for politicians and political participation have encouraged voting (Aldrich and Simon 1986; Straughn and Andriot 2011). Individualism has underlain e-activity (Chak and Leung 2004). Religiousness has constituted donation and spiritual activity (Hall and Edwards 2002; Peifer 2010; Wang and Graddy 2008).

National human development reduced personal organizational and strike participation, possibly through the deterministic mechanism of analytical functionalism.

Table 8.20 Standardized effects of national characteristics on participation in environmental demonstration

Predictor	(1)	(2)
Wave	0.014**	0.007
Democracy	0.122***	0.128***
Human development	−0.115***	−0.096***
Population	−0.017**	−0.001
Technology	−0.013*	−0.008
Wave × democracy		0.124***
Wave × human development		−0.106***
Nigeria		0.035***
Mexico		0.029***
Philippines		−0.024***
Japan		−0.024***
Turkey		−0.018***
Brazil		−0.015**
Egypt		−0.012*
R^2	0.027	0.055

*$p < 0.05$, **$p < 0.01$, ***$p < 0.001$

These mechanisms are feasible because of the function of human development to escalate people's capability, motivation, and satisfaction (Castles 2000; Inglehart and Welzel 2005).

Applying the indirect deterministic mechanism of framing, national human development frames ideas to influence personal practice with the voluntaristic mechanism of idea consistency. Ideas framed have consisted in people's civility, obedience, responsibility, self-direction, support for privatization, and trust (Bond and Lun 2014; Jakobsen 2010; Fridberg and Kangas 2008b). These ideas have weakened organizational and strike participation (Bagherior et al. 2009; Litor 2019). Conversely, national human development has diminished ideas based on personal communitarianism or group orientation and extremity (Davis and Robinson 2006; He et al. 2014). Such weakening has alleviated organizational and strike participation (Healy and Kirton 2013).

Leveraging the indirect deterministic mechanism of incentivizing, national human development shapes the utility of personal practice to affect the practice through the voluntaristic mechanism of utility optimization. The utility of organizational and strike participation has declined when national human development has raised personal health, life satisfaction, other forms of well-being, and perception of corruption such as in the organization (Basabe et al. 2002; Eikemo et al. 2008; Meulemann 2010; Uslaner 2008). This decline has withdrawn organizational and strike participation (Dixon et al. 2004; Nussio 2019).

National prosperity raised personal e-activity and diminished personal risk aversion. These effects reflect the function of national prosperity to sustain personal

Table 8.21 Standardized effects on green donation

Predictor	(1)	(2)	(3)
Wave	−0.015**	0.005	0.030***
China	−0.072***	−0.021**	−0.005
Philippines	0.050***	0.044***	0.029***
US	0.044***	0.041***	0.039***
Pakistan	0.041***	0.042***	0.043***
Germany	0.031***	0.036***	0.032***
Russia	−0.031***	−0.025***	−0.030***
Egypt	−0.028***	−0.01***	−0.020***
Nigeria	0.024***	0.012*	0.001
Mexico	0.023***	0.031***	0.035***
Brazil	−0.018***	−0.009	−0.007
Turkey	−0.011*	−0.012**	−0.016**
Acquiescence		0.093***	0.116***
Creative work		0.079***	0.079***
Supervision		0.042***	0.048***
Independent work		−0.041***	−0.042***
Education		0.036***	0.049***
Nonprofit organization employment		−0.035***	−0.003
Family income		0.034***	0.026***
Part-time employment		0.027***	0.017**
Homemaking		0.026***	0.031***
Private business employment		−0.025***	0.034***
Earner		0.025***	0.022***
Age		0.023**	0.030***
Irreligious		−0.021**	−0.015*
Retired		−0.020***	0.010
Student		0.017**	0.020***
Full-time employment		0.016**	0.047***
Female		0.015**	0.015**
Public employment		−0.014**	0.015**
Self-employment		0.013*	0.025***
Living with parents		0.012**	0.007
Father immigrant		0.010*	0.008
Graduation age		0.009	0.005
Kid		−0.007	−0.012*
Interest		0.006	0.006

(continued)

Table 8.21 (continued)

Predictor	(1)	(2)	(3)
Divorced		−0.005	−0.003
Age squared		0.005	−0.001
Married		−0.003	−0.004
Widowed		0.003	0.003
Earner employed		0.003	0.000
Cohabited		−0.001	0.002
Separated		0.000	0.000
Wave × acquiescence			0.111***
Wave × education			0.057***
Wave × nonmanual work			0.051***
Wave × supervision			0.048***
Wave × private business employment			0.034***
Wave × family income			0.028***
Wave × idleness			−0.026***
Wave × age			0.025***
Wave × earner			0.025***
Wave × irreligious			−0.022***
Wave × full-time employment			0.019***
Wave × female			0.017**
Wave × homemaking			0.016**
Wave × married			−0.015**
Wave × orthodox			−0.014**
Wave × Islam			−0.014**
Wave × Catholic			0.013*
Wave × graduation age			0.011*
Wave × father immigrant			0.009*
R^2	0.017	0.043	0.076

*$p < 0.05$, **$p < 0.01$, ***$p < 0.001$

dignity, efficiency, and compensation for loss to meet the challenge of modernity (Bourguignon et al. 2007; Deller and Maher 2009; Fukuyama 1995; Peet and Hatwick 2009). As such, national prosperity functions for a better life, meeting needs, avoiding crises, fostering emancipation, and boosting consumption and satisfaction by enhancing technology for the person (Hunt 1989; Peet and Hatwick 2009; Wolff and Resnick 2012). This function obtains through the deterministic mechanism of analytical functionalism.

Activating the indirect deterministic mechanism of empowering, national prosperity raises power for personal practices through the voluntaristic mechanism of

Table 8.22 Standardized effects of national characteristics on green donation

Predictor	(1)	(2)
Wave	−0.002	−0.007
Liberty	0.087***	0.105***
Income inequality	−0.046***	−0.077***
Phone	−0.044***	−0.059***
Population	−0.034***	0.001
Land	−0.025***	−0.006
Wave × democracy		0.098***
Wave × income inequality		−0.067***
Wave × phone		−0.028***
Wave × land		−0.018***
Philippines		0.037***
R^2	0.012	0.025

*$p < 0.05$, **$p < 0.01$, ***$p < 0.001$

power realization. Power raised has consisted in health, knowledge, and self-efficacy as opposed to hardship and illness (Corcoran et al. 2011; Fridberg and Kangas 2008; Norris 2011). The power has rested on the bases of education raised by national prosperity (Baldacci et al. 2003). These power and power bases have driven e-activity and risk confrontation as opposed to aversion (Brown and Zoorob 2022; Chen 2015; Khang et al. 2014; Loader 2007).

Leveraging the indirect deterministic mechanism of incentivizing, national prosperity hikes the utility of personal practice to attract the personal through the voluntaristic mechanism of utility optimization. The utility has rested on the values of emancipation, imagination, and independence (Fjellvang 2011; Welzel 2013). These values characterize the function of e-activity (Caldwell 2020; Fuchs 2008). Furthermore, national prosperity has reduced personal perception of risk and threat (Schneider 2007; Schwartz and Melech 2000). Such reduction has discouraged risk aversion (Custers et al. 2017; Lee-Baggley et al. 2004; Ruiter et al. 2003). Accordingly, national prosperity dwindles the utility of risk aversion.

Applying the indirect deterministic mechanism of framing, national prosperity frames ideas to rationalize and sustain personal practice through the voluntaristic mechanism of idea consistency. Such framed ideas have consisted in cosmopolitanism, liberalism, postmaterialism, postmodernism, tolerance, and trust (Inglehart and Baker 2000; Pichler 2009; Tov and Diener 2008; Traunmuller 2011; Yuchtman-Yaar and Alkalay 2007). These ideas have underlain e-activity and discouraged risk aversion (Gardner and Schmitt 2001; Hardy et al. 2009; Levontin and Bardi 2019; Peter and Valkenburg 2007).

National bank credit raised personal organizational participation and appealing. Such raising reflects the function of national bank credit to circulate economic resources for activity, thus removing people's alienation and loneliness (Haiven

2014). This activation stands on raising autonomy, creativity, freedom, imagination, and individuality by national bank credit (Haiven 2014). The activation benefits from the deterministic mechanism of empowering in analytical functionalism to fulfill the function. Specifically, national bank credit has been economically empowering to uplift people's economic power or resources to boost practice (Chang et al. 2008). Notably, economic resources meet organizational participation and appeal requirements (Bagherior et al. 2009; Grasso 2014; Meyer 2004; Opp 2009; Van Zomeren 2009). For instance, economic resources enhance people's ability to appeal and participate in organizations (Corcoran et al. 2011). Moreover, national bank credit has provided funding to enable organizational activity (Kilburn and Maume 2000; King et al. 2000). Such activity has engaged people's participation and mobilized their appealing (Gillham et al. 2019; Giugni and Grasso 2019; Guillen et al. 2011; Klandermans and de Weerd 2000; Somma et al. 2020).

National income inequality diminished personal learning and raised personal voting. These impacts manifest the inequality as dysfunction depriving, exploiting, and thus activating the demand for change, such as redistribution (Fein 2012; Grover 2011; Neckerman and Toche 2007; Suchweh 2012). Such manifestation hinges on the deterministic mechanisms of analytical functionalism.

With the direct deterministic mechanism, national inequality has diminished practice collectively to reduce personal practice successively through sharing privately or publicly or vicariously. National inequality has eroded national education or learning collectively (Maurer 2011). Education has been an essential basis for learning (Chou 2003). Thus, the reduction, in turn, would attenuate personal learning opportunities privately or vicariously.

Activating the indirect deterministic mechanism of empowering or disempowering, national inequality reduces personal power for practice and thus the practice through the voluntaristic mechanism of power realization. Power reduced has rested on functionality, health, self-direction, and social capital (Bond and Lun 2014; Kim and Kawachi 2007; Portes and Vickstrom 2011). National inequality has also dampened such power bases as homeownership and wealth (Martin 2000; Nilson 1981). Such reduction has deactivated learning (Chou 2003).

Leveraging the indirect deterministic mechanism of incentivizing, national inequality lifts the utility of personal voting through the direct mechanism of utility optimization. The utility has laid in the perceptions and experiences of problems, disadvantage, anomie, corruption, illness, injustice, social exclusion, unfairness, and violence, which call for voting and political action (Jones et al. 2015; Oishi et al. 2011; Portes and Vickstrom 2011; Reardon and Bischoff 2011; Eriksson et al. 2015; Teymoori et al. 2016; Uslaner 2008; Wilkinson and Pickett 2009). Moreover, national inequality has raised the personal practices of crime and violence (Ousey and Lee 2013; van Wilsem 2007). Likewise, national inequality has boosted crime, depression, gambling, health problems, risk, schizophrenia, and violence collectively (Hipp et al. 2009; Hughes et al. 2015; Knack 2002; Wilkinson and Pickett 2017). These practices would translate into personal perceptions and experiences about others. Furthermore, national inequality has instigated the personal desire for opportunity and need for income (McCall and Kenworthy 2009; Winkelmann and Winkelmann

2010). Herein, voting functions as a political action to tackle needs and problems (Chaney 2014). As such, voting has responded to needs and problems perceived or experienced (Aytac and Stokes 2019; Schwartz et al. 2010).

Using the indirect deterministic mechanism of framing, national inequality frames ideas affecting personal practice through the voluntaristic mechanism of idea consistency. Accordingly, national inequality has eroded personal cohesion, self-direction, and trust (Bond and Lun 2014; Green et al. 2003; Oishi et al. 2011). National inequality has also mitigated trust collectively (Knack 2002; Uslaner 2002). Such erosion has discouraged communication or learning (Onu et al. 2016; Kanar and Bouckenooghe 2022; Littlejohn et al. 2017).

National land share per capita raised personal learning and alleviated personal spiritual activity. Land share functions to sustain a living and the community (Biggs and Knauss 2012; Evans and Saegert 2000). The functioning benefits from the deterministic mechanisms of analytical functionalism.

Activating the indirect deterministic mechanism of empowering, national land share raises power to enable personal practice through the voluntaristic mechanism of power realization. Such power has rested on health as opposed to illness (Pattie et al. 2004). This power has enabled learning (Chou 2003).

Leveraging the indirect deterministic mechanism of incentivizing or disincentivizing, national land share reduces the utility of spiritual activity and hence the activity through the voluntaristic mechanism of utility optimization. The utility reduction has arisen from reducing depression, illness, and risk by national land share (Oliver 2003; Pattie et al. 2004). This reduction has eroded spiritual activity (Medvedovski and Allison 2017; Miller 1995). Herein, spiritual activity has helped reduce depression, illness, and risk (Coffe and Geys 2007; Ellison et al. 2001; Muennig et al. 2013; Seidlitz et al. 2002). Spiritual activity thus holds the utility of risk diversion (Gall et al. 2005).

National population size dampens personal spirituality. The dampening reflects the function of population size to boost productivity with agglomeration or the economies of scale (Glaeser et al. 2009). This function benefits from the deterministic mechanisms of analytical functionalism.

Leveraging the indirect deterministic mechanism of incentivizing or disincentivizing, national population size reduces the utility of personal spiritual activity and thus the activity through the voluntaristic mechanism of utility optimization. Such reduction has happened with the increase in collective resources, economic growth, development, quality, or well-being as opposed to conflict by population size (Deller and Maher 2009; Frey et al. 1997; Obschonk et al. 2016; Ryckman 2019; Turner 2013). The collective increase has translated into a corresponding personal increase (Brady 2006; Fridberg and Kangas 2008; Hadden et al. 2003). This translation works through sharing privately or vicariously. Such an increase has lessened spiritual activity (Fjellvang 2011; Wuthnow 2004; Yuchtman-Yaar 2002). Herein, the increase dampens the utility and thus the function of spiritual activity to tackle deficits in resources and well-being (Day 2010; Levin and Chatters 1998).

With the indirect deterministic mechanism of framing, national population size frame ideas to discourage personal spiritual activity through the voluntaristic mechanism of idea consistency. Such ideas have concerned innovation, productivity, revolution, and science (Collier and Hoeffler 2004; Florida 2005; Foster et al. 2001; Turner 1984). These ideas have contradicted and thus lessened spiritual activity (MacDonald 2000; Saucier and Skrzypinska 2006).

National technology boosted personal voting. This boosting reflects the function of national technology to uplift communication, propaganda, and rationality, primarily through the component of information or online technology (Chen 2008; Matthewman 2011; Norris 2001; Roderick 2016; Schroeder and Swedberg 2002). The function is conducive to voting (Brennan 2011; Schecter 2009). More specifically, the function benefits from the deterministic mechanism of analytical functionalism.

Activating the indirect deterministic mechanism of empowering, national technology raises power to enable personal voting through the voluntaristic mechanism of power realization. Such power has rested on financial and online capability and resources to access inf9ormation (Florida 2005; Norris 2001; Welzel 2013). The power has also originated from employment facilitated by national technology (Goetz et al. 2011). Such power has facilitated personal voting (Anderson 2009; Aytac and Stokes 2019; Child and Nikolova 2020).

Leveraging the indirect deterministic mechanism of incentivizing, national technology raises the utility of voting for tackling problems and thus voting through the voluntaristic mechanism of utility optimization. The utility has rested on such problems as footprinting and unsustainability in the environment (Welzel 2013). Such problems have underlain personal voting (Bahry and Lipsmeyer 2001; Brown and Zoorob 2022). Herein, voting functions to urge the government to tackle problems (Fife and Breakwell 1990; Hennessy et al. 2015). In addition, the valuation of voting has elevated the voting (Aytac and Stokes 2019).

National government effectiveness reduced personal spiritual activity. Such reduction reflects building the government instead of spirituality (Holcombe 1985; McCright and Clark 2006). The building stands on the deterministic mechanism of analytical functionalism.

Activating the indirect deterministic of incentivizing, national government effectiveness affects personal practice by affecting the utility of the practice through the voluntaristic mechanism of utility optimization. Herein, national government effectiveness has generally boosted people's prosperity, equality, satisfaction, and well-being (Bohnke 2008; Bratton and Mattes 2001; Guisan 2009; Uslaner 2008). Such boosting has diminished personal spiritual activity (Fjellvang 2011; Sasaki 1979). The diminishment is attributable to the reduced utility of spiritual activity in relieving problems in inadequate prosperity, equality, and well-being (Day 2010; Hart and Goldenberg 2008; Levin and Chatters 1998). As such, effective government replaces spirituality as a relief.

Time Influences

Time affected personal practices and their susceptibility to national characteristics. Notably, time lifted personal e-activity and learning but lessened organization participation and spiritual activity. For instance, learning has increased, and spiritual activity has declined with time (Hamermesh 2019; Requena and Stanek 2014). Time also strengthened the negative effects of national population size, democracy, liberty, and human development on personal organizational participation, weapon carrying, voting, and strike participation, respectively. In addition, time strengthened the positive effect of national income inequality on strike participation. By contrast, time weakened the negative effect of national globalization and the positive effect of national democracy on personal organizational participation. These time effects apply the deterministic mechanisms of analytical functionalism.

With the indirect deterministic mechanism of empowering, time elevates power to activate personal practice through the voluntaristic mechanism of power realization. Such power has emanated from personal income from earnings, marriage, and wage, safety, social class as opposed to poverty, threat, and unemployment (Campbell and Pearlman 2013; Dekkers 2008; Francesconi and Golsch 2005; Hamermesh 2019; Lichter et al. 2002; Sahar 2008; Smith et al. 2001). Time has also increased people's development, political power, prosperity, and social integration (Hamermesh 2019; Norris 2012; M. Smith et al. 2001; Turner 2003). Such power has facilitated personal e-activity (Chen 2015; Pratt et al. 2010). The power has also boosted learning (Chou 2003; Ma et al. 2019; Wentzel 2003; Wink and Dillon 2003).

Leveraging the indirect deterministic mechanism of incentivizing or disincentivizing, time diminishes the utility of personal practice and the practice with the voluntaristic mechanism of utility optimization. Such diminished utility has rested on the rise of personal homeownership, income, and safety as opposed to threat and unemployment (Conley and Gifford 2006; Hamermesh 2019; Sahar 2008; Smith et al. 2001). The diminishment has discouraged personal organizational participation (Nussio 2019). Such diminishment has also dampened personal spiritual activity (Fjellvang 2011; Immerzeel and van Tubergen 2013; Miller 1995; Yuchtman-Yaar 2002). Herein, organization and spiritual activity hold utility for mitigating financial and social problems (Day 2010; Myers 1999; Wetterbeng 2007).

Applying the indirect deterministic mechanism of framing, time frames ideas affecting practice through the voluntaristic mechanism of idea consistency. Accordingly, time has escalated neighboring and social interaction (Smith et al. 2001). The escalation has activated e-activity and learning (Mesirow 2003; Peter and Valkenburg 2007; Wheatley and Buglass 2019). By contrast, time has diminished civic engagement (Foster et al. 2001). Such diminishment has discouraged organizational participation and spiritual activity (Wang and Graddy 2008; Wuthnow 2004).

Also, using the indirect deterministic mechanism of framing, time frames ideas affecting the impact or values of national characteristics through the voluntaristic mechanism of idea consistency. As such, time has raised the personal value of tradition (Brynin et al. 2009). Such tradition covers national population size, democracy, liberty, human development, and income inequality, which have stabilized over time (Abouharb and Cingranelli 2007; Castles 2000; Chenoweth and Stephan 2011; Dreher et al. 2008). Hence, the impacts of traditional national characteristics of liberty escalated with time. The impacts illustrate the accumulation, familiarization, or stabilization effect of time to augment the effects of stable national characteristics. The accumulation, familiarization, or stabilization of national characteristics magnify their impacts. Conversely, national globalization is emerging and new rather than stabilized and traditional (Reese et al. 2019; Sirgy et al. 2004). The impact of national globalization thereby declined with time. Meanwhile, national government legitimacy has declined with time (Harper and Leicht 2011). Government legitimacy has been germane to personal public rather than private practice (Klandermans and de Weerd 2000; Van Zomeren 2009). Thus, the influence of national democracy on personal organizational participation also declined with time.

Overall, the time effect manifests individualization in advancing private, self-reliant practice in e-activity and learning and diminishing public or self-effacing practice in organizational participation and spiritual activity (Morody and Giza-Poleszczuk 2018). Herein, individualization sustains e-activity and learning with the development of cyberspace, media, and the knowledge economy, which popularizes information and knowledge (Bauman 2001; Burgess 2018). Individualization also diverts organizational participation and spiritual activity by instituting personal agency, autonomy, choice, detachment, disembeddedness, disengagement, disintegration, emancipation, independence, liberty, and self-determination (Bauman 2001; Beck and Beck-Gernsheim 2002; Krys et al. 2019). Conversely, individualization defuses bonding and obligation (Burgess 2018). These features reject the higher power of the organization or outside source from organizational participation or spiritual activity (Gorsuch and Miller 1999; Yahne and Miller 1999).

Summary

The five private life practices and the five public life practices (with green demonstrating and green donation as one) were notably predictable by various personal and national characteristics and selectively by the global characteristic of time. The prediction embodies the voluntaristic and deterministic mechanisms of analytical functionalism to fulfill the functions of the characteristics and practices.

E-activity appreciably grew with creative work, supervisory work, family income, national democracy, national prosperity, and time. The activity hinges on power, utility, norms, and ideas to achieve the functions to mobilize and normalize connection or networking, decentralization, democracy, flexibility, identity, individualization, rights, social capital, and teamwork personally and collectively (Bargh and McKenna 2004; Caldwell 2020; Dan et al. 2011; Fuchs 2008; Livingstone et al. 2007; Mesch and Coleman 2007; Norris 2001; Wallace 2016; Y. Wong et al. 2010).

For the functions, e-activity thus benefits from power, utility, norms, and ideas toward the functions. Regarding this benefit, creative work, supervisory work, and family income would provide power for e-activity to achieve its functions with the voluntaristic mechanism of power realization. National prosperity also offers power to enable personal e-activity through the indirect deterministic mechanism of empowering and voluntaristic mechanism of power realization successively. National democracy is congruous with the function of e-activity for democracy, thus contributing to the activity through the indirect deterministic mechanism of framing and voluntaristic mechanism of idea consistently successively. Similarly, individualization with time is congruous with the function of e-activity for individualization, and thus the time effect would realize the cascading mechanisms of the indirect deterministic mechanism of framing and voluntaristic mechanism of idea consistency.

Learning from friends and media increased with education, national income equality, national liberty, and national land share. The functions of learning are to raise certainty and rationality in the runaway world (Robert and Bukodi 2005). Learning benefits from power and ideas emitted from education for learning to achieve the functions, according to the voluntaristic mechanisms of power realization and idea consistency. Herein, education enhances power and rationality for fulfilling the functions of learning (Papastephanon 2015; Sotirovic 2001; Straughn and Andriot 2011; Teodoro 2003). Indirectly, learning benefits from power or opportunities given by national income equality, liberty, and land share through the deterministic mechanism of empowering and the voluntaristic mechanism of power realization successively. Alternatively, national land share indicates social underdevelopment, isolation, and thus uncertainty (Obschonk et al. 2016). The share would thus prompt the need for or utility of learning to activate learning through the indirect deterministic mechanism of incentivizing and the voluntaristic mechanism of utility optimization successively. In addition, learning increases with time, possibly thanks to the growth of knowledge society with time (Burgess 2018). Such growth would empower and incentivize learning, considering the indirect deterministic mechanisms of empowering and incentivizing.

Spiritual activity declined with nonprofit organization employment, national populations size, national land share, national government effectiveness, and time but rose with national democracy. The decline reflects incongruity between spiritual activity or its function and its negative predictors. Accordingly, spiritual activity and its functions seek to achieve individuality, sacredness, and even transcendence beyond the person (Hill and Pargament 2003; Miller and Thoresen 2003; Seidlitz et al. 2002). These functions are incongruous with the organization, community, and government. The negative effects would thereby rest on the pair of indirect deterministic mechanism of framing and the voluntaristic mechanism of idea consistency in national influence, and the pair of the indirect deterministic mechanism of standardizing and the voluntaristic mechanism of norm conformity in organizational influence. Conversely, national democracy respects individuality (Galston 2005; Ringen 2007). This respect is congruous with spirituality and thus encourages personal spiritual activity. Alternatively, national land share per capita lessens environmental and thus living problems (Stretesky and Lynch 2009). This lessening would reduce the utility of personal spiritual activity to relieve the problems. The reduction builds on the indirect deterministic mechanism of incentivizing and the voluntaristic mechanism of utility optimization.

Risk aversion decreased with national prosperity. The aversion functions as a response to risk or threat (Makhanova and Shepherd 2020). National prosperity has reduced risk or threat (Fridberg and Kangas 2008; Schwartz and Melech 2000). Such reduction means the reduced utility of risk aversion. The decrease would ensue from the indirect deterministic mechanism of incentivizing and the voluntaristic mechanism of utility optimization successively.

Organizational participation increased with nonprofit organization employment, national bank credit, and national democracy but declined with national human development and time. These influences reflect the functional match between organizational participation and the predictors. On the one hand, organizational participation functions to build engagement and social capital (Palmer et al. 2011; Wang and Graddy 2008). The participation would benefit from power, norms, and ideas generated for the organization from employment and credit given to the organization. This benefit arises from the paired mechanisms of empowering and power realization, standardizing and norm conformity, and framing and idea consistency. Simply put, organizational input generates organizational output. Moreover, national democracy favors organizing voluntarily (Dryzek and Dunleavy 2009; Tan 2003). The democracy would also encourage personal organization participation through the indirect deterministic mechanism of framing and voluntaristic mechanism of idea consistency successively. Conversely, national human development and time breed individualization (Bond and Lun 2014; de Graaf et al. 2001). The characteristics are incongruous with organizational participation.

Appealing rose with national bank credit and liberty. The rise reflects the functional match between appealing and national characteristics. On the one hand, appealing functions to sustain organization and liberty (Buechler 2011; S. Lo 2021; Stewart et al. 2012; S. Wright 2010). Appealing thereby benefits from power and ideas emanating from national bank credit and liberty for the organization. The benefit builds on the indirect deterministic mechanisms of empowering and framing and the voluntaristic mechanisms of power realization and idea consistency.

Strike participation increased with national liberty but diminished with national human development. The increase reflects the contribution of the framed idea of liberty from national liberty to the liberalization function of strike participation. Accordingly, at least among employees, strike participation functions to buttress liberty (Litor 2019). The contribution thus builds on the indirect deterministic mechanism of framing and the voluntaristic mechanism of idea consistency successively. Meanwhile, national human development would lessen the utility of strike participation with the indirect deterministic mechanism of incentivizing and voluntaristic mechanism of utility optimization. The lessening happens as national human development affords economic and health adequacy and satisfaction (Castles 2000; Eikemo et al. 2008). Attaining such adequacy is the function of strike participation (Litor 2019).

Table 8.23 Substantiation of hypothesized effects on practices

Predictor	E-act	Learn	Spirit	Avert	Weapon	Organ	Appeal	Strike	Vote	Donate
Wave	⊕	⊕	◇+	+	–	⊖	+	+	–	–
Personal										
Irreligious	+	–	–	+	+	–	–	–	–	–
Family income	⊕	+	+	–	–	+	–	–	+	+
Female	–	–	–	+	–	–	–	–	–	–
Age	–	–	+	+	–	+	–	–	+	+
Age squared	+	–	+	+	+	+	+	+	–	–
Married	–	–	–	+	–	–	–	–	+	+
Cohabited	–	–	–	+	–	–	–	–	+	+
Divorced	+	+	+	–	+	+	+	+	–	–
Separated	+	+	+	–	+	+	+	+	–	–
Widowed	+	+	+	–	+	+	+	+	–	–
Kid	–	–	–	+	–	–	–	–	–	–
Mother immigrant	–	–	–	+	+	–	–	–	–	–
Father immigrant	–	–	–	+	+	–	–	–	–	–
Education	+	⊕	+	+	–	+	–	–	+	+

(continued)

Table 8.23 (continued)

Predictor	E-act	Learn	Spirit	Avert	Weapon	Organ	Appeal	Strike	Vote	Donate
Graduation age	+	+	+	+	–	+	–	–	+	+
Interest	+	+	+	–	–	+	+	+	+	+
Living with parents	–	–	–	+	–	–	–	–	–	–
Full-time employment	+	–	–	–	–	–	–	+	+	+
Part-time employment	+	–	–	–	–	–	–	+	+	+
Self-employment	+	–	–	–	–	–	–	–	+	+
Retired	–	–	+	+	–	+	–	–	–	–
Homemaking	–	–	–	+	–	–	–	–	–	–
Student	+	+	–	–	+	–	+	–	–	–
Unemployed	–	–	–	+	+	–	+	–	–	–
Public employment	+	–	–	–	–	–	–	+	+	+
Private business employment	+	–	–	–	–	–	–	+	+	+
Nonprofit organization employment	+	–	⊖	–	–	◇–	–	+	◇+	+

(continued)

Table 8.23 (continued)

Predictor	E-act	Learn	Spirit	Avert	Weapon	Organ	Appeal	Strike	Vote	Donate
Intellectual work	+	–	–	–	–	–	–	+	+	+
Creative work	⊕	–	–	–	–	–	–	+	+	⊕
Independent work	+	–	–	–	–	–	–	+	+	+
Supervision	⊕	–	–	–	–	–	–	+	+	+
Earner	+	–	–	–	–	–	–	+	+	+
Earner employed	+	–	–	–	–	–	–	+	+	+
National										
Population	–	–	⊖	+	+	–↑	–	–	–	–
Phone	+	+	+	–	+	+	+	+	–	–
Land	–	◇-	⊖	–	+	–	–	–	–	–
Technology	+	+	–	–	–	–	+	+	◇-	–
Credit	+	+	–	+	+	◇-	⊕	+	–	–
Prosperity	⊕	+	+	⊖	–	+	–	–	–	–

(continued)

Table 8.23 (continued)

Predictor	E-act	Learn	Spirit	Avert	Weapon	Organ	Appeal	Strike	Vote	Donate
Income inequality	−	⊖	+	−	+	−	+	+	◇− ↑	−
Globalization	+	+	−	−	−	−↓	+	+	−	+
Government effectiveness	−	−	⊖	−	−	−	−	−	−	−
Democracy	◇+	+	◇−	−	(−)↑	⊕↓	+	+	⊕	⊕
Liberty	+	⊕	−	−	−	−	⊕	⊕	(−)↑	−
Human development	+	+	−	−	−	⊖	−	⊖↑	+	◇+
Human capital	+	+	−	−	−	−	−	−	+	+
CO_2	−	−	−	+	+	−	+	+	−	−

Note Circle: notable and agreeing with the hypothesis; Diamond: notable but contrary to the hypothesis; Bracket: contrary to hypothesis; upward arrow: notably more positive with time; downward arrow: notably more negative with time

Voting increased with national democracy, technology, and income inequality and decreased with nonprofit organization employment. The susceptibility benefits from the functional match between voting and its predictors. Voting fulfills functions for citizenship, democracy, and addressing issues (Abelson et al. 1992; Claassen and Povtak 2010; Joslyn and Cigler 2001). Voting thus results from the deterministic and voluntaristic mechanisms of analytical functionalism. With the indirect deterministic mechanism of empowering, national democracy provides the structure to dictate personal voting (Norris 2002). National technology would also mobilize voting with the indirect deterministic mechanism of empowering and voluntaristic mechanism of power realization successively. Meanwhile, national income inequality would raise the utility of voting to tackle the inequality, considering the coupling of the indirect deterministic mechanism of incentivizing and the voluntaristic mechanism of utility optimization. Conversely, nonprofit organization disseminates the social norm for tackling issues by the organization rather than the government (Sanyal 2006). This norm would discourage voting through the voluntaristic mechanism of norm conformity.

Green activism, comprising green demonstration and donation, increased with creative work and national democracy and reduced with national human development. Such prediction reflects functionalist mechanisms. Accordingly, green activism functions to fabricate imagery and reflexivity about the environment and constrain development (Anderson 2010; Foss 2009; Glasson 2015; Maxton-Lee 2020). These functions align with ideas inherent in creative work and national democracy (Fairfield 2008; Zittoun and Gillespie 2016). Therefore, personal creative work and national democracy encourage personal green activism, considering the voluntaristic mechanism of idea consistency and the indirect deterministic mechanism of framing. Conversely, the functions contradict national human development. Hence, national human development discourages personal green activism, considering the cascading mechanisms of framing and idea consistency (Table 8.23).

Chapter 9
Conclusions

For the average person in the world, the production of life quality appraisals, experiences, and practices stand on the static framework of analytical functionalism and the dynamics of social change. Life quality appraisals involve health, life satisfaction, delight, and non-worry. Social life experiences concern economic hardship, neighborhood nuisance, victimization, security, and family saving. Life practices include the private practices of e-activity, learning, spiritual activity, risk aversion, and weapon carrying, and the public practices of appealing, organizational participation, spiritual activity, political voting, and green activism. The static framework of analytical functionalism differentiates personal voluntaristic mechanisms and contextual deterministic mechanisms to fulfill the requisite functions of goal attainment, adaptation, integration, and latency. Voluntaristic mechanisms hinge on power realization, utility optimization, norm conformity, and idea consistency. Deterministic mechanisms work directly through sharing privately or publicly and indirectly through empowering, incentivizing, standardizing, and framing. Social change dynamics rest on denaturalization, globalization, individualization, modernization, and postmodernization.

Within the static analytical-functionalist mechanisms, power realization, utility optimization, norm conformity, and idea consistency respectively rely on personal power to drive, utility perceived to gravitate, norms perceived to assimilate, and ideas to rationalize. Meanwhile, the context applies indirect deterministic mechanisms to raise personal power, utility, norms, and ideas respectively through empowering, incentivizing, standardizing, and framing. The context also exerts the direct deterministic mechanism to influence directly through sharing privately and publicly without the media of power, utility, norms, and ideas. By this mechanism, for instance, contextual life quality induces personal life quality directly. More specifically, the wealthy context shares wealth with people privately by giving or publicly or communally such that people take others' wealth vicariously.

C. Cheung, *Production Dynamics for Life Quality in the Incipient 21st Century*,
https://doi.org/10.1007/978-981-19-3827-6_9

The dynamic framework applies to social change across time, denaturalization, globalization, individualization, modernization, and postmodernization. Denanturalization means the increasing impacts of artificial factors, including emission, information, and technology. Globalization means the increasing impacts of global factors and conversely the decreasing impacts of local or national factors. Individualization means the increasing impacts of private factors and conversely the decreasing impacts of collective, group, organizational, or social factors. Modernization means the increasing impacts of the rational factors of utility and ideas. Postmodernization means the decreasing impacts of all factors or decreasing predictability.

Statics

Life quality appraisals appreciably rose with independent work, the life experiences of family saving and security, national bank credit, national carbon dioxide emission, national human development, and declined with age, the life experience of economic hardship, and the life practice of risk aversion. Among these predictors, family saving and security indicate personal power, and age indicates the lack of personal power, considering the voluntaristic mechanism of power realization. National bank credit and human development represent national power, considering the indirect deterministic mechanism of empowering. Independent work and security register personal ideas consistent with and rationalizing life quality, considering the voluntaristic mechanism of idea consistency. Conversely, economic hardship and risk aversion give personal ideas contradicting life quality, considering the voluntaristic mechanism of idea consistency. National carbon dioxide emission proffers a national idea about development conducive to life quality, considering the indirect deterministic mechanism of framing. Herein, the emission signifies development or modernization and its elements of prosperity and urbanization (Kick and McKinney 2014; Rudel et al. 2011). This signification is consonant with life quality, which embraces development and modernization (Galtung 2005; Huta 2014; Nevarez 2011). Notably, no life practice contributed to life quality appraisals appreciably. Personal practice, including five private and five public practices, thus fails to produce personal life quality appraisal substantially. The failure implies that the practices are not directly and successfully functional to life quality, as the practices can meet with frustration.

Economic hardship, as a life experience inhibiting life quality appraisal, appreciably slid with education, nonprofit organization employment, national bank credit, national human development, and time, and rose with family income and national democracy. Among the predictors, education, national bank credit, and national human development generate power to counter economic hardship, considering the voluntaristic mechanism of power realization and the indirect deterministic mechanism of empowering. The nonprofit organization transmits a norm to devalue profit and thus dispel the experience of economic hardship, considering the voluntaristic mechanism of norm conformity. Similarly, time suggests ideas about development and prosperity (Hamermesh 2019; Norris 2012). The idea contradicts and thus lessens the experience of economic hardship, considering the indirect deterministic mechanism of framing and the voluntaristic mechanism of idea consistency. Conversely, family income represents a standard for comparison to generate an idea about personal deficiency, thus raising the experience of economic hardship, considering the voluntaristic mechanism of idea consistency. Broadly speaking, social comparison has bred the idea of deficiency (Fujita 2008). This idea has fomented the experience of hardship (Whelan and Maitre 2013). Likewise, national democracy carries ideas about agonism, appealing, argument, competition, contest, and struggle (Dryzek and Dunleavy 2009; Moller and Skaaning 2013; Pappas 2019; Tracy and Hughes 2014). These ideas have been conducive to the experience of hardship (Robila 2006). Hence, national democracy induces the experience of economic hardship—through the indirect deterministic mechanism of framing and voluntaristic mechanism of idea consistency.

As a salutary life experience, security appreciably rose with creative work, independent work, nonprofit organization employment, national bank credit, and national government effectiveness, and slid with student status and national population size. Among these predictors, creative work and independent work exhibit ideas of autonomy, controlling, problem-solving, and self-efficacy (Afsar and Masood 2018; Fontenot 1993; Morrison et al. 1999). These ideas have been conducive to the experience of security (La Guardia et al. 2000; Valera and Guardia 2014). Hence, such work contributes to the experience, considering the voluntaristic mechanism of idea consistency. Meanwhile, national government effectiveness provides power and ideas about effectiveness, harmony, legitimacy, justice, living standards, and problem-solving (Mizrahi 2016; Wolfe et al. 2016; Wong and Wan 2011). Such power and ideas lift personal experience about security (Carter and Wolfe 2021; La Guardia et al. 2000; Sacks and Levi 2010; Salehi 2012). Therefore, national government effectiveness contributes to the experience, considering the indirect deterministic mechanisms of empowering and framing, coupled with the voluntaristic mechanisms of power realization and idea consistency.

As a salutary life experience, family saving appreciably rose with family income and personal education. Family income furnishes the economic basis for saving, considering the voluntaristic mechanism of power realization. Similarly, education is power functional to wealth accumulation (Bullock 2021; Schnittker and Behrman 2012). Education thus facilitates family saving, considering the power realization mechanism.

Neighborhood nuisance, an experience not notably impairing life quality, appreciably rose with national human capital and declined with nonprofit organization employment, creative work, national technology, national bank credit, and national liberty. The rise of neighborhood nuisance by national human capital may stem from increasing public activities empowered by human capital (Teorell 2003; Van Dyke and Dixon 2013). Such activities and their noise are the sources of neighborhood nuisance (Parkes et al. 2002). Thus, national talent or human capital raises personal experience about neighborhood nuisance, considering the indirect deterministic mechanism of empowering. Conversely, creative work is conducive to problem solving and avoidance (Fontenot 1993). The work thus represents the power to avoid neighborhood nuisance, considering the voluntaristic mechanism of power realization. Likewise, national technology and bank credit provide resources to mitigate neighborhood problems (Haiven 2014; Welzel 2013). They thus reduce personal experience about neighborhood nuisance through the coupled mechanisms of empowering and power realization. Similarly, the nonprofit organization propagates a norm for resolving neighborhood problems (Aligica 2015; Milligan and Fyfe 2005). This norm adopted through employment in the organization would abate the experience of neighborhood nuisance, considering the voluntaristic mechanism of norm conformity. Meanwhile, national liberalism frames ideas about autonomy, empowerment, and tolerance as opposed to interference (Delanty 2009; Kinna et al. 2019; Scruton 2014; Yoos 2007). Such framing counters the experience of neighborhood nuisance (Greenberg 1999). Therefore, national liberty diminishes the experience through the coupled mechanisms of framing and idea consistency.

Victimization, an experience not remarkably impairing life quality, appreciably rose with national population size. Such size heightens interpersonal exposure and conflict (Turner 2003; Yagci 2017). Interpersonal exposure and conflict underlie victimization (Madero-Hernandez and Fisher 2013; Mishna 2012). Therefore, national population size provides opportunities to raise personal victimization through the indirect deterministic mechanism of empowering and the voluntaristic mechanism of power realization successively.

Risk aversion, notably detrimental to life quality, appreciably decreased with national prosperity. National prosperity dampens risks (Fridberg and Kangas 2008; Schwartz and Melech 2000). Such dampening would reduce the utility of risk aversion, considering the indirect deterministic mechanism of incentivizing or disincentivizing. Herein, risk aversion has lower utility when the risk is less.

Though not notably affecting life quality, e-activity appreciably grew with creative work, supervisory work, family income, national democracy, and national prosperity. Creative work, supervisory work as social status, and family income provide power, including knowledge and resources, for activity (Afsar and Masood 2018; Keltener et al. 2008; Shin 2012). Hence, they raise e-activity with the voluntaristic mechanism of power realization. Similarly, national prosperity enhances power, knowledge, or resources (Baldacci et al. 2003; Booth and Richard 1998). National prosperity hence activates personal e-activity through the indirect deterministic mechanism of empowering and the voluntaristic mechanism of power realization. Meanwhile, national democracy frames ideas for personal agency or activity and individualism (Fairfield 2008; Shin 2012). Such ideas have been conducive to e-activity (Chak and Leung 2004). Therefore, national democracy lifts personal e-activity by the indirect deterministic mechanism of framing and the voluntaristic mechanism of idea consistency.

Though not notably affecting life quality, learning appreciably increased with education, national income equality, national liberty, and national land share. Education is the power base and necessary condition for learning (Chou 2003; Pallas 2002). The contribution of education draws on the voluntaristic mechanism of power realization. National land share sustains an environment for people's learning, free of others' interference. Accordingly, a spacious, quiet, isolated, and self-regulated environment is conducive to people's learning (Schunk and Usher 2019; Tanggaard 2009). This sustenance reflects the indirect deterministic mechanism of empowering and the voluntaristic mechanism of power realization successively. Alternatively, national liberty and income equality incentivize people's learning, according to the indirect deterministic mechanism of incentivizing and voluntaristic mechanism of utility optimization. Accordingly, the national conditions sustain the utility of learning that fits one's autonomy and interest without compulsion and worry of unfairness (Hagger and Hamilton 2018; Tanggaard 2009). More broadly, inequality has discouraged and deactivated constructive action (Green et al. 2003; Lipford and Yandle 2009).

Spiritual activity, though not notably affecting life quality, appreciably declined with nonprofit organization employment, national populations size, national land share, and national government effectiveness but rose with national democracy. National population size, national land share, and national government effectiveness would reduce the utility of spiritual activity and thus the activity, considering the indirect deterministic mechanism of incentivizing or disincentivizing and the voluntaristic mechanism of utility optimization. Accordingly, these conditions facilitate people's obtaining help from the government and other people as opposed to exposure to their stress (Guisan 2009; Oliver 2003; Pattie et al. 2004; Phan et al. 2009; Glaeser and Gottlieb 2006). That is, spiritiual activity represents self-helping (Kalkstein and Tower 2009; Seidlitz et al. 2002). Similarly, the nonprofit organization dissemination the norm for organizational support (Islam and William 2012; Milligan and Fyfe 2005). This norm, fostered with employment in the organization, would reduce the utility of spiritual activity. Hence, nonprofit organization employment dampens spiritual activity, considering the voluntaristic mechanism of norm conformity. Conversely, national democracy frames ideas for self-helping, as in agency and individualism (Caprara and Vecchione 2017; Shin 2012). This framing encourages spiritual activity through the indirect deterministic mechanism of framing and the voluntaristic mechanism of idea consistency.

Though not notably affecting life quality, organizational participation appreciably increased with nonprofit organization employment, national bank credit, and national democracy and declined with national human development. National bank credit raises economic resources to sustain organizational activity (Haiven 2014). The raising would empower personal participation in the organization through the indirect deterministic mechanism of empowering and the voluntaristic mechanism of power realization. Similarly, national democracy fosters the idea for a free organization to counterbalance the government (Dryzek and Dunleavy 2009). The idea would rationalize and encourage organization participation through the indirect deterministic mechanism of framing and the voluntaristic mechanism of idea consistency. Meanwhile, the nonprofit organization cultivates a norm for the organization (Fric 2008). The cultivation through employment in the organization would sustain organizational participation with the voluntaristic mechanism of norm conformity. Conversely, national human development lessens reliance on organizational support and thus the utility of organizational participation (Davis and Robinson 2006). The lessening reflects the indirect deterministic mechanism of incentivizing or disincentivizing and the voluntaristic mechanism of utility optimization successively.

Though not notably affecting life quality, Appealing appreciably rose with national bank credit and liberty. National bank credit and liberty afford organizing for appealing without repression by the authority (Bavetta et al. 2014; Haiven 2014). This affording works with the indirect deterministic mechanism of empowering and the voluntaristic mechanism of power realization. Furthermore, national liberty fosters the idea for free activity (Rasmussen and Den Uyl 2005). The idea encourages appealing, considering the indirect deterministic mechanism of framing and the voluntaristic mechanism of idea consistency.

Though not notably affecting life quality, Strike participation appreciably increased with national liberty but diminished with national human development. National liberty provides rights or power as opposed to resistance to strike participation (Moller and Skaaning 2014; Rasmussen and Den Uyl 2005). Hence, national liberty activates personal strike participation through the indirect deterministic mechanism of empowering and the voluntaristic mechanism of power realization. Similarly, national liberty frames the idea for rights to strike participation (Moller and Skaaning 2014; Rasmussen and Den Uyl 2005). The contribution of national liberty to personal strike participation thus also rests on the indirect deterministic mechanism of framing and the voluntaristic mechanism of idea consistency. As indicated by national resources, welfare, and other economic alternatives, national human development lessens the gain from strike participation (Dixon and Roscigno 2003). Therefore, the lessening builds on the indirect deterministic mechanism of incentivizing or disincentivizing and the voluntaristic mechanism of utility optimization. Moreover, national human development has championed the idea of civility (Bond and Lun 2014). The idea has discouraged strike participation (Born et al. 2013). Thus, national human development also diverts personal strike participation through the indirect deterministic mechanism of framing and the voluntaristic mechanism of idea consistency.

Though not notably affecting life quality, voting appreciably increased with national democracy, technology, and income inequality and decreased with nonprofit organization employment. National democracy and technology, such as information and media technology, furnish the basis, ease, or power for voting (Brennan 2011; Shockley and Fairdosi 2015). The contribution of the basis or power represents the indirect deterministic mechanism of empowering and the voluntaristic mechanism of power realization. National income inequality poses the utility of voting to address the issue of the inequality (Schwartz et al. 2010). Thus, the contribution of the inequality to personal political voting reflects the indirect deterministic mechanism of incentivizing and the voluntaristic mechanism of utility optimization. Conversely, the nonprofit organization advocates a norm for tackling social problems by the organization instead of the government (Aligica 2015; Sanyal 2006). The norm received through employment in the organization thus discounts political voting through the indirect deterministic mechanism of standardizing and the voluntaristic mechanism of norm conformity.

Although not notably affecting life quality, Green activism appreciably increased with creative work and national democracy and reduced with national human development. Creative work conveys the idea of problem-solving (Kozbelt et al. 2010;

Metzl and Morrell 2008). This idea underlies green activism to resolve environmental problems (Lalander and Merimaa 2018). Hence, creative work contributes to green activism through the voluntaristic mechanism of idea consistency. Meanwhile, national democracy upholds ideas for agency and activism (Brennan 2016; Caprara and Vecchione 2017). These ideas also constitute green activism (Bertuzzi 2019; Truelove et al. 2019). Therefore, national democracy raises personal green activism through the indirect deterministic mechanism of framing and the voluntaristic mechanism of idea consistency.

Dynamics

Dynamics transpire from time (i.e., wave) effects on life quality appraisal, experiences, practices, and the impacts or values of personal and national characteristics. Essentially, time did not generate an appreciable effect on life quality appraisal. Its negative effect on delight was slight. Instead, time appreciably reduced economic hardship, spiritual activity, and organizational participation. By contrast, time appreciably increased e-activity and learning. Meanwhile, time appreciably weakened the impacts of national government effectiveness, national globalization, religious faith, and organizational participation on life quality. Furthermore, time appreciably weakened the impacts of family income, education, national population size, national bank credit, and national human development on life experiences. By contrast, time appreciably strengthened the impact of appealing on life quality. Time also appreciably strengthened the impacts of full-time employment, student status, and unemployment on life experiences. In addition, time appreciably weakened the impact of national globalization on life practice. By contrast, time appreciably strengthened the impacts of national population size, income inequality, liberty, and human development on life practices.

Time slightly reduced delight. The reduction is a case of life quality decline with time (Gil-Lacruz et al. 2019; Sarracino 2010). This decline reflects individualization, particularly its personal growth in aspiration or demand and risk and its reflexivity (Bauman 2001; Burgess 2018; de Graaf et al. 2001; Elliott 2003). Herein, individualization emphasizes the person and his or her growth and thus downplays growth outside the person (Fuchs 2015; Krys et al. 2019). The emphasis boosts aspirations, demand, narcissism, or self-culture (Burgess 2018; Krys et al. 2019). Such boosting means the idea of personal deficiency (Harrison and Waller 2018). The idea, in turn, weakens well-being (Chesters et al. 2021; Ganesh and McAllum 2010). The lowering thus reflects the indirect deterministic mechanism of framing and the voluntaristic mechanism of idea consistency. In addition, individualization also magnifies personal risk and awareness or reflexivity about risk (Bauman 2001; Burgess 2018). Risk is detrimental to life quality materially and idealistically, respectively, depriving power and morale (Chesters et al. 2021; Van Haaften et al. 2004; Zotti et al. 2016). The time effect thus reflects the indirect deterministic mechanisms of empowering or disempowering and framing respectively through the voluntaristic mechanisms of power realization and idea consistency.

Individualization also underlies the negative time effects on organizational participation and spiritual activity (including religious activity), the impacts of weakened effects of national government effectiveness, national globalization, religious faith, and organizational participation on life quality, the impacts of family income, national population size, national bank credit, and national human development on life experiences, and the negative effect of national globalization on life practice. That is, organizational practice and influence and national influence declined with time (Burgess 2018). Conversely, the impact of national liberty on life practice strengthened with time. Liberalization also characterizes individualization (Krys et al. 2019).

Modernization, alternatively, is responsible for the negative time effects on economic hardship and spiritual activity and the impact of religious faith on life quality, and the positive time effects on e-activity and learning, the impacts of full-time employment, student status, and unemployment on life experiences, and the impacts of national liberty and human development on life practices. Accordingly, growth in e-activity, employment, human development, learning, and liberty as opposed to hardship and religion characterize modernization (Inglehart 2018; Sorensen and Christiansen 2013; Zhang 1999). Contradictory to modernization, however, the impacts of national government effectiveness and organizational participation on life quality and the impacts of education, family income, national bank credit, and national human development on life experiences weakened with time. Such factors are also the features of modernization (Dioale and Seda 2001; Martinelli 2005; Steinhardt and Delhey 2020). Hence, modernization is not a wholly successful social change factor.

However, globalization, possibly as a form of modernization, was less influential on life experience and practice with time. Nevertheless, the impact of national government effectiveness as a non-global factor also diminished with time. Hence, globalization does not register a consistent social change factor.

Denaturalization does not explain the appreciable time effects. Accordingly, environmental and technological influences did not grow with time.

Postmodernization explains the negative time effects on the impacts of national government effectiveness, national globalization, religious faith, and organizational participation on life quality, the impacts of family income, education, national population size, national bank credit, and national human development on life experiences, and the impact of national globalization on life practice. Distinctly, postmodernization explains the weakened impacts of education and national population size with time. However, postmodernization contradicts the strengthened impacts of appealing, national population size, income inequality, liberty, and human development with time. Hence, postmodernization does not go unchallenged.

To conclude, individualization fares as the best social change dynamic underlying the appreciable time effects without contradiction. Essentially, individualization buttresses the negative time effect on delight as a life quality appraisal.

Summary

The average person in the world appreciably maintains life quality appraisal with young age, the experiences of family saving and security as opposed to economic hardship, risk non-aversion, national bank credit, carbon dioxide emission, and human development. According to the voluntaristic mechanism of power realization, young age affords power to sustain life quality. Notably, young age has sustained cognitive and physical power or abilities (Gerstorf et al. 2006; Herd et al. 2008). Moreover, family savings and security experience afford such power as financial, physical, and social capital (Brisson 2009; Curley 2010; Muffels and Fouarge 2004). Such power has facilitated life quality (Hill 2019; Michalos et al. 2000). The power also emanates from national bank credit, human development, and even carbon dioxide emission to represent economic, educational, interpersonal, and organizational support through the indirect deterministic mechanism of empowering. These national economic or productive factors have been empowering (Norris 2011; Ross et al. 2000; Schaie 2013). By contrast, economic hardship and risk aversion, carrying ideas about hardship and risk, contradict and thus weaken life quality based on the voluntaristic mechanism of idea consistency. Such adverse ideas have jeopardized life quality appraisal (Bellani and D'Ambrosio 2011; Chesters et al. 2021; Gudmundsdottir 2013; van Praag and Frijters 1999; Zotti et al. 2016). Conversely, their reverse ideas about adaptation, courage, hardiness, and optimism have been salutary (DeNeve and Cooper 1998; Diener et al. 2009; Holliman et al. 2021; Magaletta and Oliver 1999). This idea consistency mechanism also underlies the salutary effects of experiences of security and family saving. The ideas of security and saving have been salutary (Baumeister et al. 2013; Muffels and Fouarge 2004; Obucina 2013; van Praag et al. 2003).

Nevertheless, private and public practices other than risk aversion failed to exhibit substantial impacts on life quality. These practices are e-activity, learning, spiritual activity, weapon carrying, appealing, strike participation, organizational participation, political voting, and environmental activism. The failure illustrates that the practices do not function well for the voluntaristic mechanisms of power realization and idea consistency to advance life quality. Not affording the power realization mechanism, the practices do not principally aim or function to generate life quality. Similarly, the practices do not induce ideas conducive to life quality through the idea consistency mechanism. Instead, the practices involve cost, energy or resource depletion, or exhaustion, thus offsetting their salutary effects through realization and consistency mechanisms. Besides risk aversion, therefore, practices such as arguing, avoidance, childcare, isolation, reflection, searching, and television watching have downgraded life quality (Battersby and Phillips 2016; Baumeister et al. 2013; Van Haaften et al. 2004). The failure of personal practices to raise life quality reveals the limitation of self-production in life quality, as the production is personally costly. By contrast, one's life quality benefits from others' production, such as enhancing savings, security, and other resources.

Delight as a component of life quality slightly diminished with time. This decline reflects the dynamic of individualization in raising aspirations, demand, and risk and its concern (Bauman 2001; Burgess 2018; de Graaf et al. 2001; Elliott 2003; Krys et al. 2019). Risk is debilitating according to the indirect deterministic mechanism of empowering or disempowering. In addition, the indirect deterministic mechanism of framing indicates that aspiration, demand, and concern are ideas contradicting and thus discouraging life quality.

The impacts of education, family income, national population size, national bank credit, and national human development on life quality appreciably declined with time, whereas the impact of appealing on life quality rose with time. These declines reflect the dynamics of postmodernization about unpredictability (Gibbins and Reimer 1999). The declines in national impacts register the dynamic of globalization downplaying the country specifically (O'Byrne and Hensby 2011). Meanwhile, the rise in the appealing impact illustrates the dynamics of individualization regarding agency and assertiveness (Krys et al. 2019).

References

Abbott, Pamela, and Roger Sapsford. 2006. Life-Satisfaction in Post-Soviet Russia and Ukraine. *Journal of Happiness Studies* 7: 251–287.

Abbott, Pamela, Claire Wallace, and Roger Sapsford. 2011. Surviving the Transformation: Social Quality in Central Asia and the Caucuses. *Journal of Happiness Studies* 12: 199–223.

Abel, Millicent H. 2002. Humor, Stress, and Coping Strategies. *Humor* 15 (4): 365–381.

Abelson, Robert P., Elizabeth F. Loftus, and Anthony G. Greenwald. 1992. Attempts to Improve the Accuracy of Self-Reports of Voting. In *Questions about Questions: Inquiries into the Cognitive Bases of Surveys*, 138–153, ed. Judith M. Tanur. New York: Russell Sage.

Abizadeh, Arash. 2002. Does Liberal Democracy Presuppose a Cultural Nation? Four Arguments. *American Political Science Review* 96 (3): 495–509.

Abouharb, M. Rodwan., and David Cingranelli. 2007. *Human Rights and Structural Adjustment*. Cambridge, UK: Cambridge University Press.

Abrahms, Max. 2008. What Terrorists Really Want: Terrorist Motives and Counterterrorism Strategy. *International Security* 32 (4): 78–105.

Achilov, Dilshod. 2016. Revisiting Political Islam: Explaining the Nexus between Political Islam and Contentious Politics in the Arab World. *Social Science Quarterly* 97 (2): 252–270.

Achterberg, Peter, and Dick Houtman. 2009. Ideologically Illogical? Why Do the Lower-educated Dutch Display so Little Value Coherence? *Social Forces* 87 (3): 1649–1670.

Acker, Gila M., and Dorothea Lawrence. 2009. Social Work and Managed Care: Measuring Competence, Burnout, and Role Stress of Workers Providing Mental Health Servies in a Managed Care Era. *Journal of Social Work* 9 (3): 269–283.

Ackerman, Frank, David Kiron, Neva R. Goodwin, Jonathan M. Harris, and Kevin Gallegher. 1997. *Human Well-Being and Economic Goals*. Washington, DC: Island.

Ackerman, Phillip L., and Stacey D. Wolman. 2007. Determinants and Validity of Self-estimates of Abilities and Self-concept Measures. *Journal of Experimental Psychology. Applied* 13 (2): 57–78.

Adams, Matthew. 2007. *Self and Social Change*. London, CA: Sage.

Adams, Philippe, John R. Z. Abela, Randy Auerbach, and Steven Skitch. 2009. Self-Criticism, Dependency, and Stress Reactivity: An Experience Sampling Approach to Testing Blatt and Zuroff's (1992) Theory of Personality Predispositions to Depression in High-Risk Youth. *Personality & Social Psychology Bulletin* 35 (11): 1440–1451.

Adely, Fida Issa J., Ankushi Mitra, Menatalla Mohamed, and Adam Shaham. 2021. Poor Education, Unemployment and the Promise of Skills: The Hegemony of the "Skills Mismatch" Discourse. *International Journal of Educational Development* 82: 102381.

C. Cheung, *Production Dynamics for Life Quality in the Incipient 21st Century*,
https://doi.org/10.1007/978-981-19-3827-6

Adeola, Francis O. 2000. Endangered Community, Enduring People: Toxic Contamination, Health, and Adaptive Responses in a Local Context. *Environment & Behavior* 32 (2): 209–249.

Adler, Mitchel G., and N.S. Fegley. 2005. Appreciation: Individual Differences in Finding Value and Meaning as a Unique Predictor of Subjective Well-Being. *Journal of Parenting* 73 (1): 79–114.

Adnanes, Marian. 2004. Exit and/or Voice? Youth and Post-communist Citizenship in Bulgaria. *Political Psychology* 25 (5): 795–815.

Adsera, Alicia. 2003. Changing Fertility Rates in Developed Countries: The Impact of Labor Market Institutions. *Journal of Population Economics* 17: 17–43.

Afifi, Walid A., and Stephanie Robbins. 2015. Theory of Motivated Information Management: Struggles with Uncertainty and Its Outcomes. In *Engaging Theories in Interpersonal Communication: Multiple Perspectives*, 143–156, ed. Dawn O. Braithwaite and Paul Schrodt. Thousand Oaks, CA: SAGE.

Afsar, Bilal, and Mariam Masood. 2018. Transformational Leadership, Creative Self-efficacy, Trust in Supervisor, Uncertainty Avoidance, and Innovative Work Behavior of Nurses. *The Journal of Applied Behavioral Science* 54 (1): 36–61.

Ager, Alustair, and J. Ager. 2011. Faith and the Discourse of Secular Humanitarianism. *Journal of Refugee Studies* 24 (3): 456–472.

Agha, Nadia. 2016. Kinship in Rural Pakistan: Consanguineous Marriages and Their Implications for Women. *Women's Studies International Forum* 54: 1–10.

Agnew, Robert, and Timothy Brezina. 2010. Strain Theories. In *The SAGE Handbook of Criminological Theory*, 96–113, ed. Eugene McLaughlin and Tim Newburn. London, UK: SAGE.

Ahern, Melissa M., and Michael S. Hendryx. 2003. Social Capital and Trust in Providers. *Social Science & Medicine* 57: 1195–1203.

Ahmad, Fahad, and Jeffrey Monaghan. 2019. Mapping Criminological Engagements within Radicalization Studies. *British Journal of Criminology* 59 (6): 1288–1308.

Ahnquist, Johanna, Sarah P. Wamala, and Martin Lindstrom. 2012. Social Determinants of Health: A Question of Social or Economic Capital? Interaction Effects of Socioeconomic Factors on Health Outcomes. *Social Science & Medicine* 74 (6): 930–939.

Aishwarya, C.S., Indranil Samanta, and Puja Dudeja. 2019. Psychosocial Determinants of Stress among Adolescents in an Urban Slum in a City of Western Maharashtra: A Cross-Sectional Study. *International Journal of Adolescent Medicine Health* 33 (2): 20180139.

Akers, Caroline, and Catherine Kaukinen. 2009. The Public Reporting Behavior of Intimate Partner Violence Victims. *Journal of Family Violence* 24: 159–171.

Akinboade, Oludele Akinloye, Mandisa Putuma Mokwena, and Emilie Chanceline Kinfack. 2014. Protesting for Improved Public Service Delivery in South Africa's Sedibeng District. *Social Indicators Research* 119 (1): 1–23.

Akiyama, Hiroko, and Toni Antonucci. 2002. Gender Differences in Depressive Symptoms: Insights from a Life Span Perspective on Life Stages and Social Networks. *Advnaces in Medical Sociology* 8: 343–358.

Akkus, Birol, Tom Postmes, Katherine Stroebe, and Gamze Baray. 2020. Cultures of Conflict: Protests, Violent Repression, and Community Values. *British Journal of Social Psychology* 59 (1): 49–65.

Albrecht, Gary L. 2005. The Sociology of Health and Illness. In *The SAGE Handbook of Sociology*, 267–283, ed. Craig Calhoun, Chris Rojek, and Bryan Turner. London, UK: SAGE.

Aldrich, John H. 1993. Rational Choice and Turnout. *American Journal of Political Science* 37 (1): 246–278.

Aldrich, John H., and Dennis M. Simon. 1986. Turnout in American National Elections. *Research in Micropolitics* 1: 271–301.

Alea, Nicole, Susan Bluck, and Angelania B. Semegon. 2004. Young and Older Adults' Experience of Emotional Experience: Do Autobiographical Narratives Tell a Different Story? *Journal of Adult Development* 11 (4): 235–250.

Alesina, Alberto, and George-Marios. Angeletos. 2005. Fairness and Redistribution. *American Economic Review* 95 (4): 960–980.

Alessio, John C. 2011. *Social Problems and Inequality: Social Responsibility through Progressive Sociology*. Farnham, UK: Ashgate.

Alexander, Jeffrey C. 1997. The Paradoxes of Civil Society. *International Sociology* 12 (2): 115–133.

Alexander, Jeffrey C. 1998. *Neofunctionalism and After*. Malden, MA: Blackwell.

Aligica, Paul Dragos. 2015. Addressing Limits to Mainstream Economic Analysis of Voluntary and Nonprofit Organizations. *Nonprofit & Voluntary Sector Quarterly* 44 (5): 1025–1040.

Al-krenawi, Alean, John R. Graham, and Fakir Al Gharaibeh. 2011. A Comparison Study of Psychological, Family Function Marital and Life Satisfactions of Polygamous and Monogamous Women in Jordan. *Community Mental Health Journal* 47 (5): 594–602.

Allmer, Thomas. 2015. *Critical Theory and Social Media: Between Emancipation and Commodification*. Abingdon, UK: Routledge.

Allwood, Maureen A., and Cathy Spatz Widom. 2013. Child Abuse and Neglect, Developmental Role Attainment, and Adult Arrests. *Journal of Research in Crime and Delinquency* 50 (4): 551–578.

Alnsour, Jamal, and Julia Meaton. 2009. Factors Affecting Compliance with Residential Standards in the City of Old Salt, Jordan. *Habitat International* 33: 301–309.

Aloia, Lindsey Susan, and Denise Haunani Solomon. 2015. The Physiology of Argumentative Skill Deficiency: Cognitive Ability, Emotional Competence, Communication Qualities, and Responses to Conflict. *Communication Monographs* 82 (3): 315–338.

Alonso-Arbiol, Itziar, Nekane Baluerka, and Phillip R. Shaver. 2007. A Spanish Version of the Experiences in Close Relationships (ECR) Adult Attachment Questionnaire. *Personal Relationships* 14: 45–63.

Altman, Andrew, and Christopher Heath Wellman. 2009. *A Liberal Theory of International Justice*. Oxford, UK: Oxford University Press.

Alvarado, Felix. 1996. Concerning Postmodernity and Organizations in the Third World: Opening a Debate and Suggestions for a Research Agenda. *Organization Science* 7 (6): 667–681.

Alvesson, Mats, and Stanley Deetz. 2000. *Doing Critical Management Research*. London: Sage.

Alvesson, Mats. 2002. *Postmodernism and Social Research*. Buckingham, UK: Open University Press.

Amato, Paul R., and Jacob Chendle. 2005. The Long Reach of Divorce: Divorce and Child Well-Being Across Three Generations. *Journal of Marriage & Family* 67: 191–206.

Ambrey, Christopher L., and Christopher M. Fleming. 2014. Valuing Ecosystem Diversity in South East Queensland: A Life Satisfaction Approach. *Social Indicators Research* 115: 45–65.

Amiot, Catherine E., Winnifred R. Louis, Sarah Bourdeau, and Oulma Maalouf. 2017. Can Harmful Intergroup Behaviors Truly Represent the Self? The Impact of Harmful and Prosocial Normative Behaviors on Intra-individual Conflict and Compartmentalization. *Self & Identity* 16 (6): 703–731.

An, Weihua, and Christopher Winship. 2017. Causal Inference in Panel Data with Application to Estimating Race-of-Interviewer Effects in the General Social Survey. *Sociological Methods & Research* 46 (1): 68–102.

Anciaes, Paulo Rui, Paul James Metcalfe, and Chris Heywood. 2017. Social Impacts of Road Traffic: Perceptions and Priorities of Local Residents. *Impact Assessment & Project Appraisal* 35 (2): 172–183.

Andersen, Jorgen Goul. 1999. Changing Labour Markets, New Social Divisions and Welfare State Support. In *The End of the Welfare State? Responses to State Retrenchment*, 13–33, ed. Stefan Svallfors and Peter Taylor-Gooby. London: Routledge.

Anderson, C. Leigh., and Neil Nevitte. 2006. Teach Your Children Well: Values of Thrift and Saving. *Journal of Economic Psychology* 27: 247–261.

Anderson, Jon. 2010. From Zombies to Coyotes: Environmentalism Where We Are. *Environmental Politics* 19 (6): 973–991.

Anderson, Mary R. 2009. Beyond Membership: A Sense of Community and Political Behavior. *Political Behavior* 31 (4): 603–627.

Anderson, Steven G., and Mary Keegan Eamon. 2005. Stability of Health Care Coverage among Low-income Working Women. *Health & Social Work* 30 (1): 7–17.

Anderson-Butcher, Dawn, Angela Oliver Khairallah, and Janis Race-Bigelow. 2004. Mutual Support Groups for Long-term Recipients of TANF. *Social Work* 49 (1): 131–140.

Anderson-Connolly, Richard. 2002. Is Lean Mean? Workplace Transformation and Employee Well-Being. *Work, Employment & Society* 16 (3): 389–413.

Andersson, Eva. 2004. From Valley of Sadness to Hill of Happiness: The Significance of Surroundings for Socioeconomic Career. *Urban Studies* 40 (3): 641–659.

Andreeva, Elena, Yuliya Myslyakova, Pavel Glukhikh, and Artem Ratner. 2017. Economic and Social Impact of Modernization on Cultural Values. *Journal of International Studies* 10 (1): 193–208.

Andreoletti, Carrie, Leslie A. Zebrowitz, and Margie E. Lachman. 2001. Physical Appearance and Control Beliefs in Young, Middle-aged and Older Adults. *Personality & Social Psychology Review* 27 (8): 969–981.

Andrews, Frank M., and Stephen B. Withey. 1976. *Social Indicators of Well-Being: Americans' Perceptions of Life Quality*. New York: Plenum.

Andrews, Kenneth T., Kraig Beyerlein, and Tuneka Tucker Farnum. 2015. The Legitimacy of Protest: Explaining White Southerners' Attitudes Toward the Civil Rights Movement. *Social Forces* 94 (3): 1021–1044.

Andrews, Rhys, et al. 2009. Students' Attitudes Toward History: Does Self-identity Matter? *Educational Research* 51 (3): 365–377.

Angelusz, Robert, and Robert Tardos. 2001. Change and Stability in Social Network Resources: The Case of Hungary under Transformation. In *Social Capital: Theory and Research*, 297–323, ed. Nan Lin, Karen Cook, and Ronald S. Burt. New York: Aldine de Gruyter.

Angelusz, Robert, and Robert Tardos. 2008. Assessing Social Capital and Attainment Dynamics: Position Generator Applications in Hungary, 1989–2003. In *Social Capital: An International Research Program*, 394–420, ed. Nan Lin and Bonnie H. Erickson. Oxford, UK: Oxford University Press.

Anson, Ofra. 1988. Living Arrangements and Women's Health. *Social Science & Medicine* 26 (2): 201–208.

Anton, Charis E., and Carmen Lawrence. 2014. Home is Where The Heart Is: The Effect of Place of Residence on Place Attachment and Community Participation. *Journal of Environmental Psychology* 40: 451–461.

Antonakis, John, and Joerg Dietz. 2011. Looking for Validity or Testing It? The Perils of Stepwise Regression, Extreme-score Analysis, Heteroscedasticity, and Measurement Error. *Personality & Individual Differences* 50: 409–415.

Anusic, Ivana, Stevie C.Y.. Yap, and Richard E. Lucas. 2014. Does Personality Moderate Reaction and Adaptation to Major Life Events? Analysis of Life Satisfaction and Affect in an Australian National Sample. *Journal of Research in Personality* 51: 69–77.

Apinunmahakul, Amornat, and Rose Anne Devlin. 2008. Social Networks and Private Philanthropy. *Journal of Public Economics* 92: 309–328.

Appleton, Simon, and Lina Song. 2008. Life Satisfaction in Urban China: Components and Determinants. *World Development* 36 (11): 2335–2340.

Arai, Susan M., and Alison M. Pedlar. 1997. Building Communities Through Leisure: Citizen Participation in a Healthy Communities Initiative. *Journal of Leisure Research* 29 (2): 167–182.

Aral, Sinan, and Dylan Walker. 2012. Identifying Influential and Susceptible Members of Social Networks. *Science* 337 (6092): 337–341.

Arguedas, Amy A. Ross 2020. Can Naughty Be Healthy? Healthism and Its Discontents in News Coverage of Orthorexia Nervosa. *Social Science & Medicine* 246: 112784.

Ariza-Montes, Antonio, and Ana María Lucia-Casademunt. 2016. Nonprofit Versus for-Profit Organizations: A European Overview of Employees' Work Conditions. *Human Service Organizations, Management, Leadership & Governance* 40 (4): 334–351.

Armon, Cheryl, and Theo Linda Dawson. 2003. The Good Life: A Longitudinal Study of Adult Value Reasoning. In *Handbook of Adult Development*, 271–300, ed. Jack Demick and Carrie Andreoletti. New York: Kluwer Academic.

Armon, Cheryl. 1984. Ideals of the Good Life and Moral Judgment: Ethical Reasoning across the Lifespan. In *Beyond Formal Operation: Late Adolescent and Adult Cognitive Development*, 357–380, ed. Michael L. Commons, Francis A. Richards and Cheryl Armon. New York: Praeger.

Armony, Ariel C., and Victor Armony. 2005. Indictments, Myths, and Citizen Mobilization in Argentina: A Discourse Analysis. *Latin American Politics & Society* 47 (4): 27–54.

Arnau, Randolph C. 2018. Hope and Anxiety. In *The Oxford Handbook of Hope*, 221–231, ed. Matthew W. Gallagher and Shane J. Lopez. New York, NY: Oxford University Press.

Arnett, Jeffrey Jensen. 2002. The Psychology of Globalization. *American Psychologist* 57 (10): 774–783.

Arnett, Jeffrey Jensen. 2018. Happily Stressed: The Complexity of Well-Being in Midlife. *Journal of Adult Development* 25 (4): 270–278.

Arsandaux, Julie, Ilaria Montagni, Mélissa. Macalli, Nathalie Texier, Mathilde Pouriel, Raphaël Germain, Adel Mebarki, Shérazade. Kinouani, Marie Tournier, Stéphane. Schuck, and Christophe Tzourio. 2021. Mental Health Condition of College Students Compared to Non-students During Covid-19 Lockdown: The CONFINS Study. *British Medical Journal Open* 11 (8): e053231.

Arthaud-Day, Marne L., and Janet P. Near. 2005. The Wealth of Nations and the Happiness of Nations: Why Accounting Matters. *Social Indicators Research* 74: 511–548.

Asogwa, Chika Euphemia. 2020. Internet-Based Communications: A Threat or Strength to National Security? *SAGE Open* 10 (2): 215824402091458 (\d12–5.17).

Ateca-Amestoy, Victoria, Alexandra Cortes Aguilar, and Ana L. Moro-Egido. 2014. Social Interacting and Life Satisfaction: Evidence from Latin America. *Journal of Happiness Studies* 15: 527–554.

Atkeson, Lonna Rae, and Cherie D. Maestas. 2012. *Catastrophic Politics: How Extraordinary Events Redefine Perceptions of Government*. New York: Cambridge University Press.

Atkins, Judi. 2008. How Virtue-theoretic Arguments May Be Used in the Justification of Policy. *Politics* 28 (3): 129–137.

Atkinson, Giles, Andrew Healey, and Susana Mourato. 2005. Valuing the Costs of Violent Crime: A Stated Preference Approach. *Oxford Economic Papers* 57 (4): 559–585.

Atkinson, Will. 2008. Not All that Was Social Has melted into Air (or Liquid): A Critique of Bauman in Individualization and Class in Liquid Modernity. *Sociological Review* 56 (1): 1–17.

Atkinson, Will. 2013. Class Habitus and Perception of the Future: Recession, Employment Insecurity and Temporality. *British Journal of Sociology* 64 (4): 643–661.

Au, Kevin, and Mike W.L.. Cheung. 2004. Intra-cultural Variation and Job Autonomy in 42 Countries. *Organization Studies* 25 (8): 1339–1362.

Aucoin, Peter. 1990. Administrative Reform in Public Management: Paradigms, Principles, Paradoxes, and Pendulums. *Governance* 3 (2): 115–137.

Auerbach, Randy P., Christian A. Webb, Meghan Schreck, Chad M. McWhinnie, Moon-Ho Ringo. Ho, Xiongzhao Zhu, and Shuqiao Yao. 2011. Examining the Pathway through Which Intrinsic and Extrinsic Aspirations Generate Stress and Subsequent Depressive Symptoms. *Journal of Social & Clinical Psychology* 30 (8): 856–886.

Austin, Erica Weintraub, and Bruce E. Pinkleton. 1999. The Relation between Media Content Evaluations and Political Disaffection. *Mass Communication & Society* 2 (3/4): 105–122.

Axford, Barrie. 2013. *Theories of Globalization*. Cambridge, UK: Polity.

Ayala, Louis J. 2000. Trained for Democracy: The Differing Effects of Voluntary and Nonvoluntary Organizations on Political Participation. *Political Research Quarterly* 53 (1): 99–115.

Ayalon, Hanna, Eliezer Ben-Rafael, and Abraham Yogev. 1993. *Community in Transition: Mobility, Integration, and Conflict*. Westport, CT: Greenwood.

Ayanian, Arin H., and Nicole Tausch. 2016. How Risk Perception Shapes Collective Action Intentions in Repressive Contexts: A Study of Egyptian Activists During the 2013 Post-coup Uprising. *British Journal of Social Psychology* 55 (4): 700–721.

Ayob, Abu H. 2020. An Exploratory Study of Societal Values in Social Participation across Nations. *Social Science Journal* 57 (3): 310–325.

Aytac, Isik A., Bruce H. Rankin, and Arda Ibikoglu. 2008. The Social Impact of the 2008 Global Economic Crisis on Neighborhoods, Households, and Individuals in Turkey. *Social Indicators Research* 124 (1): 1–19.

Aytac, Isik A., and Bruce H. Rankin. 2009. Economic Crisis and Marital Problems in Turkey: Testing the Family Stress Model. *Journal of Marriage & Family* 71: 756–767.

Aytac, I.şık A., Bruce H. Rankin, and Arda İbikoğlu. 2015. The Social Impact of the 2008 Global Economic Crisis on Neighborhoods, Households, and Individuals in Turkey. *Social Indicators Research* 124 (1): 1–19.

Aytac, S. Esdem., and Susan C. Stokes. 2019. *Why Bother? Rethinking Participation in Elections and Protests*. Cambridge, UK: Cambridge University Press.

Baba, Vishwanath V., Louise Tourigny, Xiaoyun Wang, Terri Lituchy, and Silvia Inés Monserrat. 2013. Stress Among Nurses: A Multi-nation Test of the Demand-Control-Support Model. *Cross Cultural Management* 20 (3): 301–320.

Backman, Olof, and Anders Nilsson. 2011. Pathways to Social Exclusion: A Life-course Study. *European Sociological Review* 27 (1): 107–123.

Bagherior, Reza, A.S. Bahaman, A.S. Asnarulkhadi, and A. Shamsudain. 2009. A Social Exchange Approach to People's Participation in Watershed Management Programs in Iran. *European Journal of Scientific Research* 34 (3): 428–441.

Baharumshah, Ahmad Z. 2003. Determinants of Gross National Saving in Malaysia: A Macroeconomic Analysis 1960–2000. *Savings & Development* 27 (4): 421–440.

Bahr, Howard M., and Kathleen S. Bahr. 2001. Families and Self-sacrifice: Alternative Models and Meanings for Family Theory. *Social Forces* 79 (4): 1231–1258.

Bahry, Donna, and Christine Lipsmeyer. 2001. Economic Adversity and Public Mobilization in Russia. *Electoral Studies* 20 (3): 371–398.

Bailey, Stephen J. 2004. *Strategic Public Finance*. Houndmills, UK: Palgrave.

Baker, Joseph O., and Buster G. Smith. 2009. Growing up in Context: The Nones: Social Characteristics of the Religiously Unaffiliated. *Social Forces* 87 (3): 1251–1263.

Baldacci, Emanuele, Maria Teresa Guin-Siu, and Luiz de Mello. 2003. More on the Effectiveness of Public Spending on Health Care and Education: A Covariance Structure Model. *Journal of International Development* 15: 709–725.

Baldus, Bernd. 2017. *Origins of Inequality in Human Societies*. New York, NY: Routledge.

Ball, Michael. 2004. Co-operation with the Community in Property-led Urban Regeneration. *Journal of Property Research* 21 (2): 119–142.

Banse, Rainer, and Cludia Kowalick. 2007. Implicit Attitudes Towards Romantic Partners Predict Well-Being in Stress Life Conditions: Evidence from the Antenatal Maternity Ward. *International Journal of Psychology* 42 (3): 149–157.

Barber, Larissa K., Patricia G. Bagsby, and David C. Munz. 2010. Affect Regulation Strategies for Promoting (or Preventing) Flourishing Emotional Health. *Personality & Individual Differences* 49: 663–666.

Bardeen, Joseph R., Thomas A. Fergus, and Holly K. Orcutt. 2016. Examining the Specific Dimensions of Distress Tolerance that Prospectively Predict Perceived Stress. *Cognitive Behaviour Therapy* 46 (3): 1–13.

Bargh, John A., and Katelyn Y.A.. McKenna. 2004. The Internet and Social Life. *Annual Review of Psychology* 55: 573–590.

Barker, David C., and James D. Tinnick, III. 2006. Competing Visions of Parental Roles and Ideological Constraint. *American Political Science Review* 100 (2): 249–263.

Barker, David, Kimberly Nalder, and Jessica Newham. 2021. Clarifying the Ideological Asymmetry in Public Attitudes toward Political Protest. *American Politics Research* 49 (2): 157–170.

Barlow, Anne. 2004. Regulation of Cohabitation, Changing Family Policies and Social Attitudes: A Discussion of Britain within Europe. *Law & Policy* 26 (1): 57–86.

Barnawi, Fatima Hamza. 2017. Prevalence and Risk Factors of Domestic Violence against Women Attending a Primary Care Center in Riyadh, Saudi Arabia. *Journal of Interpersonal Violence* 32 (8): 1171–1186.

Barnett, Rosalind Chait, and Janet Shibley Hyde. 2001. Women, Men, Work, and Family: An Expansionist Theory. *American Pyschologist* 56 (10): 781–796.

Baron, Lois. 2007. *Contemporary Issues in Youth Sports*. New York, NY: Nova.

Barr, Michael. 2012. Nation Branding as Nation Building: China's Image Campaign. *East Asia* 29: 81–94.

Barrett, Anne E. 1999. Social Support and Life Satisfaction among the Never Married. *Research on Aging* 21 (1): 46–72.

Bartels, Larry M. 1993. Messages Received: The Political Impact of Media Exposure. *American Political Science Review* 87 (2): 267–285.

Bartsch, Anne, and Mary Beth Oliver. 2017. Appreciation of Meaningful Entertainment Experiences and Eudaimonic Well-Being. In *The Routledge Handbook of Media Use and Well-being: International Perspectives on Theory and Research on Positive Media Effects*, 80–105, ed. Leonard Reinecke and Mary Beth Oliver. New York, NY: Routledge.

Basabe, Nekane, Dario Paez, Jose Valencia, Jose Luis Gonzalez, Bernard Rime, and Ed Diener. 2002. Cultural Dimensions, Socioeconomic Development, Climate, and Emotional Hedonic Level. *Cognition & Emotion* 16 (1): 103–125.

Bask, Miia. 2005. Welfare Problems and Social Exclusion among Immigrants in Sweden. *European Sociological Review* 21 (1): 73–89.

Baslevent, Cem, and Hasan Kirmanoglu. 2011. Discerning Self-interested Behaviour in Attitudes towards Welfare State Responsibilities across Europe. *International Journal of Social Welfare* 20: 344–352 (\105-47).

Bassani, Cherylynn. 2008. The Influence of Financial, Human and Social Capital on Japanese Men's and Women's Health in Single- and Two-parent Family Structures. *Social Indicators Research* 85: 191–209.

Bassoli, Matteo, and Lara Monticelli. 2018. What about the Welfare State? Exploring Precarious Youth Political Participation in The Age of Grievances. *Acta Politica* 53 (2): 204–230.

Basu, Santonu, and Sushanta Mallick. 2008. When Does Growth Trickle down to the Poor? The Indian Case. *Cambridge Journal of Economics* 32: 461–477.

Bates, Robert H., and Irene Yackovkev. 2002. Ethnicity, Capital Formation, and Conflict: Evidence from Africa. In *The Role of Social Capital in Development: An Empirical Assessment*, 300–340, ed. Christiaan Grootaert and Thierry van Bastelaer. Cambridge, UK: Cambridge University Press.

Batta, Anna. 2011. Statism. In *21st Century Political Science: A Reference Handbook*, 91–98, ed. John T. Ishiyama and Marijke Breuning. Thousand Oaks, CA: SAGE.

Battersby, Annabel, and Lisa Phillips. 2016. In the End It All Makes Sense Meaning in Life at Either End of the Adult Lifespan. *International Journal of Aging & Human Development* 83 (2): 184–204.

Bauer, Jack J., Dan P. McAdams, and April R. Sakaeda. 2005. Interpreting the Good Life: Growth Memories in the Lives of Mature, Happy People. *Journal of Personality & Social Psychology* 88 (1): 203–217.

Baum, Scott, Patrick Mullins, Robert Stimson, and Kevin O'Connor. 2002. Communities of the Postindustrial City. *Urban Affairs Review* 37 (3): 322–357.

Bauman, Zygmunt. 2001. *The Individualized Society*. Cambridge, UK: Polity.

Baumann, Shyon, Athena Engman, and Josee Johnston. 2015. Political Consumption, Conventional Politics, and High Cultural Capital. *International Journal of Consumer Studies* 39 (5): 413–421.

Baumeister, Roy F., Kathleen D. Vohs, Jennifer L. Aaker, and Emily N. Garbinsky. 2013. Some Key Differences between a Happy Life and a Meaningful Life. *Journal of Positive Psychology* 8 (6): 505–516.

Bavetta, Sebastiano, Pietro Navarra, and Dario Maimone. 2014. *Freedom and the Pursuit of Happiness: An Economic and Political Perspective*. New York, NY: Cambridge University Press.

Baylis, Nick. 2005. Relationship with Reality and Its Role in the Well-being of Young Adults. In *The Science of Well-being*, 241–272, ed. Felica A. Huppert, Nick Baylis and Barry Keverne. Oxford, UK: Oxford University Press.

Beasley, Margaret, Ted Thompson, and John Davidson. 2003. Resilience Response to Life Stress: The Effects of Coping Style and Cognitive Hardiness. *Personality & Individual Differences* 34: 77–95.

Beasley, Ryan K., and Mark R. Joslyn. 2001. Cognitive Dissonance and Post-decision Attitude Change in Six Presidential Elections. *Political Psychology* 22 (3): 521–540.

Beaudoin, Christopher E. 2009. Bonding and Bridging Neighborliness: An Individual-Level Study in the Context of Health. *Social Science & Medicine* 68 (12): 2129–2136.

Beaudoin, Christopher, and Esther Thorson. 2006. The Social Capital of Blacks and Whites: Differing Effects of the Mass Media in the United States. *Human Communication Research* 32: 157–177.

Bebbington, A.J., D. Mittin, J. Mogaladi, M. Scurrah, and C. Bielcih. 2010. Decentring Poverty, Reworking Government: Social Movements and States in the Government of Poverty. *Journal of Development Studies* 46 (7): 1304–1326.

Becchetta, Leonardo. 2010. The Money-Happiness Relationships in Transition Countries: Evidence from Albania. *Transition Studies Review* 17: 39–62.

Beck, Aaron T., and Gary Emery. 1985. *Anxiety Disorders and Phobias: A Cognitive Perspective.* New York: Basic Books.

Beck, Ulrich, and Elisabeth Beck-Gernsheim. 2002. *Individualization: Institutionalized Individualism and Its Social and Political Consequences.* London: Sage.

Beck, Ulrich, Anthony Giddens, and Scott Lash. 1994. *Reflexive Modernization: Politics, Tradition and Aesthetics in the Modern Social Order.* Cambridge, UK: Polity.

Becker, Thomas E., Robert S. Billings, Daniel M. Eveleth, and Nicole W. Gilbert. 1997. Validity of Scores on Three Attachment Style Scales: Exploratory and Confirmatory Evidence. *Educational & Psychological Measurement* 57 (3): 477–493.

Beckfield, Jason. 2004. Does Income Inequality Harm Health: New Cross-national Evidence. *Journal of Health & Social Behavior* 45 (3): 231–248.

Bednall, Timothy C., Liliana L. Boveb, Ali Cheethamb, and Andrea L. Murray. 2013. A Systematic Review and Meta-Analysis of Antecedents of Blood Donation Behavior and Intentions. *Social Science & Medicine* 96 (13): 86–94.

Behr, Dorothee, Michael Braun, Lars Kaczmirek, and Wolfgang Bandilla. 2014. Item Comparability in Cross-national Surveys: Results from Asking Probing Questions in Cross-national Web Surveys about Attitudes Towards Civil Disobedience. *Quality & Quantity* 48: 127–148.

Beinc, Miehcel, Frederic Docquier, and Hillel Rapoport. 2001. Brain Drain and Economic Growth: Theory and Evidence. *Journal of Development Economics* 64: 275–289.

Bekker, Marrie H.J.., Judit Arends-Toth, and Marcel A. Croon. 2011. Autonomy-Connectedness, Acculturation, and Independence-Interdependence Among Various Cultural Groups in a Multicultural Society. *International Journal of Intercultural Relations* 35 (3): 368–376.

Bekkers, Rene, and Woods Boisman. 2009. The Relationship between Confidence in Charitable Organizations and Volunteering Revisited. *Nonprofit & Voluntary Sector Quarterly* 38 (5): 884–897.

Belanger, Jocelyn J., Birga M. Schumpe, Noemie Nociti, Manuel Moyano, Stephane Dandeneau, Pier-Eric. Chamberland, and Robert J. Vallerand. 2019. Passion and Moral Disengagement: Different Pathways to Political Activism. *Journal of Personality* 87 (6): 1234–1249.

Bell, Duncan. 2010. Political Realism and the Limits of Ethics. In *Ethics and World Politics*, 93–110, ed. Duncan Bell. Oxford, UK: Oxford University Press.

Bell, Margret E., Lisa A. Gordman, and Mary Ann Dutton. 2007. The Dynamics of Staying and Leaving: Implications for Battered Women's Emotional Well-being and Experiences of Violence at the End of a Year. *Journal of Family Violence* 22: 413–428.

Bellair, Paul E., and Vincent J. Roscigno. 2000. Local Labor-Market Opportunity and Adolescent Delinquency. *Social Forces* 78 (4): 1509–1538.

Bellani, Luna, and Conchita, D'Ambrosio. 2011. Deprivation, Social Exclusion and Subjective Well-Being. *Social Indicators Research* 104: 67–86.

Belli, Robert F., Michael W. Traugott, Margaret Young, and Kathrine A. McGonagle. 1999. Reducing Vote Overreporting in Surveys: Social Desirability, Memory Failure, and Source Monitoring. *Public Opinion Quarterly* 63 (1): 90–108.

Bellingtier, Jennifer A., Marcus Mund, and Cornelia Wrzus. 2022. The Role of Extraversion and Neuroticism for Experiencing Stress During the Third Wave of the Covid-19 Pandemic. *Current Psychology*.

Belliotti, Raymond A. 1993. *Good Sex: Perspectives on Sexual Ethics*. Lawrence, KA: University Press of Kansas.

Belzil, Christian, and Jörgen. Hansen. 2020. The Evolution of the Us Family Income-Schooling Relationship and Educational Selectivity. *Journal of Applied Econometrics* 35 (7): 841–859.

Bendixsen, Synnøve. 2018. Differentiation of Rights in the Norwegian Welfare State: Hierarchies of Belonging and Humanitarian Exceptionalism. *Social Inclusion* 6 (3): 162–171.

Benford, Robert D., and David A. Snow. 2000. Framing Processes and Social Movements: An Overview and Assessment. *Annual Review of Sociology* 26: 611–639.

Bengtson, Vern L., Robert A. Harootyan, Karl Kronebusch, Leora Lawton, Mark Schlesinger, Merril Silverstein, and Robert E. Vorek. 1994. *Intergenerational Linkages: Hidden Connections in American Society*. New York: Springer.

Ben-Ner, Avner, and Ting Ren. 2015. Comparing Workplace Organization Design Based on Form of Ownership. *Nonprofit & Voluntary Sector Quarterly* 44 (2): 340–359.

Bennett, Stephen Earl, and David Resnick. 1990. The Implications of Nonvoting for Democracy in the United States. *American Journal of Political Science* 34 (3): 771–802.

Bennett, Stephen Earl, Staci L. Rhine, and Richard S. Flickinger. 2000. Reading's Impact on Democratic Citizenship in America. *Political Behavior* 22 (3): 167–195.

Benson, Michael L., John Wooldredge, Amy B. Thistlethwaite, and Greer Litton Fox. 2004. the Correlation Between Race and Domestic Violence Is Confounded with Community Context. *Social Problems* 51 (3): 326–342.

Benstock, Michael. 2008. Deconstructing the Sibling Correlation: How Families Increase Inequality. *Journal of Family & Economic Issues* 29: 325–345.

Benton, Richard A. 2016. Uniters or Dividers? Voluntary Organizations and Social Capital Acquisition. *Social Networks* 44: 209–218.

Bentrovato, Denise, and Marie Nissanka. 2018. Teaching Peace in the Midst of Civil War: Tensions Between Global and Local Discourses in Sri Lankan Civics Textbooks. *Global Change, Peace & Security* 30 (3): 353–372.

Ben-Zur, Hasida. 2002. Coping, Affect and Aging: The Roles of Mastery and Self-esteem. *Personality & Individual Differences* 32 (2): 357–372.

Berger, Lawrence M. 2005. Income, Family Characteristics, and Physical Violence toward Children. *Child Abuse & Neglect* 29 (2): 107–133.

Berger, Mark T. 2003. Decolonisation, Modernisation and Nation-Building: Political Development Theory and the Appeal of Communism in Southeast Asia, 1945–1975. *Journal of Southeast Asian Studies* 34 (3): 421–448.

Berman, Shuyler L., and Michele A. Wittig. 2004. An Intergroup Theories Approach to Direct Political Action among African Americans. *Group Processes & Intergroup Relations* 7 (1): 19–34.

Bernstein, Jeffrey L. 2001. Linking Presidential and Congressional Approval during Unified and Divided Governments. In *What Is It about Government that Americans Dislike?* 98–117, ed. John R. Hibbing and Elizabeth Theiss-Morse. Cambridge, UK: Cambridge University Press.

Berry, Helen Louise, and Jennifer A. Welsh. 2010. Social Capital and Health in Australia: An Overview from the Household Income and Labour Dynamics in Australia Survey. *Social Science & Medicine* 70: 588–596.

Berry, John W., and Colette Sabatier. 2010. Acculturation, Discrimination, and Adaptation among Second Generation Immigrant Youth in Montreal and Paris. *International Journal of Intercultural Relations* 34: 191–207.

Bertuzzi, Niccolò. 2019. Political Generations and the Italian Environmental Movement(S): Innovative Youth Activism and the Permanence of Collective Actors. *American Behavioral Scientist* 63 (11): 1556–1577.

Besic, Nejra, and Margaret Kerr. 2009. Punks, Goths, and Other Eye-Catching Peer Crowds: Do They Fulfill a Function for Shy Youths? *Journal of Research on Adolescence* 19 (1): 113–121.

Best, Samuel J., and Brian Krueger. 2002. New Approach to Assessing Opinion: The Prospects for Electronic Mail Surveys. *International Journal of Public Opinion Research* 14 (1): 72–92.

Best, Samuel J., and Brian S. Krueger. 2010. Government Monitoring and Political Participation in the United States: The Distinct Roles of Anger and Anxiety. *American Politics Research* 39 (1): 85–117.

Best, Steven, and Douglas Kellner. 2001. *The Postmodern Adventure: Science, Technology, and Cultural Studies at the Third Millennium*. New York: Guilford.

Bettencurt, B. Ann., and Kennon Sheldon. 2001. Social Roles as Mechanisms for Psychological Need Satisfaction within Social Groups. *Journal of Personality & Social Psychology* 81 (6): 1131–1143.

Betz, Diana E., Laura R. Ramsey, and Denise Sekaquaptewa. 2013. Gender Stereotype Threat among Women and Girls. In *The SAGE Handbook of Gender and Psychology*, 428–449, ed. Michelle K. Ryan and Myla R. Branscombe. London, UK: SAGE (BF692.2S24).

Bhatia, Aditi. 2009. The Discourses of Terrorism. *Journal of Pragmatics* 41 (2): 279–289.

Bhavnani, Ravi, Karsten Donnay, Dan Miodownik, Maayan Mor, and Dirk Helbing. 2014. Group Segregation and Urban Violence. *.American Journal of Political Science* 58 (1): 226–245.

Bian, Yanjie, Ronald Breiger, Deborah Davis, and Joseph Galashkiewicz. 2005. Occupation, Class, and Social Networks in Urban China. *Social Forces* 83 (4): 1443–1468.

Bianchi, Suzanne, Philip N. Cohen, Sara Raley, and Kei Nomaguchi. 2004. Inequality on Parental Investment in Child-rearing: Expenditures, Time, and Health. In *Social Inequality*, 189–219, ed. Kathryn M. Neckerman. New York: Russell Sage.

Biggs, Michael, and Steven Knauss. 2012. Explaining Membership in the British National Party: A Multilevel Analysis of Contact and Threat. *European Sociological Review* 28 (5): 633–646.

Billett, Stephen. 2011. Subjectivity, Self and Personal Agency in Learning through and for Work. In *The SAGE Handbook of Workplace Learning*, 60–72, ed. Margaret Malloch, Len Cairns, Karen Evans and Bridget N. O'Connor. London, UK: SAGE.

Billiet, Jaak, Bart Maddens, and Roeland Beerten. 2003. National Identity and Attitude Toward Foreigners in a Multinational State: A Replication. *Political Psychology* 24 (2): 241–257.

Bills, David B. 2005. Participation in Work-related Education: Variations in Skill Enhancement among Workers, Employers, and Occupational Closure. *Research in Social Stratification & Mobility* 23: 67–102.

Birman, Dina, Edison Trickett, and Rebecca M. Buchanan. 2005. A Tale of Two Cities: Replication of a Study on the Acculturation and Adaptation of Immigrant Adolescents from the Former Soviet Union in a Different Community Context. *American Journal of Community Psychology* 35 (1/2): 83–101.

Bish, Alison, and Susan Michie. 2010. Demographic and Attitudinal Determinants of Protective Behaviors During Pandemic: A Review. *British Journal of Health Psychology* 15: 797–824.

Bishop, Michael A. 2015. *The Good Life: Unifying the Philosophy and Psychology of Well-Being*. New York: Oxford University Press.

Bjarnegard, Elin, Karen Brounéus, and Erik Melander. 2019. Violent Boyhoods, Masculine Honor Ideology, and Political Violence: Survey Findings from Thailand. *Journal Interpersonal Violence* 36 (15–16): 7136–7160.

Bjerk, David. 2009. How Much Can We Trust Causal Interpretations of Fixed-effects Estimators in the context of Criminality? *Journal of Quantitative Criminology* 25: 391–417.

Bjorgo, Tore. 2016. Counter-Terrorism as Crime Prevention: A Holistic Approach. *Behavioral Sciences of Terrorism & Political Aggression* 8 (1): 25–44.

Bjornberg, Ulla, and Hans Ekbrand. 2008. Financial and Practical Kin Support in Sweden: Normative Guidelines and Practice. *Journal of Comparative Family Studies* 39 (1): 73–95.

Bjornskov, Christian, and Martin Paldam. 2012. The Spirits of Capitalism and Socialism: A Cross-country Study of Ideology. *Public Choice* 150 (3): 469–498.

Bjornskov, Christian. 2003. The Happy Few: Cross-country Evidence on Social Capital and Life Satisfaction. *Kyklos* 56: 3–16.

Bjornskov, Christian. 2005. Does Political Ideology Affect Economic Growth? *Public Choice* 123: 133–146.

Black, Richard, W. Neil Adger, Nigel W. Arnell, Stefan Dercon, Andrew Geddes, and David Thomas. 2011. The Effect of Environmental Change on Human Migration. *Global Environmental Change* 21 (SUPPL. 1): S3–S11.

Blackshaw, Tony. 2005. *Zygmunt Bauman*. Abingdon, UK: Routledge.

Blackshaw, Tony. 2017. *Re-imaging Leisure Studies*. Abingdon, UK: Routledge.

Blackwell, Brenda Sims, and Sarah Eschholz. 2002. Sex Differences and Rational Choice: Traditional Tests and New Directions. In Rational Choice and Criminal Behavior: Recent Research and Future Challenges, 109–135, ed. Alex R. Piquero and Stephen G. Tibbetts. New York: Routledge.

Blackwell, David, Carrie Leaman, Rose Tramposch, Ciera Osborne, and Miriam Liss. 2017. Extraversion, Neuroticism, Attachment Style and Fear of Missing out as Predictors of Social Media Use and Addiction. *Personality & Individual Differences* 116: 69–72.

Blain, Michael. 2015. Social Science Discourse and the Biopolitics of Terrorism. *Sociological Compass* 9 (3): 161–179.

Blair, John M. 2005. Community Indicator Programs: Their Construction, Logic and Consistency Based on a Program Evaluation of the Santa Monica CIP, California. *Journal of Environmental Policy & Management* 7 (4): 597–617.

Blair, Margaret M. 2011. An Economic Perspective on the Notion of Human Capital. In *The Oxford Handbook of Human Capital*, 49–70, ed. Alan Burton-Jones and J.C. Spender. Oxford, UK: Oxford University Press.

Blakely, Tony A., Bruce P. Kennedy, and Ichiro Kawachi. 2001. Socioeconomic Inequality in Voting Participation and Self-rated Health. *American Journal of Public Health* 91 (1): 99–104.

Blalock, Susan J. 2007. Predictors of Calcium Intake Patterns: A Longitudinal Analysis. *Health Psychology* 26 (3): 251–258.

Blanchflower, David, and Andrew J. Oswald. 2000. The Rising Well-being of the Young. In *Youth Employment and Joblessness in Advanced Countries*, 289–328, ed. David G. Blanchflower and Richard B. Freeman. Chicago, IL: University of Chicago Press.

Blokker, Paul. 2018. Democracy and Democratization: Theory and Research. In *The SAGE Handbook of Political Sociology*, 622–636, ed. William Outhwaite and Stephen Turner. London, UK: SAGE.

Blomberg, Helena, and Christian Kroll. 1999. Do Structural Contents Matter? Macro-sociological Factors and Popular Attitudes Towards Public Welfare Services. *Acta Sociologica* 42: 319–335.

Bluhm, William T., and Robert A. Heineman. 2007. *Ethics and Public Policy: Methods and Cases*. Upper Saddle River, NJ: Pearson.

Bock, Dora E., Judith Anne Garretson. Folse, and William C. Black. 2016. When Frontline Employee Behavior Backfires. *Journal of Service Research* 19 (3): 322–336.

Boehnke, Klaus, and Becky Wong. 2011. Adolescent Political Activism and Long-term Happiness: A 21-Year Longitudinal Study on the Development of Micro- and Macrosocial Worries. *Personality & Social Psychology Bulletin* 37 (3): 435–447.

Boeri, Tito, Gordon Hanson, and Barry McCormick. 2002. *Immigration Policy and the Welfare System*. Oxford, UK: Oxford University Press.

Bogg, Tim. 2008. Conscientiousness, the Transtheoretical Model of Change, and Exercise: A Neo-socioanalytic Integration of Trait and Social-Cognitive Frameworks in the Prediction of Behavior. *Journal of Personality* 76 (4): 775–802.

Bohnke, Petra. 2008. Does Society Matter? Life Satisfaction in the Enlarged Europe. *Social Indicators Research* 87: 189–210.

Boiney, John, and David L. Paletz. 1991. In Search of the Model: Political Science versus Political Advertising Perspectives on Voter Decision Making. In *Television and Political Advertising, Vol.1: Psychological Processes*, 3–25, ed. Frank Biocca. Hillsdale, NJ: Lawrence Erlbaum.

Boje, David M. 1995. Stories of the Storytelling Organization: A Postmodern Analysis of Disney as Tamara-Land. *Academy of Management Journal* 38 (4): 997–1035.

Bonaiuto, Marino, Antonio Aiello, Marco Perugini, Mirilia Bonnes, and Anna Parla Ercolani. 1999. Multidimensional Perception of Residential Environment Quality and Neighbourhood Attachment in the Urban Environment. *Journal of Environmental Psychology* 19: 331–352.

Bond, Michael Harris, and Vivian Miu-Chi. Lun. 2014. Citizen-Making: The Role of National Goals for Socializing Children. *Social Science Research* 44: 75–85.

Bonin-Scaon, Sylvie, Maria Teresa-Munoz. Sastre, Gerard Chasseigne, Paul C. Sorum, and Etienne Mullet. 2009. End-of-Life Preferences: A Theory-Driven Inventory. *International Journal of Aging & Human Development* 68 (1): 1–26.

Bonke, Jens, and Peter Fallesen. 2010. The Impact of Incentives and Interview Methods on Response Quantity and Quality in Diary- and Booklet-Based Surveys. *Survey Research Methods* 4 (2): 91–101.

Booth, John A., and Patricia Bayer Richard. 1998. Civil Society and Political Context in Central America. *American Behavioral Scientist* 42 (1): 33–46.

Booysen, Frederik. 2002. An Overview and Evaluation of Composite Indices of Development. *Social Indicators Research* 59: 115–151.

Borbath, Endre, and Theresa Gessler. 2020. Different Worlds of Contention? Protest in Northwestern, Southern and Eastern Europe. *European Journal of Political Research* 59 (4): 910–935.

Borch, Christian. 2013. Crowd Theory and the Management of Crowds: A Controversial Relationship. *Current Sociology* 61 (5–6): 584–601.

Borgonovi, Francesca. 2008. Doing Well by Doing Good: The Relationships Between Formal Volunteering and Self-reported Health and Happiness. *Social Science & Medicine* 66: 2321–2334.

Borjas, George. 1999. *Heaven's Door: Immigration Policy and the American Economy*. Princeton, NJ: Princeton University Press.

Born, Marieke, Agnes Akkerman, and René Torenvlied. 2013. Trust Your Boss or Listen to the Union?: Information, Social Identification, Trust, and Strike Participation. *Mobilization* 18 (2): 161–178.

Borne, Gregory. 2009. Achieving Sustainable Lifestyles or Encouraging a Counter-reflexivity: Exploratory Motivations for Sustainability in a Mediated Risk Society. *Local Environment* 14 (1): 93–107.

Bornstein, Robert F. 2006. The Complex Relationship Between Dependency and Domestic Violence: Converging Psychological Factors and Social Forces. *American Psychologist* 62 (7): 709–711.

Bosi, Lorenzo, and Donatella Della Porta. 2012. Micro-mobilization into Armed Groups: Ideological, Instrumental and Solidaristic Paths. *Qualitative Sociology* 35: 361–383.

Bosma, Anouk, Maarten Kunst, Joni Reef, Anja Dirkzwager, and Paul Nieuwbeerta. 2016. Prison-Based Rehabilitation. *Crime & Delinquency* 62 (8): 1095–1120.

Bossy, Sophie. 2014. The Utopias of Political Consumerism: The Search of Alternatives to Mass Consumption. *Journal of Consumer Culture* 14 (2): 179–198.

Bostrom, Ann, Robert E. O'Connor, Gisela Böhm, Daniel Hanss, Otto Bodi, Frida Ekström, Pradipta Halder, Sven Jeschke, Birgit Mack, Qu. Mei, Lynn Rosentrater, Anethe Sandve, and Ingrid Sælensminde. 2012. Causal Thinking and Support for Climate Change Policies: International Survey Findings. *Global Environmental Change* 22 (1): 210–222.

Bottici, Chiara, and Benvit Chall. 2010. *The Myth of the Clash of Civilizations*. Milton Park, UK: Routledge.

Boudon, Raymond. 2011. Ordinary Rationality: The Case of Analytical Sociology. In *Analytical Sociology and Social Mechanisms*, 33–49, ed. Pierre Demeulenaere. Cambridge, UK: Cambridge University Press.

Bourguignon, Francois, Francisco H. G. Ferreira, and Michael Walton. 2007. Equity, Efficiency and Inequality Traps: A Research Agenda. *Journal of Economic Inequality* 5: 235–256.

Bouton, Mark E., Susan Mineka, and David H. Barlow. 2001. A Modern Learning Theory Perspective on the Etiology of Panic Disorder. *Psychological Review* 108 (1): 4–32.

Bowker, Matthew H. 2016. *Ideologies of Experience: Trauma, Failure, Deprivation, and the Abandonment of the Self*. New York, NY: Routledge.

Bowman, Nicholas, A., Julie J. Park, and Nida Denson. 2015. Student Involvement in Ethnic Student Organizations: Examining Civic Outcomes 6 Years After Graduation. *Research in Higher Education* 56 (2): 127–145.

Box, Richard C. 2008. *Making a Difference: Progressive Values in Public Administration*. Armonk, NY: Sharpe.

Boyd, Richard. 2006. The Value of Civility? *Urban Studies* 43 (5/6): 863–878.

Boyes, Mark E., Thea M. Carmody, Patrick J. F. Clarke, and Penelope A. Hasking. 2017. Emotional Reactivity and Perseveration: Independent Dimensions of Trait Positive and Negative Affectivity and Differential Associations with Psychological Distress. *Personality & Individual Differences* 105: 70–77.

Bozeman, Berry. 2007. *Public Values and Public Inerest: Counterbalancing Economic Individualism*. Washington, DC: Georgetown University Press.

Braaten, Jane. 1991. *Habermas's Critical Theory of Society*. New York: State University of New York Press.

Brady, David, Jason Beckfield, and Wei Zhao. 2007. The Consequences of Economic Globalization for Affluent Democracies. *Annual Review of Sociology* 33: 313–334.

Brady, David. 2005. The Welfare State and Relative Poverty in Rich Western Democracies, 1967–1997. *Social Forces* 83 (4): 1329–1364.

Brady, David. 2006. Structural Theory and Relative Poverty in Rich Western Democracies, 1969–2000. *Research in Social Stratification & Mobility* 24: 153–175.

Braithwaite, Valerie. 1997. Harmony and Security Value Orientations in Political Evaluation. *Personality & Social Psychology Bulletin* 23 (4): 401–414.

Braithwaite, Valerie. 1998. Communal and Exchange Trust Norms: Their Value Base and Relevance to Institutional Trust. In *Trust and Governance*, 46–74, ed. Valerie Braithwaite and Margaret Levi. New York; Russell Sage.

Bramley, Glen, and James Morgan. 2003. Building Competitiveness and Cohesion: The Role of New Housebuilding in Central Scotland's Cities. *Housing Studies* 18 (4): 447–471.

Brand, Peter. 1999. The Environment and Postmodern Spatial Consciousness: A Sociology of Urban Environmental Agendas. *Journal of Environmental Planning & Management* 42 (5): 631–648.

Brannstrom, Inger, and Ingar Britt Lindblad. 1994. Mass Communication and Health Promotion: The Power of the Media and Public Opinion. *Health Communication* 6 (1): 21–36.

Bratton, Michael, and Robert Mattes. 2001. Support for Democracy in Africa: Intrinsic or Instrumental. *British Journal of Political Science* 31: 447–474.

Braun, Jerome. 2011. *To Break Our Chains: Social Cohesiveness and Modern Democracy*. Leiden, Netherlands: Brill.

Braun, Robert, and Rens Vliegenthart. 2008. The Contentious Fans: The Impact of Repression, Media Coverage, Grievances and Aggressive Play on Supporters?? Violence. *International Sociology* 23 (6): 796–818.

Brayne, Sarah. 2014. Surveillance and System Avoidance: Crimnal Justice Contact and Institutional Attachment. *Amnerican Sociological Review* 79 (3): 367–391.

Brennan, Jason. 2011. *The Ethics of Voting*. Princeton, NJ: Princeton University Press.

Brennan, Robert T., Rosalind Chart Barnett, and Karen C. Gareis. 2001. When She Earns More than He Does: A Longitudinal Study of Dual-Earner Couples. *Journal of Marriage & Family* 63: 168–182.

Brewer, Noel T., Gretchen B. Chapman, Frederick X. Gibbons, Meg Gerrard, Kevin D. McCaul, and Neil D. Weinstein. 2007. Meta-Analysis of the Relationship between Risk Perception and Health Behavior: The Example of Vaccination. *Health Psychology* 26 (2): 136–145.

Brewer, Paul R., and Lee Sigelman. 2002. Trust in Government: Personal Ties that Bind? *Social Science Quarterly* 83 (2): 624–631.

Brigg, Morgan. 2018. Humanitarian Symbolic Exchange: Extending Responsibility to Protect through Individual and Local Engagement. *Third World Quarterly* 39 (5): 838–853.

Briscoe, Michael D., Jennifer E. Givens, Shawn Olson Hazboun, and Richard S. Krannich. 2019. At Home, in Public, and in Between: Gender Differences in Public, Private and Transportation Pro-environmental Behaviors in the US Intermountain West. *Environmental Sociology* 5 (4): 374–392.

Brisson, Daniel. 2009. Testing the Relationship of Formal Bonding, Informal Bonding, and Formal Bridging Social Capital on Key Outcomes for Females in Low Income Neighborhoods. *Journal of Sociology & Social Welfare* 36 (1): 167–183.

Brockmann, Hilke, Jan Delhey, Christian Welzel, and Hao Yuan. 2009. The China Puzzle: Falling Happiness in a Rising Economy. *Journal of Happiness Studies* 10: 387–405.

Brolis, Olivier, and Marthe Nyssens. 2020. Does the Mission of an Organization Affect the Quality of Low-Skilled Jobs in Quasi-Markets? A Comparison between Social Enterprises and for-Profit Organizations. *VOLUNTAS: International Journal of Voluntary and Nonprofit Organizations* 31 (3): 533–549.

Brooks, Clem, and Jeff Manza. 2006. Social Policy Responsiveness in Developed Democracies. *American Sociological Review* 71 (3): 474–494.

Brooks, John, and Charles Prysby. 1999. Contextual Effects on Retrospective Economic Evaluations: The Impact of the State and Local Economy. *Political Behavior* 21 (1): 1–16.

Brooks, Rachel. 2013. The Social Construction of Young People within Education Policy: Evidence from the UK's Coalition Government. *Journal of Youth Studies* 16 (3): 318–333.

Broom, Alexander, K.R. David Sibbritt, Pamela Nilan Nayar, and Emma Kirby. 2013. What Factors Predict Exposure to Caste, Political and Religious Violence in India? A Cross-Sectional Survey of 1000 Indian Men. *Asian Social Science* 9 (1): 1–8.

Brotchie, Janet, Caroline Meyer, Alex Copello, Robert Kidney, and Glenn Waller. 2004. Cognitive Representations in Alcohol and Opiate Abuse: The Role of Core Beliefs. *British Journal of Clinical Psychology* 43: 337–342.

Brown, David K. 2001. The Social Sources of Educational Credentialism: Status Cultures, Labor Markets, and Organizations. *Sociology of Education* Extra Issues: 19–34.

Brown, Eleanor, and James M. Ferris. 2007. Social Capital and Philanthropy: An Analysis of the Impact of Social Capital on Individual Giving and Volunteering. *Nonprofit & Voluntary Sector Quarterly* 36 (1): 85–99.

Brown, Graham, Barbara B. Brown, and Douglas D. Perkins. 2004. New Housing as Neighborhood Revitalization: Place Attachment and Confidence among Residents. *Environment & Behavior* 36 (6): 749–775.

Brown, Jacob R. and Michael Zoorob. 2022. Resisting Broken Windows. *Political Behavior*.

Brown, Jessica. 2016. Social Support and Crime: A State-Level Analysis of Social Support Policies. *Journal of Sociology & Social Welfare* 43 (2): 135–156.

Brown, Kevin M., Russell Hoye, and Matthew Nicholson. 2014. Generating Trust? Sport and Community Participation. *Journal of Sociology* 50 (4): 437–457.

Brown, Olivia K., and Douglas K. Symons. 2016. My Pet Has Passed: Relations of Adult Attachment Styles and Current Feelings of Grief and Trauma after the Event. *Death Studies* 40 (4): 247–255.

Brown, Ralph B., Shawn F. Dorius, and Richard S. Krannich. 2005. The Boom-Bust Recovery Cycle: Dynamics of Change in Community Satisfaction and Social Integration in Delta, Utah. *Rural Sociology* 70 (1): 28–49.

Brown, Rebecca C. H. 2018. Resisting Moralisation in Health Promotion. *Ethical Theory & Moral Practice* 21 (4): 997–1011.

Brown, Richard P.C., and John Connell. 2004. The Migration of Doctors and Nurses from South Pacific Island Nations. *Social Science & Medicine* 58: 2193–2210.

Brown, Stephanie L., and R. Michael Brown. 2006. Selective Investment Theory: Recasting the Functional Significance of Class Relationships. *Psychological Inquiry* 17 (1): 1–29.

Browning, Christopher R., Seth L. Feinberg, and Robert D. Dietz. 2004. the Paradox of Social Organization: Networks, Collective Efficacy and Violent Crime in Urban Neighboroods. *Social Forces* 83 (2): 503–534.

Browning, Don S., and Terry D. Cooper. 2004. *Religious Thought and the Modern Psychologies*. Minneapolis, MN: Fortress.

Bruch, Sarah K., Myra Marx Ferree, and Joe Soss. 2010. From Policy to Polity: Democracy, Paternalism, and the Incorporation of Disadvantaged Citizens. *American Sociological Review* 75 (2): 205–226.

Brulle, Robert J. 2000. *Agency, Democracy, and Nature: The U.S. Environmental Movement from a Critical Theory Perspective*. Cambridge, MA: MIT Press.

Brusting, Suzanne, and Tom Postmes. 2002. Social Movement Participation in the Digital Age: Predicting Offline and Online Collective Action. *Small Group Research* 33 (5): 525–554.

Bryce, Herrington J. 2009. Trust in Government: A By-product of NGO Intervention in Public Policy. *International Journal of Public Administration* 32 (11): 951–969.

Brynin, Malcolm, Alvaro Martinez Perez, and Simonetta Longhi. 2009. How Close Are Couples? In *Changing Relationships*, 93–108, ed. Malcolm Brynin and John Ermisch. New York: Routledge.

Buck, Nick. 2001. Identifying Neighbourhood Effects on Social Exclusion. *Urban Studies* 38 (12): 2251–2275.

Buechler, Steven M. 2011. *Understanding Social Movements: Theories from the Classical Era to the Present. Boulder*, CO: Paradigm.

Bull, S., M. Salyers, L. Lloyd. McFarlane, and C. Rietmeijer. 2004. The Process of Seeking Sex Partners Online and Implications for STD/HIV Prevention. *AIDS Care* 16 (8): 1012–1020.

Bullock, John G. 2021. Education and Attitudes Toward Redistribution in the United States. *British Journal of Political Science* 51 (3): 1230–1250.

Bulmahn, Thomas. 2000. Modernity and Happiness: The Case of Germany. *Journal of Happiness Studies* 1: 375–400.

Bunge, Mario. 1996. *Finding Philosophy in Social Science*. New Haven, CT: Yale University Press.

Burchardt, Tania. 2005. Are One Man's Rag Another Man's Riches? Identifying Adaptive Expectation Using Panel Data. *Social Indicators Research* 74: 57–102.

Burgess, Adam. 2018. Individualization Revisited: Global Family Developments, Uncertainty and Risk. *Journal of Risk Research* 21 (1): 83–95.

Burke, Peter J. 2008. Identity, Social Status, and Emotion. In *Social Structure and Emotion*, 75–93, ed. Jody Clay-Warner and Dawn Robinson. Amsterdam, Netherlands: Academic.

Burke, Peter J., and Jan E. Stets. 1999. Trust and Commitment Through Self-verification. *Social Psychology Quarterly* 62 (4): 347–360.

Burke, Peter J., and Jan E. Stets. 2009. *Identity Theory*. New York: Oxford University Press.

Burnett, Simon. 2012. *The Happiness Agenda: A Modern Obsession*. New York, NY: Palgrave.

Burningham, Kate. 1998. A Noisy Road or Noisy Resident? A Demonstration of the Utility of Social Constructionism for Analyzing Environmental Problems. *Sociological Review* 46 (3): 536–563.

Burns, Richard Andrew, and Michael Anthony Machin. 2012. Moving beyond the Pleasure Principle within and between Occasion Effects of Employee Eudaimonia within School Organizational Climate Context. *Journal of Vocational Behavior* 80: 118–128.

Bynner, John, and Sheena Ashford. 1994. Politics and Participation: Some Antecedents of Young People's Attitudes to the Political System and Political Activity. *European Journal of Social Psychology* 24: 225–236.

Byrd, Stephanie Ellen. 2009. The Social Construction of Marital Commitment. *Journal of Marriage & Family* 71: 318–336.

Cabanas, Edgar. 2016. Rekindling Individualism, Consuming Emotions: Constructing Psytizens in the Age of Happiness. *Cultural & Psychology* 22 (3): 467–480.

Cabelkova, Inna, and Jan Honousek. 2004. The Power of Negative Thinking: Corruption, Perception and Willingness to Bribe in Ukraine. *Applied Economics* 36: 383–397.

Cai, Shaohan, Xiaoyan Wang, Xinyue Zhou, Michael R. Hyman, and Zhilin Yang. 2021. Political and Community Logics Jointly Affect 'Social Distancing' Compliance. *Sustainable Cities & Society* 74: 103200.

Cairney, Paul. 2012. *Understanding Public Policy: Theories and Issues*. Houndmills, UK: Palgrave.

Caldwell, David. 2020. Sounds of the Game: An Interpersonal Discourse Analysis of on Field Language in Sports Media. *Discourse, Context & Media* 33: 100363.

Calloni, Marina. 2016. Images of Fear in Political Philosophy and Fairy Tales: Linking Private Abuse to Political Violence in Human Rights Discourse. *Journal of International Political Theory* 12 (1): 67–87.

Cameron, Gary. 2002. Motivation to Join and Benefits from Participation in Parent Mutual Aid Organizations. *Child Welfare* 81 (1): 33–57.

Camfield, Laura, and Monica Guillen-Royo. 2010. Wants, Needs and Satisfaction: A Comparative Study in Thailand and Bangladesh. *Social Indicators Research* 96: 183–203.

Campbell, Colin, and Jessica Pearlman. 2013. Period Effects, Cohort Effects, and the Narrowing Gender Wage Gap. *Social Science Research* 42 (6): 1693–1711.

Campbell, Heidi A., Katherine Arredondo, Katie Dundas, and Cody Wolf. 2018. The Dissonance of "Civil" Religion in Religious-Political Memetic Discourse During the 2016 Presidential Elections. *Social Media + Society* 4 (2): 205630511878267.

Cano, Annmarie, and Dina Vivian. 2003. Are Life Stressors Associated with Marital Violence? *Journal of Family Psychology* 17 (3): 302–314.

Cantor, Nancy, and Catherine A. Sanderson. 1999. Life Task, Participation and Well-being: The Importance of Taking Part in Daily Life. In *Well-being: The Foundations of Hedonic Psychology*, 230–243, ed. Daniel Kahneman, Ed Diener and Norbert Schwarz. New York: Russell Sage.

Cantzler, Julia Miller. 2007. Environmental Justice and Social Power Rhetoric in the Morale Battle Over Whaling. *Sociological Inquiry* 77 (3): 483–512.

Caplan, Leslie J., and Carmi Schooler. 2006. Household Work Complexity, Intellectual Functioning, and Self-esteem in Men and Women. *Journal of Marriage & Family* 68: 883–900.

Caplan, Leslie J., and Carmi Schooler. 2007. Socioeconomic Status and Financial Coping Strategies: The Mediating Role of Perceived Control. *Social Psychology Quarterly* 70 (1): 43–58.

Caprara, Gian Vittorio, and Michele Vecchione. 2017. *Personalizing Politics and Realizing Democracy*. New York, NY: Oxford University Press.

Caprara, Gian Vittorio, and Patrizia Steca. 2005. Self-efficacy Beliefs as Determinants of Prosocial Behavior Conducive to Life Satisfaction Across Ages. *Journal of Social & Clinical Psychology* 24 (2): 191–217.

Caputo, Richard K. 2003. The Effects of Socioeconomic Status, Perceived Discrimination and Mastery on Health Status in a Youth Cohort. *Social Work in Health Care* 37 (2): 17–42.

Carbery, Julie, and Duane Buhrmester. 1998. Friendship and Need Fulfillment during Three Phases of Young Adulthood. *Journal of Social & Personal Relationships* 15 (3): 393–409.

Carle, Adam C., Kurt J. Bauman, and Kathleen Short. 2009. Assessing the Measurement and Structure of Material Hardship in the United States. *Social Indicators Research* 92: 35–51.

Carley, Kathleen M., and David Krackhardt. 1996. Cognitive Inconsistencies and Non-symmetric Friendship. *Social Networks* 18: 1–27.

Carli, Linda L. 2004. Gender Effects on Social Influence. In *Perspectives and Persuasion, Social Influence, and Compliance Gaining*, 133–148, ed. John S. Seiter and Robert H. Gass. Boston, MA: Pearson.

Carli, Linda L., and Alice E. Eagly. 2011. Gender and Leadership. In *The SAGE Handbook of Leadership*, 103–117, ed. Alan Bryman, David Collinson, Keith Grint, Brad Jackson and Mary Uhl-Bien. London: SAGE.

Carli, Linda L., and Panuta Bukatko. 2000. Gender, Communication, and Social Influence: A Developmental Perspective. In *The Developmental Social Psychology of Gender*, 295–331, ed. Thomas Eckes and Hannes M. Trautner. Mahwah, NJ: Lawrence Erlbaum.

Carlsen, Benedicte. 2003. Professional Support of Self-help Groups: A Support Group Project for Chronic Fatigue Syndrome Patients. *British Journal of Guidance & Counselling* 31 (3): 289–302.

Carlton, Eric. 2006. *Politeia: Visions of the Just Society*. Cranbury, NJ: Associated University Presses.

Carmeli, Abraham, Stephen Brammer, Emanuel Gomes, and Shlomo Y. Tarba 2017. An Organizational Ethic of Care and Employee Involvement in Sustainability-Related Behaviors: A Social Identity Perspective. *Journal of Organizational Behavior* 38 (9): 1380–1395.

Carollo, Luca, and Luca Solari. 2019. Discourses of Professionalism in Front-Line Service Work: Insights from a Case Study in an Italian Bank. *Work, Employment & Society* 33 (5): 829–845.

Carpiano, Richard M. 2008. Actual or Potential Neighborhood Resources and Access to Them: Testing Hypotheses of Social Capital for the Health of Female Caregivers. *Social Science & Medicine* 67: 568–582.

Carr, Deborah, and Debra Umberson. 2013. The Social Psychology of Stress, Health, and Coping. In *Handbook of Social Psychology*, 465–487, ed. John Delamater and Amanda Ward. Dordrecht, Netherlands: Springer.

Carr, Deborah, and Michael A. Friedman. 2005. Is Obesity Stigmatizing? Body Weight, Perceived Discrimination and Psychological Well-Being in the United States. *Journal of Health & Social Behavior* 46 (3): 244–259.

Carr, E. Summerson. 2004. Accessing Resources, Transforming Systems: Group Work with Poor and Homeless People. In *Handbook of Social Work with Groups*, 360–383, ed. Charles D. Garoin Lorraine M. Gutierrez, and Maeda J. Galinsky. New York: Guilford.

Carreras, Miguel. 2018. Why No Gender Gap in Electoral Participation? A Civic Duty Explanation. *Electoral Studies* 52: 36–45.

Carrieri, Vincenzo. 2012. Social Comparison and Subjective Well-Being: Does the Health of Others Matter? *Bulletin of Economic Research* 64 (1): 31–55.

Carson, Thomas L. 2000. *Value and the Good Life*. Notre Dame, IN: University of Notre Dame Press.

Carter, Travis M., and Scott E. Wolfe. 2021. Explaining the Relationship Between Neighborhood Disorder and Crime Fear: The Perceptual Role of Neighbors and the Police. *Journal of Criminal Justice* 77: 101867.

Cassino, Dan, and Yasemin Besen-Cassino. 2020. Sometimes (but Not This Time), a Gun Is Just a Gun: Masculinity Threat and Guns in the United States, 1999–2018. *Sociological Forum* 35 (1): 5–23.

Castells, Manuel. 2000. *End of Millennium*. Oxford, UK: Blackwell.

Castillo, Juan Carols. 2011. Legitimacy of Inequality in Highly Unequal Context: Evidence from the Chilean Case. *Social Justice Research* 24: 314–340.

Castles, Francis G. 2000. Putting the Economy First: Or Does Postmodernization Really Matter? *Political Studies* 48 (1): 38–50.

Catley, Bob. 2001. The Bush Administration and Changing Geopolitics in the Asia-Pacific Region. *Contemporary Southeast Asia* 23 (1): 149–167.

Cattell, Vicky. 2004. Having a Laugh and Mucking in Together: Using Social Capital to Explore Dynamics Between Structure and Agency in the Context of Declining and Regenerated Neighbourhoods. *Sociology* 38 (5): 945–963.

Celso, B.G., D.J. Ebener, and E.J. Burkhead. 2003. Humor coping, Health Status, and Life Satisfaction among Older Adults Residing in Assisted Living Facilities. *Aging & Mental Health* 7 (6): 438–445.

Cepulic, Dominik-Borna, Giovanni A. Travaglino, Stavroula Chrona, Ena Uzelac, Alma Jeftić, Cecilia Reyna, and Marta Kowal. 2022. Iron Fists and Velvet Gloves: Investigating the Associations between the Stringency of Governments' Responses to Covid-19, Stress, and Compliance in the Early Stages of the Pandemic. *British Journal of Social Psychology*.

Cerin, Ester, and Eva Leslie. 2008. How Socio-economic Status Contributes to Participation in Leisure-Time Physical Activity. *Social Science & Medicine* 66: 2596–2609.

Ceva, Emanuela, and Federico Zuolo. 2013. A Matter of Respect: On Majority-Minority Relations in a Liberal Democracy. *Journal of Applied Psychology* 30 (3): 239–253.

Chaffee, Steven H., Xinshu Zhao, and GlennLeshner. 1994. Political Knowledge and the Campaign Media of 1992. *Communication Research* 21 (3): 305–324.

Chaitin, Julia, Shoshana Steinberg, and Sharon Steinberg. 2017. Polarized Words: Discourse on the Boycott of Israel, Social Justice and Conflict Resolution. *International Journal of Conflict Management* 28 (3): 270–294.

Chak, Katherine, and Louis Leung. 2004. Shyness and Locus of Control as Predictors of Internet Addiction and Internet Use. *CyberPsychology & Behavior* 7 (5): 559–570.

Chakrabarty, Debaj Yoti, Hajime Katayama, and Hanna Maslen. 2008. Why Do the Rich Save More? A Theory and Australian Evidence. *Economic Record* 84: S32–S44.

Chan, Elaine. 2014. Are Informal Connections a Functional Alternative to Associational Life in Enhancing Social Cohesion? Findings from Hong Kong. *Social Indicators Research* 119 (2): 803–821.

Chan, Joseph M., and Francis L. F. Lee. 2007. Media and Large-Scale Demonstrations: The Pro-Democracy Movement in Post-Handover Hong Kong. *Asian Journal of Communication* 17 (2): 215–228.

Chen, Ying-Keung., and Rance Pui-Leung Lee. 2006. Network Size, Social Support and Happiness in Later Life: A Comparative Study of Beijing and Hong Kong. *Journal of Happiness Studies* 7: 87–112.

Chaney, Paul. 2014. Party Politicisation and the Formative Phase of Environmental Policy-Making in Multi-Level Systems: Electoral Discourse in UK Meso-Elections 1998–2011. *Political Studies* 62 (2): 252–272.

Chang, Kurtis Ko-Li., Pi-Shan. Hsu, and Chieh-Peng. Lin. 2009a. A Qualitative Integration of Self-determination Theory and Expectation-Confirmation Theory Using Physical Education as an Example. *Quality & Quantity* 43: 977–981.

Chang, Roberto, Linda Kaltani, and Norman V. Loayza. 2008. Openness Can Be Good for Growth: The Role of Policy Complementarities. *Journal of Development Economics* 90 (1): 33–49.

Chang, Shu-Sen., David Gynnell, Jonathan A.C.. Sterne, Lu. Tsung-Hsueh, and Andrew T.A.. Cheng. 2009b. Was the Economic Crisis 1997–1998 Responsible for Rising Suicide Rates in East/Southeast Asia? A Time Trend Analysis for Japan, Hong Kong, South Korea, Taiwan, Singapore and Thailand. *Social Science & Medicine* 68: 1322–1331.

Chang, Wen-Chun. 2009. Social Capital and Subjective Happiness in Taiwan. *International Journal of Social Economics* 36 (8): 844–868.

Chapman, Jenny. 1985. Marital Status, Sex and the Formation of Political Attitudes in Adult Life. *Political Studies* 33: 592–609.

Chappell, Neena L., and Michael J. Prince. 1997. Reasons Why Canadian Seniors Volunteers. *Canadian Journal on Aging* 16 (2): 336–353.

Charke, Valerie A., et al. 2000. Unrealistic Optimism and the Health Belief Models. *Journal of Behavioral Medicine* 23 (4): 367–376.

Charles, Matthew. 2011. *Development and Religion: Theology and Practice.* Cheltenham, UL: Elgar.

Charles, Susan T., and Laura L. Carstensen. 2009. Social and Emotional Aging. *Annual Review of Psychology* 61: 383–409.

Charles, Susan Turk, and Laura L. Carstensen. 2008. Unpleasant Situations Elicit Different Emotional Responses in Younger and Older Adults. *Psychology and Aging* 23 (3): 495–504.

Charles, Susan Turk. 2010. Strength and Vulnerability Integration: A Model of Emotional Well-Being Across Adulthood. *Psychological Bulletin* 136 (6): 1068–1091.

Charrad, Mounira M., and Nicholas E. Reith. 2019. Local Solidarities: How the Arab Spring Protests Started. *Sociological Forum* 34: 1174–1196.

Chatterjee, Santanu, and Stephen J. Turnovsky. 2012. Infrastructure and Inequality. *European Economic Review* 56: 1730–1745.

Chatwin, J., and P. Tovey. 2004. Complementary and Alternative Medicine (CAM), Cancer and Group-Based Action: A Critical Review of the Literature. *European Journal of Cancer Care* 13: 210–218.

Chen, Chih-Kai. 2008. Causal Modeling of Knowledge-Based Economy. *Management Decision* 46 (3): 501–514.

Chen, Jie, and Yang Zhong. 1998. Defining the Political System of Post-Deng China: Emerging Public Support for a Democratic Political System. *Problems of Post-Communism* 45 (4): 30–42.

Chen, Jie, and Yang Zhong. 2002. Why Do People Vote in Semicompetitive Elections in China? *Journal of Politics* 64 (1): 178–197.

Chen, Jinqi, Michael P. Dunne, and Ping Han. 2004. Child Sexual Abuse in China: A Study of Adolescents in Four Provinces. *Child Abuse & Neglect* 28: 1171–1186.

Chen, Sheying. 1996. *Social Policy of the Economic State and Community Care in Chinese Culture: Aging, Family, Urban Change, and the Socialist Welfare Pluralism.* Aldershot, UK: Avebury.

Chen, Sylvia Xiashua, and Winnie W.S.. Mak. 2008. Seeking Professional Help: Etiology Beliefs about Mental Illness Across Cultures. *Journal of Counseling Psychology* 55 (4): 442–450.

Chen, Xinjie, Hoi Yan Cheung, Xitao Fan, and Wu. Joseph. 2018. Factors Related to Resilience of Academically Gifted Students in The Chinese Cultural and Educational Environment. *Psychology in the Schools* 55 (2): 107–119.

Cheng, Cecilia, and Aik-kwang Ng. 2006. Psychosocial Factors Predicting SARS-Preventive Behaviors in Four Major SARS-Affected Regions. *Journal of Applied Social Psychology* 36 (1): 222–247.

Cheng, Cecilia, and Mike W.L.. Cheung. 2005. Psychological Responses to Outbreak of Severe Acute Respiratory Symptom: A Prospective, Multiple Time-Point Study. *Journal of Personality* 73 (1): 261–285.

Cheng, Cecilia, Hsin-Yi. Wang, Leif Sigerson, and Chor-Lam. Chau. 2019. Do the Socially Rich Get Richer? A Nuanced Perspective on Social Network Site Use and Online Social Capital Accrual. *Psychological Bulletin* 145 (7): 734–764.

Cheng, Cecilia. 2003. Cognitive and Motivational Processes Underlying Coping Flexibility: A Dual Process Model. *Journal of Personality & Social Psychology* 84 (2): 425–438.

Cheng, Qijin, Tim Mh Li, Chi-Leung. Kwok, Tingshao Zhu, and Paul Siu-fai Yip. 2017. Assessing Suicide Risk and Emotional Distress in Chinese Social Media: A Text Mining and Machine Learning Study. *Journal of Medical Internet Research* 19 (7): e243.

Chenoweth, Erica. 2021. *Civil Resistance: What Everyone Needs to Know*. New York, NY: Oxford University Press.

Chesters, Graeme, and Ian Welsh. 2005. Complexity and Social Movement(s): Process and Emergence in Planetary Action Systems. *Theory, Culture & Society* 22 (5): 187–211.

Chesters, Jenny, Jehane Simona, and Christian Suter. 2021. Cross-National Comparison of Age and Period Effects on Levels of Subjective Well-Being in Australia and Switzerland During Volatile Economic Times (2001–2016). *Social Indicators Research* 154 (1): 361–391.

Cheung, Chau-kiu, and Kwan-kwok Leung. 2011.6. Neighborhood Homogeneity and Cohesion in Sustainable Community Development. *Habitat International 35*: 564–572.

Child, Travers Barclay, and Elena Nikolova. 2020. War and Social Attitudes. *Conflict Management & Peace Science* 37 (2): 152–171.

Chilton, Paul. 2004. *Analysing Political Discourse: Theory and Practice.* London: Routledge.

Chiricos, Ted, Kathy Padgett, and Marc Gertz. 2000. Fear, TV News, and the Reality of Crime. *Criminology* 38 (3): 755–785.

Chirkov, Valery, Richard M. Ryan, Youngmee Kim, and Ulas Kaplan. 2003. Differentiating Autonomy from Individualism and Independence: A Self-determination Theory Perspective on Internalization of Cultural Orientations and Well-Being. *Journal of Personality & Social Psychology* 84 (1): 97–110.

Chisholm, Marie A., Henry Cobb, Lori Duke, Charles McDuffie, and William K. Kennedy. 2006. Development of an Instrument to Measure Professionalism. *American Journal of Pharmaceutical Education* 70 (4): 1–6.

Cho, Seo-Young., Axel Dreher, and Eric Neumayer. 2013. Does Legalized Prostitution Increase Human Trafficking? *World Development* 41 (1): 67–82.

Cho, Young Ho, and Injeong Hwang. 2021. Democratization Who Defends Democracy and Why? Explaining the Participation in the 2016–2017 Candlelight Protest in South Korea. *Democratization* 28 (3): 625–644.

Choi, Chonghyun, and Dongwook Kim. 2019. The Determinants of Anti-government Protests in Asia. *Journal of East Asian Studies* 19 (3): 315–338.

Choi, Jiyoung, David W. Johnson, and Roger Johnson. 2011. Relationships among Cooperative Learning Experiences, Social Interdependence, Children's Aggression, Victimization, and Prosocial Behaviors. *Journal of Applied Social Psychology* 41 (4): 976–1003.

Chongatera, Godfred. 2013. Hate-Crime Victimization and Fear of Hate Crime among Racially Visible People in Canada: The Role of Income as a Mediating Factor. *Journal of Immigrant & Refugee Studies* 11 (1): 44–64.

Chou, K.L., A.H.Y. Ho, and I. Chi. 2006. Living Alone and Depression in Chinese Older Adults. *Aging & Mental Health* 10 (6): 583–591.

Chou, Kee-Lee. 2003. Interest in Formal Learning among Soon-to-be-Aged Adults in Hong Kong. *Educational Gerontology* 29: 723–737.

Chow, Alice S. Y., Irene N. Y. Cheng, and Lewis T. O. Cheung. 2019. Self-determined Travel Motivations and Ecologically Responsible Attitudes of Nature-Based Visitors to the Ramsar Wetland in South China. *Annals of Leisure Research* 22 (1): 42–61.

Chow, Sy.-miin, Fumiaki Hamagami, and John R. Nesselroade. 2007. Age Differences in Dynamical Emotion-cognition Linkages. *Psychology & Aging* 22 (4): 765–780.

Christensen, Henrik Serup. 2016. All the Same? Examining the Link between Three Kinds of Political Dissatisfaction and Protest. *Comparative European Politics* 14 (6): 781–801.

Christian, Elliott, Martin Sellbom, and Ross B. Wilkinson. 2017. Clarifying the Associations between Individual Differences in General Attachment Styles and Psychopathy. *Personality Disorders: Theory, Research, & Treatment* 8 (4): 329–339.

Christians, Clifford G., Theodore L. Glasser, Denis McQuail, Kaarle Nordenstreng, and Robert A. White. 2009. *Normative Theories of the Media: Journalism in Democratic Societies*. Urbana, IL: University of Illinois Press.

Christoph, Bernhard. 2010. The Relation between Life Satisfaction and the Material Situation: A Re-evaluation Using Alternative Measures. *Social Indicators Research* 98: 475–499.

Christopher, Michael S., Paul Norris, June B. D'Souza, and Kristin A. Tiernan. 2012. A Test of the Multidimensionality of the Self-Construal Scale in Thailand and the United States. *Journal of Cross-Cultural Psychology* 43 (5): 758–773.

Chu, Godwin C. 2001. The Changing Concept of Zhong (Loyalty): Emerging New Chinese Political Culture. In *Chinese Political Culture*, 1989–2000, 42–69, ed. Shiping Hua. Armonk, NY: Sharpe.

Chuang, Yao-Chia. 2005. Effects of Interaction Pattern in Family Harmony and Well-Being: Test of Interpersonal Theory, Relational Models Theory, and Confucian Ethics. *Asian Journal of Social Psychology 8*: 272–291.

Chulef, Ada S., Stephen J. Read, and David A. Walsh. 2001. A Hierarchical Taxonomy of Human Goal. *Motivation & Emotion* 25 (3): 191–230.

Chumbler, Neale R., Ashley Foster, James W. Grimm, and Philip Williams. 2000. The Influence of Mid-life Adult Status and Functional Health Status on Health Lifestyles". *Research in the Sociology of Health Care* 18: 249–267.

Church, A. Timothy. 2010. Measurement Issues in Cross-cultural Research. In *The SAGE Handbook of Measurement*, 151–175, ed. Geoffrey Walford, Eric Tucker, and Madhu Viswanathan. London, UK: SAGE.

Cialdini, Robert B. 2012. The Focus Theory of Normative. In *Handbook of Theories of Social Psychology*, vol. 2, 295–312, ed. Paul A.M. Van Lange, Arie W. Kruglanski and E. Tory Higgins. London, CA: SAGE.

Cichy, Kelly E., Karen L. Fingerman, and Eva S. Lefkowitz. 2007. Age Differences in Types of Interpersonal Tensions. *International Journal of Aging & Human Development* 64 (2): 171–193.

Claassen, Ryan L. 2008. Testing the Reciprocal Effects of Campaign Participation. *Political Behavior* 30: 277–296.

Claassen, Ryan L., and Andrew Povtak. 2010. The Christian Right Thesis: Explaining Longitudinal Change in Participation Among Evangelical Christians. *Journal of Politics* 72 (1): 2–15.
Clain, Suzanne Heller. 2007. How Living Wage Legislation Affect U.S. Poverty Rates. *Journal of Labor Research* 29: 205–218.
Clark, Andrew E., Paul Frijters, and Michael A. Shields. 2008. Relative Income Happiness and Utility: An Explanation for the Easterlin Paradox and Other Puzzles. *Journal of Economic Literature* 46 (1): 95–144.
Clark, Christopher F., Matthew J. Kotchen, and Michael R. Moore. 2003a. Internal and External Influences on Pro-environmental Behavior: Participation in a Green Electricity Program. *Journal of Environmental Psychology* 23: 237–246.
Clark, Terry D., Ernest Goss, and Larisa B. Kosova. 2003b. Economic Well-Being and Popular Support for Market Reform in Russia. *Economic Development & Cultural Change* 51 (3): 753–768.
Clark, Terry Nichols, and Ronald Inglehart. 1998. The New Political Culture: Changing Dynamics of Support for the Welfare State and Other Policies in Postindustrial Societies. In *The New Political Culture*, 9–72, ed. Terry Nichols Clark and Vincent Hoffmann-Martinot. Boulder, CO: Westview.
Clausen, John A. 1986. *The Life Course: A Sociological Perspective*. Englewood, NJ: Prentice-Hall.
Cleary, Paul D., and Ronald Angel. 1984. The Analysis of Relationships Involving Dichotomous Dependent Variables. *Journal of Health & Social Behavior* 25: 334–348.
Clemence, Alain. 2001. Social Positioning and Social Representations. In *Representations of the Social: Bridging Theoretical Traditions*, 83–95, ed. Kay Deaux and Gina Philogene. Oxford, UK: Blackwell.
Clune, Michael S. 1998.The Fiscal Impacts of Immigrants: A California Case Study. In *The Immigration Debate: Studies on the Economic, Demographic, and Fiscal Effects of Immigration*, 120–182, ed. James P. Smith and Barry Edmonston. Washington, DC: National Academy Press.
Coburn, David. 2004. Beyond the Income Inequality Hypothesis: Class, Neo-liberalism, and Health Inequalities. *Social Science & Medicine* 58: 41–56.
Cochran, John K., Mitchell B. Chamlin, Leonard Beeghley, and Melissa Fenwick. 2004. Religion, Religiosity, and Nonmarital Sexual Conduct: An Application of Reference Group Theory. *Sociological Inquiry* 74 (1): 102–127.
Cochrane, Allan. 2007. *Understanding Urban Policy: A Crucial Approach*. Malden, MA: Blackwell.
Coffe, Hilde, and Benny Geys. 2007. Participation in Bridging and Bonding Associations and Civic Attitudes: Evidence from Flanders. *VOLUNTAS: International Journal of Voluntary and Nonprofit Organizations* 18: 385–406.
Coffey, John K., Laura Wray-Lake, Debra Mashek, and Brittany Branand. 2016. A Multi-study Examination of Well-Being Theory in College and Community Samples. *Journal of Happiness Studies* 17 (1): 187–211.
Cohen, Allan S., and David M. Bolt. 2005. A Mixture Model Analysis of Differential Item Functioning. *Journal of Educational Measurement* 42 (2): 133–148.
Cohen, Joseph R., Benjamin L. Hankin, Brandon E. Gibb, Constance Hammen, Nicholas A. Hazel, Denise Ma, Shuqiao Yao, Xiong Zhao Zhu, and John R. Z. Abela. 2013. Negative Attachment Cognitions and Emotional Distress in Mainland Chinese Adolescents: A Prospective Multiwave Test of Vulnerability-Stress and Stress Generation Models. *Journal of Clinical Child & Adolescent Psychology* 42 (4): 531–544.
Cohen, Mark A., Rolad T. Rust, and Sara Steen. 2006. Prevention, Crime Control or Cash? Public Preferences towards Criminal Justice Spending Priorities. *Justice Quarterly* 23 (3): 317–335.
Cohn, Ellen G., James Rotton, Amy G. Peterson, and Deborah B. Tarr. 2004. Temperature, City Size, and the Southern Subculture of Violence: Support for Social Escape/Avoidance Theory. *Journal of Applied Social Psychology* 34 (8): 1652–1674.
Cole, Brenda S., and Kenneth I. Pargament. 1999. Spiritual Surrender: A Paradoxical Path to Control. In *Integrating Spirituality into Treatment: Resources for Practitioners*, 179–198, ed. William R. Miller. Washington, DC: American Psychological Association.

Cole, Mike. 2003. Might It Be in the Practice That It Fails to Succeed? A Marxist Critique of Claims for Postmaterialism and Poststructuralism as Forces for Social Change and Social Justice. *British Journal of Sociology of Education* 24 (4): 487–500.

Coleman, James S. 1988. Social Capital in the Creation of Human Capital. *American Journal of Sociology* 94 (Supplement): S95–S120.

Coleman, Major G., Willaim A. Darity, Jr., and Rhonda V. Sharpe. 2008. Are Reports of Discrimination Valid? Considering the Moral Hazard Effect. *American Journal of Economics & Sociology* 67 (2): 149–175.

Coleman, Stephen, and Julie Firmstone. 2014. Contested Meanings of Public Engagement: Exploring Discourse and Practice within a British City Council. *Media, Culture, & Society* 36 (6): 826–844.

Coley, Jonathan S., Dakota K. T. Raynes, and Dhruba Das. 2020. Are Social Movements Truly Social? The Prosocial and Antisocial Outcomes of Social Movements. *Sociology Compass* 14 (8): e12820.

Collier, Paul, and Anke Hoeffler. 2004. Gre4ed and Grievance in Civil War. *Oxford Economic Papers* 56: 563–595.

Collier, Paul. 2002. Social Capital and Poverty: A Microeconomic Perspective. In *The Role of Social Capital in Development: An Empirical Assessment*, 19–41, ed. Christiaan Grootaert and Thierry van Bastelaer. Cambridge, UK: Cambirdge University Press.

Collins, Nancy L., and Brooke C. Feeney. 2004. Working Models of Attachment Shape Perceptions of Social Support: Evidence from Experimental and Observational Studies. *Journal of Personality & Social Psychology* 87 (3): 363–383.

Collins, R. Lorraine., Brian Quigley, and Kenneth E. Leonard. 2007. Women's Physical Aggression in Bars: An Event-Based Examination of Precipitants and Predictors of Severity. *Aggressive Behavior* 33 (4): 304–313.

Collins, Randall. 2000. Situational Stratification: A Micro-macro Theory of Ineqaulity. *Sociological Theory* 18 (1): 17–43.

Collins, Randall. 2001. Civilizations as Zones of Prestige and Social Contact. *International Sociology* 16 (3): 421–437.

Collins, Randall. 2008. *Violence: A Micro-sociological Theory*. Princeton, NJ: Princeton University Press.

Comartin, Erin, Victoria Nelson, Nanci Hambrick, Sheryl Kubiak, Emily Sightes, and Bradley Ray. 2020. Comparing for-Profit and Nonprofit Mental Health Services in County Jails. *Journal of Behavioral Health Services & Research* 48 (2): 320–329.

Combes, Jean-Louis., Mahamat Hamit-Haggar, and Sonia Schwartz. 2018. A Multilevel Analysis of the Determinants of Willingness to Pay to Prevent Environmental Pollution across Countries. *Social Sience Journal* 55 (3): 284–299.

Comor, Edward. 2010. Contextualizing and Critiquing the Fantastic Prosumer: Power, Alienation and Hegemony. *Critical Sociology* 37 (3): 309–327.

Conard, Maureen A., and Russell A. Matthews. 2008. Modeling the Stress Process: Personality Eclipses Dysfunctional Cognitions and Workload in Predicting Stress. *Personality & Individual Differences* 44 (1): 171–181.

Congdon, Peter. 2010. A Multiple Indicator, Multiple Cause Method for Representing Social Capital with an Application to Psychological Distress. *Journal of Geographical Systems* 12 (1): 1–23.

Conger, Rand D., and Katherine J. Conger. 2002. Resilience in Midwestern Families: Selected Findings from the First Decade of a Prospective, Longitudinal Study. *Journal of Marriage & Family* 64 (2): 361–373.

Conley, Dalton, and Brian Gifford. 2006. Home Ownership, Social Insurance, and the Welfare State. *Sociological Forum* 21 (1): 55–82.

Conley, Dalton. 2001. Decomposing the Black-White Wealth Gap: The Role of Parental Resources, Inheritance, and Investment Dynamics. *Sociological Inquiry* 71 (1): 39–66.

Connor, Brian T., and Long Doan. 2021. Government and Corporate Surveillance: Moral Discourse on Privacy in the Civil Sphere. *Information, Communication & Society* 24 (1): 52–68.

Connors, Gerard J., Radka T. Toscova, and J. Scott Tonigan. 1999. Serenity. In *Integrating Spirituality into Treatment: Resources for Practitioners*, 235–250, ed. William R. Miller. Washington, DC: American Psychological Association.

Consedine, Nathan S. 2011. Emotion, Regulation, and Learning across the Adult Lifespan: Implications from Developmental Functionalism. In *The Oxford Handbook of Reciprocal Adult Development Learning*, 132–154, ed. Carol Hoare, New York: Oxford University Press.

Constantino, Michael J., Keely R. Wilson, Leonard M. Horowitz, and Elizabeth C. Pinel. 2006. The Direct and Stress-buffering Effects of Self-organization on Psychological Adjustment. *Journal of Social & Clinical Psychology* 25 (3): 333–360.

Conway, Anne M., Michele M. Tugade, Lahnna I. Catalino, and Barbara L. Fredrickson. 2014. The Broaden-and-Build Theory of Positive Emotions: Form, Function, and Mechanisms. In *The Oxford Handbook of Happiness*, 17–34, ed. Susan A. David, Ilona Boniwell and Amanda Conley Ayers. Oxford, UK: Oxford University Press.

Conway, Lucian Gideon, III, and Mark Schaller. 2002. On the Verifiability of Evolutionary Psychological Theories: An Analysis of the Psychology of Scientific Persuasion. *Personality & Social Psychology Review* 6 (2): 152–166.

Cook, Deborah. 2001. The Two Faces of Liberal Democracy in Habermas. *Philosophy Today* 45 (1): 95–104.

Cook, Karen S., Coye Cheshire, Eric R.W. Rice, and Sandra Nakagawa. 2013. Social Exchange Theory. In *Handbook of Social Psychology*, 61–88, ed. John DeLamater and Amanda Ward. Dordrecht, Netherlands: Springer.

Cooke, Richard, and Pascheal Sheeran. 2004. Moderation of Cognition-intention and Cognition-behavior Relations: A Meta-analysis of Properties of Variables from the Theory of Planned Behavior. *British Journal of Social Psychology* 43: 159–186 (\88–92).

Copen, Casey E., and Merril Silverstein. 2008. The Transmission of Religious Beliefs across Generations: Do Grandparents Matter? *Journal of Comparative Family Studies* 39 (1): 59–71.

Corcoran, Katie E., David Pettinicchio, and Jacob T.N.. Young. 2011. The Context of Control: A Cross-National Investigation of the Link Between Political Institutions Efficacy, and Collective Action. *British Journal of Social Psychology* 50: 575–605.

Corcoran, Mang, and Terry Adams. 1997. Race, Sex, and the Intergenerational Transmission of Poverty. In *Consequences of Growing Up Poor*, 461–517, ed. Greg J. Duncan and Jeanne Brooks-Gunn. New York: Russell Sage.

Cornelis, Ilse, Alain Van Hiel, Arne Roets, and Malgorzata Kossowska. 2009. Age Differences in Conservatism: Evidence on the Mediating Effects of Personality and Cognitive Style. *Journal of Personality* 77: 51–87.

Cornell, Agnes, and Marcia Grimes. 2015. Institutions as Incentives for Civic Action: Bureaucratic Structures, Civil Society, and Disruptive Protests. *Journal of Politics* 77 (3): 664–678.

Cornwall, Benjamin. 2009. Good Health and the Bridging of Structural Holes. *Social Networks* 31: 92–103.

Corral-Vergugo, Victor. 2002. A Structural Model of Proenvironmental Competency. *Environment & Behavior* 34 (4): 531–549.

Correll, Shelley J. 2004. Constraints into Preferences: Gender Status, and Emerging Career Aspirations. *American Sociological Review* 69 (1): 93–113.

Corrigan, Michael W., Ann Higgins-D'Alessandro, and Philip Brown. 2013. The Case of Adding Prosocial Education to Current Education Policy: Preparing Students for the Test of Life, Not Just a Life of Tests. *KEDI Journal of Educational Policy Special Issue* 2013: 37–50.

Corrigan, Patrick W., Natalie Slopen, Gabriela Gracia, Sean Phelan, Cornelius B. Keogh, and Lorraine Keck. 2005. Some Recovery Processes in Mutual-Help Groups for Persons with Mental Illness, II: Qualitative Analysis of Participant Interviews. *Community Mental Health Journal* 41 (6): 721–735.

Corstange, Daniel, and Erin A. York. 2018. Sectarian Framing in the Syrian Civil War. *American Journal of Political Science* 62 (2): 441–455.

Cosculluela, Victor. 1995. *The Ethics of Suicide*. New York, NY: Garland.

Costigan, Catherine L., Martha Cox, and AnaMari Cauce. 2003. Work-Parenting Linkages Among Dual-Earner Couples at the Transition to Parenthood. *Journal of Family Psychology* 17 (1): 397–408.

Cote, James E. 2000. *Arrested Adulthood: The Changing Nature of Maturity and Identity*. New York: New York University Press.

Cote, Stéphane., Jennifer E. Stellar, Robb Willer, Rachel C. Forbes, Sean R. Martin, and Emily C. Bianchi. 2021. The Psychology of Entrenched Privilege: High Socioeconomic Status Individuals from Affluent Backgrounds Are Uniquely High in Entitlement. *Personality & Social Psychology Bulletin* 47 (1): 70–88.

Cotter, David A., JoAnn DeFiore, Joan M. Hermsen, Brenda Marsteller Kowalewsa, and Reeve Vanneman. 1998. The Demand for Female Labor. *American Journal of Sociology* 103 (6): 1673–1712.

Cotterell, John. 2007. *Social Networks in Youth and Adolescence*, 2nd ed. London: Routledge.

Cowen, Emory L., and Ryan P. Kilmer. 2002. Positive Psychology: Some Pulses and Some Open Issues. *Journal of Community Psychology* 30 (4): 440–460.

Cox, Gary. 2012. *The Existentialist's Guide to Death, the Universe and Nothingness*. London: Continuum.

Cox, Martha J., and Blair Paley. 1997. Families as Systems. *Annual Review of Psychology* 48: 243–267.

Craig, C. Samuel, and Susan P. Douglas. 2012. Culture and Consumer Behavior: Contextual and Compositional Components. In *Handbook of Developments in Consumer Behavior*, 47–82, ed. Victoria Wells and Gordon Foxall. Cheltenham, UK: Elgar.

Cramer, Phebe. 2000. Development of Identity: Gender Makes a Difference. *Journal of Research in Personality* 34: 42–72.

Cramm, J.M., V. Moller, and A.P. Nieboer. 2012. Individual- and Neighbourhood-level Indicators of Subjective Well-Being in a Small and Poor Eastern Cape Township: The Effect of Health, Social Capital, Marital Status, and Income. *Social Indicators Research* 105 (3): 581–593.

Crandall, Christian S., and Ryan K. Beasley. 2001. A Perceptual Theory of Legitimacy: Politics, Prejudice, Social Institutions, and Moral Value. In *The Psychology of Legitimacy: Emerging Perspectives on Ideology, Justice, and Intergroup Relations*, 77–102, ed. John T. Jost and Brenda Major. Cambridge, UK: Cambridge University Press.

Cronin, Tracey, Stephen Reysen, and Nyla R. Branscombe. 2012. Wal-Mart's Conscientious Objectors: Perceived Illegitimacy, Moral Anger, and Retaliatory Consumer Behavior. *Basic & Applied Social Psychology* 34 (4): 322–335.

Crook, Stephen, Jan Pakulski, and Malcolm Waters. 1992. *Postmodernization: Change in Advanced Society*. London: Sage.

Cropanzano, Russell, Jordan H. Stein, and Thierry Nadisic. 2011. *Social Justice and the Experience of Emotion*. New York: Routledge.

Crosnoe, Robert. 2001. Academic Orientation and Parental Involvement in Education During High School. *Sociology of Education* 74 (3): 210–230.

Crossley, Nick. 2012. Global Anti-corporate Struggle: A Preliminary Analysis. *British Journal of Sociology* 53 (4): 667–691.

Crossley, Noele. 2020. Consistency, Protection, Responsibility: Revisiting the Debate on Selective Humanitarianism. *Global Governance* 26 (3): 473.

Crowder, Kyle, Scott J. South, and Erick Chavez. 2006. Wealth, Race, and Inter-neighborhood Migraiton. *American Sociological Review* 71: 72–94.

Crowe, Jessica. 2010. Community Attachment and Satisfaction: The Role of a Community's Social Network Structure. *Journal of Community Psychology* 38 (5): 622–644.

Cummins, Robert A. 2000. Objective and Subjective Quality of Life: An Interactive Model. *Social Indicators Research* 52: 55–72.

Cummins, Robert A. 2005. Moving from the Quality of Life Concept to a Theory. *Journal of Intellectual Disability Research* 49 (10): 699–706.

Cummins, Robert A. 2010. Subjective Wellbeing: Homeostatically Protected Mood and Depression: A Synthesis. *Journal of Happiness Studies* 11: 1–17.
Cummins, Robert A. 2016. Happiness is the Right Metric to Measure Good Societal Functioning. *Society* 53 (3): 273–277.
Cummins, Robert A., Anna A.L.D.. Lau, David Mellor, and Mark A. Stokes. 2009. Encouraging Governments to Enhance the Happiness of Their Nation: Encouraging Governments to Enhance the Happiness of Their Nation: Step 1: Understand Subjective Wellbeing. *Social Indicators Research* 91: 23–36.
Cummins, Robert A., Richard Eckersley, Julie Pallant, Jackie van Vugt, and Roseanne Misajon. 2003. Developing a National Index of Subjective Wellbeing: The Australian Unity. *Social Indicators Research* 64: 159–190.
Cump, Brooks B., and James A. Kulik. 1997. Stress, Affiliation, and Emotional Contagion. *Journal of Personality & Social Psychology* 72 (2): 305–319.
Cundiff, Jenny M., Timothy W. Smith, Jonathan Butner, Kenneth L. Critchfield, and Jill Nealey-Moore. 2015. Affiliation and Control in Marital Interaction Interpersonal Complementarity Is Present but Is Not Associated with Affect or Relationship Quality. *Personality & Social Psychology Bulletin* 41 (1): 35–51.
Curley, Alexandra M. 2005. Theories of Urban Poverty and Implications for Public Housing Policy. *Journal of Sociology & Social Welfare* 32 (2): 97–119.
Curley, Alexandra M. 2010. Relocating the Poor: Social Capital and Neighborhood Resources. *Journal of Urban Affairs* 32 (1): 79–103.
Curney, Stacie, and William G. Gale. 2001. Asset Accumulation among Low-income Households. In *Assets for the Poor: The Benefits of Spreading Asset Ownership*, 165–205, ed. Thomas M. Shapiro and Edward N. Wolff. New York: Russell Sage.
Curry, Philip, and Michael F. O'Connell. 2000. Postmaterialist Values and Political Preferences: Some Unlikely Findings from Northern Ireland. *European Journal of Political Research* 37: 17–30.
Curtin, Nicola, Abigail J. Stewart, and Lauren E. Duncan. 2010. What Makes the Political Personal? Openness, Personal Political Salience, and Activism. *Journal of Personality* 78 (3): 943–968.
Curtis, Allan, and Michael Lockwood. 2000. Landcare and Catchment Management in Australia: Lessons for State-Sponsored Community Participation. *Society & Natural Resources* 13 (1): 61–72.
Cutler, David M., and Adriana Lleras-Muney. 2008. "Education and Health: Evaluating Theories and Evidence. In *Making American Healthier: Social and Economic Policy as Health Policy*, 29–60, ed. Robert F. Schoeni, James S. House, George A. Kaplan, and Harold Pollack. New York: Russell Sage.
Cyranowski, Jill M., and Barbra L. Andersen. 1998. Schemes, Sexuality, and Romantic Attachment. *Journal of Personality & Social Psychology* 74 (5): 1364–1379.
Dafoe, Allan. 2015. On Technological Determinism. *Science, Technology, & Human Values* 40 (6): 1047–1076.
Dahl, Espen. 1993. Social Inequality in Health: The Role of the Healthy Work Effect. *Social Science & Medicine* 36 (8): 1077–1086.
Dahlberg, Lincoln. 2007. The Internet, Deliberative Democracy, and Power: Radicalizing the Public Sphere. *International Journal of Media & Cultural Politics* 3 (1): 47–64.
Dahlberg, Stefan, Sören Holmberg, Bo Rothstein, Natalia Alvarado Pachon, and Richard Svensson. 2018. *The Quality of Government Basic Dataset* (Version Jan 18). University of Gothenburg: Quality of Government Institute, http://www.qog.pol.gu.se. https://doi.org/10.18157/QoGBasJan18
Dalby, P. 2006. Is There a Process of Spiritual Change in Development Associated with Ageing? A Critical Review of Research. *Ageing & Mental Health* 10 (1): 4–12.
Dalton, Russell, Alix Van Sickle, and Steven Weldon. 2010. The Individual-Institutional Nexus of Protest Behaviour. *British Journal of Political Science* 40 (1): 51–73.

Dan, Zhongdang, Wenjie Yan, Gang Jing, and Jiawen Zheng. 2011. Exploring Structured Inequality in Internet Use Behavior. *Asian Journal of Communication* 21 (2): 116–132.

Dant, Tim. 2006. Material Civilization: Things and Society. *British Journal of Sociology* 57 (2): 289–308.

Daraei, Minor, and Artmiz Mohajery. 2013. The Impact of Socioeconomic Status on Life Satisfaction. *Social Indicators Research* 112 (1): 69–81.

Darnell, Simon C. 2012. Olympism in Action, Olympic Hosting and the Politics of 'Sport for Development and Peace': Investigating the Development Discourses of Rio 2016. *Sport in Society* 15 (6): 869–887.

Datler, Georg, Wolfgang Jagodzinski, and Peter Schmidt. 2013. Two Theories on the Test Bench: Internal and External Validity of the Theories of Ronald Inglehart and Shalom Schwartz. *Social Science Research* 42: 906–925.

Davidson, Elsa. 2008. Marketing the Self: The Politics of Aspiration among Middle-class Silicon Valley Youth. *Environment & Planning A* 40: 2814–2830.

Davies, Lynn. 2008. *Educating against Extremism*. Stoke on Trent, UK: Trentham.

Davis, Darren W., and Christian Davenport. 1999. Assessing the Validity of the Postmaterialism Index. *American Political Science Review* 93 (3): 649–664.

Davis, Nancy J., and Robert V. Robinson. 1999. Their Brothers' Keepers? Orthodox Religionists, Modernists, and Economic Justice in Europe. *American Journal of Sociology* 104 (6): 1631–1665.

Davis, Nancy J., and Robert V. Robinson. 2001. Theological Modernism, Cultural Libertarianism and Laissez-faire Economics in Contemporary European Societies. *Sociology of Religion* 62 (1): 23–50.

Davis, Nancy J., and Robert V. Robinson. 2006. The Egalitarian Face of Islamic Orthodoxy: Support for Islamic Law and Economic Justice in Seven Muslim-Majority Nations. *American Sociological Review* 71 (2): 167–190.

Day, James M. 2011. Religious, Spiritual, and Moral Development and Learning in the Adult Years: Classical and Contemporary Questions, Cognitive-developmental and Complementary Paradigms, and Prospects for Future Research. In *The Oxford Handbook of Reciprocal Adult Development Learning*, 318–345, ed. Carol Hoare, New York: Oxford University Press.

Day, James. 2010. Religion, Spirituality, and Positive Psychology in Adulthood: A Developmental View. *Journal of Adult Development* 17 (4): 215–229.

Day, Jennifer. 2013. Effects of Involuntary Residential Relocation on Household Satisfaction in Shanghai, China. *Urban Policy & Research* 31 (1): 93–117.

Dayton, Bruce W. 2000. Policy Frames, Policy Making, and the Global Climate Change Discourse. In *Social Discourse and Environmental Policy: An Application of Q Methodology*, 71–99, ed. Helen Addams. Cheltenham, UK: Edward Elgar.

Backer, De., J.S. Charlotte, Mark Nelissen, Patrick Vyncke, Johan Braeckman, and Francis T. McAndrew. 2007. Celebrities: From Teachers to Friends: A Test of Two Hypotheses on the Adaptiveness of Celebrity Gossip. *Human Nature* 18 (4): 334–354.

de Beer, Paul, and Ferry Kostere. 2009. *Sticking Together or Falling Apart? Solidarity in an Era of Individualization and Globalization*. Amsterdam, Netherlands: Amsterdam University Press.

de Bruin, Boudewijn. 2016. *Ethics and the Global Financial Crisis: Why Incompetence Is Worse than Greed*. Cambridge, UK: Cambridge University Press.

Carlo, De., Damiano Girardi Alessandro, Alessandra Falco, Laura Dal Corso, and Annamaria Di Sipio. 2019. When Does Work Interfere with Teachers? Private Life? An Application of the Job Demands-Resources Model. *Frontiers in Psychology* 10: 1121.

de Costa, Ravi. 2006. Identity, Authority, and the Moral Worlds of Indigenous Petitions. *Comparative Studies in Society & History* 48 (3): 669–698.

de Coster, Stacy. 2005. Depression and Law Violation: Gendered Responses to Gendered Stresses. *Sociological Perspectives* 48 (2): 155–187.

de Graaf, Nan, Anthony Heath Dirk, and Ariana Need. 2001. Declining Cleavages and Political Choices: The Interplay of Social and Political Factors in the Netherlands. *Electoral Studies* 20: 1–15.

De Graaf, Nan Dirk. 2013. Secularization: Theoretical Controversies Generating Empirical Research. In *The Handbook of Rational Choice Social Research*, 322–354, ed. Rafael Wittek, Tom A. H. Snijders, and Victor Nee. Stanford, CA: Stanford University Press.

de Graaf, Paul M., and Matthijs Kalmijn. 2003. Alternative Routes in the Remarriage Market: Competing-Risk Analyses of Union Formation After Divorce. *Social Forces* 81 (4): 1459–1498.

de Jonge, Jan. 2012. *Rethinking Rational Choice theory: A Companion on Rational and Moral Action*. Houndmills, UK: Palgrave.

Moortel, De., Laia Palenciab Deborah, Lucia Artazcoz, Carme Borrell, and Christophe Vanroelen. 2015. Neo-Marxian Social Class Inequalities in the Mental Well-Being of Employed Men and Women: The Role of European Welfare Regimes. *Social Science & Medicine* 128: 188–200.

de Oliver, Miguel. 1999. Attitudes and Inaction: A Case Study of the Manifest Demographics of Urban Water Conservation. *Environment & Behavior* 31 (3): 372–394.

de Ruijter, Esther. 2004. Trends in the Outsourcing of Domestic Work and Childcare in the Netherlands: Compositional or Behavioral Change? *Acta Sociologica* 47 (3): 219–234.

de Witte, Hans, Elsy Verhofstadt, and Eddy Omey. 2007. Testing Karasek's Learning and Strain Hypothesis on Young Workers in Their First Job. *Work & Stress* 21 (2): 131–141.

de Zuniga, Homero Gil, Sebastián Valenzuela, and Brian E. Weeks. 2016. Motivations for Political Discussion: Antecedents and Consequences on Civic Engagement. *Human Communication Research* 42 (4): 533–552.

Dean, Mitchell. 2015. The Malthus Effect: Population and the Liberal Government of Life. *Economy & Society* 44 (1): 18–39.

Deaton, Angus, Jane F Ortson, and Robert Tortora. 2010. Life (Evaluation), HIV/AIDS, and Death in Africa. In *International Differences in Well-being*, 105–136, ed. Ed Diener, John F. Helliwell and Daniel Kahneman. New York: Oxford University Press.

Deci, Edward L., and Richard M. Ryan. 2008. Facilitating Optimal Motivation and Psychological Well-Being Across Life Domains. *Canadian Psychology* 49 (1): 14–23.

Deci, Edward L., Jennifer G. La Guardia, Arlen C. Moller, Marc J. Scheiner, and Richard M. Ryan. 2006. On the Benefits of Giving as Well as Receiving Autonomy Support: Mutuality in Close Friendships. *Personality & Social Psychology Bulletin* 32 (3): 313–327.

Degenne, Alain, Marie-Odile Lebeaux, and Yannick Lemel. 2004. Does Social Capital Offset Social and Economic Inequalities? Social Capital in Everyday Life. In *Creation and Returns of Social Capital: A New Research Program*, 51–73, ed. Henk Flap and Beate Volker. London: Routledge.

Dekkers, Gijs J.M.. 2008. Are You Unhappy? Then You Are Poor? Multi-dimensional Poverty in Belgium. *International Journal of Sociology & Social Policy* 28 (11/12): 502–545.

Delang, Claudio O., and Ho Cheuk Lung. 2010. Public Housing and Poverty Concentration in Urban Neighbourhoods: The Case of Hong Kong in the 1990s. *Urban Studies* 47 (7): 1391–1413.

Delanty, Gerard. 2009. *The Cosmopolitan Imagination: The Renewal of Critical Social Theory*. Cambridge, UK: Cambridge University Press.

Delbosc, Alexa, and Graham Currie. 2011. Exploring the Relative Influences of Transport Disadvantage and Social Exclusion on Well-Being. *Transport Policy* 18: 555–562.

DeLeon, Richard E., and Katherine C. Naff. 2004. Identity Politics and Local Political Culture: Some Comparative Results from the Social Capital Benchmark Survey. *Urban Affairs Review* 39 (6): 689–719.

Delgado, Melvin, and Lee Staples. 2008. *Youth-Led Community Organizing: Theory and Action*. New York: Oxford University Press.

Delhey, Jan. 2010. From Materialist to Post-materialist Happiness? National Affluence and Determinants of Life Satisfaction in Cross-National Perspective. *Social Indicators Research* 97: 65–84.

Fave, Delle, Ingrid Brdar Antonella, Teresa Freire, Dianne Vella-Brodrick, and Marie P. Wissing. 2011. The Eudaimonic and Hedonic Components of Happiness: Qualitative and Quantitative Findings. *Social Indicators Research* 100: 185–207.

Deller, Steven, and Craig Maher. 2009. Government, Effectiveness, Performance, and Local Property Values. *International Journal of Public Administration* 32 (13): 1182–1212.

Carpini, Delli, and X. Michael. 1986. Work and Politics: A Decomposition of the Concept of Work and an Investigation of Its Impact on Political Attitudes and Actions. *Political Psychology* 7 (1): 117–140.

Dell'Oro, Roberto. 2002. Theological Discourse and the Postmodern Condition: The Case of Bioethics. *Medicine, Health Care, & Philosophy* 5 (2): 127–136.

DeLuca, Kevin Michael, and Jennifer Peeples. 2002. From Public Sphere to Public Screen: Democracy, Activism, and the Violence of Seattle. *Critical Studies in Media Communication* 19 (2): 125–151.

DeMaris, Alfred, Michael L. Benson, Greer L. Fox, Terrence Hill, and Judy Van Wyk. 2003. Distal and Proximal Factors in Domestic Violence: A Test of an Integrated Model. *Journal of Marriage & Family* 65: 652–667.

Demerath, Loren. 2012. *Explaining Culture: The Social Pursuit of Subjective Order*. Lanham, MD: Lexington.

Demerath, Nicholas J., III. 2002. A Sinner among the Saints: Confessions of a Sociologist of Culture and Religion. *Sociological Forum* 17 (1): 1–19.

Demers, Christiane. 2007. *Organizational Change Theories: A Synthesis*. Thousand Oaks, CA: Sage.

Demertzis, Nicolas. 2020. *The Political Sociology of Emotions: Essays on Trauma and Ressentiment*. Abingdon, UK: Routledge.

Demo, David H., and Cheryl Buehler. 2013. "theoretical Approaches to Studying Divorce. In *Handbook of Family Theories: A Content-Based Approach*, 263–279, ed. Mark A. Fine and Frank D. Fincham. New York: Routledge.

DeNeve, Kristina M., and Harris Cooper. 1998. The Happy Personality: A Meta-analysis of 137 Personality Traits and Subjective Well-Being. *Psychological Bulletin* 124 (2): 197–229.

Derks, Anton. 2004. Are the Underprivileged Really that Economically Leftist? Attitudes towards Economic Redistribution and the Welfare State in Flanders. *European Journal of Political Research* 43: 509–521.

Derrick, Jaye L., Shira Gabriel, and Kurt Hugenberg. 2009. Social Surrogacy: How Favored Television Programs Provide the Experience of Belonging. *Journal of Experimental Social Psychology* 45 (2): 352–362.

Devine, Joel A., Charles J. Brody, and James D. Wright. 1997. Evaluating an Alcohol and Drug Treatment Program for the Homeless: An Econometric Approach. *Evaluation & Program Planning* 20 (2): 205–215.

Devos, Thierry, Dario Spini, and Shalom H. Schwartz. 2002. Conflicts Among Human Values and Trust in Institutions. *British Journal of Social Psychology* 41: 481–494.

Dickson, Eric S., Sanford C. Gordon, and Gregory A. Huber. 2009. Enforcement and Compliance in an Uncertain World: An Experimental Investigation. *Journal of Politics* 71 (4): 1307–1378.

Dieckhoff, Martina. 2007. Does It Work? The Effect of Continuing Training on Labour Market Outcomes: A Comparative Study of Germany, Denmark, and the United Kingdom. *European Sociological Review* 23 (3): 295–308.

Diener, Ed, and Eunkook Mark Suh. 1999. National Differences in Subjective Well-being. In *Well-Being: The Foundations of Hedonic Psychology*, 434–450, ed. Daniel Kahneman, Ed Diener and Norbert Schwarz. New York: Russell Sage.

Diener, Ed, and Frank Fujita. 1995. Resources, Personal Strivings, and Subjective Well-being: A Nomothetic and Idiographic Approach. *Journal of Personality & Social Psychology* 68 (5): 926–935.

Diener, Ed, and William Tov. 2012. National Accounts of Well-Being. In *Handbook of Social Indicators and Quality of Life Research*, 137–157, ed. Kenneth C. Land, Alex C. Michalos, and M. Joseph Sirgy. Dordrecht, Netherlands: Springer.

Diener, Ed, Daniel Kahneman, William Tov, and Raksha Arora. 2010. Income's Association with Judgments of Life versus Feelings. In *International Differences in Well-Being*, 3–15, ed. Ed Diener, John F. Helliwell and Daniel Kahneman. New York: Oxford University Press.

Diener, Ed, Eunkook M. Suh, Richard E. Lucas, and Heidi L. Smith. 1999. Subjective Well-Being: Three Decades of Progress. *Psychological Bulletin* 125 (2): 276–302.

Diener, Ed, Richard E. Lucas, Ulrich Schimmack, and John F. Helliwell. 2009. *Well-Being for Public Policy*. Oxford, UK: Oxford University Press.

Diener, Ed., and Richard E. Lucas. 1999. Personality and Subjective Well-Being. In *Well-Being: The Foundations of Hedonic Psychology*, 213–229, ed. Daniel Kahneman, Ed Diener and Norbert Schwarz. New York: Russell Sage.

Diener, Ed., and Robert Biswas-Diener. 2002. Will Money Increase Subjective Well-being? *Social Indicators Research* 57: 119–169.

Dietz, Thomas, Linda Kalof, and Paul C. Stern. 2002. Gender Values, and Environmentalism. *Social Science Quarterly* 83 (1): 353–364.

Diez-Nicolas, Juan. 2002. Two Contradictory Hypotheses on Globalization: Societal Convergence or Civilization Differentiation and Clash. *Comparative Sociology* 1 (3–4): 465–493.

Dillard, James, Price. 2015. Goals-plan-action Theory of Message Production: Making Influence Messages. In *Engaging Theories in Interpersonal Communication: Multiple Perspectives*, 63–74, ed. Dawn O. Braithwaite and Paul Schrodt. Thousand Oaks, CA: SAGE.

Dillon, James J. 2019. Humanistic Psychology and the Good: A Forgotten Link. *Humanistic Psychologist* 2019: 7.

Dioale, William, and Albert Seda. 2001. Modernization as Changes in Cultural Complexity: New Cross-Cultural Measurements. *Cross-Cultural Research* 35 (2): 129–153.

DiRenzo, Gordon J. 1990. Socialization for Citizenship in Modern Democratic Society. In *Political Socialization, Citizenship, Education, and Democracy*, 25–46, ed. Orit Ichilov. New York: Teachers College.

Distante, Roberta. 2013. Subjective Well-Being, Income and Relative Concerns in the UK. *Social Indicators Research* 113: 81–105.

Dittman, Joerg, and Jan Goebel. 2010. Your House Your Car, Your Education: The Socioeconomic Situation of the Neighborhood and Its Impact on Life Satisfaction in Germany. *Social Indicators Research* 96: 497–513.

Dixon, Marc, and Vincent J. Roscigno. 2003. Status, Networks, and Social Movement Participation: The Case of Striking Workers. *American Journal of Sociology* 108 (6): 1292–1327.

Dixon, Marc, Vincent J. Roscigno, and Randy Hodson. 2004. Unions, Solidarity, and Striking. *Social Forces* 83 (1): 3–33.

Djupe, Paul A., and Andrew R. Lewis. 2015. Solidarity and Discord of Pluralism: How the Social Context Affects Interest Group Learning and Belonging. *American Politics Research* 43 (3): 394–424.

Doane, Woody. 2017. Humanist Sociology. In *The Cambridge Handbook of Sociology, Vol. 2: Specialty and Interdisciplinary Studies*, 322–329, ed. Kathleen Odell Korgen. New York, NY: Cambridge University Press.

Dobewall, Henrik, Anu Realo, Juri Allik, Tonu Esko, and Andres Metspalu. 2013. Self-other Agreement in Happiness and Life-satisfaction: The Role of Personality Traits. *Social Indicators Research* 114: 479–492.

Dodson, Kyle. 2016. Economic Threat and Protest Behavior in Comparative Perspective. *Sociological Perspectives* 59 (4): 873–891.

Doerner, William G., and Steven P. Lab. 2012. *Victimology*. Burlington, MA: Anderson.

Doff, Wnda, and Reinout Kleinhans. 2011. Residential Outcomes of Forced Relocation: Lifting a Corner of the Veil on Neighbourhood Selection. *Urban Studies* 48 (4): 661–680.

Dolton, Peter, Ros Levacic, and Anna Vignoles. 2004. The Economic Impact of Schooling Resources. In *Human Capital over the Life Cycle: A European Perspective*, 36–52, ed. Catherine Sofer. Cheltenham, UK: Edward Elgar.

Domina, Tanya, and Kathryn Koch. 2002. Convenience and Frequency of Recycling: Implications for Including Textiles in Carbide Recycling Programs. *Environment & Behavior* 34 (2): 216–238.

Donahue, Michael J. 1985. Intrinsic and Extrinsic Religiousness: Review and Meta Analysis. *Journal of Personality & Social Psychology* 48 (2): 400–419.

Donnellan, M. Brent, Monica J. Martin, Katherine J. Conger, and Rand D. Conger. 2013. Economic Distress and Poverty in Families. In *Handbook of Family Theories: A Content-based Approach*, 338–355, ed. Mark A. Fine and Frank D. Fincham. New York: Routledge.

Donnelly, Gabrielle. 2013. Reading the Signs of the Times: Centering Religion and Development. *Canadian Journal of Developmental Studies* 34 (2): 189–202.

Donohew, Lewis, J.D. Philip Palmgreen, and I.I. Rayburn. 1987. Social and Psychological Origins of Media Use: A Lifestyle Analysis. *Journal of Broadcasting & Electronic Media* 31 (3): 255–278.

Donovan, Todd, and Jeffrey A. Karyn. 2006. Popular Support for Direct Democracy. *Party Politics* 12 (5): 671–688.

Dooley, David, and Joann Prause. 2004. *The Social Costs of Underemployment: Inadequate Employment as Disguised Unemployment*. Cambridge, UK: Cambridge University Press.

Dorff, Cassy. 2017. Violence, Kinship Networks, and Political Resilience: Evidence from Mexico. *Journal of Peace Research* 54 (4): 558–573.

Dosman, Donna M., Wiktor L. Adamowicz, and Steve E. Hrudey. 2001. Socioeconomic Determinants of Health- and Food Safety-related Risk Perceptions. *Risk Analysis* 21 (2): 307–317.

Dovidio, John F., Jane Allyn Piliavin, David Al Schroeder, and Louis A. Penner. 2006. *The Social Psychology of Prosocial Behavior*. Mahwah, NJ: Lawrence Erlbaum.

Dowling, Robyn, Rowland Atkinson, and Pauline McGuirk. 2010. Privatism, Privatisation and Social Distinction in Master-Planned Residential Estates. *Urban Policy Research* 28 (4): 391–410.

D'raven, L. Lambert., and N. Pasha-Zaidi. 2016. Using the PERMA Model in the United Arab Emirates. *Social Indicators Research* 125: 905–933.

Dreher, Axel, Noel Gaston, and Pim Martens. 2008. *Measuring Globalisation: Gauging Its Consequences*. New York: Springer.

Dressler, William W. 1991. *Stress and Adaptation in the Context of Culture: Depression in a Southern Black Community*. Albany, NY: State University of New York Press.

Drope, Jeffrey, and Abdur Chowdhury. 2014. The Puzzle of Heterogeneity in Support for Free Trade. *Business & Politics* 16 (3): 453–479.

Drury, John. 2002. When the Mobs Are Looking for Witches to Burn, Nobody's Safe: Talking about the Reactionary Crowd. *Discourse & Society* 13 (1): 41–73.

Drus, Marina, Aaron Kozbelt, and Robert R. Hughes. 2014. Creativity, Psychopathology, and Emotion Processing: A Liberal Response Bias for Remembering Negative Information is Associated with Higher Creativity. *Creativity Research Journal* 26 (3): 251–262.

Dryzek, John S. 1997. *The Plitics of the Earth: Environmental Discourses*. Oxford, UK: Oxford University Press.

Dryzek, John S. 2006. *Deliberative Global Politics: Discourse and Democracy in a Divided World*. Cambridge, UK: Polity.

Dryzek, John S., and Patrick Dunleavy. 2009. Theories of the Democratic State. Houndmills, UK: Palgrave.

Duberstein, P.R., Y. Conwell, K.R. Conner, S. Eberly, J.S. Evinger, and E.D. Caine. 2004. Poor Social Integration and Suicide: Fact or Artifact? A Case-Control Study. *Psychological Medicine* 34: 1331–1337.

Dugan, Laura, and Erica Chenoweth. 2012. Moving Beyond Deterrence. *American Sociological Review* 77 (4): 597–624.

Duncan, Grant. 2014. Politics, Paradoxes and Pragmatics of Happiness. *Culture, Theory & Critique* 55 (1): 79–95.

Duncan, Lauren E. 1999. Motivation for Collective Action: Group Consciousness as Mediator of Personality, Life Experiences, and Women's Rights Activism. *Political Psychology* 20 (3): 611–635.

Durbin, Daniel T. 2020. From Plato to St. Paul: Ancient Sport as Performative Public Discourse. *Journal of the Philosophy of Sport* 47 (3): 403–418.

Dutton, Courtney E., Sasha M. Rojas, Christal L. Badour, Sonya G. Wanklyn, and Matthew T. Feldner. 2016. Posttraumatic Stress Disorder and Suicidal Behavior: Indirect Effects of Impaired Social Functioning. *Archives of Suicide Research* 20 (4): 567–579.

Dutton, William H. 2013. Internet Studies: The Foundations of a Transformative Field. In *The Oxford Handbook of Internet Studies*, 1–23, ed. William H. Dutton. Oxford, UK: Oxford University Press.
Duxbury, Linda, and Michael Halinski. 2018. It's not all about Guns and Gangs: Role Overload as a Source of Stress for Male and Female Police Officers. *Policing & Society* 28 (8): 930–946.
Dweck, Carol S. 2012. Implicit Theories. In *Handbook of Theories of Social Psychology*, vol. 2, 43–61, ed. Paul A.M. Van Lange, Arie W. Kruglanski and E. Tory Higgins. London, CA: SAGE.
Dyck, Joshua J., and Edward L. Lascher, Jr. 2009. Direct Democracy and Political Efficacy Reconsidered. *Political Behavior* 31: 401–427.
Dy-Liacco, Gabriel S., Ralph L. Piedmont, Nichole A. Murray-Swank, Thomas E. Rodgerson, and Martin F. Sherman. 2009. Spirituality and Religiosity as Cross-Cultural Aspects of Human Experience. *Psychology of Religion & Spirituality* 1 (1): 35–52.
Eagly, Alice H., and Wendy Wood. 2012. Social Role Theory. In *Handbook of Theories of Social Psychology*, vol. 2, 458–476, ed. Paul A.M. Van Lange, Arie W. Kruglanski and E. Tory Higgins. London, CA: SAGE.
Eatough, Virginia, and Jonathan A. Smith. 2008. Interpretative Phenomenological Analysis. In *The Sage Handbook of Qualitative Research in Psychology*, 179–214, ed. Carla Willig and Wendy Stainton-Rogers. Los Angeles, CA: Sage.
Eccles, Jacquelynne S., and Allan Wigfield. 2002. Motivational Beliefs, Values, and Goals. *Annual Review of Psychology* 53: 109–132.
Eccles, Jacquelynne S., and Bonnie L. Barber. 1999. Student Council, Volunteering, Basketball, or Marching Band: What Kind of Extracurricular Involvement Matters? *Journal of Adolescent Res4earch* 14 (1): 10–43.
Echabe, A. Echebarria, D. Paez Rovira, and J.F. Valencia Garate. 1988. Testing Ajzen and Fishbein's Attitudes Model: The Predicting of Voting. *European Journal of Social Psychology* 18: 181–189.
Economou, Marina, Elias Angelopoulos, Lily Evangelia Peppou, Kyriakos Souliotis, Chara Tzavara, Konstantinos Kontoangelos, Michael Madianos, and Costas Stefanis. 2016. Enduring Financial Crisis in Greece: Prevalence and Correlates of Major Depression and Suicidality. *Social Psychiatry and Psychiatric Epidemiology* 51 (7): 1015–1024.
Eddy, J. Mark, Jean Schumer, Joann Wu Shortt, Deborah M. Caldi, Stacey S. tiberio, and Sabina Low. 2018. A Life-course Model for the Development of Intimate Partner Violence. In *The Cambridge Handbook of Violent Behavior and Aggression*, 52–64, ed. Alexander T. Vazsonyi, David J. Flannery and Matt DeLisi. Cambridge, UK: Cambridge University Press.
Eder, Klaus. 2015. Social Movements in Social Theory. In *Oxford Handbook of Social Movements*, 31–49, ed. Donatella della Porta and Mario Diani. Oxford, UK: Oxford University Press.
Edyvane, Derek. 2017. The Passion for Civility. *Political Studies Review* 15 (3): 344–354.
Egerton, Muriel, and Mike Savage. 2000. Age Stratification and Class Formation: A Longitudinal Study of the Social Mobility of Young Men and Women, 1971–1991. *Work, Employment & Society* 14 (1): 23–49.
Ehrensuft, Miriam K., Patricia Cohen, Jocelyn Brown, Elizabeth Smailes, Henian Chen, and Jeffrey G. Johnson. 2003. Intergenerational Transmission of Partner Violence: A 20-Year Prospective Study. *Journal of Consulting & Clinical Psychology* 71 (4): 741–753.
Eibner, Christine E., and William N. Evans. 2004. The Income-health relationship and the Role of Relative Deprivation. In *Social Inequality*, 545–568, ed. Kathryn M. Neckerman. New York: Russell Sage.
Eikemo, Terje Andreas, Arne Matekaasa, and Kristen Ringdal. 2008. Health and Happiness. In *Nordic Social Attitudes in a European Perspective*, 48–64, ed. Heikki Ervasti, Torben Fridberg, Mikael Hjerm, and Kristen Ringdal. Cheltenham, UK: Edward Elgar.
Eitle, Tamela McNutlty., and David J. Eitle. 2002. Race, Cultural Capital, and the Educational Effects of Participation in Sports. *Sociology of Education* 75 (2): 123–146.
Elchardus, Mark, and Kobe De Keere. 2013. Social Control and Institutional Trust: Reconsidering the Effect of Modernity on Social Malaise. *Social Science Journal* 50 (1): 101–111.

Eldersveld, Samuel J., Lars Stromberg, and Wim Derksen. 1995. *Local Elites in Western Democracies: A Comparative Analysis of Urban Political Leaders in the U.S., Sweden, and the Netherlands*. Boulder, CO: Westview.

Elder-Vass, Dave. 2010. *The Causal Power of Social Structures: Emergence, Structure and Agency*. Cambridge, UK: Cambridge University Press.

Eliason, Grafton T., Jeff L. Samide, George Williams, and Mark F. Lepore. 2010. Existential Theory and Our Search for Spirituality. *Journal of Spirituality in Mental Health* 12 (2): 86–111.

Ellemers, Naomi, and S. Alexander Haslam. 2012. Social Identity Theory. In *Handbook of Theories of Social Psychology*, vol. 2, ed. Paul A.M. Van Lange, Arie W. Kruglanski and E. Tory Higgins. London, CA: SAGE.

Elliott, Anthony. 2003. *Critical Visions: New Directions in Social Theory*. Lanham, MD: Rowman & Littlefield.

Ellison, Christopher G. 1991. Identification and Separatism: Religious Involvement and Racial Orientation among Black Americans. *Sociological Quarterly* 22 (3): 477–494.

Ellison, Christopher G., Jaswon D. Boardman, David R. Williams, and James S. Jackson. 2001. Religious Involvement, Stress, and Mental Health: Findings from the 1995 Detroit Area Study. *Social Forces* 80 (1): 215–249.

Ellwood, David T., and Christopher Jencks. 2004. The Uneven Spread of Sing-parent Families: What Do We Know? Where Do We Look for Answers? In *Social Inequality*, 3–78, ed. Kathryn M. Neckerman. New York: Russell Sage.

Elmore, Richard F. 2009. Schooling Adolescents. In *Handbook of Adolescent Psychology, Vol.2: Contextual Influences and Adolescent Development*, 193–227, ed. Richard M. Lerner and Laurence Steinberg. Hoboken, NJ: Wiley.

Elster, Jon. 2000. Rationality, Economy, and Society. In *The Cambridge Companion to Weber*, 21–41, ed. Stephen Turner. Cambridge, UK: Cambridge University Press.

Elster, Jon. 2011. Indeterminancy of Emotional Mechanisms. In *Analytical Sociology and Social Mechanisms*, 50–63, ed. Pierre Demeulenaere. Cambridge, UK: Cambridge University Press.

Elster, Jon. 2015. *Explaining Social Behavior: More Nuts and Bolts for the Social Sciences*. Cambridge, UK: Carmbridge University Press.

Emery, Clifton R., and Wu. Shali. 2020. A Tale of Two Confucian Capitals: The Role of Friends and Secrecy in Beijing and Seoul. *Violence against Women* 26 (5): 458–481.

Emjaian, Brian, Sarah Beth Bell, Zachary Whitt, and C. Nathan De Wall. 2018. Social-cognitive Processes in the Development of Antisocial and Violent Behavior. In *The Cambridge Handbook of Violent Behavior and Aggression*, 259–277, ed. Alexander T. Vazsonyi, David J. Flannery and Matt DeLisi. Cambridge, UK: Cambridge University Press. Pinker, Steven. 2011. *The Better Angels of Our Nature: Why Violence Has Declined*. New York: Viking.

Emler, Nicholas, and Elizabeth Frazer. 1999. Politics: The Education Effect. *Oxford Review of Education* 25 (1/2): 251–273.

Enders, Adam M. 2022. The Relationship between Social Media Use and Beliefs in Conspiracy Theories and Misinformation. *Political Behavior.*

Engel, Uwe, and Manuela Potschke. 1998. Willingness to Pay for the Environment: Social Structure Value Orientations and Environmental Behavior in a Multilevel Perspective. *Innovation* 11 (3): 315–332.

Engels, Christian Archer, and Susan K. Jacobson. 2007. Evaluating Long-Term Effects of the Golden Lion Tarmarin Environmental Education Program in Brazil. *Journal of Environmental Education* 38 (3): 3–14.

Erickson, Bonnie. H. 2004. The Distribution of Gendered Social Capital in Canada. In *Creation and Returns of Social Capital: A New Research Program*, 27–50, ed. Henk Flap and Beate Volker. London: Routledge.

Erickson, Bruce. 2020. Anthropocene Futures: Linking Colonialism and Environmentalism In An Age Of Crisis. *Environment & Planning D: Society & Space* 38 (1): 111–128.

Erickson, Rebecca J., and Christian Ritter. 2001. Emotional Labor, Burnout, and Inauthenticity: Does Gender Matter? *Social Psychology Quarterly* 64 (2): 146–163.

Erickson, Sarah J., and Sarah W. Feldstein. 2007. Adolescent Humor and Its Relationship to Coping, Defense Strategies, Psychological Distress, and Well-Being. *Child Psychiatry & Human Development* 37: 255–271.

Eriksson, Kimmo, Ali Kazemi, and Kjell Tornblom. 2015. A New Look at Individual Differences in Perceptions of Unfairness: The Theory of Maximally Unfair Allocations in Multiparty Situations. *Social Justice Research* 28 (4): 401–414.

Ervasti, Heikki. 2008. The Meaning and Implications of Religiosity. In *Nordic Social Attitudes in a European Perspective*, 231–248, ed. Heikki Ervasti, Torben Fridberg, Mikael Hjerm, and Kristen Ringdal. Cheltenham, UK: Edward Elgar.

Esaisason, Peter. 2014. Nimbyism: A Reexamination of a Phenomenon. *Social Science Research* 48: 185–195.

Evans, Gary W., and Susan Saegert. 2000. Residential Crowding in the Context of Inner City Poverty. In *Theoretical Perspectives in Environment-behavior Research: Underlying Assumptions, Research, Problems, and Methodologies*, 247–267, ed. Seymour Wapner, Jack Demick, Takiji Yamamoto and Hirofumi Minami. New York: Kluwer.

Evans, Geoffrey. 1993. The Decline of Class Divisions in Britain? Class and Ideological Preferences in the 1960s and the 1980s. *British Journal of Sociology* 44: 449–471.

Evans, M.D.R., and Jonathan Kelley. 2004. Effect of Family Structure on Life Satisfaction: Australian Evidence. *Social Indicators Research* 69: 303–349.

Evans, M.D.R., Jonathan Kelley, and Clayton D. Peoples. 2010. Justifications of Inequality: The Normative Basis of Pay Differentials in 31 Nations. *Social Science Quarterly* 91 (5): 1405–1431.

Evans, Tony, and John Harris. 2004. Street-Level Bureaucracy, Social Work and the (exaggerated) Death of Discretion. *British Journal of Social Work* 34: 871–895.

Evers, Adalbert. 2009. Civicness and Civility: Their Meanings for Social Services. *VOLUNTAS: International Journal of Voluntary and Nonprofit Organizations* 20: 239–259.

Evetts, Julia. 2003. The Construction of Professionalism in New and Existing Occupational Contexts: Promoting and Facilitating Occupational Change. *International Journal of Sociology & Social Policy* 23 (4–5): 22–35.

Ewing, Reid, Shima Hamidi, and James B. Grace. 2016. Compact Development and Vmt—Environmental Determinism, Self-Selection, or Some of Both? *Environment & Planning.*

Exelmans, Liese, and Jan Van den Bulck. 2021. "Glued to the Tube": The Interplay between Self-Control, Evening Television Viewing, and Bedtime Procrastination. *Communication Research* 48 (4): 594–616.

Extremera, Natalio, Anxiliadora Duran, and Lourades Rey. 2007. Perceived Emotional Intelligence and Dispositional Optimism-pessimism: Analyzing Their Roles in Predicting Psychological Adjustment among Adolescents. *Personality & Individual Differences* 42: 1069–1079.

Fagan, Jeffrey, Deanna L. Wilinson, and Garth Davies. 2007. Social Contagion of Violence. In *The Cambridge Handbook of Violent Behavior and Aggression*, 688–723, ed. Daniel J. Flannery, Alexander T. Vazsonyi and Irwin D. Waldman. Cambridge, UK: Cambridge University Press.

Fahmy, Eldin. 2006. *Young Citizens: Young People's Involvement in Politics and Decision Making*. Aldershot, UK: Ashgage.

Fairfield, Paul. 2008. *Why Democracy?* Albany, NY: State University of Neew York Press.

Fairris, David, and Mark Brenner. 2001. Workplace Transformation and the Rise in Cumulative Trauma Disorders: Is There a Connection? *Journal of Labor Research* 22 (1): 15–28.

Fall, Kevin A., Janice Miner Holden, and Andre Marquis. 2004. *Theoretical Models of Counseling and Psychotherapy*. New York: Brunner-Routledge.

Falola, Toyin, and Adam Paddock. 2012. *Environment and Economics in Nigeria*. Abington, UK: Routledge.

Fan, Shenggen, Linxiu Zhang, and Xiaobo Zhang. 2004. Reforms, Investment, and Poverty in Rural China. *Economic Development & Cultural Change* 52 (2): 395–421.

Fang, Yu-Hui., Chia-Ying. Li, Ghulam Ali Arain, and Zeeshan Ahmed Bhatti. 2019. How Does Participation and Browsing Affect Continuance Intention in Virtual Communities? An Integration of Curiosity Theory and Subjective Well-Being. *Behaviour & Information Technology* 40 (3): 221–239.

Fanning, Bryan, Trutz Haase, and Neil O'Boyle. 2011. Well-being, Cultural Capital and Social Inclusion: Immigrants in the Republic of Ireland. *International Migration & Integration* 12: 1–24.

Fararo, Thomas J. 2001. *Social Action Systems: Foundation and Synthesis in Sociological Theory*. Westport, CT: Praeger.

Farla, Kristine. 2015. Industrial Policy for Growth. *Journal of Industry, Competition & Trade* 15 (3): 257–282.

Farone, Diane Weise, Tanya R. Fitz Patrick, and Suzanne Y. Bushfield. 2008. Hope, Locus of Control, and Quality of Health among Elder Latina Cancer Survivors. *Social Work in Health Care* 46 (2): 51–70.

Farran, Carol J., Eleanora Keane-Hagerty, Sandra Salloway, Sylvia Kupferer, and Carolyn S. Wilkin. 1991. Finding Meaning: An Alternative Paradigm for Alzheimer's Disease Family Caregivers. *The Gerontologist* 31 (4): 483–489.

Farrington, David P. 2007. Origins of Violent Behavior Over the Life Span. In *The Cambridge Handbook of Violent Behavior and Aggression*, 19–48, ed. Daniel J. Flannery, Alexander T. Vazsonyi and Irwin D. Waldman. Cambridge, UK: Cambridge University Press.

Farrington, David P. 2018. "Origins of Violent Behavior over the Life Span. In *The Cambridge Handbook of Violent Behavior and Aggression*, 3–30, ed. Alexander T. Vazsonyi, David J. Flannery and Matt DeLisi. Cambridge, UK: Cambridge University Press (\113-96).

Fasakin, J.O. 2000. Willingness to Pay for the Services of Commercial Motorcycles in Akure, Nigera. *Cities* 17 (6): 447–452.

Faunce, William A. 2003. *Work, Status, and Self Esteem: Theory of Selective Self Investment*. Lanham, MD: University Press of America.

Fawcett, Barbara. 2012. Mental Health. In *The SAGE Handbook of Social Work*, 515–530, ed. Mel Gray, James Midgley and Stephen A. Webb. London, UK: SAGE.

Fei, Jingyi, and William J. Zakrzewski. 2021. Institutional Imbalance as a Force of Direction: The Implication of Institutional Anomie Theory in Stream Analogy of Lethal Violence. *Sociological Quarterly* 62 (1): 161–186.

Fein, Melvyn L. 2015. *Evolution versus Revolution: The Paradoxes of Social Change*. New Brunswick, NJ: Transaction.

Fein, Melvyn. 2012. *Human Hierarchies: A General Theory*. New Brunswick, NJ: Transaction.

Feingold, Alan. 1994. Gender Differences in Personality: A Meta-Analysis. *Psychological Bulletin* 116 (3): 429–456.

Feldman, David B. 2006. Can Suicide Be Ethical? A Utilitarian Perspective on the Appropriateness of Choosing to Die. *Death Studies* 30: 529–538.

Felson, Richard B., and Maureen C. Outlaw. 2007. The Control Motive and Marital Violence. *Violence & Victims* 22 (4): 387–407.

Femia, Joseph V. 1993. *Marxism and Democracy*. Oxford, UK: Oxford University Press.

Fenwick, Rudy, and Mark Tausig. 1994. The Macroeconomic Context of Job Stress. *Journal of Health & Social Behavior* 35: 266–282.

Fernandes, April. 2018. Red Lights and Handcuffs: The Effect of Arrests on the Fear of Crime. *Social Science Quarterly* 99 (4): 1390–1408.

Fernandes-Jesus, Maria, Maria Luísa Lima, and José-Manuel. Sabucedo. 2020. "Save the Climate! Stop the Oil": Actual Protest Behavior and Core Framing Tasks in the Portuguese Climate Movement. *Journal of Social & Political Psychology* 8 (1): 426–452.

Ferraro, Kenneth F., and Melissa M. Farmer. 1999. Utility of Health Data from Social Surveys: Is There a Gold Standard for Measuring Morbidity. *American Sociological Review* 64: 303–315.

Ferriss, Abbott L. 2002. Studying and Measuring Civility: A Framework, Trends, and Scale. *Sociological Inquiry* 72 (3): 376–392.

Ferssizidis, Patty, Leah M. Adams, Todd B. Kashdan, Christine Plummer, Anjali Mishra, and Joseph Ciarroch. 2010. Motivation for and Commitment to Social Values: The Roles of Age and Gender. *Motivation & Emotion* 34 (4): 354–362.

Fife-Schaw, Chris, and Glynis M. Breakwell. 1990. Predicting the Intention Not to Vote in Late Teenage: A U.K. Study of 17- and 18-Year-Olds. *Political Psychology* 11 (4): 739–755.

Fillieule, Olivier. 2015. Demobilization and Disengagement in a Life Course Perspective. In *Oxford Handbook of Social Movements*, 275–288, ed. Donatella della Porta and Mario Diani. Oxford, UK: Oxford University Press.

Fine, Ben. 2010. *Theories of Social Capital: Researchers Behaving Badly*. London: Pluto.

Finegan, Joan E. 2000. The Impact of Person and Organizational Values on Organizational Commitment. *Journal of Occupation & Organizational Psycholgy* 73 (2): 149–169.

Finegold, Kenneth, and Elaine Kl.. Swigt. 2001. What Works? Competitive Strategies of Major Parties out of Power. *British Journal of Political Science* 31: 95–120.

Fingerman, Karen L., B. Bradford Brown, and Rosemary Blieszner. 2011. Informal Ties across the Life Span: Peers, Consequential Stangers, and People We Encounter in Daily Life. In *Handbook of Life-Development*, 487–511, ed. Karen L. Fingerman, Cynthia A. Berg, Jacque Smith and Toni C. Antonucci. New York: Springer.

Finke, Roger, Matt Bakr, and Christopher P. Scheitle. 2006. Toward Explaining Congregational Giving. *Social Science Research* 35: 620–641.

Finkel, Steven E. 1995. Reciprocal Effects of Participation, and Political Efficacy: A Panel Analysis. *American Journal of Political Science* 29: 891–913.

Finn, Dan. 1999. Job Guarantees for the Unemployed: Lessons from Australian Welfare Reform. *Journal of Social Policy* 28 (1): 53–71.

Finseraas, Henning. 2010. What If Robin Hood is a Social Conservative? How the Political Response to Increasing Inequality Depends on Party Polarization. *Socio-Economic Review* 8: 283–306.

Firebaugh, Glenn, and Matthew B. Schroeder. 2009. Does Your Neighbor's Income Affect Your Happiness? *American Journal of Sociology* 115 (3): 805–831.

Fischer, Agneta, and Catharine Evers. 2013. The Social Basis of Emotion in Men and Women. In *The SAGE Handbook of Gender and Psychology*, 183–215, ed. Michelle K. Ryan and Myla R. Branscombe. London, UK: SAGE.

Fischer, Claude S., Michael Hout, Martin Sanchez Jankowski, Samuel R. Lucas, Ann Swindler, and Kim Voss. 1996. *Inequality by Design: Cracking the Bell Curve Myth*. Princeton, NJ: Princeton University Press.

Fishbein, Martin, and Icek Ajzen. 2010. *Predicting and Changing Behavior: The Reasoned Action Approach*. New York, NY: Psychology.

Fisher, Dana R., and William R. Freudenburg. 2004. Postindustrialization and Environmental Quality: An Empirical Analysis of the Environmental State. *Social Forces* 83 (1): 157–188.

Fisher, Jeffrey D., and William A. Fisher. 2002. The Information-Motivation-Behavioral Skills Model. In *Emerging Theories in Health Promotion Practice and Research Strategies for Improving Public Health*, 40–70, ed. Ralph J. DiClemente, Richard A. Crosby, and Michelle C. Kegler. San Francisco, CA: Jossey-Bass.

Fiske, Susan, Richard R. Lau, and Richard A. Smith. 1990. On the Varieties and Utilities of Political Expertise. *Social Cognition* 8 (1): 31–48.

Fjellvang, Tormod. 2011. Socialization Values, Cultural-Religious Zones and Modernization Theory. *European Sociological Review* 27 (2): 196–211.

Flam, Helena. 2015. Micro-mobilization and Emotions. In *Oxford Handbook of Social Movements*, 264–276, ed. Donatella della Porta and Mario Diani. Oxford, UK: Oxford University Press.

Flanagan, Scott C., and Aie-Rie. Lee. 2000. Value Change and Democratic Reform in Japan and Korea. *Comparative Political Studies* 33 (5): 626–659.

Flap, Henk, and Beate Volker. 2013. Social Capital. In *The Handbook of Rational Choice Social Research*, 220–251, ed. Rafael Wittek, Tom A. H. Snijders, and Victor Nee. Stanford, CA: Stanford University Press.

Flavin, Patrick, and Michael J. Keane. 2011. Life Satisfaction and Political Participation: Evidence from the United States. *Journal of Happiness Studies* 13 (1): 63–78.
Flinkfeldt, Marie. 2020. Respecifying 'Worry': Service and Emotion in Welfare Encounters. *Qualitative Research in Psychology* 17 (3): 372–395.
Flint, Courtney G., and A.E. Luloff. 2007. Community Activeness in Response to Forest Disturbance in Alaska. *Society & Natural Resources* 20 (5): 431–450.
Flogheraiter, Fabio, and Annalisa Pasini. 2009. Self-help Groups and Social Capital: New Directions in Welfare Policies? *Social Work Education* 28 (3): 253–267.
Flogie, Andrej, Andreja Barle Lakota, and Boris Aberšek. 2018. The Psychosocial and Cognitive Influence of ICT on Competences of Stem Students. *Journal of Baltic Science Education* 17 (2): 267–276.
Flores, Rene, and Edward Telles. 2012. Social Stratification in Mexico: Disentangling Color, Ethnicity, and Class. *American Sociological Review* 77 (3): 486–494.
Florida, Richard, and Gary Gates. 2004. Technology and Tolerance: The Importance of Diversity to High-Technology Growth. *Research in Urban Policy* 9: 199–219.
Florida, Richard. 2005. *Cities and the Creative Class*. New York: Routledge.
Flouri, Eirini, and Ann Buchanan. 2002. The Protective Role of Parental Involvement in Adolescent Suicide. *Crisis* 23 (1): 17–22.
Flouri, Eirini. 2003. Parental Socialization in Childhood and Offspring Materialist and Postmaterialist Values in Adult Life. *Journal of Applied Social Psychology* 33 (10): 2106–2122.
Floyd, Donna L., Steven Prentice-Dunn, and Ronald W. Rogers. 2000. A Meta-Analysis of Research on Protection Motivation Theory. *Journal of Applied Social Psychology* 30 (2): 407–429.
Floyd, Kory. 2019. *Affectionate Communication in Close Relationships*. Cambridge, UK: Cambridge University Press.
Fontenot, Nancy A. 1993. Effects of Training in Creativity and Creative Problem Solving Upon Business People. *Journal of Social Psychology* 133 (1): 11–22.
Forester, Summer. 2019. Protecting Women, Protecting the State: Militarism, Security Threats, and Government Action on Violence against Women in Jordan. *Security Dialogue* 50 (6): 475–492.
Forgas, Joseph P., Janos Laszlo, Istvan Siklaki, and Stephanie J. Moylan. 1995. Images of Politics: A Multidimensional Analysis of Implicit Representations of Political Parties in a Newly Emerging Democracy. *European Journal of Social Psychology* 25: 481–496.
Forsyth, James. 2003. *Psychological Theories of Religion*. Upper Saddle River, NJ: Prentice Hall.
Forte, Jams A. 2001. *Theories for Practice: Symbolic Interactionist Translations*. Lanham, MD: University Press of America.
Foschi, Renato, and Marco Lauriola. 2014. Does Sociability Predict Civic Involvement and Political Participation? *Journal of Personality & Social Psychology* 106 (2): 339–357.
Foshee, Vangie A., Thad S. Benefield, Heath Luz McNaughton. Reyes, Susan T. Ennett, Robert Faris, Ling-Yin. Chang, Andrea Hussong, and Chirayath M. Suchindran. 2013. The Peer Context and the Development of the Perpetration of Adolescent Dating Violence. *Journal of Youth & Adolescence* 42 (4): 471–486.
Foss, Jeffrey E. 2009. *Beyond Environmentalism: A Philosophy of Nature*. Hoboken, NJ: Wiley.
Foster, Dennis M., Alex Braithwaite, and David Sobek. 2013. There Can Be No Compromise: Institutional Inclusiveness, Fractionalization and Domestic Terrorism. *British Journal of Political Science* 43 (3): 541–557.
Foster, Vivien, Susana Mourato, David Pearce, and Ece Ozdemiroglu. 2001. *The Price of Virtue: The Economic Value of the Charitable Sector*. Cheltenham, UK: Edward Elgar.
Fragnon, Julien. 2019. 'We Are at War': Continuity and Rupture in French Anti-terrorist Discourse. *Media, War & Conflict* 12 (2): 131–152.
Fraley, R. Chris., Marie E. Heffernan, Amanda M. Vicary, and Claudia Chloe Brumbaugh. 2011. The Experiences in Close Relationships-Relationship Structures Questionnaire: A Method for Assessing Attachment Orientations Across Relationships. *Psychological Assessment* 23 (3): 615–625.

Francesconi, Marco, and Katrin Golsch. 2005. "The Process of Globalization and Transitions to Adulthood in Britain. In *Globalization, Uncertainty and Youth in Society*, 249–276, ed. Hans-Peter Blossfeld, Erik Klijzing, Melinda Mills and Karin Kurz. London: Routledge.

Frank, Christine, Christopher G., Davis, and Frank J. Elgar. 2014. Financial Strain, Social Capital, and Perceived Health during Economic Recession: A Longitudinal Survey in Rural Canada. *Anxiety, Stress, & Coping* 27 (4): 422–438.

Frank, David John, and John M. Meyer. 2002. The Profusion of Individual Roles and Identities in the Postwar Period. *Sociological Theory* 20 (1): 86–105.

Frank, Lawrence Douglas, Brian E. Saelems, Ken E. Powell, and James E. Chapman. 2007. Stepping towards Causation: Do Built Environments or Neighborhood and Travel Preferences Explain Physical Activity, Driving, and Obesity. *Social Science & Medicine* 65: 1898–1914.

Franklin, Leanne. 2012. *Gender*. Houndmills, UK: Palgrave.

Franklin, Mark N. 1996. Electoral Participation. In *Comparing Democracies: Elections and Voting in Global Perspective*, 216–235, ed. Lawrence LeDuc, Richard G. Niemi, and Pippa Norris. Thousand Oaks, CA: Sage.

Franks, Bradley, Adrian Bangerter, and Martin W. Bauer. 2013. Conspiracy Theories as Quasi-Religious Mentality: An Integrated Account from Cognitive Science, Social Representations Theory, and Frame Theory. *Frontiers in Psychology* 4: 424.

Frantz, Gilda. 2013. Aging and Individuation. *Psychological Perspectives* 56 (2): 129–132.

Franzen, Axel, and Dominik Hangartner. 2006. Social Networks and Labour Market Outcomes: The Non-monetary Benefits of Social Capital. *European Sociological Review* 22 (4): 353–368.

Franzen, Axel, and Dominikus Vogl. 2013. Acquiescence and the Willingness to Pay for Environmental Protection: A Comparison of the ISSP, WVS, and EVS. *Social Science Quarterly* 94 (3): 637–659.

Franzese, Alexis T. 2013. Motivation, Motives, and Individual Agency. In *Handbook of Social Psychology*, 281–318, ed. John Delamater and Amanda Ward. Dordrecht, Netherlands: Springer.

Franzini, Luisa, Margaret Cauphy, William Spears, and Maria Eugenia Fernandez. Esquer. 2005. Neighborhood Economic Conditions, Social Processes, and Self-rated Health in Low-Income Neighborhoods in Texas: A Multilevel Latent Variables Model. *Social Science & Medicine* 61: 1135–1150.

Franzosi, Roberto. 1998. Narrative Analysis or Why (and How) Sociologists Should be Interested in Narrative. *Annual Review of Sociology* 24: 517–554.

Frazer, Elizabeth. 1999. *The Problems of Communitarian Politics: Unity and Conflict*. Oxford, UK: Oxford University Pres.

Frazier, Kathryn E., and Rachel Joffe Falmagro. 2014. Empowered Victims? Women's Contradictory Positions on the Discourse of Violence Prevention. *Feminism & Psychology* 24 (4): 479–499.

Frazier, Leslie D., Frederick L. Newman, and James Jaccard. 2007. Psychosocial Outcomes in Later Life: A Multivariate Model. *Psychological & Aging* 22 (4): 676–689.

Frederick, David A., Gaganjyot Sandhu, Patrick J. Morse, and Viren Swami. 2016. Correlates of Appearance and Weight Satisfaction in a U.S. National Sample: Personality, Attachment Style, Television Viewing, Self-Esteem, and Life Satisfaction. *Body Image* 17: 191–203.

Fredrickson, Barbara L. 2008. Promoting Positive Affect. In *The Science of Subjective Well-Being*, 449–468, ed. Michael Eid and Randy J. Larsen. New York: Guilford.

Fredrickson, Barbara L., and Marcial F. Losada. 2005. Positive Affect and the Complex Dynamics of Human Flourishing. *American Psychologist* 60 (7): 678–686.

Fredrickson, Barbara. 2001. The Role of Positive Emotions in Positive Psychology: The Broaden-and-Build Theory of Positive Emotions. *American Psychologist* 56 (3): 218–226.

Freeman, Richard B. 2004. What, Me Vote? In *Social Inequality*, 703–728, ed. Kathryn M. Neckerman. New York: Russell Sage.

Frei, Andreas, Kay W. Axhausen, and Timo Ohnmacht. 2009. Mobilities and Social Network Geography: Size and Spatial Disperson: The Zurich Case Study. In *Mobilities and Inequality*, 99–120, ed. Timo Ohnmacht, Hanja Maksim, and Marfred Max Bergman. Farnham, UK: Ashgate.

Frenk, Steven M., Yang Claire Yang, and K.C. Land. 2013. Assessing the Significance of Cohort and Period Effects in Hierarchical Age-Period-Cohort Models: Applications to Verbal Test Scores and Voter Turnout in U.S. Presidential Elections. *Social Forces* 92 (1): 221–248.

Freund, Alexandra M. 2006. Age-Differential Motivational Consequences of Optimization Versus Compensation Focus in Younger and Older Adults. *Psychology & Aging* 21 (2): 240–252.

Freund, Anat. 2005. Work Attitudes of Social Workers Across Three Sectors of Welfare Organization: Public, for-Profit, and Third Sector. *Journal of Social Service Research* 31 (3): 69–92.

Frey, Bruno S., and Alois Stutzer. 2000. Happiness, Prospers in Democracy. *Journal of Happiness Studies* 1: 79–102.

Frey, Bruno S., and Alois Stutzer. 2005. Happiness Research: State and Prospects. *Review of Social Economy* 62 (2): 207–228.

Frey, Bruno S., Christine Benesch, and Alois Stutzer. 2007. Does Watching TV Make Us Happy. *Journal of Economic Psychology* 28: 283–313.

Frey, R. Scott., and Fengxiang Song. 1997. Human Well-Being in Chinese Cities. *Social Indicators Research* 42: 77–101.

Fric, Pavol. 2008. The Uneasy Partnership of the State and the Third Sector in the Czech Republic. In *The Third Sector in Europe: Prospects and Challenges*, 230–253, ed. Stephen P. Osborne. Oxon, UK: Routledge.

Fridberg, Torben and Olli Kangas. 2008b. Social Capital. In *Nordic Social Attitudes in a European Perspective*, 65–85, ed. Heikki Ervasti, Torben Fridberg, Mikael Hjerm, and Kristen Ringdal. Cheltenham, UK: Edward Elgar.

Friedman, Mark D. 2011. *Nozick's Libertarian Project: An Elaboration and Defense*. London: Continuum.

Friedman, Maurice. 1992. *Religion and Psychology: A Dialogical Approach*. New York: Paragon House.

Fritsche, Immo, Eva Jonas, Daniela Niesta Kayser, and Nicholas Koranyi. 2010. Existential Threat and Compliance with Pro-environmental Norms. *Journal of Environmental Psychology* 30: 67–79.

Frohlich, Katherine L., Louise Potvin, Patrick Chabot, and Ellen Corin. 2002. A Theoretical and Empirical Analysis of Context: Neighborhoods, Smoking and Youth. *Social Science & Medicine* 54: 1401–1417.

Fromhold-Eisebith, Martina. 2004. "Innovative Milieu, and Social Capital—Complementary or Redundant Concepts of Collaboration-Based Regional Development? *European Planning Studies* 12 (6): 747–765.

Frosh, Stephen. 1991. *Identity Crisis: Modernity, Psychoanalysis and the Self*. Houndmills, England: Macmillan.

Frye, Victoria. 2007. The Informal Social Control of Intimate Partner Violence against Women: Exploring Personal Attitudes and Perceived Neighborhood Social Cohesion. *Journal of Community Psychology* 35 (8): 1001–1018.

Fuchs, Christian. 2008. *Internet and Society: Social Theory in the Information Age*. New York: Routledge.

Fuchs, Martin. 2015. Processes of Religious Individualisation: Stocktaking and Issues for the Future. *Religion* 45 (3): 330–343.

Fuchs, Stephan. 2001. What Makes Sciences Scientific? In *Handbook of Sociological Theory*, 21–35, ed. Jonathan H. Turner. New York: Kluwer.

Fujii, Satoshi, Ryuichi Kitamura, and Hideo Suda. 2004. Contingent Valuation Method Can Increase Procedural Justice. *Journal of Economic Psychology* 25: 877–889.

Fujisawa, Yoshikazu, Tsuyashi Hamano, and Shogo Takegama. 2009. Social Capital and Perceived Health in Japan: An Ecological and Multilevel Analysis. *Social Science & Medicine* 69: 500–505.

Fujita, Frank. 2008. The Frequency of Social Comparison and Its Relation to Subjective Well-Being." In *The Science of Subjective Well-Being*, 239–257, ed. Michael Eid and Randy J. Larsen. New York: Guilford.

Fukuyama, Francis. 1992. *The End of History and the Last Man*. London: Penguin (D16.8F85).

Fukuyama, Francis. 1995. *Trust: The Social Virtues and the Creation of Prosperity*. New York: Free Press.

Fukuyama, Francis. 2003. *Our Posthuman Future: Consequences of the Biotechnology Revolution*. London: Profile.

Fukuyama, Francis. 2018b. Why National Identity Matters. *Journal of Democracy* 29 (4): 5–15 (\99–304).

Fullwood, Chris. 2019. Impression Management and Self-presentation Online. In *The Oxford Handbook of Cyberpsychology*, 45–56, ed. Alison Attrill-Smith, Chris Fullwood, Melanie Keep and Daria J. Kuss. Oxford, UK: Oxford University Press.

Fumagalli, Matteo. 2007. Framing Ethnic Minority Mobilisation in Central Asia: The Cases of Uzbeks in Kyrgyzstan and Tajikistan. *Europe-Asia Studies* 59 (4): 567–590.

Fung, Anthony, and Eric Ma. 2000. Formal vs. Informal Use of Television and Sex-Role Stereotyping in Hong Kong. *Sex Roles* 42 (1/2): 57–81.

Fung, Helene H., and Siu-Kei. Ng. 2006. Age Differences in the Sixth Personality Factor: Age Differences in Interpersonal Relatedness among Canadians and Hong Kong Chinese. *Psychology & Aging* 21 (4): 810–814.

Fung, Helene H., Derek M. Isaacowitz, Alice Y. Lu, Heather A. Wadlinger, Deborah Goren, and Hugh R. Wilson. 2008. Age-Related Positivity Enhancement Is Not Universal: Older Chinese Look away from Positive Stimuli. *Psychology & Aging* 23 (2): 440–446.

Furnham, Adrian, and Helen Cheng. 2000. Lay Theories of Happiness. *Journal of Happiness Studies* 1: 227–246.

Furnham, Adrian. 1997. Lay Theories of Work Stress. *Work Stress* 11 (1): 68–78 (\d12-6.21).

Furstenberg, Frank F., Jr., and Mary Elizabeth Hughes. 1995. Social Capital and Successful Development among At-risk Youth. *Journal of Marriage and the Family* 57 (3): 580–592.

Fyall, Rachel, and Beth Gazley. 2015. Applying Social Role Theory to Gender and Volunteering in Professional Associations. *Voluntas: International Journal of Voluntary & Nonprofit Organizations* 26 (1): 288–314.

Gadsden, Vivian L. 2008. The Arts and Education: Knowledge Generation, Pedagogy, and the Discourse of Learning. *Review of Research in Education* 32 (1): 29–61.

Gadzella, Bernadette M., and Elizabeth Penland. 1995. Is Creativity Related to Scores on Critical Thinking. *Psychological Reports* 77: 817–818.

Gagne, Marylene, and Edward L. Deci. 2005. Self-determination Theory and Work Motivation. *Journal of Organizational Behavior* 26: 331–362.

Gahlawat, Neha, Rina S. Phogat, and Subhash C. Kundu. 2019. Evidence for Life Satisfaction among Dual-Career Couples: The Interplay of Job, Career, and Family Satisfaction in Relation to Workplace Support. *Journal of Family Issues* 40 (18): 2893–2921.

Gaines, N. Susan., and James C. Garand. 2010. Morality Equality or Locality: Analyzing the Determinants of Same-Sex Marriage. *Political Research Quarterly* 63 (3): 553–567.

Gainsborough, Juliet F. 2008. A Tale of Two Cities: Civic Culture and Public Policy in Miami. *Journal of Urban Affairs* 30 (4): 419–435.

Gaitan-Rossi, Pablo, and Ce. Shen. 2018. Fear of Crime in Mexico: The Impacts of Municipality Characteristics. *Social Indicators Research* 135 (1): 373–399.

Gall, Terry Lynn, Claire Charbonneau, Neil Henry Clarke, Karen Grant, Anjali Joseph, and Lisa Shouldice. 2005. Understanding the Nature and Role of Spirituality in Relation to Coping and Heath: A Conceptual Framework. *Canadian Psychology* 46 (2): 88–104.

Gallego, Aina. 2009. Where Else Does Turnout Decline Come From? Education, Age, Generation and Period Effects in Three European Countries. *Scandinavian Political Studies* 32 (1): 23–44.

Gallie, Duncan, and Serge Paugam. 2000. The Experience of Unemployment in Europe: The Debate. In *Welfare Regimes and the Experience of Unemployment in Europe*, 1–22, ed. Duncan Gallie and Serge Paugam. Oxford, UK: Oxford University Press.

Gallie, Duncan, Michael White, Yuan Cheng, and Mark Tomlinson. 1998. *Restructuring the Employment Relationship*. Oxford, UK: Clarendon.

Gallie, Duncan. 2004. Unemployment, Marginalization Risks and Welfare Policy. In *Resisting Marginalization: Unemployment Experience and Social Policy and the European Union*, 1–33, ed. Duncan Gallie. Oxford, UK: Oxford University Press.

Galston, William A. 2005. *The Practice of Liberal Pluralism.* Cambridge, UK: Cambridge University Press.

Galtung, Johan. 2005. Meeting Basic Needs: Peace and Development. In *The Science of Well-Being*, 475–501, ed. Felica A. Huppert, Nick Baylis and Barry Keverne. Oxford, UK: Oxford University Press.

Gamble, Hilary. 2019. Acquiescing to the Script: A Panel Study of College Students' Sexual Media Habits, Endorsement of Heteronormative Scripts, and Their Hesitance toward Resisting Unwanted Hookups. *Sex Roles* 80 (11–12): 707–723.

Gan, Yiqun, Ying Liu, and Yiling Zhang. 2004. Flexibility Coping Resources to Severe Acute Respiratory Syndrome-related and Daily Life Stressful Events. *Asian Journal of Social Psychology* 77: 55–66.

Gandjour, Afschin, and Karl Wilhelm Lauterbach. 2003. Utilitarian Theories Reconsidered: Common Misconceptions, More Recent Developments, and Health Policy Implications. *Health Care Analysis* 11 (3): 229–244.

Ganesh, Shiv, and Kirstie McAllum. 2010. Well-Being as Discourse: Potentials and Problems for Studies of Organizing and Health Inequalities. *Management Communication Quarterly* 24 (3): 491–498.

Gani, Azmat, and Michael D. Clemes. 2006. Information and Communications Technology: A Non-income Influence on Economic Well Being. *International Journal of Social Economics* 33 (9): 649–663.

Gans, Chaim. 1992. *Philosophical Anarchism and Political Disobedience.* Cambridge, UK: Cambridge Univesity Press.

Gao, Qin, Irwin Garfinkel, and Fuhua Zhai. 2009. Anti-poverty Effectiveness of the Minimum Living Standard Assistance Policy in Urban China. *Review of Income & Wealth* 55 (S1): 630–655.

Garcia, Danilo, Fredrik Ryberg, Ann-Christine Andersson. Arnten, Trevor Archer, and Ali Al Nima. 2017. Autonomy and Responsibility as a Dual Construct. *International Journal of Police Science & Management* 19 (3): 195–204.

Gardner, Philip D., and Neal Schmitt. 2001. The Racial Digital Divide: Motivational, Affective and Cognitive Correlates of Internet Use. *Journal of Applied Social Psychology* 31 (10): 2019–2046.

Garfin, Dana Rose, E. Alison Holman, and Roxane Cohen Silver. 2015. Cumulative Exposure to Prior Collective Trauma and Acute Stress Responses to the Boston Marathon Bombings. *Psychological Science* 26 (6): 675–683.

Garred, Michelle G. 2013. The Power of Mindsets: Bridging, Bonding, and Associational Change in Deeply Divided Mindanao. *Journal of Civil Society* 9 (1): 21–40.

Gartman, David. 1998. Postmodernism or the Cultural Logic of Post-Fordism? *Sociological Quarterly* 39 (1): 119–137.

Gattino, Silvia, Chiara Rollero, and Norma De Piccoli. 2015. The Influence of Coping Strategies on Quality of Life from a Gender Perspective. *Applied Research in Quality of Life* 10 (4): 689–701.

Gaus, Gerald. 2011. *The Order of Public Reason: A Theory of Freedom and Morality in Diverse and Bounded World.* New York: Cambridge University Press.

Gavrilova, Natalia S., Victoria G. Semyonova, Galina N. Evdokashkina, and Leonid Gavrilov. 2000. The Response of Violent Mortality to Economic Crisis in Russia. *Population Research & Policy Review* 19: 397–419.

Gay, David A., and John P. Lynxwiler. 2009. The Impact of Race on Denominational Variations in Social Attitudes: The Issue and Its Dimensions. *Sociological Spectrum* 30 (1): 110–127.

Gears, Andrew L., and G. Daniel Lassiter. 2002. Effects of Affective Expectations on Affective Experience: The Moderating Role of Optimism-pessimism. *Personality & Social Psychology Bulletin* 28 (8): 1026–1039.

Gebbia, Melissa I., and Andrea Honigsfeld. 2012. Learner Developmental Outcomes and Intellectual Styles. In *Handbook of Intellectual Styles: Preferences in Cognition, Learning, and Thinking*, 251–271. New York: Springer.

Geerts, Robbe, Frédéric. Vandermoere, and Stijn Oosterlynck. 2020. The Functionality of Dissimilarity: Pro-environmental Behavior Through Heterogenous Networks. *Social Sciences* 9 (12): 221–316.

Gehring, Kai. 2013. Who Benefits from Economic Freedom? Unraveling the Effect of Economic Freedom on Subjective Well-Being. *World Development* 50: 74–90.

Gelade, Garry A. 1999. Creativity in Conflict: The Personality of the Commercial Creative. *Journal of Genetic Psychology* 158 (1): 67–78.

Gelissen, John. 2002. *Worlds of Welfare, Worlds of Consent? Public Opinion on the Welfare State.* Leiden, Netherlands: Brill.

Gelles, Richard J. 2007. Family Violence. In *The Cambridge Handbook of Violent Behavior and Aggression*, 403–417, ed. Daniel J. Flannery, Alexander T. Vazsonyi and Irwin D. Waldman. Cambridge, UK: Cambridge University Press.

George, Login S., and Crystal L. Park. 2013. Are Meaning and Purpose Distinct? An Examination of Correlates and Predictors. *Journal of Positive Psychology* 8 (5): 365–375.

George, Paul, Gordon Lawrence, and Donna Bushnell. 1998. *Handbook for Middle School Teaching.* New York: Longman.

Gerrard, Gary. 2002. *The New Social Contract: Beyond Liberal Democracy.* Lanham, MD: University Press of America.

Gershuny, Jonathan. 2000. *Changing Times: Work and Leisure in Postindustrial Society.* Oxford, UK: Oxford University Press.

Gerstorf, Denis, Jacqui Smith, and Paul B. Baltes. 2006. A Systemic-Wholistic Approach to Differential Aging: Longitudinal Findings from the Berlin Aging Study. *Psychology & Aging* 21 (4): 645–663.

Gerteis, Joseph, and Mike Savage. 1998. The Salience of Class in Britain and American: A Comparative Analysis. *British Journal of Sociology* 49 (2): 252–274.

Gerxhani, Klarita, and Arthur Schram. 2006. Tax Evasion and Income Source: A Comparative Experimental Study. *Journal of Economic Psychology* 27: 402–422.

Gerxhani, Klarita. 2012. I Am Not Alone: Understanding Public Support for The Welfare State. *International Sociology* 27 (6): 768–787.

Geser, Hans. 1998. Toward a One-Dimensional Ideological Culture: Evidence from Swiss Local Parties. In *The New Political Culture*, 235–259, ed. Terry Nichols Clark and Vincent Hoffmann-Martinot. Boulder, CO: Westview.

Geys, Benny. 2012. Association Membership and Generalized Trust: Are Connections between Associations Losing their Value? *Journal of Civil Society* 8 (1): 1–15.

Ghazali, Ezlika M., Dilip S. Mutum, and Nanang Ariswibowo. 2018. Impact of Religious Values and Habit on an Extended Green Purchase Behaviour Model. *International Journal of Consumer Studies* 42 (6): 639–654.

Gibbins, John R. 1998. Postmodernism, Poststructuralism and Social Policy. In *Postmodernity and the Fragmentation of Welfare*, 31–48, ed. John Carter. London, Routledge.

Gibbins, John R., and Bo Reimer. 1999. *The Politics of Postmodernity: An Introduction to Contemporary Politics and Culture.* London, UK: SAGE.

Gibson, James L. 2013. Measuring Political Tolerance and General Support for Pro-civil Liberties Policies. *Public Opinion Quarterly* 77 (S1): 45–68.

Giddens, Anthony. 1984. *The Constitution of Society: Outline of the Theory of Structuration.* Berkeley, CA: University of California Press.

Giele, Janet Zollinger. 2008. Homemaker or Career Woman: Life Course Factors and Racial Influences Among Middle Class. *American Journal of Comparative Family Studies* 39 (3): 393–411.

Giffords, Elissa D. 2009. An Examination of Organizational Commitment and Professional Commitment and the Relationship to Work Environment, Demographic and Organizational Factors. *Journal of Social Work* 9 (4): 386–404.

Gil de Zuniga, K. Homero, Matthew Barnidge, and Andrés Scherman. 2017. "Social Media Social Capital, Offline Social Capital, and Citizenship: Exploring Asymmetrical Social Capital Effects. *Political Communication* 34 (1): 44–68.

Gilberbloom, John I., and John Po. Markham. 1995. The Impact of Homeownership on Political Beliefs. *Social Forces* 73 (4): 1589–1607.

Gilbert, Jeremy. 2008. Against the Commodification of Everything. *Cultural Studies* 22 (5): 551–566.

Giles, Howard, and Gordan Soliz. 2015. Communication Accommodation theory: A Situated Framework for Relational, Family, and Intergroup Dynamics. In *Engaging Theories in Interpersonal Communication: Multiple Perspectives*, 161–173, ed. Dawn O. Braithwaite and Paul Schrodt. Thousand Oaks, CA: SAGE.

Gill, Anthony. 2004. Weber in Latin America: Is Protestant Growth Enabling the Consolidation of Democratic Capitalism? *Democratization* 11 (4): 42–65.

Gil-Lacruz, Marta, María I. Saz-Gil, and Ana I. Gil-Lacruz. 2019. Benefits of Older Volunteering on Wellbeing: An International Comparison. *Frontiers in Psychology* 10: 2647.

Gillath, Omri, Phillip R. Shaver, Mario Mikulineer, Rachel E. Nitzberg, Ayelet Erez, and Marinus H. van Izendoorr. 2005. Attachment, Caregiving, and Volunteering: Placing Volunteerism in an Attachment-theoretical Framework. *Personal Relationships* 12: 425–466.

Gilley, Bruce. 2009. *The Right to Rule: How States Win and Lose Legitimacy*. New York: Columbia University Press.

Gillham, Patrick F., Nathan C. Lindstedt, Bob Edwards, and Erik W. Johnson. 2019. The Mobilizing Effects of Economic Threats and Resources on the Formation of Local Occupy Wall Street Protest Groups in 2011. *Sociological Perspectives* 62 (4): 433–454.

Ginev, Dimitri. 2018. *Toward a Hermeneutic Theory of Social Practices: Between Existential Analytic and Social Theory*. Abingdon, UK: Routledge.

Giridharan, R., S.S.Y. Lau, S. Ganesan, and B. Givoni. 2007. Urban Design Factors Influencing Heat Island Intensity in High-Rise High-Density Environments of Hong Kong. *Building & Environment* 42: 3669–3684.

Gitterman, Alex. 2005. Building Mutual Support in Groups. *Social Work with Groups* 28 (3/4): 91–106.

Gitto, Lara, Yong-Hwan. Noh, and Antonio Rodríguez Andrés. 2020. Have Lifestyle Factors Led to Perceiving a Higher Level of Stress? Implications for Mental Health Policies from an Econometric Analysis for South Korea. *Journal of Asian Public Policy* 13 (3): 257–276.

Giugni, Marco, and Maria T. Grasso. 2019. *Street Citizens: Protest Politics and Social Movement, Activism in the Age of globalization*. Cambridge, UK: Cambridge University Press.

Glaeser, Andreas. 2016. Action in Society: Reflexively Conceptualizing Activities. In *Handbook of Contemporary Sociological Theory*, 63–83, ed. Seth Abrutyn. Cham, Switzerland: Springer.

Glaeser, Edward L., and Joshua D. Gottlieb. 2006. Urban Resurgence and the Consumer City. *Urban Studies* 43 (8): 1275–1299.

Glaeser, Edward L., and Joshua D. Gottlieb. 2009. The Wealth of Cities: Agglomeration Economies and Spatial Equilibrium in the United States. *Journal of Economic Literature* 47 (4): 983–1028.

Glaeser, Edward l., David Laibson, and Bruce Sacerdote. 2002. An Economic Approach to Social Capital. *Economic Journal* 112: F437–F458.

Glanville, Jennifer L. 1999. Political Socialization or Selection? Adolescent Extracurricular Participation and Political Activity in Early Adulthood. *Social Science Quarterly* 80 (2): 279–290.

Glasson, Benjamin. 2015. Subversive Rearticulation between Radicalism and Reform: The Case of Ecologism. *Journal of Political Ideologies* 20 (2): 156–178.

Glendinning, Anthony, Mark Nuttall, Leo Hendry, Marion Kloep, and Sheila Wood. 2003. Rural Communities and Well-Being: A Good Place to Grow Up? *Sociological Review* 51 (1): 129–156.

Glennie, Paul. 1998. Consumption, Consumerism, and Urban Form: Historical Perspectives. *Urban Studies* 35 (5/6): 927–951.

Glicken, Morley D. 2004. *Using the Strengths Perspective in Social Work Practice: A Positive Approach for the Helping Professions*. Boston, MA: Pearson.

Godoy, Richardo A., Michael Gurven, Elizabeth Byron, Victoria Reyes-Garcia, James Keough, Vincent Vadez, David Witkie, William R. Leonard, Lillian Apaza, Tomas Huanca, and Eddy Perez. 2004. Do Markets Worsen Economic Inequalities? Kuznets in the Bush. *Human Ecology* 32 (3): 339–364.

Godoy, Richardo, Victoria Reyes-Garcia, Tomas Huanca, William R. Leonard, Ramona G. Olvera, Jonathan Bauchet, Zhao Ma, Jonathan St, Marisa Miodowski John, Oscar Zapata Rios, Vincent Vadez, and Craig Seyfried. 2007. The Role of Community and Individuals in the Formation of Local Capital. *Human Ecology* 35: 709–721.

Goel, M. Lal. 1980. Conventional Political Participation. In *Participation in Social and Political Activities: A Comprehensive Analysis of Political Involvement, Expressive Leisure Time, and Helping Behavior*, 108–132, ed. David Horton Smith, Jacqueline Macaulay and Associates. San Francisco, CA: Jossey-Bass.

Goerres, Achim. 2007. Why are Older People More Likely to Vote? The Impact of Ageing on Electoral Turnout in Europe. *British Journal of Politics & International Relations* 9 (1): 90–121.

Goetz, Edward G. 2011. Where Have All the Towers Gone? The dismantling of Public Housing in U.S. Cities. *Journal of Urban Affairs* 33 (3): 267–287.

Goetz, Stephan J., Mark D. Partridge, Dan S. Rickman, and Shibalee Majumdar. 2011. Sharing the Gains of Local Economic Growth: Race-to-the-Top Versus Race-to-the Bottom Economic Development. *Environment & Planning C: Government & Policy* 29: 428–456.

Goidel, Robert K., and Todd G. Shields. 1994. The Vanishing Marginals, the Bandwagon, and the Mass Media. *Journal of Politics* 56 (3): 802–810.

Goldberg, Abbie E., and Mauren Perry-Jenkins. 2004. Division Off Labor and Working-Class Women's Well-Being Across the Transition to Parenthood. *Journal of Family Psychology* 18 (1): 225–236.

Goldberg, Gertrude Schaffner. 2012. Economic Inequality and Economic Crisis: A Challenge for Social Workers. *Social Work* 57 (3): 211–224.

Goldberg, Steven. 1993. *Why Men Rule: A Theory of Male Dominance*. Chicago, IL: Open Court.

Goldblatt, David. 1996. *Social Theory and the Environment*. Cambridge, UK: Polity.

Goldstein, Kenneth M., and Matthew Holleque. 2010.Getting up off the Canvass: Rethinking the Study of Mobilization. In *The Oxford Handbook of American Elections and Political Behavior*, 577–594, ed. Jan E., Leighley. Oxford, UK: Oxford University Press.

Gomez-Roman, Cristina, and Jose-Manuel. Sabucedo. 2014. The Importance of Political Context: Motives to Participate in a Protest Before and After the Labor Reform in Spain. *International Sociology* 29 (6): 546–564.

Gonzalez, Oscar, David P. MacKinnon, and Felix B. Muniz. 2021. Extrinsic Convergent Validity Evidence to Prevent Jingle and Jangle Fallacies. *Multivariate Behavioral Reseacrh* 56 (1): 3–19.

Gore, Jonathan S. 2014. The Influence of Close Others in Daily Goal Pursuit. *Journal of Social & Personal Relationships* 31 (1): 71–92.

Goren, Paul. 2000. Political Expertise and Principal Thought. *Political Research Quarterly* 53 (1): 117–136.

Goren, Paul. 2005. Party Identification and Core Political Values. *American Journal of Political Science* 49 (4): 881–896.

Gorman, Ryan R. 2010. War and the Virtues in Aquinas's Ethical Thought. *Journal of Military Ethics* 9 (3): 245–261.

Gorsuch, Richard L. 1994. Toward Motivational Theories of Intrinsic Religious Commitment. *Journal of the Scientific Study of Religion* 33 (4): 315–325.

Gorsuch, Richard L., and William R. Miller. 1999. Assessing Spirituality. In *Integrating Spirituality into Treatment: Resources for Practitioners*, 47–64, ed. William R. Miller. Washington, DC: American Psychological Association.

Gotzsche-Astrup, Oluf. 2020. Pathways to Violence: Do Uncertainty and Dark World Perceptions Increase Intentions to Engage in Political Violence? *Behavioral Sciences of Terrorism & Political Aggression* 13 (2): 142–159.

Goulding, Christina. 2000. The Commodification of the Past, Postmodern Pastiche, and the Search for Authentic Experiences at Contemporary Heritage Attraction. *European Journal of Marketing* 34 (7): 835–853.

Gountas, John, Sandra Gountas, Robert A. Reeves, and Lucy Moran. 2012. Desire for Fame: Scale Development and Association with Personal Goals and Aspirations. *Psychology & Marketing* 29 (9): 680–689.

Graddy, Elizabeth, and Lili Wang. 2009. Community Foundation Development and Social Capital. *Nonprofit & Voluntary Sector Quarterly* 30 (1): 392–412.

Graham, Carol, and Stefano Pettinato. 2002. *Happiness and Hardship: Opportunity and Insecurity in New Market Economies*. Washington, DC: Brookings.

Graham, Carol, Soumya Chattopadhyay, and Mario Picon. 2010. The Easterlin and Other Paradoxes: Why Both Sides of the Debate May Be Correct. In *International Differences in Well-Being*, 247–288, ed. Ed Diener, John F. Helliwell and Daniel Kahneman. New York: Oxford University Press.

Graham, Gordon. 2008. *Ethics and International Relations*. Malden, MA: Blackwell.

Graham, Rlspeth, Peggy Tee, Brenda S.A.. Yeoh, and Susan Levy. 2002. Reproducing the Asian Family across the Generations: Tradition, Gender, and Expectations in Singapore. *Asia-Pacific Population Journal* 17 (2): 61–86.

Granzin, Kent L., and Janeen E. Olsen. 1998. Americans' Choice of Domestic over Foreign Products: A Matter of Helping Behavior? *Journal of Business Research* 43: 39–54.

Granzin, Kent L., and Lois M. Haggard. 2000. An Integrative Explanation for Quality of Life: Development and Test of a Structural Model. In *Advances in Quality of Life Theory and Research*, 31–64, ed. Ed Diener and Don R. Rahtz. Dordrecht, Netherlands: Kluwer Academic.

Grasner, Aviva Twersky. 2013. Lonnie Athens Revisited: The Social Construction of Violence. *Aggression & Violent Behavior* 18: 281–285.

Grasso, Maria T. 2014. Age, Period and Cohort Analysis in A Comparative Context: Political Generations and Political Participation Repertoires in Western Europe. *Electoral Studies* 33: 63–76.

Grasso, Maria T., and Marco Giugni. 2016. Protest Participation and Economic Crisis: The Conditioning Role of Political Opportunities. *European Journal of Political Research* 55: 663–680.

Grayling, A.C. 2013. *The God Argument: The Case Against Religion and for Humanism*. New York: Bloomsbury.

Graziano, William O., and Renee M. Tobin. 2009. Agreeableness. In *Handbook of Individual Differences in Social Behavior*, 46–61, ed. Mark R. Leary and Rick H. Hoyle. New York, NY: Guilford.

Grcic, Joseph. 2000. *Ethics and Political Theory*. New York: Lanham.

Green, Andy, John Preeton, and Ricardo Sabates. 2003. Education, Equality and Social Cohesion: A Distributional Approach. *Compare* 33 (4): 453–470.

Green, Eva G. T., Lotte Thomsen, Jim Sidanius, Christian Staerklé, and Polina Potanina. 2009. Reactions to Crime as a Hierarchy Regulating Strategy: The Moderating Role of Social Dominance Orientation. *Social Justice Research* 22 (4): 416–436.

Green, Michael J., Colin A. Espie, and Michael Benzeval. 2014. Social Class and Gender Patterning of Insomnia Symptoms and Psychiatric Distress: A 20-year Prospective Cohort Study. *BMC Psychiatry* 14 (1): 263–280.

Greenberg, David F. 1999. Punishment, Division of Labor and Solidarity. *Advances in Criminological Theory* 8: 283–361.

Greenberg, Joshua. 2004. Tories, Teachers and the Media Politics of Education Reform: News Discourse and the 1997 Ontario Teachers' Strike. *Journalism Studies* 5 (3): 353–371.

Greene, Roberta R. 1999. *Human Behavior Theory and Social Work Practice*. New York: Aldine de Gruyter.

Greenfield, Liah, and Jonathan Eastwood. 2005. Nationalism in Comparative Perspective. In *The Handbook of Political Sociology: States, Civil Societies, and Globalization*, 247–265, ed. Thomas Janoski, Robert Alford, Alexander Hicks, and Mildred A. Schwartz. Cambridge, UK: Cambridge University Press.

Greenfield, Patricia M. 2009. Linking Social Change and Developmental Change: Shifting Pathways of Human Development. *Developmental Psychology* 45 (2): 401–418.

Grenier, Paola, and Karen Wright. 2006. Social Capital in Britain. *Policy Studies* 27 (1): 27–53.

Gries, Peter Hays, H. Michael Crowson, and Todd Sandel. 2010. The Olympic Effect on American Attitudes Towards China Beyond Personality, Ideology, and Media Exposure. *Journal of Contemporary China* 19 (64): 213–231.

Griffin, Christine, Andrew Bengry-Howell, Sarah Riley, Yvette Morey, and Isabelle Szmigin. 2018. We Achieve the Impossible: Discourses of Freedom and Escape at Music Festivals and Free Parties. *Journal of Consumer Culture* 18 (4): 477–496.

Griffiths, Mark. 2000. Excessive Internet Use: Implications for Sexual Behavior. *CyberPsychology & Behavior* 3 (4): 537–552.

Grimes, Marcia. 2006. Organizing Consent: The Role of Procedural Fairness in Political Trust and Compliance. *European Journal of Political Research* 45: 285–315.

Grimmelikhuijsen, Stephan G., and Albert J. Meijer. 2015. Does Twitter Increase Perceived Police Legitimacy? *Public Administration Review* 75 (4): 598–607.

Grindstaff, Laura, and Joseph Turow. 2006. Video Culture: Television Sociololgy in the New TV Age. *Annual Review of Sociology* 32: 103–125.

Groot, Wim, and Henriette Maassen Van Den. Brink. 2003. Sympathy and the Value of Health. *Social Indicators Research* 61: 97–120.

Groot, Wim, Henriette Maassen van den Brink, and Bernard van Praag. 2007. The Compensating Income Variation of Social Capital. *Social Indicators Research* 82: 189–207.

Grootaert, Christiaan, and Thierry van Bastelaer. 2002. *Understanding and Measuring Social Capital: A Multidisciplinary Tool for Practitioners*. Washington, DC: World Bank.

Gross, Michael L. 1995. Moral Judgment, Organizational Incentives and Collective Action: Participation in Abortion Politics. *Political Research Quarterly* 48 (3): 507–534.

Gross, Neil. 2009. A Pragmatist Theory of Social Mechanisms. *American Sociological Review* 74 (3): 358–379.

Gross, Revital, and Shuli Brammli-Greenberg. 2004. Evaluating the Effect of Regulatory Prohibitions against Risk Selection by Health Status on Supplemental Insurance Ownership in Israel. *Social Science & Medicine* 58: 1609–1622.

Grover, Chris. 2011. Social Protest in 2011: Material and Cultural Aspects of Economic Inequalities. *Sociological Research Online* 16 (4): 18.

Growiec, Katarzyna, and Jakub Growiec. 2010. Bridging Social Capital and Individual Earnings: Evidence for an Inverted U. *Social Indicators Research* 127 (2): 601–631.

Grych, John H., and Kristen M. Kinsfogel. 2010. Exploring the Role of Attachment Style in the Relation between Family Aggression and Abuse in Adolescent Dating Relationships. *Journal of Aggression, Maltreatment & Trauma* 19 (6): 624–640.

Grzywacz, Joseph G., and David M. Almeida. 2008. Stress and Binge Drinking: A Daily Process Examination of Stressor Pile-up and Socioeconomic Stress on Affect Regulation. *International Journal of Stress Management* 15 (4): 364–380.

Grzywacz, Joseph G., and Nadine F. Marks. 2000. Reconceptualizing the Work-family Interface: An Ecological Perspective on the Correlates of Positive and Negative Spillover Between Work and Family. *Journal of Occupational Health Psychology* 5 (1): 111–126.

Guardia, Joan, and Enric Pol. 2002. A Critical Study of Theoretical Models of Sustainability through Structural Equation Systems. *Environment & Behavior* 34 (1): 137–149.

Guardiola, Jorge, and Teresa Garcia-Munoz. 2011. Fulfilment of Basic Needs from a Subjective Point of View in Rural Guatemala. *International Journal of Social Welfare* 20 (4): 393–403.

Gudmundsdottir, Dora Gudrun. 2013. The Impact of Economic Crisis on Happiness. *Social Indicators Research* 110 (3): 1083–1101.

Guillen, Laura, Lluis Coromina, and Willem E. Saris. 2011. Measurement of Social Participation and Its Place in Social Capital Theory. *Social Indicators Research* 100 (2): 331–350.

Guillen-Royo, Monica. 2008. Consumption and Subjective Wellbeing: Exploring Basic Needs, Social Comparison, Social Integration and Hedonism in Peru. *Social Indicators Research* 89: 535–555.

Guimond, Serge, Armand Chatard, and Fabio Lorenzi-Cloldi. 2013. The Social Psychology of Gener Across Cultures. In *The SAGE Handbook of Gender and Psychology*, 216–233, ed. Michelle K. Ryan and Myla R. Branscombe. London, UK: SAGE.

Guisan, M.-C. 2009. Government Effectiveness, Education, Economic Development and Well-Being: Analysis of European Countries in Comparison with the United States and Canada, 2000–2007. *Applied Econometrics & International Development* 9 (1): 39–55.

Guiso, Luigi, Paloa Sapienza, and Luigi Zingales. 2004. The Role of Social Capital in Financial Development. *American Economic Review* 94 (3): 526–536.

Gundersen, Craig, and James P. Ziliak. 2004. Poverty and Macroeconomic Performance across Space, Race, and Family Structure. *Demography* 41 (1): 61–86.

Guneratne, Arjun. 2008. The Cosmopolitanism of Environmental Activists in Sri Lanka. *Nature + Culture* 3 (1): 98–114.

Gunter, Barrie. 2013. The Study of Online Relationships and Dating. In *The Oxford Handbook of Internet Studies*, 173–194, ed. William H. Dutton. Oxford, UK: Oxford University Press.

Guo, Baorong, and Jin Huang. 2005. Marital and Sexual Satisfaction in Chinese Families: Exploring the Moderating Effects. *Journal of Sex & Marital Therapy* 31: 21–29.

Guo, Xiaohui, Seth J. Schwartz, and Brian E. McCabe. 2008. Aging, Gender, and Self: Dimensionality and Measurement Invariance Analysis in Self-construal. *Self & Identity* 7 (1): 1–24.

Gurak, Douglas T., and Mary M. Kritz. 2000. The Interstate Civilization of U.S. Immigrants: Individual and Contextual Determinants. *Social Forces* 78 (3): 1017–1039.

Gutmann, David. 1987. *Reclaimed Powers: Toward a New Psychology of Men and Women in Later Life*. New York: Basic.

Guven, Cahit, and Bent E. Sorensen. 2012. Subjective Well-Being: Keeping up with the Perception of the Joneses. *Social Indicators Research* 109: 439–469.

Guven, Cahit. 2012. Reversing the Question: Does Happiness Affect Consumption and Savings Behavior? *Journal of Economic Psychology* 33: 701–717.

Ha, Eunyoung. 2012. Globalization, Government Ideology and Income Inequality in Development Countries. *Journal of Politics* 74 (2): 541–557.

Haapanen-Niemi, Nina, Seppo Miilunpalo, Ilkka Nuori, Matti Pasanen, and Pekka Oja. 1999. The Impact of Smoking, Alcohol Consumption, and Physical Activity on Use of Hospital Services. *American Journal of Public Health* 989 (5): 691–698.

Haar, Jarrod, Albert Sune, Marcello Russo, and Ariane Ollier-Malaterre. 2019. A Cross-National Study on the Antecedents of Work?Life Balance from the Fit and Balance Perspective. *Social Indicators Research* 142 (1): 261–282.

Habb, M.A.R. 2011. *Literary Criticism from Plato to the Present: An Introduction*. Chichester, UK: Wiley.

Hadden, Wilbur C., Gregory Pappas, and Abdul Qayyum Khan. 2003. Social Stratification Development and Health in Pakistan: An Empirical Exploration of Relationships in Population-based National Health Examination Survey Data. *Social Science & Medicine* 57: 1863–1874.

Haddorff, David W. 2000. Religion and the Market Opposition, Absorption, or Ambiguity. *Review of Social Economy* 58 (4): 483–503.

Hadjar, Andreas, and Robin Samuel. 2015. Does Upward Social Mobility Increase Life Satisfaction? A Longitudinal Analysis Using British and Swiss Panel Data. *Research in Social Stratification and Mobility* 39: 48–58.

Hafner, By Rebecca, David Elmes, Daniel Read, and Mathew P. White. 2019. Exploring the Role of Normative, Financial and Environmental Information in Promoting Uptake of Energy Efficient Technologies. *Journal of Environmental Psychology* 63: 26–35.

Hagan, John, Susanne Rippl, Klaus Boehnke, and Hans Merkens. 1999. The Interest in Evil: Hierarchic Self-interest and Right-wing Extremism among East and West German Youth. *Social Science Research* 28: 162–183 (\a00-7.27).

Hagerty, Michael R. 1998. Unifying Livability and Comparison Theory: Cross-national Time-Series Analysis of Life Satisfaction. *Social Indicators Research* 47: 343–356.

Hagerty, Michael R. 2000. Social Comparison of Income in One's Community: Evidence from National Surveys of Income and Happiness. *Journal of Personality & Social Psychology* 78 (4): 764–771.

Hagerty, Michael R. 2003. Was Life Better in the Good Old Days? Intertemporal Judgments of Life Satisfaction. *Journal f Happiness Studies* 4: 115–139.

Hagger, Martin S., and Kyra Hamilton. 2018. Motivational Predictors of Students' Participation in out-of-School Learning Activities and Academic Attainment in Science: An Application of the Trans-Contextual Model Using Bayesian Path Analysis. *Learning & Individual Differences* 67: 232–244.

Hagopian, Frances. 2000. Political Development, Revisited. *Comparative Political Studies* 33 (6/7): 880–911.

Hagquist, Curt, and David Andrich. 2004. Measuring Subjective Health among Adolescents in Sweden. *Social Indicators Research* 68: 201–220.

Hahn, Elisabeth, Wendy Johnson, and Frank M. Spinath. 2013. Beyond the Heritability of Life Satisfaction: The Roles of Personality and Twin-Specific Influences. Journal of Research in Personality 47: 757–767 (\116-231).

Haidt, Jonathan. 2012. *The Righteous Mind: Why Good People Are Divided by Politics and Religion.* New York: Pantheon.

Hair, M., K.V. Renaud, and J. Ramsay. 2007. The Influence of Self-esteem and Locus of Control on Perceived Email-Related Stress. *Computers in Human Behavior* 23 (6): 2791–2803.

Haivas, Simona, Joeri Hofmans, and Roland Pepermans. 2012. Self-determination Theory as a Framework for Exploring the Impact of the Organizational Context on Volunteer Motivation. *Nonprofit & Voluntary Sector Quarterly* 41 (6): 1195–1214.

Haiven, Max. 2014. *Cultures of Finacialization: Fictitious Capital in Popular Culture and Everyday Life.* Houndmills, UK: Palgrave.

Hakhverdian, Armen, and Quinton Mayne. 2012. Institutional Trust, Education, and Corruption: A Micro-Macro Interactive Approach. Journal of Politics 74 (3): 1739–1750 (\88-265).

Hakim, Catherine. 2006. Women, Careers, and Work-Life Preferences. *British Journal of Guidance & Counselling* 34 (3): 279–294.

Halasz, Jacek. 2018. About the Right to Be Ill. *Medicine, Health Care, & Philosophy* 21 (1): 113–123.

Hall, Deborah L., David C. Matz, and Wendy Wood. 2010. Why Don't We Practice What We Preach? A Meta-Analytic Review of Religious Racism. *Personality & Social Psychology Review* 14 (1): 126–139.

Hall, Todd W., and Keith J. Edwards. 2002. The Spiritual Assessment Inventory: A Theistic Model and Measurement for Assessing Spiritual Development. *Journal of the Scientific Study of Religion* 41 (2): 341–357.

Haller, Max, and Markus Hadler. 2006. How Social Relations and Structures Can Produce Happiness and Unhappiness: An International Comparative Analysis. *Social Indicators Research* 75: 169–216.

Haller, Max. 2002. Theory and Method in the Comparative Study of Values: Critique and Alternative to Inglehart. *European Sociological Review* 1892: 139–158.

Hallerod, Bjorn. 2006. Sour Grapes: Relative Deprivation Adaptive Preferences and the Measurement of Poverty. *Journal of Social Policy* 35 (3): 371–390.

Halvari, Ann E., Hallgeir Halvari Munster, Gunnar Bjornebeckk, and Edward L. Deci. 2010. Motivation and Anxiety for Dental Treatment: Testing a Self-determination Theory, Model of Oral Self-care Behavior and Dental Clinic Attendance. *Motivation & Emotion* 34: 15–33.

Halvari, Anne E. Munster, and Hallgeir Halvari. 2006. Motivational Predictors of Change in Oral Health: An Experimental Test of Self-determination Theory. *Motivation & Emotion* 30: 295–306.

Hamann, Darla J., and Nicole T. Foster. 2014. An Exploration of Job Demands, Job Control, Stress, and Attitudes in Public, Nonprofit, and for-Profit Employees. *Review of Public Personnel Administration* 34 (4): 332–355.

Hamermesh, David S. 2019. *Spending Time: The Most Valuable Resource*. New York, NY: Oxford University Press.

Hamilton, Andy. 2008. J.S. Mill's Elitism: A Classical Liberal's Response to the Rise of Democracy. In *Anti-democratic Thought*, 49–66, ed. Erich Kofmel. Exeter, UK: Imprint Academic.

Hammond, Matthew D., Chris G. Sibley, and Nickola C. Overall. 2014. The Allure of Sexism. *Social Psychological & Personality Science* 5 (4): 422–429.

Hammond, Michelle, Jeanette N. Cleveland, John W. O'Neill, Robert S. Stawski, and April Jones Tate. 2015. Mediators of Transformational Leadership and the Work-Family Relationship. *Journal of Managerial Psychology* 30 (4): 454–469.

Hampton, Keith N. 2016. Why Is Helping Behavior Declining in the United States but Not in Canada? Ethnic Diversity, New Technologies, and Other Explanations: The Decline of Helping Behavior. *City & Community* 15 (4): 380–399.

Han, Sang-Jin., and Young-Hee. Shim. 2010. Redefining Second Modernity for East Asia: A Critical Assessment. *British Journal of Sociology* 61 (3): 465–488.

Han, Sungil, and Nadine M. Connell. 2020. The Effects of School Police Officers on Victimization, Delinquency, and Fear of Crime: Focusing on Korean Youth. *International Journal of Offender Therapy & Comparative Criminology* 65 (12): 1356–1372.

Han, Ziqiang, Ivan Y. Sun, and Hu. Rong. 2017. Social Trust, Neighborhood Cohesion, and Public Trust in the Police in China. *Policing* 40 (2): 380–394.

Hanewinkel, Reiner, and Gudrun Wiborg. 2006. Initial Evaluation of a Real-World Self-help Smoking Cessation Programme for Adolescents and Young Adults. *Addictive Behavior* 31: 1939–1945.

Hansen, Eric R., and Andrew Tyner. 2019. Educational Attainment and Social Norms of Voting. *Political Behavior* 43 (2): 711–735.

Hansen, Thomas, Britt Slagsvold, and Reidun Ingebretsen. 2012. The Strains and Gains of Caregiving: An Examination of the Effects of Providing Personal Care to a Parent on a Range of Indicators of Psychological Well-Being. *Social Indicators Research* 114 (2): 323–343.

Hansen-Nord, Nete, Sloth Mette Skar, Finn Kjaerulf, Juan Almendarez, Sergio Bohr, Oscar Sosa, Julio Castro, Anne-Marie Nybo. Andersen, and Jens Modvig. 2014. Social Capital and Violence in Poor Urban Areas of Honduras. *Aggression & Violent Behavior* 19 (6): 643–648.

Hanser, Amy. 2010. Uncertainty and The Problem of Value: Consumers, Culture and Inequality in Urban China. *Journal of Consumer Culture* 10 (3): 307–332.

Hanson, Rochelle F., Genelle K. Sawyer, Angela M. Begle, and Prace S. Hubel. 2010. The Impact of Crime Victimization on Quality of Life. *Journal of Traumatic Stress* 23 (2): 189–197.

Hantula, Donald A. 2012. Consumer Are Foragers, Not Rational Actors: Toward a Behavioral Ecology of Consumer Choice. In *Handbook of Developments in Consumer Behavior*, 549–577, ed. Victoria Wells and Gordon Foxall. Cheltenham, UK: Elgar.

Hardy, Bruce W., Kathleen Hall Jamieson, and Kenneth Winneg. 2009. Wired to Fact: The Role of the Internet in Identifying Deception during the 2004 US. Presidential Campaign. In *Routledge Handbook of Internet Politics*, 139–143, ed. Andrew Chadwick and Philip N. Howard. Abingdon, UK: routledge.

Harkema, Beverly. 2022. Autonomy in Philanthropy: A Model for Nonprofit Organizations. *Public Integrity*.

Harkhess, Susan. 2007. Social and Political Indicators of Human Well-being. In *Human Well-Being: Concept and Measurement*, 88–112, ed. Mark McGillivray. Houndmills, UK: Palgrave.

Harper, Charles L., and Kevin T. Leicht. 2011. *Exploring Social Change: America and the World*. Boston, MA: Prentice Hall.

Harring, Niklas. 2014. Corruption, Inequalities and The Perceived Effectiveness of Economic Pro-environmental Policy Instruments: A European Cross-National Study. *Environmental Science & Policy* 39: 119–128.

Harrington, Maureen, and Simone Fullagar. 2013. Challenges for Active Living Provision in an Era of Healthism. *Journal of Policy Research in Tourism, Leisure & Events* 5 (2): 139–157.

Harris, David R. 2001. Why Are Whites and Blacks Averse to Black Neighbors? *Social Science Research* 30: 100–116.

Harris, Frederick C. 1994. Something Within: Religion as a Mobilizer of African-American Political Activism. *Journal of Politics* 56 (1): 42–68.

Harrison, Denis, and Murielle Laberge. 2002. Innovation, Identification and Resistance: The Social Construction of an Innovation Network. *Journal of Management Studies* 59 (4): 497–521.

Harrison, Neil, and Richard Waller. 2018. Challenging Discourses of Aspiration: The Role of Expectations and Attainment in Access to Higher Education. *British Educational Research Journal* 44 (5): 914–938.

Hart, Joshua, and Jamie L. Goldenberg. 2008. A Terror Management Perspective on Spirituality and the Problem of the Body. In *Existential and Spiritual Issues in Death Attitudes*, 91–113, ed. Adrian Tomer, Grafton T. Eliason and Paul T.P. Wong. New York: Lawrence Erlbaum.

Hart, Randle J. 2008. Practicing Birchism: The Assumption and Limits of Idiocultural Coherence in Framing Theory. *Social Movement Studies* 7 (2): 121–147.

Harter, James K., and Raksha Arora. 2010. The Impact of Time Spent Working and Job Fit onn Well-being around the World. In *International Differences in Well-Being*, 398–435, ed. Ed Diener, John F. Helliwell and Daniel Kahneman. New York: Oxford University Press.

Harvey, David. 2016. *The Ways of the World*. New York, NY: Oxford University Press.

Harvie, Peter, and Tonoy Manzis. 2011. Interpreting Multi-agency Partnership: Ideology, Discourse and Domestic Violence. *Social & Legal Studies* 26 (1): 79–85.

Harwood, Jake, Miles Hewstone, Stefania Padini, and Alberto Voci. 2005. Grandparent-Grandchild Contact and Attitudes Toward Older Adults: Moderators and Mediators Effects. *Personality & Social Psychology Bulletin* 31 (3): 393–406.

Hasenfeld, Yeheskel, and Lisa Evans Powell. 2004. The Role of Non-profit Agencies in the Provision of Welfare-to-Work Services. *Administration in Social Work* 28 (3/4): 91–110.

Haskell, John. 2001. *Direct Democracy or Representative Government? Dispelling the Populist Myth*. Boulder, CO: Westview.

Hassan, Riaz. 1995. *Suicide Explained: The Australian Experience*. Victoria, Australia: Melbourne University Press.

Hassenzahl, Marc, Annika Wiklund-Engblom, Anette Bengs, Susanne Hägglund, and Sarah Diefenbach. 2015. Experience-Oriented and Product-Oriented Evaluation: Psychological Need Fulfillment, Positive Affect, and Product Perception. *International Journal of Human-Computer Interaction* 31 (8): 530–544.

Hassler, Tabea, Özden Melis Uluğ, Mariska Kappmeier, and Giovanni A. Travaglino. 2021. Intergroup Contact and Social Change: An Integrated Contact-Collective Action Model. *Journal of Social Issues* 77 (1): 217–241.

Hatch, Stephani L. 2007. Economic Stressors, Social Integration, and Drug Use among Women in an Inner-city Community. *Journal of Drug Issues* 37: 257–280.

Hatcher, William, and Augustine Hammond. 2018. Nonprofit Economic Development Organizations and the Institutional Arrangement of Local Economic Development. *Journal of Public & Nonprofit Affairs* 4 (1): 21–40.

Hathaway, Andrew D. 2003. Cannabis Effects and Dependency Concerns in Long-term Frequent Users: A Missing Piece of the Public Health Puzzle. *Addiction Research & Theory* 11 (6): 441–458.

Hattery, Angela, and Earl Smith. 2012. *The Social Dynamics of Family Violence*. Boulder, CO: Westview.

Hatzidimitriadou, Eleni. 2002. Political Ideology, Helping Mechanisms and Empowerment of Mental Health Self-help/Mutual Aid Groups. *Journal of Community & Applied Social Psychology* 12: 271–285.

Hausermann, Silja. 2006. Changing Coalitions in Social Policy Reforms: The Politics of New Social Needs and Demands. *Journal of European Social Policy* 16 (1): 5–21.

Haustein, Jorg. 2021. Development as a Form of Religious Engineering? Religion and Security in Development Discourse. *Religion* 51 (1): 19–39.

Havinga, Tetty. 2002. The Effects and Limits of Anti-discrimination Law in the Netherlands. *International Journal of the Sociology of Law* 30: 75–90.

Haybron, Daniel M. 2008. Philosophy and the Science of Subjective Well-being. In *The Science of Subjective Well-Being*, 17–43, ed. Michael Eid and Randy J. Larsen. New York: Guilford.

Haynes, Jo., and Raphaël Nowak. 2021. We Were Never Cool: Investigating Knowledge Production and Discourses of Cool in the Sociology of Music. *British Journal of Sociology* 72 (2): 448–462.

Hayo, Bernd. 2004. Public Support for Creating a Market Economy in Eastern Europe. *Journal of Comparative Economics* 32: 720–744.

Hays, Bernd, and Wolfgang Seifert. 2003. Subjective Economic Well-Being in Eastern Europe. *Journal of Economic Psychology* 24: 329–348.

Hays, R. Allen., and Alexandra M. Kogl. 2007. Neighborhood Attachment, Social Capital Building, and Political Participation: A Case Study of Low- and Moderate-Income Residents of Waterloo, Iowa. *Journal of Urban Affairs* 29 (2): 181–205.

He, Jia, Dave Bartram, Ilke Inceoglu, and Fons J. R. van de Vijver. 2014. Response Styles and Personality Traits: A Multilevel Analysis. *Journal of Cross-Cultural Psychology* 45 (7): 1028–1045.

Headey, Bruce, and Markus M. Grabka. 2007. Pets and Human Health in Germany and Australia: National Longitudinal Results. *Social Indicators Research* 80 (2): 297–311.

Headey, Bruce, Fu. Na, and Richard Zheng. 2001. Pet Dogs' Benefit Owners' Health: A Natural Experiment in China. *Social Indicators Research* 87: 481–493.

Healy, Geraldine, and Gill Kirton. 2013. The Early Mobilization of Women Union Leaders: A Comparative Perspective. *British Journal of Industrial Relations* 51 (4): 709–732.

Heaphy, Brian. 2007. *Late Modernity and Sociual Change: Reconstructing Social and Personal Life*. Abingdon, UK: Routledge.

Heath, Anthony, Roger Jowell, John Curtice, Geoff Evans, Julia Field, and Sharon Witherspoon. 1991. *Understanding Political Change: The British Voter 1964–1987*. Oxford: Pergamon.

Heatherington, Marc J., and Suzanne Globetti. 2002. Political Trust and Racial Policy Preferences. *American Journal of Political Science* 46 (2): 253–295.

Hechter, Michael. 2004. From Class to Culture. *American Journal of Sociology* 110 (2): 400–445.

Hedstrom, Peter. 2005. *Dissecting the Social: On the Principles of analytical Sociology*. Cambridge, UK: Cambridge University Press.

Hegre, Håvard., John R. Oneal, and Bruce Russett. 2010. Trade Does Promote Peace: New Simultaneous Estimates of the Reciprocal Effects of Trade and Conflict. *Journal of Peace Research* 47 (6): 763–774.

Heidemeier, Heike, and Ursula M. Staudinger. 2012. Self-evaluation Process in Life Satisfaction: Uncovering Measurement Non-equivalence and Age-Related Differences. *Social Indicators Research* 105: 39–61.

Heinrich, Carolyn J. 2000. Organizational Form and Performance: An Empirical Investigation of Nonprofit and for-Profit Job-Training Service Providers. *Journal of Policy Analysis & Management* 19 (2): 233–261.

Heinz, Walter R. 2002. Self-socialization and Post-traditional Society. *Advances in Life Course Research* 7: 41–64.

Heise, David R. 1999. Controlling Affective Experience Interpersonally. *Social Psychology Quarterly* 62 (1): 4–16.

Heitmeyer, Wilhelm, and Reimund Anhut. 2008. Disintegration, Recognition, and Violence: A Theoretical Perspective. *New Directions for Youth Development* 119: 25–37.

Held, Virginia. 2008. *How Terrorism is Wrong: Morality and Political Violence*. New York: Oxford University Press.

Heller, Agnes. 2009. *A Theory of Feelings*. Lanham, MD: Lexington.

Heller, Patrick. 2020. The Age of Reaction: Retrenchment Populism in India and Brazil. *International Sociology* 35 (6): 590–609.

Hellerod, Bjorn. 2004. What I need and What the Poor Deserve: Analyzing the Gap between the Minimum Income Needed for Oneself and the View of an Adequate Norm for Social Assistance. *Social Forces* 83 (1): 35–60.

Hellevik, Ottar. 2003. Economy, Values and Happiness in Norway. *Journal of Happiness Studies* 4: 243–283.

Hellinger, Moshe. 2008. The Criticism of Democracy in Rabbi E.E.M. Shach's Thought. In *Anti-democratic Thought*, 123–139, ed. Erich Kofmel. Exeter, UK: Imprint Academic.

Helliwell, John F. 2003. Do Borders Matters for Social Capital? Economic Justice and Civic Culture in U.S. States and Canadian Provinces. In *Economic Implications of Social Cohesion*, 19–42, ed. Lars Osberg. Toronto, Canada: University of Toronto Press.

Helliwell, John F. 2006. Well-Being and Social Capital: Does Suicide Pose a Puzzle? *Social Indicators Research* 81: 455–496.

Helliwell, John F., and Robert D. Putnam. 2005. The Social Context of Well-Being. In *The Science of Well-Being*, 435–459, ed. Felica A. Huppert, Nick Baylis and Barry Keverne. Oxford, UK: Oxford University Press.

Helliwell, John F., Chris Burrington-Leigh, Anthony Harris, and Haifang Huang. 2010. International Evidence on the Social Context of Well-Being. In *International Differences in Well-Being*, 291–327, ed. Ed Diener, John F. Helliwell and Daniel Kahneman. New York: Oxford University Press.

Helson, Ravenna, and Sanjay Srivastava. 2001. Three Paths of Adult Development: Conservers, Seekers, and Achievers. *Journal of Personality & Social Psychology* 80 (6): 995–1010.

Henderson, Sheila J. 2004. Product Inventors and Creativity: The Finer Dimensions of Enjoyment. *Creativity Research Journal* 16 (2–3): 293–312.

Hendry, Leo B., Janet Shucksmith, John G. Love, and Anthony Glendinning. 1993. *Young People's Leisure and Lifestyles*. London, UK: Routledge.

Hengeveld, Rob. 2012. *Wasted World: How Our Consumption Challenges the Planet*. Chicago, IL: Univeristy of Chicago Press.

Hennessy, Michael, Michael X. Delli, Michael B. Carpini, Kenneth Winneg Blank, and Kathleen Hall Jamieson. 2015. Using Psychological Theory to Predict Voting Intentions. *Journal of Community Psychology* 43 (4): 466–483.

Henretta, John C. 1987. Family Transitions, Housing Market Context and First Home Purchase by Young Married Households. *Social Forces* 26: 520–536.

Henricks, Thomas S. 2012. *Selves, Societies, and Emotions: Understanding the Pathways of Experience*. Boulder, CO: Paradigm.

Henry, Carolyn S., Andy L. Stephenson, Michelle Fryer Hanson, and William Harzett. 1993. Adolescent Suicide and Families: An Ecological Approach. *Adolescence* 28 (110): 291–308.

Herd, Pamela, James S. House, and Robert F. Schoeni. 2008. Income Support Policies and Health Among the Elderly. In *Making American Healthier: Social and Economic Policy as Health Policy*, 97–121, ed. Robert F. Schoeni, James S. House, George A. Kaplan, and Harold Pollack. New York: Russell Sage.

Herda-Rapp, Ann. 2003. The Social Construction of Local School Violence Threats by the News Media and Professional Organizations. *Sociological Inquiry* 73 (4): 545–574.

Herian, Mitchel N., Louis Tay, Joseph A. Hamm, and Ed Diener. 2014. Social Capital, Ideology, and Health in the United States. *Social Science & Medicine* 105: 30–37.

Herman, Lise Esther. 2021. Can Partisans Be Pluralist? A Comparative Study of Party Member Discourse in France and Hungary. *British Journal of Politics & International Relations* 23 (1): 22–42.

Hess, Thomas M., Nicole L. Osowski, and Christina M. Leclerc. 2005. Age and Experience Influences on the Complexity of Social Inferences. *Psychology & Aging* 20 (3): 447–459.

Hewitt, John P. 1991. *Self and Society: A Symbolic Interactionist Social Psychology*. Boston, MA: Allyn and Bacon.

Heyman, Richard E., and Amy M. Smith Slep. 2007. Therapeutic Treatment Approaches to Violent Behavior. In *The Cambridge Handbook of Violent Behavior and Aggression*, 602–617, ed. Daniel J. Flannery, Alexander T. Vazsonyi and Irwin D. Waldman. Cambridge, UK: Cambridge University Press.

Hicks, Darrin, Carl Larson, Christopher Nelson, David Olds, and Erik Johnston. 2008. The Influence of Collaboration on Program Outcomes: The Colorado Nurse-Family Partnership. *Evaluation Review* 32 (5): 453–477.

Hicks, Sarah, and Sarah Brown. 2013. Perceptions of Risk: A Review of the Effects of Individual and Community-Level Variables on Perceptions of Risk. *International Review of Victimology* 19 (3): 249–267.

Higgins, E. Tony. 1998. Promotion and Prevention: Regulatory Focus as Motivational Principle. *Advances in Experimental Social Psychology* 30: 1–46.

Higgins-Desbiolles, Freya. 2010. The Elusiveness of Sustainability in Tourism: The Culture-Ideology of Consumerism and Its Implications. *Tourism & Hospitality Research* 10 (2): 116–129.

Hightower, Eugene. 1988. Four Illustrations of Healthy Personality: A Prescription for Living the Good Life. *Journal of Clinical Psychology* 44: 527–535.

Hilbert, Richard A. 1986. Anomie and the Moral Regulation of Reality: The Durkheimian Tradition in Modern Relief. *Sociological Theory* 4: 1–19.

Hill, Charles T. 2019. *Intimate Relationships Across Cultures: A Comparative Study*. Cambridge, UK: Cambridge University Press.

Hill, Peter C., and Kenneth I. Pargament. 2003. Advances in the Conceptualization and Measurement of Religion and Spirituality: Implications for Physical and Mental Health Research. *American Psychologist* 58 (1): 64–74.

Hill, Sarah E., and David M. Buss. 2008. Evolution and Subjective Well-Being. In *The Science of Subjective Well-Being*, 62–93, ed. Michael Eid and Randy J. Larsen. New York: Guilford.

Himes, Kenneth R. 2007. Consumerism and Christian Ethics. *Theological Studies* 68: 132–153.

Hintsanen, Mirka, Markus Jokela, Laura Pulkki-Råback, Jorma S. A. Viikari, and Liisa Keltikangas-Järvinen. 2010. Associations of Youth and Adulthood Body-Mass Index and Waist-Hip Ratio with Attachment Styles and Dimensions. *Current Psychology* 29 (3): 257–271.

Hipp, John R., George E. Tita, and Lyndsay N. Boggess. 2009. Iintergroup and Intragroup Violence: Is Violent Crime an Expression of Group Conflict or Social Disorganization? *Criminology* 47 (2): 521–564.

Hirono, Miwa. 2013. Three Legacies of Humanitarianism in China. *Disasters* 37 (S2): S202–S220.

Hirsch, Eric L. 1993. Protest Movements and Urban Theory. *Research in Urban Sociology* 3: 159–180.

Hjelm, Titus. 2014. Religion, Discourse and Power: A Contribution Towards a Critical Sociology of Religion. *Critical Sociology* 40 (6): 855–872.

Ho, Jeffrey C. F. and Ryan Ng. 2022. Perspective-Taking of Non-Player Characters in Prosocial Virtual Reality Games: Effects on Closeness, Empathy, and Game Immersion. *Behaviour & Information Technology*.

Ho, Lok San. 1998. A Model of Human Nature and Personal Development. *Journal of Socio-Economics* 27 (2): 271–277.

Hobfoll, Steven E., and Jeremiah A. Schumm. 2002. Conservation of Resources Theory: Application to Public Health Promotion. In *Emerging Theories in Health Promotion Practice and Research Strategies for Improving Public Health*, 285–312, ed. Ralph J. DiClemente, Richard A. Crosby, and Michelle C. Kegler. San Francisco, CA: Jossey-Bass.

Hobolt, Sara Binzer, and Robert Klemmemsen. 2005. Responsive Government? Public Opinion and Government Policy Preferences in Britain and Denmark. *Political Studies* 53: 379–402.

Hocking, Elise C., Raluca M. Simons, and Renata J. Surette. 2016. Attachment Style as a Mediator Between Childhood Maltreatment and the Experience of Betrayal Trauma as an Adult. *Child Abuse & Neglect* 52: 94–101.

Hodges, Ernest V.E.., and David G. Perry. 1999. Personal and Interpersonal Antecedents and Consequences of Victimization by Peers. *Journal of Personality & Social Psychology* 76 (4): 677–685.

Hodson, Randy. 1996. Dignity in the Workplace under Participative Management: Alienation and Freedom Revisited. *American Sociological Review* 61 (5): 719–738.

Hodson, Randy. 1997. Individual Voice on the Shop Floor: The Role of Unions. *Social Forces* 75 (4): 1183–1212.

Hoekstra, Erin. 2021. "Not a Free Version of a Broken System:" Medical Humanitarianism and Immigrant Health Justice in the United States. *Social Science & Medicine* 285: 114287.

Hoffman, Kristi L., and John N. Edwards. 2004. An Integrated Theoretical Model of Sibling Violence and Abuse. *Journal of Family Violence* 19 (3): 185–200.

Hoffman, Louis, Nathaniel Granger, Lisa Vallejos, and Michael Moats. 2016. An Existential-Humanistic Perspective on Black Lives Matter and Contemporary Protest Movements. *Journal of Humanistic Psychology* 56 (6): 595–611.

Hoffman, Michael, and Hannah E. Bagdanov. 2020. Defensive Minoritarianism: Support for Democracy among Lebanese Christians. *Religion, State & Society* 48 (5): 378–397.

Hofmann, Wilhelm, Roy F. Baumeister, Georg FÖRster, and Kathleen D. Vohs. 2012. Everyday Temptations: An Experience Sampling Study of Desire, Conflict, and Self-control. *Journal of Personality & Social Psychology* 102 (6): 1318–1335.

Hofstetter, C. Richard., David Barker, James T. Smith, Gina M. Zari, and Thomas A. Ingrassia. 1999. Information, Misinformation, and Political Talk Radio. *Political Research Quarterly* 52 (2): 353–369.

Hogg, Michael A., and Janice Adelman. 2013. Uncertainty-Identity Theory: Extreme Groups, Radical Behavior, and Authoritarian Leadership. *Journal of Social Issues* 69 (3): 436–454.

Holbrook, Allyson L., Melanie C. Green, and Jon A. Krosnick. 2003. Telephone versus Face-to-face Interviewing of National Probability Samples with Long Questionnaires: Comparisons of Respondent Satisficing and Social Desirability Response Bias. *Public Opinion Quarterly* 67: 79–125.

Holcombe, Randall G. 1985. *An Economic Analysis of Democracy*. Carbondale, IL: Southern Illinois University Press.

Holliday, Ian, and Waikeung Tam. 2001. Social Capital in Hong Kong. *East Asia: An International Quarterly* 19 (1/2): 144–170.

Hollyer, james R., B. Peter Rosendorff, and James Raymond Vreeland. 2018. *Information, Democracy, and Autonomy: Economic Transparency and Political (In)stability*. Cambridge, UK: Cambridge University Press.

Holman, E. Alison., Rachel G. Lucas-Thompson, and Lu. Tammy. 2011. Social Constraints, Genetic Vulnerability, and Mental Health Following Collective Stress. *Journal of Traumatic Stress* 24 (5): 497–505.

Holstein, James A., and Jaber F. Gubrium. 2000. *Constructing the Life Course*, 2nd ed. Dix Hills, NY: General Hall.

Holzel, Lars, Martin Harter, Christina Reese, and Levente Kriston. 2011. Risk Factors for Chronic Depression: A Systematic Review. *Journal of Affective Disorders* 129 (1–3): 1–13.

Homant, Robert J. 2013. Risky Altruism, Criminal Victimization, Fear of Crime, and Security Mindedness. *Journal of Applied Security Research* 8 (2): 203–221.

Homer, Melissa M., Patti A. Freeman, Raomn B. Zabriskie, and Dennis L. Eggett. 2007. Rituals and Relationships: Examining the Relationship Between Family of Origin Rituals and Young Adult Attachment. *Marriage & Family Review* 42 (1): 5–28.

Hommerich, Carola, and Tim Tiefenbach. 2018. Analyzing the Relationship between Social Capital and Subjective Well-Being: The Mediating Role of Social Affiliation. *Journal of Happiness Studies* 19 (4): 1091–1114.

Hong, Fang, Amanda R. Tarullo, Andrea E. Mercurio, Siyu Liu, Qiyue Cai, and Kathleen Malley-Morrison. 2018. Childhood Maltreatment and Perceived Stress in Young Adults: The Role of Emotion Regulation Strategies, Self-efficacy, and Resilience. *Child Abuse & Neglect* 86: 36–146.
Hood, Albert B., and David L. Deopere. 2002. The Relationship of Cognitive Development to Age When Education and Intelligence Are Controlled for. *Journal of Adult Development* 9 (3): 229–234.
Hooghe, Marc, and Anna Kern. 2015. Party Membership and Closeness and the Development of Trust in Political Institutions: An Analysis of the European Social Survey, 2002–2010. *Party Politics* 21 (6): 944–956.
Hooghe, Marc, Ruth Dassonneville, and Sofie Marien. 2015. The Impact of Education on the Development of Political Trust: Results from a Five-Year Panel Study among Late Adolescents and Young Adults in Belgium. *Political Studies* 63 (1): 123–141.
Hooghe, Marc. 2003. Participation in Voluntary Associations and Value Indicators: The Effect of Current and Previous Participation Experiences. *Nonprofit and Voluntary Sector Quarterly* 32 (1): 47–69.
Hopcroft, Rosemary L. 2016. *Evolution and Gender: Why It Matters for Contemporary Life*. New York: Routledge.
Hope, Ann, and Deirdre Morgan. 2011. A Profile of Self-reported Alcohol-Related Violence in Ireland. *Contemporary Drug Problems* 38 (2): 237–258.
Hordern, Joshua. 2013. *Political Affections: Civil Participation and Moral Theology*. Oxford, UK: Oxford University Press.
Horell, Harold D. 2014. On Learning to See the World Religiously: Moral Awareness, Faith, and Public Moral Discourse. *Religious Education* 109 (4): 424–439.
Horn, Robert V. 1993. *Statistical Indicators for the Economics and Social Sciences*. Cambridge, UK: Cambridge University Press.
Horowitz, Jonathan. 2018. Relative Education and the Advantage of a College Degree. *American Sociological Review* 83 (4): 771–801.
Hossain, Sayed, and Ming Yu Cheng. 2003. *An Introduction to Knowledge Economy: Concepts and Issues*. Kuala Lumper, Malaysia: McGraw Hill.
Hostetler, Andrew J., Stephen Sweet, and Phyllis Moen. 2007. Gendered Career Paths: A Life Course Perspective on Returning to School. *Sex Roles* 56: 85–103.
Hou, Wai Kai, Brian J. Halld, Daphna Canettig, Kam Man Laua, Sin Man Nga, and Stevan E. Hobfoll. 2015. Threat to Democracy: Physical and Mental Health Impact of Democracy Movement in Hong Kong. *Journal of Affective Disorders* 186 (1): 74–82.
Hounknatin, Hilda Osafo, Alex M. Wood, Christopher J. Boyce, and Graham Dunn. 2014. An Existiential-Humanistic View of Personality Change: Co-occurring Change with Psychological Well-Being in a 10 Year Cohort Study. *Social Indicators Research* 121 (2): 455–470.
Hounkpatin, Hilda Osafo, Alex M. Wood, Christopher J. Boyce, and Graham Dunn. 2015. An Existential-Humanistic View of Personality Change: Co-occurring Changes with Psychological Well-Being in a 10 year Cohort Study. *Social Indicators Research* 121 (2): 455–470.
Houtman, Disk. 2000. the Working Class and the Welfare State Support for Economic Redistribution, Tolerance for Nonconformity and the Conditionality of Solidarity with the Unemployed. *Netherlands' Journal of Social Sciences* 36 (1): 37–55.
Hovden, Jorid. 2012. Discourses and Strategies for the Inclusion of Women in Sport—The Case of Norway. *Sport in Society* 15 (3): 287–301.
Howe, Paul. 2010. *Citizens Adrift: The Democratic Disengagement of Young Canadians*. Vancouver, Canada: UBC Press.
Howell, Jude. 2012. Civil Society, Corporatism and Capitalism in China. *Journal of Comparative Asian Development* 11 (2): 271–297.
Howell, Ryan T., and Colleen J. Howell. 2008. The Relation of Economic Status to Subjective Well-being in Developing Countries: A Meta analysis. *Psychological Bulletin* 134 (4): 536–560.
Hraba, Joseph, Rehan Mullick, Frederick Lorenz, and Jiri Vecernik. 2001. Age and Czechs' Attitudes Toward the Postcommunist Economic Reforms. *Sociological Quarterly* 42 (3): 421–435.

Hsieh, Chang-Ming. 2002. Trends in Financial Satisfaction: Does Poverty Make a Difference? *International Journal of Aging & Human Development* 54 (1): 15–30.

Hsu, Han-Yu., Li.-Li. Huang, and Kwang-Kuo. Hwang. 2019. Liberal–Conservative Dimension of Moral Concerns Underlying Political Faction Formation in Taiwan. *Asian Journal of Social Psychology* 22 (3): 301–315.

Hu, Shaohua. 2015. Small State Foreign Policy: The Diplomatic Recognition of Taiwan. *China: An International Journal* 13 (2): 1–23 (\93-236).

Hu, Yiliang. 2005. *Guanxi Community*. Beijing, China: People.

Huang, Chien-chung. 2002. The Impact of Child Support Enforcement on Nonmarital and Marital Births: Does It Differ by Racial and Age Groups? *Social Service Review* 275–300.

Hubbard, Phil. 2003. Fear and Loathing at the Multiplex: Everyday Anxiety in the Post-industrial City. *Capital & Class* 80: 51–75.

Huber, Brigitte, Manuel Goyanes, and Homero Gil de Zúñiga. 2022. Linking Extraversion to Collective and Individual Forms of Political Participation: The Mediating Role of Political Discussion. *Social Science Quarterly*.

Huber, Matthew. 2012. Refined Politics: Petroleum Products, Neoliberalism, and the Ecology of Entrepreneurial Life. *Journal of American Studies* 46 (2): 295–312.

Huddy, Leonie, and Nadia Khatib. 2007. American Patriotism, National Identity, and Political Involvement. *American Journal of Political Science* 51 (1): 63–77.

Hudson, John, and Philip Jones. 2005. Public Goods: An Exercise in Calibration. *Public Choice* 24: 267–282.

Hughes, Gerard J. 2001. *Aristotle on Ethics*. London: Routledge.

Hughes, Lorine A., Lonnie M. Schaible, and Benjamin R. Gibbs. 2015. Economic Dominance, the American Dream, and Homicide: A Cross-National Test of Institutional Anomie Theory. *Sociological Inquiry* 85 (1): 100–128.

Hui, Eddie Chi Man, and Ka Hung Yu. 2009. Residential Mobility and Aging Population in Hong Kong. *Habitat International* 33: 10–14.

Huinink, Johannes, and Michaela Kreyenfeld. 2006. Family Formation in Times of Abrupt Social and Economic Change. In *After the Fall of the Wall: Life Courses in the Transformation of East Germany*, 170–190, ed. Martin Diewald, Anne Goedicke and Karl Ulrich Mayer. Stanford, CA: Stanford University Press.

Hultgren, John. 2018. 21st Century American Environmental Ideologies: A Re-evaluation. *Journal of Political Ideologies* 23 (1): 54–79.

Humphrey, Mathew. 2010. Green Political Theory. In *Ethics and World Politics*, 181–199, ed. Duncan Bell. Oxford, UK: Oxford University Press. Ojala, Maria. 2005. "Adolescents' Worries about Environmental Risks: Subjective Well-being, Values, and Existential Dimensions." *Journal of Youth Studies* 8 (3):331–347.

Hunt, Diana. 1989. *Economic Theories of Development: An Analysis of Competing Paradigms*. New York: Harvester Wheatsheaf.

Hunter, Bronwyn A., Leonard A. Jason, and Christopher B. Keys. 2013. Factors of Empowerment for Women in Recovery from Substance Use. *American Journal of Community Psychology* 51 (1–2): 91–102.

Hunter, Lance Y. 2016. Terrorism, Civil Liberties, and Political Rights: A Cross-National Analysis. *Studies in Conflict & Terrorism* 39 (2): 165–193.

Huntington, Samuel P. [1993] 1997. *The Clash of Civilization and the Remaking of World Order*. Taipei, Taiwan: Linking.

Huta, Veronika. 2017. An Overview of Hedonic and Eudaimonic Well-being concepts. In *The Routledge Handbook of Media Use and Well-being: International Perspectives on Theory and Research on Positive Media Effects*, 14–33, ed. Leonard Reinecke and Mary Beth Oliver. New York, NY: Routledge.

Hutcheson, John D., Jr., and James E. Prather. 1981. Interpreting the Effects of Missing Data in Survey Research. *South-Eastern Political Review* 9 (2): 129–143.

Hutchings, Vincent L. 2003. *Public Opinion and Democratic Accountability: How Citizens Learn about Politics*. Princeton, NJ: Princeton University Press.
Hyesun, Hwang, and Kee-Ok. Kim. 2015. Social Media as a Tool for Social Movements: The Effect of Social Media Use and Social Capital on Intention to Participate in Social Movements. *International Journal of Consumer Studies* 39 (5): 478–488.
Hwang, Eui-Gab., Edmund F. McGarrell, and Bruce L. Benson. 2005. Public Satisfaction with the South Korean Police: The Effect of Residential Location in a Rapidly Industrializing Nation. *Journal of Criminal Justice* 33: 585–599.
Hyggen, Christer. 2006. Risks and Resources: Social Capital among Social Assistance Recipients in Norway. *Social Policy & Administration* 40 (5): 493–508.
Hyland, James L. 1995. *Democratic Theory: The Philosophical Foundations*. Manchester, UK: Manchester University Press.
Ibrahim, Yousaf. 2011. Political Distinction in the British Anti-capitalist Movement. *Sociology* 45 (2): 318–334.
Iceland, John, and Josh Kim. 2001. Poverty among Working Families: New Insights from an Improved Poverty Measure. *Social Science Quarterly* 82 (2): 253–266.
Iida, Takeshi, and Tetsuya Matsubayashi. 2010. Constitutions and Public Support for Welfare Policies. *Social Science Quarterly* 91 (1): 42–62.
Imbroscio, David L. 1997. *Reconstructing City Politics: Alternative Economic Development and Urban Regimes*. Thousand Oaks, CA: Sage.
Immerzeel, Tim, and Frank van Tubergen. 2013. Religion as Reassurance? Testing the Insecurity Theory in 26 European Countries. *European Sociological Review* 29 (2): 359–372.
Inglehart, Ronald F. 2010. Faith and Freedom: Traditional and Modern Ways to Happiness. in *International Differences in Well-Being*, 351–397, ed. Ed Diener, John F. Helliwell and Daniel Kahneman. New York: Oxford University Press.
Inglehart, Ronald, and Christian Welzel. 2005. *Modernization, Cultural Change, and Democracy: The Human Development Sequence*. New York: Cambridge University Press.
Inglehart, Ronald, and Hans-Dieter Klingemann. 2000. Genes, Culture, Democracy, and Happiness. In *Culture and Subjective Well-Being*, 165–183, ed. Ed Diener and Eunkook M. Suh. Cambridge, MA: MIT.
Inglehart, Ronald, and Pippa Norris. 2003. *Rising Tide: Gender Equality and Cultural Change around the World*. Cambridge, UK: Cambridge University Press.
Inglehart, Ronald, and Wayne E. Baker. 2000. Modernization, Cultural Change, and the Persistence of Traditional Values. *American Sociological Review* 65: 1–51.
Inglehart, Ronald. 1990. Values, Ideology, and Cognitive Mobilization in New Social Movements. In *Challenging the Political Order: New Social and Political Movements in Western Democracies*, 43–66, ed. Russell J. Dalton and Manfred Kuechler. Cambridge: Polity Press.
Inglehart, Ronald. 1997. *Modernization and Postmodernization: Cultural, Economic, and Political Change in 43 Societies*. Princeton, NJ: Princeton University Press.
Inglehart, Ronald. 1999. Postmodernization Erodes Respect for Authority, but Increases Support for Democracy. In *Critical Citizens: Global Support for Democratic Government*, 236–256, ed. Pippa Norris. Oxford, UK: Oxford University Press.
Inglehart, Ronald. 2000. Globalization and Postmodern Values. *Washington Quarterly* 23 (1): 215–228.
Inglehart, Ronald. 2003. Modernization and Volunteering. In *The Values of Volunteering: Cross-Cultural Perspectives*, 55–70, ed. Paul Dekker and Loek Halman. New York: Kluwer.
Inglehart, Ronald. 2018. *Cultural Evolution: People's Motivations are Changing and Reshaping the World*. Cambridge, UK: Cambridge University Press.
Ingrams, Alex. 2017. Connective Action and the Echo Chamber of Ideology: Testing a Model of Social Media Use and Attitudes toward the Role of Government. *Journal of Information Technology & Politics* 14 (1): 1–15.

Inthorn, Sanna, and Tammy Boyce. 2010. 'It's Disgusting How Much Salt You Eat!: Television Discourses of Obesity, Health and Morality. *International Journal of Cultural Studies* 13 (1): 83–100.

Irwin, Anthea. 2011. Social Constructionism. In *The SAGE Handbook of Sociolinguistics*, 100–112, ed. Ruth Wodak, Barbara Johnstone and Paul Kerswill. London, UK: SAGE.

Isaac, Larry, and Lars Christiansen. 2002. How the Civil Rights Movement Revitalized Labor Militancy. *American Sociological Review* 67: 722–746.

Isaacowitz, Derek M., George E. Vaillant, and Martin E.P.. Seligman. 2003. Strengths and Satisfaction across the Adult Lifespan. *International Journal of Aging & Human Development* 57 (2): 181–201.

Ishio, Yoshito. 2010. Social Bases of American Patriotism: Examining Effects of Dominant Social Statuses and Socialization. *Current Sociology* 58 (1): 67–93.

Ishoy, Glen A. 2017. Exploring Morality as a Mediator of the Association between Parenting Practices and Violent and Property Offending among a Sample of Juvenile Delinquents. *Crime & Delinquency* 63 (2): 113–136.

Islam, Jonathan, Jane Kolodinsky, and Garrett Kimberly. 2006. The Effects of Volunteering for Nonprofit Organizations on Social Capital Formation: Evidence from a Statewide Survey. *Nonproft & Voluntary Sector Quarterly* 35 (3): 367–383.

Islam, M. Rezaul., and J. Morgan William. 2012. Non-Governmental Organizations in Bangladesh: Their Contribution to Social Capital Development and Community Empowerment. *Community Development Journal* 47 (3): 369–385.

Israelstam, Ken. 2007. Creativity and Dialectical Phenomena: From Dialectical Edge to Dialectical Space. *International Journal of Psychoanalysis* 88 (3): 591–607.

Itzhaky, Haya, and Alan S. York. 2000. Empowerment and Community Participation: Does Gender Make a Difference? *Social Work Research* 24 (4): 225–234.

Iwasaki, Yoshitaka, Jennifer Mactavish, and Kelly MacKay. 2005. Building in Strengths and Resilience: Leisure as a Stress Survival Strategy. *British Journal of Guidance & Counselling* 33 (1): 81–100.

Iyengar, Shanto. 1987. Television News and Citizens' Explanations of National Affairs. *American Political Science Review* 81 (3): 815–832.

Iyengar, Shanto. 1990. Shortcuts to Political Knowledge: The Role of Selective Attention and Accessibility. In *Information and Democratic Processes*, 160–185, ed. John A. Ferejohn and James H. Kuklinski. Urbana, IL: University of Illinois Press.

Izquierdo, Honorio Martin, and Almudena Moreno Minguez. 2003. Sociological Theory of education in the Dialectical Perspective. In *The International Assessment of New Research and Theory*, 21–41, ed. Carlos Alberto Torres and Ari Antikainen. Lanham, MD: Rowman.

Jackman, Robert W. 1993. Rationality and Political Participation. *American Journal of Political Science* 37 (1): 279–290.

Jackson, Richard, and Gareth Hall. 2016. Talking About Terrorism: A Study of Vernacular Discourse. *Politics* 36 (3): 292–307.

Jacobs, Lawrence R., Fay Lomax Cook, and Michael X. Delli. Carpini. 2009. *Talking Together: Public Deliberative and Political Participation in America*. Chicago, IL: University of Chicago Press.

Jacoby, Mario. 1990. *Individuation and Narcissism: The Psychology of Self in Jung and Kohut*. London, UK: Routledge.

Jacques, Jeffrey M. 1998. Changing Marital and Family Patterns: A Test of the Post-Modern Perspective. *Sociological Perspectives* 41 (2): 381–413.

Jaeger, Wiliam K. 2004. Status Seeking and Social Welfare: Is There Virtue in Vanity? *Social Science Quarterly* 85 (2): 361–379.

Jagendorf, Jana, and Andrew Malekoff. 2000. Groups-on-the-Go: Spontaneously Formed Mutual Aid Groups for Adolescents in Distress. *Social Work with Groups* 22 (4): 15–32.

Jakimow, Tanya. 2009. Non-Government Organisations, Self-Help Groups and Neo-Liberal Discourses. *South Asia* 32 (3): 469–484.

Jakobsen, Tor Georg. 2010. Public versus Private: The Conditional Effect of State Policy and Institutional Trust on Mass Opinion. *European Sociological Review* 26 (3): 307–318.

James, Rachel K., and Ye. Luo. 1999. The Culture of Poverty and African-American Culture: An Empirical Assessment. *Sociological Perspectives* 42 (3): 439–458.

James, Spencer L., and Paul R. Amato. 2013. Self-esteem and the Reproduction of Social Class. *Social Science Quarterly* 94 (4): 933–955.

Janack, Marianne. 2012. *What We Mean by Experience.* Stanford, CA: Stanford University Press.

Jang, Hyewon. 2016. Identifying 21st Century STEM Competencies Using Workplace Data. *Journal of Science Education & Technology* 25 (2): 284–301.

Janoski, Thomas, and Fengjuan Wang. 2005. The Politics of Immigration and National Integration. In *The Handbook of Political Sociology: States, Civil Societies, and Globalization*, 630–654, ed. Thomas Janoski, Robert Alford, Alexander Hicks, and Mildred A. Schwartz. Cambridge, UK: Cambridge University Press.

Janoski, Thomas, and John Wilson. 1995. Pathways to Voluntarism: Family Socialization and Studies Transmission Models. *Social Forces* 74 (1): 271–292.

Jasper, James M. 2005. Culture, Knowledge, Politics. In *The Handbook of Political Sociology: States, Civil Societies, and Globalization*, 115–134, ed. Thomas Janoski, Robert Alford, Alexander Hicks, and Mildred A. Schwartz. Cambridge, UK: Cambridge University Press.

Jasper, James M., Kevn Moran, and Marisa Tramontano. 2015. Strategy. In *Oxford Handbook of Social Movements*, 399–409, ed. Donatella della Porta and Mario Diani. Oxford, UK: Oxford University Press.

Jasso, Guillermina. 2001. Comparison Theory. In *Handbook of Sociological Theory*, 669–698, ed. Jonathan H. Turner. New York: Kluwer.

Jasso, Guillermina. 2002. Seven Secrets of Doing Theory. In *New Directions in Contemporary Sociological Theory*, 317–342, ed. Joseph Berger and Morris Zelditch, Jr. Lanham, MY: Rowman & Littlefield.

Jasso, Guillermina. 2015. Thinking, Saying, Doing in the World of Distributive Justice. *Social Justice Research* 28 (4): 435–478.

Jaye, Chrystal, Jessica Young, Richard Egan, Rebecca Llewellyn, Wayne Cunningham, and Peter Radue. 2018. The Healthy Lifestyle in Longevity Narratives. *Social Theory & Health* 16 (4): 361–378.

Jencks, Christopher. 2002. Does Inequality Matter? *Daedalus* 13 (1): 49–65.

Jenkins, J. Craig., and Michael Wallace. 1996. The Generalized Action Potential of Protest Movements: The New Class, Social Trends, and Political Exclusion Explanations. *Sociological Forum* 11 (2): 183–207.

Jenkins, J. Craig, and William Form. 2005. Social Movements and Social Change. In *The Handbook of Political Sociology: States, Civil Societies, and Globalization,* 331–349, ed. Thomas Janoski, Robert Alford, Alexander Hicks, and Mildred A. Schwartz. Cambridge, UK: Cambridge University Press.

Jenkins, Mikayla, and Marko Dragojevic. 2011. Explaining the Process of Resistance to Persuasion: A Politeness Theory-Based Approach. *Communication Research* 40 (4): 559–590.

Jenkins, Stephen P., Christian Schluter, and Gert G. Wagner. 2003. The Dynamics of Child Poverty: Britain and Germany Compared. *Journal of Comparative Family Studies* 34 (3): 337–355.

Jenkins-Smith, Hank C., and Kerry G. Herron. 2009. Rock and a Hard Place: Public Willingness to Trade Civil Rights and Liberties for Greater Security. *Politics & Policy* 37 (5): 1095–1129.

Jennings, Freddie J., and Frank M. Russell. 2019. Civility, Credibility, and Health Information: The Impact of Uncivil Comments and Source Credibility on Attitudes About Vaccines. *Public Understanding of Science* 28 (4): 417–432.

Jennings, M. Kent., and Vicki Zeitner. 2003. Internet Use and Civic Engagement: A Longitudinal Analysis. *Public Opinion Quarterly* 67 (3): 311–334.

Jewkes, Rachel, Jonathan Levin, and Loveday Penn-Kekana. 2002. Risk Factors for Domestic Violence: Findings from a South African Cross-sectional Study. *Social Science & Medicine* 55: 1603–1617.

Jiang, Shiqing, Lu. Ming, and Hiroshi Sato. 2011. Identity, Inequality, and Happiness: Evidence from Urban China. *World Development* 40 (6): 1190–1200.

Joas, Hans. 1996. *The Creativity of Action*. Chicago, IL: University of Chicago Press.

Joassart-Marcelli, Pascale. 2005. Working Poverty in Southern California: Towards an Operational Measure. *Social Science Research* 34: 20–43.

Jodl, Kathleen M., Alice Michael, Oksana Malanchuk, Jacquelynne S. Eccles, and Arnold Sameroff. 2001. Parents?? Roles in Shaping Early Adolescents?? Occupational Aspirations. *Child Development* 72 (4): 1247–1265.

Joeckel, Sven, and Leyla Dogruel. 2017. From Moral Corruption to Moral Management: Media's Influence on People's Morality and Well-Being. In *The Routledge Handbook of Media Use and Well-Being: International Perspectives on Theory and Research on Positive Media Effects*, 145–169, ed. Leonard Reinecke and Mary Beth Oliver. New York, NY: Routledge.

Johnson, Amy Janan, Kevin B. Wright, Elizabeth A. Craig, Eileen S. Gilchrist, Lindsay T. Lane, and Michel M. Haigh. 2008. A Model for Predicting Stress Levels and Marital Satisfaction for Stepmothers Utilizing a Stress and Coping Approach. *Journal of Social & Personal Relationships* 25 (1): 119–142.

Johnson, Craig. 2009. *Arresting Development: The Power of Knowledge for Social Change*. Abingdon, UK: Routledge.

Johnson, David R., and Wu. Jian. 2002. An Empirical Test of Crisis, Social Selection, and Role Explanations of the Relationship between Marital Disruption and Psychological Distress: A Pooled Time-series Analysis of Four-wave Panel Data. *Journal of Marriage & Family* 64: 211–224.

Johnson, Thomas J., and Barbara K. Kaye. 2002. Webelievability: A Path Model Examining How Convenience and Reliance Predict Online Credibility. *J&mc Quartery* 79 (3): 619–642.

Jonasson, Erik. 2012. Government Effectiveness and Regional Variation in Informal Employment. *Journal of Development Studies* 48 (4): 481–497.

Jones, Andrew W. 2001a. Caring Labor and Class Consciousness: The Class Dynamics of Gendered Work. *Sociological Forum* 16 (2): 281–299.

Jones, Antwan, Gregory D. Squires, and Cynthia Ronzio. 2015. Foreclosure Is Not an Equal Opportunity Stressor: How Inequality Fuels the Adverse Health Implications of the Nation's Financial Crisis. *Journal of Urban Affairs* 37 (5): 505–529.

Jones, Bryan D. 2001b. *Politics and the Architecture of Choice: Bounded Rationality and Governance*. Chicago, UK: University of Chicago Press.

Jones, Ellis. 2019. Rethinking Greenwashing: Corporate Discourse, Unethical Practice, and the Unmet Potential of Ethical Consumerism. *Sociological Perspectives* 62 (5): 728–754.

Jones, K. Nicole., and Melanie E. Brewster. 2017. From Awareness to Action: Examining Predictors of Lesbian, Gay, Bisexual, and Transgender (LGBT) Activism for Heterosexual People. *American Journal of Orthopsychiatry* 87 (6): 680–689.

Jones, Keely S. 2006. Giving and Volunteering as Distinct Forms of Civic Engagement: The Role of Community Integration and Personal Resources in Formal Helping. *Nonprofit & Voluntary Sector Quarterly* 35 (2): 249–266.

Jones, Michael D. 2011. Leading the Way to Compromise? Cultural Theory and Climate Change Opinion. *Political Science & Politics* 720–725.

Jones, Rachel K., and April Brayfield. 1997. Life's Greatest Joy? European Attitudes toward the Centrality of Children. *Social Forces* 75 (4): 1239–1270.

Jones, Russell, Derek Heim, Simon Hunter, and Anne Ellaway. 2014. The Relative Influence of Neighbourhood Incivilities, Cognitive Social Capital, Club Membership and Individual Characteristics on Positive Mental Health. *Health & Place* 28: 187–193.

Jonsson, Dagmar, Saga Johansson, Annika Rosengren, Georg Lappas, and Lars Wilhelmsen. 2003. Self-perceived Psychological Stress in Relation to Psychosocial Factors and Work in a Random Population Sample of Women. *Stress & Health* 19 (6): 149–162.

Jordahl, Henrik. 2009. Economic Inequality. In *Handbook of Social Capital: The Troika of Sociology, Political Science and Economics*, 323–336, ed. Gert Tinggaard Svendsen and Gunnar Linad Haase Svendsen. Cheltenham, UK: Elgar.

Jordan, Bill. 2005. Social Theory and Social Policy: Choice Order and Human Well-being. *European Journal of Social Theory* 8 (2): 149–170.

Jorgensen, Bradley S., Robert D. Jamieson, and John F. Martin. 2010. Income, Sense of Community and Subjective Well-being: Combining Economic and Psychological Variables. *Journal of Economic Psychology* 31: 612–643.

Jorgensen, Marianne, and Louise Phillips. 2002. *Discourse Analysis as Theory and Method*. London: Sage.

Jorgenson, Andrew K., Kelly Austin, and Christopher Dick. 2009. Ecologically Unequal Exchange and the Resource Consumption/Environmental Degradation Paradox. *International Journal of Comparative Sociology* 50 (3–4): 263–284.

Joseph, Mark, and Robert Chaskin. 2010. Living in a Mixed-income Development: Resident Perceptions of the Benefits and Disadvantages of Two Developments in Chicago. *Urban Studies* 47 (11): 2347–2366.

Joslyn, Mark R., and Allan Cigler. 2001. Group Involvement and Democratic Orientations: Social Capital in the Postelection Context. *Social Science Quarterly* 82 (2): 357–368.

Jost, John T. 2020. *A Theory of System Justification*. Cambridge, MA: Harvard University Press.

Jost, John T., and Jojanneke van der Toom. 2012. System Justification Theory. In *Handbook of Theories of Social Psychology*, vol. 2, 313–343, ed. Paul A.M. Van Lange, Arie W. Kruglanski and E. Tory Higgins. London, CA: SAGE.

Jost, John T., Julia Becker, Danny Osborne, and Vivienne Badaan. 2017. Missing in (Collective) Action: Ideology, System Justification, and the Motivational Antecedents of Two Types of Protest Behavior. *Current Direction of Psychological Science* 26 (2): 99–108.

Jou, Willy. 2011. How Do Citizens in East Asian Democracies Understand Left and Right? *Japanese Journal of Political Science* 12 (1): 33–55.

Judge, Timothy A., Amir Erez, Joyce E. Bono, and Carl J. Thoresen. 2002. Are Measures of Self-esteem, Neuroticism, Locus of Control, and Generalized Self-efficacy Indicators of a Common Core Construct? *Journal of Personality & Social Psychology* 83 (3): 693–710.

Jukes, Matthew C. H., Stephanie S. Zuilkowski, and Elena L. Grigorenko. 2018. Do Schooling and Urban Residence Develop Cognitive Skills at the Expense of Social Responsibility? A Study of Adolescents in the Gambia, West Africa. *Journal of Cross-Cultural Psychology* 49 (1): 82–98.

Julkunen, Ilse. 2002. Social and Material Deprivation Among Unemployed Youth in Northern Europe. *Social Policy & Administration* 36 (3): 235–253.

Just, Aida, and Christopher J. Anderson. 2014. Opinion Climates and Immigrant Political Action: A Cross-National Study of 25 European Democracies. *Comparative Political Studies* 47 (7): 935–965.

Jusufi, Islam. 2018. Reconceptualising the Security in Discourse: Inclusive Security and Popular Protests. *Journal of Multicultural Discourses* 13 (4): 362–376.

Kabakian-Khasholian, Tamar, Oona Campbell, Mona Shediac-Rizkallah, and Francoise Ghorayeb. 2000. Women's Experiences of Maternity Care: Satisfaction or Passivity. *Social Science & Medicine* 51: 103–113.

Kachadonrian, Lirig K., et al. 2013. Maladaptive Dependency Schemas, Posttraumatic Stress Hyperarousal Symptoms, and Intimate Partner Aggressive Perpetration. *Journal of Traumatic Stress* 26: 580–587.

Kagitcibasi, Cigdem. 2005. Autonomy and Relatedness in Cultural Context: Implications for Self and Family. *Journal of Cross-Cultural Psychology* 36 (4): 403–422.

Kahneman, Daniel, David A. Schkade, Calude Fishler, Alan B. Krueger, and Amy Krilla. 2010. The Structure of Well-Being in Two Cities: Life Satisfaction and Experience and Happiness in Columbus, Ohio and Rennes, France. In *International Differences in Well-being*, 16–33, ed. Ed Diener, John F. Helliwell and Daniel Kahneman. New York: Oxford University Press.

Kalkstein, Solomon, and Roni Beth Tower. 2009. The Daily Spiritual Experiences Scale and Well-Being: Demographic Comparisons and Scale Validation with Older Jewish Adults and a Diverse Internet Sample. *Journal of Religion & Health* 48: 402–417.

Kalleberg, Arne L., and Peter V. Marsden. 1995. Organizations and Wage Determination in Norway: A Multilevel Approach. *Comparative Social Research* 15: 129–165.

Kalleberg, Arne L., Barbara F. Reskin, and Ken Hudson. 2000. Bad Jobs in America: Standard and Nonstandard Employment Relations and Job Quality in the United States. *American Sociological Review* 65: 256–278.

Kam, Chester, Xiaolin Zhou, Xuan Zhang, and Man Yee Ho. 2012. Examining the Dimensionality of Self-construals and Individualistic-Collectivistic Values with Random Intercept Item Factor Analysis. *Personality and Individual Differences* 53 (6): 727–733.

Kanan, James W., and Matthew V. Pruitt. 2002. Modeling Fear of Crime and Perceived Victimization Risk: The (In)significance of Neighborhood Integration. *Sociological Inquiry* 72 (4): 527–548.

Kanar, Adam M. and Dave Bouckenooghe. 2022. Job Seekers' Self-Directed Learning Activities Explained through the Lens of Regulatory Focus. *Journal of Career Development* 49(3): 681–696.

Kane-Frieder, Rachel E., Wayne A. Hochwarter, and Gerald R. Ferris. 2013. Terms of Engagement: Political Boundaries of Work Engagement-Work Outcomes Relationships. *Human Relations* 67 (3): 357–382.

Kangas, Olli. 2003. The Grasshopper and the Ants: Popular Opinions of Just Distribution in Australia and Finland. *Journal of Socio-Economics* 31: 721–743.

Kanji, Mebs, and Neil Nevitte. 1997. Environmental Support, Concern and Action: An Exploratory Crossnational Analysis. *International Journal of Public Opinion Research* 9 (1): 66–76.

Kaplan, Howard B. 2006. Self theory and Emotions. In *Handbook of the Sociology of Emotions*, 224–253, ed. Jan E. Stets and Jonathan H. Turner. Boston, MA: Springer.

Kaplan, Howard B., and Xiaoru Liu. 2000. Social Movements as Collective Coping with Spoiled Personal Identities: Intimation from a Panel Study of Changes in the Life? Course Between Adolescence and Adulthood. In *Self, Identity, and Social Movements*, 215–238, ed. Sheldon Stryker, Timothy J. Owens, and Robert W. White. Minneapolis, MN: University of Minnesota Press.

Kapur, Kanika. 1998. The Impact of Health on Job Mobility: A Measure of Job Lock. *Industrial and Labor Relations Review* 51 (2): 282–298.

Karatzogianni, Athina, and Andrew Robinson. 2010. *Power, Reistance and Conflict on the Contemporary World: Social Movements, Networks and Hierarchical*. Abingdon, UK: Routledge.

Karger, Howard, James Midgley, Peter A. Kindle, and C. Brene Brown. 2007. *Controversial Issues in Social Policy*. Boston, MA: Pearson.

Karikari, Serwaa, Kofi Osei-Frimpong, and Nana Owusu-Frimpong. 2017. Evaluating Individual Level Antecedents and Consequences of Social Media Use in Ghana. *Technological Forecasting & Social Change* 123: 68–79.

Kasparian, Nadine A., Jordana K. McLoone, and Bettina Meiser. 2009. Skin Cancer-related Prevention and Screening Behaviors: A Review of the Literature. *Journal of Behavioral Medicine* 32: 406–428.

Kasser, Tim. 2016. Materialistic Values and Goals. *Annual Review Psychology* 67: 489–514.

Katz, James E., and Ronald E. Rice. 2002. *Social Consequences of Internet Use: Access, Involvement, and Interaction*. Cambridge, MA: MIT Press.

Katz-Gerro, Tally, and Yossi Shavit. 1998. The Stratification of Leisure and Taste: Classes and Lifestyles in Israel. *European Sociological Review* 14 (4): 369–386.

Katz-Gerro, Tally. 1999. Cultural Consumption and Social Stratification: Leisure Activities, Musical Tastes, and Social Location. *Sociological Perspectives* 42 (4): 627–646.

Katz-Schiavone, Stacey, Jill S. Levenson, and Alissa R. Ackerman. 2008. Myths and Facts about Sexual Violence: Public Perceptions and Implications for Prevention. *Journal of Criminal Justice & Popular Culture* 15 (3): 291–311.

Kaufman, Peter. 2003. Learning to Not Labor: How Working-class Individuals Construct Middle-class Identities. *Sociological Quarterly* 44 (3): 481–504.

Kaufmann, Eric, Anne Goujon, and Vegard Skirbekk. 2012. The End of Secularization in Europe? A Socio-demographic Perspective. *Sociology of Religion* 73 (1): 69–91.

Kaukinen, Catherine. 2004. Status Compatibility, Physical Violence, and Emotional Abuse in Intimate Relationships. *Journal of Marriage & Family* 66: 452–471.

Kavussanu, Maria, and Glyn C. Roberts. 2001. Moral Functioning in Sport: An Achievement Goal Perspective. *Journal of Sport & Exercise Psychology* 23: 37–54.

Kawabata, Mizuki. 2014. Childcare Access and employment: The Case of Women with Preschool-Aged Children in Tokyo. *Review of Urban & Regional Development Studies* 26 (1): 40–56.

Kawachi, Ichiro, and Lisa F. Berkman. 2001. Social Ties and Mental Health. *Journal of Urban Health* 78 (3): 458–467.

Kawachi, Ichiro, Bruce P. Kennedy, Kimbergly Lochner, and Deborah Prothrow-Stith. 1997. Social Capital, Income Inequality, and Mortality. *American Journal of Public Health* 87 (9): 1491–1498.

Kazarian, Shane S., and Rod A. Martin. 2006. Humor Styles, Culture-Related Personality, Well-being, and Family Adjustment among Armenians in Lebanon. *Humor* 19 (4): 405–423.

Kazmi, Aqdas Ali. 1993. National Savings Rates of India and Pakistan: A Macroeconometric Analysis. *Pakistan Development Review* 32 (4 Part II): 1313–1324.

Kearney, Anne R. 2006. Residential Development Patterns and Neighborhood Satisfaction: Impacts of Density and Nearby Nature. *Environment & Behavior* 38 (1): 112–139.

Kedem-Friedrich, Peri, and Maged Al-Atawneh. 2004. Does Modernity Lead to Greater Well-being? Bedoun Women Undergoing a Socio-cultural Transition. *Social Indicators Research* 67: 333–351.

Keightley, Michelle L., Gordon Winocur, Hana Burianova, Donaya Hongwanishkul, and Cheryl L. Grady. 2006. Age Effects on Social Cognition: Faces Tell a Different Story. *Psychology & Aging* 21 (3): 558–572.

Keister, Lisa A. 2003. Religion and Wealth: The Role of Religious Affiliation and Participation in Early Adult Asset Accumulation. *Social Forces* 82 (1): 175–207.

Kekes, John. 1997. *Against Liberalism*. Ithaca, NY: Cornell Univesity Press.

Kellerman, Aharon. 2014. *The Internet as Second Action Space*. Abington, UK: Routledge.

Kelly, John R., and Janice R. Kelly. 1994. Multiple Dimensions of Meaning in the Domains of Work, Family, and Leisure. *Journal of Leisure Research* 26 (3): 250–274.

Kelly, Orla. 2020. The Silver Bullet? Assessing the Role of Education for Sustainability. *Social Forces* 99 (1): 178–204.

Kelly, William E. 2002. An Investigation of Worry and Sense of Humor. *Journal of Psychology* 13 (6): 657–666.

Keltener, Dacher, Gerben A. Van Kleef, Serena Chen, and Michael W. Kraus. 2008. A Reciprocal Influence Model of Social Power: Emerging Principles and Lines of Inquiry. *Advances in Experimental Social Psychology* 40: 151–192.

Kempton, Willett, James S. Boster, and Jennifer A. Hartley. 1995. *Environmental Values in American Culture*. Cambridge, MA: MIT.

Kennamer, J. David. 1987. How Media Use During Campaign Affects the Intent to Vote. *Journalism Quarterly* 64: 291–300.

Kennamer, J. David. 1990. Comparing Predictors of the Likelihood of Voting in a Primary and a General Election. *Journalism Quarterly* 67 (4): 777–784.

Kerrissey, Jasmine, and Evan Schofer. 2013. Civic and Political Participation: Union Membership and Political Participation in the United States. *Social Forces* 91 (3): 895–928.

Kessler, Ronald C., and Kristen D. Michelson. 1997. Patterns and Correlates of Self-help Group Membership in the United States. *Social Policy* 27 (3): 27–46.

Kessler, Ronald C., Kristin D. Michelson, and David R. Williams. 1999. The Prevalence, Distribution, and Mental Health Correlates of Perceived Discrimination in the United States. *Journal of Health & Social Behavior* 40 (3): 208–230.

Keyes, Corey L.M.. 2002. Social Civility in the United States. *Sociological Inquiry* 72 (3): 393–408.

Keyes, Corey L.M. 2014. Promotion and Protectionof Positive Mental Health towards Complete Mental Health in Human Development. In *The Oxford Handbook of Happiness*, 915–925, ed.

Susan A. David, Ilona Boniwell and Amanda Conley Ayers. Oxford, UK: Oxford University Press.

Keyes, Corey L.M., and Adam D. Shapiro. 2004. Social Well-being in the United States: A Descriptive Epidemiology. In *How Healthy Are We: A National Study of Well-Being at Midlife*, 350–372, ed. Orville Gilbert Brim, Carol D. Ryff and Ronald C. Kessler. Chicago, IL: University of Chicago Press.

Khan, Rimi, Danielle Wyatt, and Audrey Yue. 2015. Making and Remaking Multicultural Arts: Policy, Cultural Difference and the Discourse of Decline. *International Journal of Cultural Policy* 21 (2): 219–234.

Khang, Hyoungkoo, Eun-Kyoung. Han, and Eyun-Jung. Ki. 2014. Exploring Influential Social Cognitive Determinants of Social Media Use. *Computers in Human Behavior* 36: 48–55.

Khatchadourian, Haig. 1999. *Community and Communitarianism*. New York: Peter Lang.

Khattab, Nabil, and Steve Fenton. 2009. What Makes Young Adults Happy? Employment and Non-work as Determinants of Life Satisfaction. *Sociology* 43 (1): 11–26.

Khoo, Shuna Shiann, Wei Xing Toh, and Hwajin Yang. 2021. Seeking Control During Uncontrollable Times: Control Abilities and Religiosity Predict Stress During Covid-19. *Personality & Individual Differences* 175: 110675.

Khoshneviss, Hadi, and Robert D. Benford. 2018. Social Movements. In *The SAGE Handbook of Political Sociology*, 828–842, ed. William Outhwaite and Stephen Turner. London, UK: SAGE.

KhosraviNik, Majid and Mohammedwesam Amer. 2022. Social Media and Terrorism Discourse: The Islamic State's (Is) Social Media Discursive Content and Practices. *Critical Discourse Studies*.

Kick, Edward L., and Laura A. McKinney. 2014. Global Context, National Interdependencies, and the Ecological Footprint. *Sociological Perspectives* 57 (2): 256–279.

Kiecolt, K. Jill. 2003. Satisfaction with Work and Family Life: No Evidence of a Cultural Reversal. *Journal of Marriage & Family* 65 (1): 23–35.

Kiecolt-Glaser, Janice, F. Lynanne McGuire, Robles Theodore, and Ronald Glaser. 2002. Emotions, Morbidity and Mortality: New Perspectives from Psychoneuroimmunology. *Annual Review of Psychology* 53: 83–107.

Kieffer, Annick, Catherine Marry, Monique Meron, and Anne Solaz. 2005. The Case of France: Family Formation in an Uncertain Labor Market. In *Globalization, Uncertainty and Youth in Society*, 105–134, ed. Hans-Peter Blossfeld, Erik Klijzing, Melinda Mills and Karin Kurz. London: Routledge.

Kiesling, Chris, Gwendolyn T. Sorell, Marilyn J. Montgomery, and Ronald K. Colwell. 2006. Identity and Spirituality: A Psychological Exploration of the Sense of Spiritual Self. *Developmental Psychology* 42 (6): 1269–1277.

Kilburn, Johnn C., Jr., and Michael O. Maume. 2000. The Paradox of Neighborhood Association Existence and Membership. *Research in Community Sociology* 10: 327–344.

Killian, Timothy, and Lawrence H. Ganong. 2002. Ideology, Context, and Obligations to Assist Older Persons. *Journal of Marriage & Family* 64 (4).

Kilminster, Richard. 2008. Narcissism or Informalization? Christopher Lasch, Norbert Elias and Social Diagnosis. *Theory, Culture & Society* 25 (3): 131–151.

Kim, Daniel, and Ichiro Kawachi. 2007. U.S. State-Level Social Capital and Health-Related Quality of Life: Multilevel Evidence of Main, Mediating, and Modifying Effects. *Annals of Epidemiology* 17 (4): 258–269.

Kim, Hansung, and Madeleine Stoner. 2008. Burnout and Turnover Intention Among Social Workers: Effects of Role Stress, Job Autonomy and Social Support. *Administration in Social Work* 32 (3): 5–25.

Kim, Jungsu, and SukJun Lee. 2020. An Emerging Online Social Network and Disaster-Induced Collective Stress. *Media Psychology* 23 (4): 521–551.

Kim, Kee Jeong, R., and D. Conger, Glen H. Elder, Jr., and Frederick O. Lorenz. 2003. Reciprocal Influences between Stressful Life Events and Adolescent Internalizing and Externalizng Problems. *Child Development* 74 (1): 127–143.

Kim, Kyung Hee, Hang Eun Lee, Ki-Byung. Chae, Lori Anderson, and Christopher Laurence. 2011. Creativity and Confucianism Among American and Korean Educators. *Creativity Research Journal* 23 (4): 357–371.

Kim, Sungmoon. 2018. *Democracy After Virtue: Toward Pragmatic Confucian Democracy*. New York, NY: Oxford University Press.

Kim, Wonik, and Jennifer Gandhi. 2010. Coopting Workers Under Dictatorship. *Journal of Politics* 72 (3): 646–658.

Kim, Young-Il., and W. Bradford Wilcox. 2013. Bonding Alone: Familism, Religion, and Secular Civic Participation. *Social Science Research* 42 (1): 31–45.

Kimiecik, Jay. 2011. Exploring the Promise of Eudaimonic Well-Being within the Practice of Health Promotion: The How Is as Important as the What. *Journal of Happiness Studies* 12 (5): 769–792.

King, Gillian, Debra Stewart, Susanne King, and Mary Law. 2000. Organizational Characteristics and Issues Affecting the Longevity of Self-help Groups for Parents of Children with Special Needs. *Qualitative Health Research* 10 (2): 225–241.

King, Laura A. 2001. The Hard Road to the Good Life: The Happy, Mature Person. *Journal of Humanistic Psychology* 41 (1): 51–72.

Kingsbury, Nancy, and John Scanzoni. 1993. Structural-Functionalism. In *Sourcebook of Family Theories and Methods: A Contextual Approach*, 195–217, ed. Pauline G. Boss, William J. Doherty, Ralph LaRossa, Walter R. Schumm, and Susanne K. Steinmetz. New York: Plenum.

Kingston, Geeta Gandhi, and John Knight. 2006. Subjective Well-Being Poverty vs. Income Poverty and Capabilities Poverty? *Journal of Development Studies* 42 (7): 1199–1224.

Kinna, Ruth, Alex Prichard, and Thomas Swann. 2019. Occupy and the Constitution of Anarchy. *Global Constitutionalism* 8 (2): 357–390.

Kiousis, Spiro. 2001. Public Trust or Mistrust? Perceptions of Media Credibility in the Informational Age. *Mass Communication & Society* 4 (4): 381–403.

Kirby, James B., and Toshiko Kaneda. 2005. Neighborhood Socioeconomic Disadvantage and Access to Health Care. *Journal of Health & Social Behavior* 46 (1): 15–31.

Kirk, David S., and Andrew V. Papachristos. 2011. Cultural Mechanisms and the Persistence of Neighborhood Violence. *American Journal of Sociology* 116 (4): 1190–1233.

Kirmanoglu, Hasan, and Cem Baslevent. 2014. Life Satisfaction of Ethnic Minority Members: An Examination of Interactions with Immigration, Discrimination, and Citizenship. *Social Indicators Research* 116: 173–184.

Kiser, Edgar, and Erin Powers. 2013. Rational Choice Approach to State-making. In *The Handbook of Rational Choice Social Research*, 443–470, ed. Rafael Wittek, Tom A. H. Snijders, and Victor Nee. Stanford, CA: Stanford University Press.

Kittel, Bernhard. 2006. A Crazy Methodology? On the Limits of Macro Quantitative Social Science Research. *International Sociology* 21 (5): 647–677.

Kivimaki, Timo A. 2012. What Generates, Constitutes and Causes Opportunity-Driven Violence? The Case of West Kalimantan. *Asian Journal of Political Science* 20 (3): 284–303.

Klandermans, Bert, and Jacquelien van Stekelenburg. 2013. Social Movements and the Dynamics of Collective Action. In *The Oxford Handbook of Political Psychology*, 774–811, ed. Leone Huddy, David O. Sears and Jack S. Levy. New York: Oxford University Press.

Klandermans, Bert, and Marga de Weerd. 2000. Group Identification and Political Protest. In *Self, Identity, and Social Movements*, 68–90, ed. Sheldon Stryker, Timothy J. Owens, and Robert W. White. Minneapolis, MN: University of Minnesota Press.

Klandermans, Bert. 2015. Motivations to Protest. In *Oxford Handbook of Social Movements*, 219–230, ed. Donatella della Porta and Mario Diani. Oxford, UK: Oxford University Press.

Kleiman, Evan M., and John H. Riskind. 2014. Negative Cognitive Style and Looming Cognitive Style Synergistically Predict Stress Generation. *Anxiety, Stress, & Coping* 27 (3): 347–359.

Klein, Ethel, Jacquelyn Campbell, Esta Soler, and Marrissa Ghez. 1997. *Ending Domestic Violence*. Thousand Oaks, CA: Sage.

Kleiner, Tuuli-Marja. 2018. Public Opinion Polarisation and Protest Behaviour. *European Journal of Political Research* 57 (4): 941–962.

Kleinhans, Reinout, Hugo Priemus, and Godfried Engbersen. 2007. Understanding Social Capital in Recently Restructured Urban Neighborhoods: Two Case Studies in Rotterdam. *Urban Studies* 44 (5/6): 1069–1091.

Kleinhans, Reinout. 2009. Does Social Capital Affect Residents' Propensity to Move from Restructured Neighborhoods? *Housing Studies* 24 (5): 629–651.

Kleinig, John, Simon Keller, and Igor Primoratz. 2015. *The Ethics of Patriotism: A Debate*. Chichester, UK: Wiley.

Kliegel, Matthias, Theodor Jager, and Louise H. Phillips. 2007. Emotional Development across Adulthood: Differential Age-Related Emotional Reactivity and Emotion-Regulation in a Negative Mood Induction Procedure. *International Journal of Aging & Human Development* 64 (3): 217–244.

Kluegal, James R., and Lawrence D. Bobo. 2001. Perceived Group Discrimination and Policy Attitudes: The Sources and Consequences of the Race and Gender Gaps. In *Urban Inequality: Evidence from Four Cities*, 163–213, ed. Alice O'Connor, Chris Tilly and Lawrence D. Bobo. New York: Russell Sage.

Kluegel, James, and Eliot R. Smith. 1986. *Beliefs about Inequality: Americans' Views of What is and What Ought to Be*. New York: Aldine de Gruyter.

Knab, Jean, Irv Garfinkel, and Sara McLanahan. 2008. The Effects of Welfare and Child Support Policies on Maternal Health and Well-being. In *Making American Healthier: Social and Economic Policy as Health Policy*, 281–303, ed. Robert F. Schoeni, James S. House, George A. Kaplan, and Harold Pollack. New York: Russell Sage.

Knack, Stephen. 2002. Social Capital, Growth, and Poverty: A Survey of Cross-Country Evidence. In *The Role of Social Capital in Development: An Empirical Assessment*, 42–84, ed. Christiaan Grootaert and Thierry van Bastelaer. Cambridge, UK: Cambirdge University Press.

Knies, Gundi. 2012. Income Comparisons Among Neighbors and Satisfaction in East and West Germany. *Social Indicators Research* 106: 471–489.

Knight, John, and Lina Song. 2005. *Towards a Labour Market in China*. Oxford, UK: Oxford University Press.

Knittila, Murray, and Wendee Kubik. 2000. *State Theories: Classical, Global, and Feminist Perspectives*. Halifax, Candada: Fernwood.

Knobloch-Westerwick, Silvia. 2015. *Choice and Preference in Media Use: Advances in Selective Exposure Theory and Research*. New York, NY: Routledge.

Koch, Jeffrey W. 1998. Political Rhetoric and Political Persuasion: The Changing Structure of Citizens' Preferences on Health Insurance during Policy Debate. *Public Opinion Quarterly* 62: 209–229.

Koch, Jeffrey W. 2000. Candidate Status, Presidential Approval, and Voting for U.S. Senates. *Electoral Studies* 19: 479–492.

Kolczyuska, Marta. 2020. Changes or Cross-National Differences? Effects of Economic Inequality on Protest Participation. *Social Science Quarterly* 101 (1): 256–268.

Kondo, Ayumi, and Kiyoshi Wada. 2009. The Effectiveness of a Mutual-Help Group Activity for Drug Users and Family Members in Japan. *Substance Use & Misuse* 44: 472–489.

Kondo, Naoki, S.V. Ichiro Kawachi, Yasuhisa Takeda Subramanian, and Zentaro Yamagata. 2008. Do Social Comparisons Explain the Association between Income Inequality and Health? Relative Deprivation and Perceived Health Among Male and Female Japanese Individuals. *Social Science & Medicine* 67 (6): 982–987.

Kongarchapatara, Boonying, George P. Moschis, and Fon Sim Ong. 2014. Understanding the Relationships Between Age, Gender, and Life Satisfaction: The Mediating Role of Stress and Religiosity. *Journal of Beliefs & Values* 35 (3): 340–358.

Koole, S.L., M.E. McCullough, J. Kuhl, and P.H.M.P. Roelofsma. 2010. Why Religion's Burdens Are Light: From Religiosity to Implicit Self-regulation. *Personality & Social Psychology Review* 14 (1): 95–107.

Koopmans, Ruud. 2007. Social Movements. In *The Oxford Handbook of Political Behavior*, 693–707,ed. Russell J. Dalton and Hans-Dieter Klingemann. New York: Oxford University Press.

Korfiatis, Konstantinos J., Tasos Hovardas, and John D. Pantis. 2004. Determinants of Environmental Behavior in Societies in Transition: Evidence form Five European Countries. *Population & Environment* 25 (6): 563–584.

Korinek, Kim, Barbara Entwisle, and Aree Jampakley. 2005. Through Think and Thin: Layers of Social Ties and Urban Settlement among Thai Migrants. *American Sociological Review* 70 (5): 779–810.

Koromeckyj-Cox, Tanya, Amy Mehraban Pienta, and Tyson H. Brown. 2007. Women of the 1950s and the Normative Life Course: The Implications of Childlessness, Fertility Timing, and Marital Status for Psychological Well-Being in Late Midlife. *International Journal of Aging & Human Development* 64 (4): 299–330.

Kosecik, Muhammet, and Isa Sagbas. 2004. Public Attitudes to Local Government in Turkey: Research on Knowledge, Satisfaction and Complaints. *Local Government Studies* 30 (3): 360–383.

Kossinets, Gueorgi, and Duncan J. Watts. 2009. Origins of Homophily in an Evolving Social Network. *American Journal of Sociology* 115 (2): 405–450.

Koven, Steven G. 2015. *Public Sector Ethics: Theory and Applications.* Boca Raton, FL: CRC.

Kovic, Marko, and Nina Hänsli. 2018. Do Millennials Care About Npos? Intergenerational Differences in Attitudes Towards Nonprofit Organizations. *VOLUNTAS: International Journal of Voluntary and Nonprofit Organizations* 29 (5): 1112–1127.

Kowalchuk, Lisa. 2005. The Discourse of Demobilization: Shifts in Activist Priorities and the Framing of Political Opportunities in a Peasant Land Struggle. *Sociological Quarterly* 46: 237–261.

Kozbelt, Aaron, Ronald A. Beghetto, and Mark A. Runco. 2010. Theories of Creativity. In *The Cambridge Handbook of Creativity*, 20–47, ed. James C. Kaufman and Robert J. Sternberg. New York, NY: Cambridge University Press.

Krahe, Barbara. 2001. *The Social Psycholoyg of Aggression.* Hove, UK: Psychology.

Kramer, Jonathan K., and Thomas Hyclak. 2002. Why Strikes Occur: Evidence from the Capital Markets. *Industrial Relations* 41 (1): 80–93.

Kravitz, David A., and Stephen L. Klineberg. 2004. Predicting Affirmative Action Attitudes: Interactions of the Effects of Individual Differences with the Strength of the Affirmative Action Plan. *Research in the Sociology of Work* 14: 107–130.

Krishman, Viuaya, and Karol J. Krotki. 1993. Life Cycle Effects on Homeownership in Canada. *Housing Studies* 8 (2): 120–127.

Kristensen, Dorthe Brogård, Ming Lim, and Søren. Askegaard. 2016. Healthism in Denmark: State, Market, and the Search for a Moral Compass. *Health* 20 (5): 485–504.

Kroll, Christian. 2011. Different Things Make Different People Happy: Examining Social Capital and Subjective Well-Being by Gender and Parental Status. *Social Indicators Research* 104: 157–177.

Kruglanski, Arie W., James Y. Shah, Antonio Pierro, and Lucia Mannetti. 2002. When Similarity Breeds Content: Need for Closure and the Allure of Homogeneous and Self-resembling Groups. *Journal of Personality & Social Psychology* 83 (3): 648–662.

Kruikemeier, S., G. van Noort, R. Vliegenthart, and C.H. de Vreese. 2014. Unraveling the Effects of Active and Passive Forms of Political Internet Use: Does It Affect Citizens' Political Involvement? *New Media & Society* 16 (6): 903–920.

Krys, Kuba, Yukiko Uchida, Shigehiro Oishi, and Ed Diener. 2019. Open Society Fosters Satisfaction: Explanation to Why Individualism Associates with Country Level Measures of Satisfaction. *Journal of Positive Psychology* 14 (6): 768–778.

Kuentzel, Walter F. 2000. Self-identity, Modernity, and the Rational Actor in Leisure Research. *Journal of Leisure Research* 32 (1): 87–92.

Kuiper, Nicholas A., and Sorrel Nicholl. 2004. Thoughts of Feeling Better? Sense of Humor and Physical Health. *Humor* 17 (1/2): 37–66.

Kunovich, Robert M. 2009. The Sources and Consequences of National Identification. *American Sociological Review* 74: 573–593.

Kuntla, Shrikant, Srinivas Goli, T.V. Sekherm and Riddhi Doshi. 2013. Consanguineous Marriages and Their Effects on Pregnancy Outcomes in India. *International Journal of Sociology & Social Policy* 33 (7/8): 437–452.

Kuppens, Toon, Matthew J. Easterbrook, Russell Spears, and Antony S. R. Manstead. 2015. Life at Both Ends of the Ladder. *Personality & Social Psychology Bulletin* 41 (9): 1260–1275.

Kurata, Toru. 2015. Support for and Opposition to Democratization in Hong Kong. *Asia-Pacific Review* 22 (1): 16–33.

Kurtz, Paul. 1988. *Forbidden Fruit: The Ethics of Humanism*. New York: Prometheus Books.

Kurz, Karin, Nikolei, Steinhage, and Katrin Golsch. 2005. Case Study Germany: Global Competition, Uncertainty and the Training to Adulthood. In *Globalization, Uncertainty and Youth in Society*, 58–81, ed. Hans-Peter Blossfeld, Erik Klijzing, Melinda Mills and Karin Kurz. London: Routledge.

Kurz, Tim, and Ngaire Donaghue. 2013. Gender and Discourse. In *The SAGE Handbook of Gender Psychology*, 61–77, ed. Michelle K. Ryan and Nyla R. Branscombe. London: SAGE.

Kutlaca, Maja, Martijn van Zomeren, and Kai Epstude. 2020. Friends or Foes? How Activists and Nonactivists Perceive and Evaluate Each Other. *PLoS ONE* 15 (4): e0230918.

Kwak, Dae-Hoon., Chaudia E. San. Miguel, and Diana L. Carreon. 2010. Political Legitimacy and Public Confidence in Police: An Analysis of Attitudes toward Mexican Police. *Policing* 35 (1): 124–146.

Kwan, Alex Yui-huen, and Beatrice Kwai-king Law. 1994. Attitudes of Student/pupil Nurses toward the Aged in Hong Kong: Implications for Nursing Education. *Hong Kong Journal of Gerontology* 8 (1): 43–51.

Kwan, Letty Y.-Y., and Chi-yue Chiu. 2018. Cultural Diversity, Fractionalization and Economic Complexity: Effects on Innovation Performance and Human Development. In *Handbook of Culture and Creativity: Basic Processes and Applied Innovations*, 105–121. New York, NY: Oxford University Press.

Kwok, Sylvia Y. C. L., Leveda Cheng, Bonnie W. Y. Chow, and Chloe C. Y. Ling. 2015. The Spillover Effect of Parenting on Marital Satisfaction Among Chinese Mothers. *Journal of Child and Family Studies* 24 (3): 772–783.

Kyle, Gerard, and Garry Chick. 2004. Enduring Leisure Involvement: The Importance of Personal Relationships. *Leisure Studies* 23 (3): 243–266.

La Grange, Adrienne, and Ngai Ming Yip. 2001. Social Belonging, Social Capital and the Promotion of Home Ownership: A Case Study of Hong Kong. *Housing Studies* 16 (3): 291–310.

Guardia, La., G. Jennifer, Richard M. Ryan, Charles E. Couchman, and Edward L. Deci. 2000. Within-person Variation in Security of Attachment: A Within-Person Variation in Security of Attachment: A Self-determination Theory Perspective on Attachment, Need, Fulfillment, and Well-being. *Journal of Personality & Social Psychology* 79 (3): 367–384.

Labigne, Anael. 2012. Civility as a Public Opinion: Theorizing Civility and Discussing an Attitude Survey-Based Research Agenda. *Journal of Civil Society* 8 (2): 123–135.

Lackey, Pat N. 1987. *Invitation to Talcott Parsons' Theory*. Houston, TX: Cap.

Ladd, Everett Corll. 1995. The 1994 Congressional Elections: The Postindustrial Realignment Continues. *Political Science Quarterly* 110 (1): 1–23.

Lahusen, Christian. 2021. *The Political Attitudes of Divided European Citizens: Public Opinion and Social Inequalities in Comparative and Relational Perspective*. Abingdon, UK: Routledge.

Lai, Johanna Hiu-wai, Michael Harris Bond, and Natalie Heung-hung Hui. 2007. The Role of Social Axioms in Predicting Life Satisfaction: A Longitudinal Study in Hong Kong. *Journal of Happiness Studies* 8: 517–535.

Lakey, Brian. 2014. Perceived Social Support and Happiness: The Role of Personality and Relational Processes. In *The Oxford Handbook of Happiness*, 847–859, ed. Susan A. David, Ilona Boniwell and Amanda Conley Ayers. Oxford, UK: Oxford University Press.

Lalander, Rickard, and Maija Merimaa. 2018. The Discursive Paradox of Environmental Conflict: Between Ecologism and Economism in Ecuador. *Forum for Development Studies* 45 (3): 485–511.

Lambert, Eric G., Hanif Qureshi, James Frank, Linda D. Keena, and Nancy L. Hogan. 2017. The Relationship of Work-Family Conflict with Job Stress Among Indian Police Officers: A Research Note. *Police Practice & Research* 18 (1): 37–48.

Lan, Lan, and James C. Kaufman. 2012. American and Chinese Similarities and Differences in Defining and Valuing Creative Products. *Journal of Creative Behavior* 46 (4): 285–306.

Land, Kenneth C., and Glenn Deane. 1992. On the Large-sample Estimation of Regression Models with Spatial-or-network Effects Terms: A Two-Stage Least Squares Approach. *Sociological Methodology* 22: 221–248.

Land, Kenneth C., Patricia L. McCall, and Daniel S. Nagin. 1996. A Comparison of Poisson, Negative Binomial, and Semiparametric Mixed Poisson Regression Models with Empirical Applications to Criminal Careers Data. *Sociological Methods & Research* 24 (4): 387–442.

Lane, Robert E. 1991. *The Market Experience*. Cambridge, UK: Cambridge University Press.

Lane, Robert E. 2000. *The Loss of Happiness in Market Democracies*. New Haven, CT: Yale University Press.

Lange, Matthaew, and Andrerw Dawson. 2009. Dividing and Ruling the World? A Statistical Test of the Effects of Colonisation on Postcolonial Civil Violence. *Social Forces* 88 (2): 785–818.

Langenderfer, Jeff, and Terence A. Shimp. 2001. Consumer Vulnerability to Scams, Swindles, and Fraud: A New Theory of Visceral Influences on Persuasion. *Psychology & Marketing* 18 (7): 763–783.

Langman, Lauren. 2005. From Virtual Public Spheres to Global Justice: A Critical Theory of Internetworked Social Movements. *Sociological Theory* 23 (1): 42–74.

Lansford, Jennifer E., and Kenneth A. Dodge. 2008. Cultural Norms for Adult Corporal Punishment of Children and Societal Rates of Endorsement and Use of Violence. *Parenting* 8: 257–270.

Larson, Reed W., David M. Hansen, and Giovanni Moneta. 2006. Differing Profiles of Developmental Experiences across Types of Organized Youth's Activities. *Developmental Psychology* 42 (5): 849–863.

Larson, Reed. 1994. Youth Organizations, Hobbies, and Sports as Developmental Contexts. In *Adolescence in Context: The Interplay of Family, School, Peers, and Work in Adjustment*, 46–65, ed. Rainer K. Silbereisen and Eberhard Todt. New York: Springer.

Laruffa, Francesco. 2020. What Is a Capability-Enhancing Social Policy? Individual Autonomy, Democratic Citizenship and the Insufficiency of the Employment-Focused Paradigm. *Journal of Human Development & Capabilities* 21 (1): 1–16.

Lasch, Christopher. 1984. *The Minimal Self: Psychic Survival in Troubled Times*. New York, NY: Norton.

Lassen, David Dreyer. 2005. The Effect of Information on Voter Turnout: Evidence from a National Experiment. *American Journal of Political Science* 49 (1): 103–118.

Lau, Joseph T.F.., Xilin Yang, H.Y. Ellie Pang, Eric Wong Tsui, and Yun Kwok Wing. 2005. SARS-Related Perceptions in Hong Kong. *Emerging Infectious Diseases* 11 (3): 417–424.

Lau, Yuk-king, Joyce L.C.. Ma, and Ying-keung Chan. 2006. Labor Force Participation of Married Women in Hong Kong: A Feminist Perspective. *Journal of Comparative Family Studies* 37 (1): 93–112.

Lauder, William, Kerry Mummery, and Siobhan Sharkey. 2006. Social Capital, Age and Religiosity In People Who Are Lonely. *Journal of Clinical Nursing* 15 (3): 334–340.

Laudet, Alexandre B., Stephen Magura, Charles M. Cleland, Howard S. Vogel, and Edward L. Knight. 2003. Addictions Services: Predictors of Retention in Dual-focus Self-help Groups. *Community Mental Health Journal* 39 (4): 281–297.

Laurence, James. 2011. The Effect of Ethnic Diversity and Community Disadvantage on Social Cohesion: A Multi-level Analysis of Social Capital and Interethnic Relations in UK Communities. *European Sociological Review* 27 (1): 70–89.

Lavis, John N., and Gregory L. Stoddart. 2003. Social Cohesion and Health. In *Economic Implications of Social Cohesion*, 121–149, ed. Lars Osberg. Toronto, Canada: University of Toronto Press.

Lavrence, Christine, and Kristin Lozanski. 2014. "This Is Not Your Practice Life": Lululemon and the Neoliberal Governance of Self. *Canadian Review of Sociology* 51 (1): 76–94.

Lavrijsen, Jeroen, and Ides Nicaise. 2017. Returns on Vocational Education over the Life Cycle: Between Immediate Labour Market Preparation and Lifelong Employability. *International Review of Education* 63 (2): 257–280.

Lawrence, Rich L., and Steven E. Daniels. 1997. Procedural Justice and Public Involvement in Natural Resource Decision Making. *Society & Natural Resources* 10 (6): 577–589.

Lawrence, Rod. 2000. Education in China: Preparation for Citizenship. *Asian Affairs* 31 (3): 273–284.

Layte, Richard, Brian Nolan, and Christopher T. Whelan. 2000. Targeting Poverty: Lessons from Monitoring Ireland's National Anti-poverty Strategy. *Journal of Social Policy* 29 (4): 553–575.

Lee, Aie-rie, and James A. Norris. 2000. Attitudes Toward Environmental Issues in East Europe. *International Journal of Public Opinion Research* 12 (4): 372–395.

Lee, Barrett A., Chad R. Farrell, and Bruce G. Link. 2004. Revisiting the Contact Hypothesis: The Case of Public Exposure to Homelessness. *American Sociological Review* 69: 40–63.

Lee, Chang-Hun., and Juyoung Song. 2012. Functions of Parental Involvement and Effects of School Climate on Bullying Behaviors among South Korean Middle School Students. *Journal of Interpersonal Violence* 27 (12): 2437–2464.

Lee, Dan, Kap-Young. Jeong, and Sean Chae. 2011. Measuring Social Capital in East Asia and Other World Regions Index of Social Capital for 72 Countries. *Global Economic Review* 40 (4): 385–407.

Lee, Francis L. F., and Joseph M. Chan. 2008. Making Sense of Particpation: The Political Culture of Pro-democracy Demonstrators in Hong Kong. *China Quarterly* 193: 84–101.

Lee, Francis L. F., and Joseph Man Chan. 2016. Digital Media Activities and Mode of Participation in a Protest Campaign: A Study of the Umbrella Movement, Information. *Communication & Society* 19 (1): 4–22.

Lee, Francis L.F.. 2012. Does Discussion with Disagreement Discourage All Topics of Political Participation? Survey Evidence from Hong Kong. *Communication Research* 39 (4): 543–562.

Lee, Francis L.F.., Zhou He, Chin-chuan Lee, Wanying Lin, and Mike Z. Yao. 2012. globalization and People's Interest in Foreign Affairs: A Comparative Survey in Hong Kong and Taipei. *International Communication Gazette* 74 (3): 221–239.

Lee, Matthew R., and Graham C. Dusey. 2011. Reconsidering the Culture and V8olence Connection: Strategies of Action in the Rural South. *Journal of Interpersonal Violence* 26 (5): 899–929.

Lee, Richard M., and Steven B. Robbins. 1998. The Relationship Between Social Connectedness and Anxiety, Self-esteem and Social Identity. *Journal of Counseling Psychology* 45 (3): 338–345.

Lee, Sang Min, M. Harry Daniels, and Daniel B. Kissinger. 2006. Parental Influences on Adolescent Adjustment: Parenting Styles versus Parenting Practices. *Family Journal* 14 (3): 253–259.

Lee, Sunwoo, and Sangwoo Lee. 2019. Relationships Among Financial Satisfaction, Life Satisfaction, and Political Action: A Comparative Study of the United States and South Korea. *Asian Social Work & Policy Review* 13 (3): 252–262.

Lee-Baggley, Dayna, Anita DeLongis, Paul Voorhoeave, and Esther Greenglass. 2004. Coping with the Threat of Severe Acute Respiratory Syndrome: Role of Threat Appraisals and Coping Responses in Health Behaviors. *Asian Journal of Social Psychology* 7: 9–12.

Lei, Chun Kwok, and Shujie Yao. 2008. On Income Convergence among China, Hong Kong and Macau. *World Economy* 345–366.

Lelieveldt, Herman. 2004. Helping Citizens Help Themselves: Neighborhood Improvement Programs and the Impact of Social Networks, Trust, and Norms on Neighborhood-oriented Forms of Participation. *Urban Affairs Review* 39 (5): 531–551.

Lelli, Sara. 2008. Operationalizing Sen's Capability Approach: The Influence of the Selected Technique. In *The Capability Approach: Concepts, Measures and Applications*, 310–361, ed. Flavio Comim, Mozaffar Qizilbash and Sabina Alinre. Cambridge, UK: Cambridge University Press.

Lemon, M.C. 2003. *Philosophy of History: A Guide for Students*. London, UK: Routledge.

Lemyre, Louise, Jennifer E.C.. Lee, Pierre Mercier, Louise Bouchard, and Daniel Krewski. 2006. The Structure of Canadians' Health Risk Perceptions, Environmental Therapeutic and Social Health Risks. *Health, Risk & Society* 8 (2): 185–195.

Lennartsson, Carin. 2010. Need and Support: Determinants of Intra-familial Financial Transfers in Sweden. *International Journal of Social Welfare* 20: 66–74.

Leonard, Peter. 1997. *Postmodern Welfare: Reconstructing an Emancipatory Project*. London: Sage.

Leonardi, Fabio, Liana Spazzafumo, and Fiorella Marcellini. 2005. Subjective Well-Being: The Constructionist Point of View: A Longitudinal Study to Verify the Predictive Power of Top-Down Effects and Bottom-Up Processes. *Social Indicators Research* 70: 53–77.

Leong, Chan-Hoong. 2008. A Multilevel Research Framework for the Analyses of Attitudes toward Immigrants. *International Journal of Intercultural Relations* 32 (2): 115–129.

Lepkowski, James M., and Mick P. Couper. 2002. Nonresponse in the Second Wave of Longitudinal Household Surveys. In *Survey Nonresponse*, 259–272, ed. Robert M. Groves, Don A. Dillman, John L. Eltinge and Roderick J.A. Little. New York: Wiley.

Lerner, Richard M., Amy E. Alberts, Pamela M. Anderson, and Elizabeth M. Dowling. 2006. On Making Humans Human: Spirituality and the Promotion of Positive Youth Development. In *The Handbook of Spiritual Development in Childhood and Adolescence*, 60–72, ed. Eugene C. Roehlkepartain, Pamela Ebstyne King, Linda Wagener and Peter L. Benson. Thousand Oaks, CA: Sage.

LeRoux, Kelly. 2007. Nonprofits as Civic Intermediaries. *Urban Affairs Review* 42 (3): 410–422.

Lessler, Judith T., Rachel A. Caspar, Michael A. Penne, and Peggy R. Barker. 2000. Developing Computer Assisted Interviewing (CAI) for the National Household Survey on Drug Abuse. *Journal of Drug Issues* 30 (1): 9–24.

Lessnoff, Michael H. 1999. *Political Philosophers of the Twentieth Century*. Oxford, UK: Blackwell.

Letki, Natalia. 2006. Investigating the Roots of Civic Morality: Trust, Social Capital, and Institutional Performance. *Political Behavior* 28: 305–325.

Letki, Natalia. 2008. Does Diversity Erode Social Cohesion? Social Capital and Race in British Neighborhoods. *Political Studies* 56 (1): 99–126.

Leu, Chao-Hsien., Ke-Mei. Chen, and Hsiu-Hui. Chen. 2016. A Multidimensional Approach to Child Poverty in Taiwan. *Children & Youth Services Review* 66: 35–44.

Leung, Angela K.-Y., and Brandon Koh. 2018. The Role of Culture in Creative Cognition. In *Handbook of Culture and Creativity: Basic Processes and Applied Innovations*, 3–31. New York, NY: Oxford University Press.

Leung, K.F., W.W. Wong, M.S.M. Tay, M.M.L. Chu, and S.S.W. Ng. 2005. Development and Validation of the Interview Version of the Hong Kong Chinese WHOQOL-BREF. *Quality of Life Research* 14: 1413–1419.

Lever, Joaquina Palomar, Nuria Lanzagorta Pinol, and Jorge Hernandez Uralde. 2005. Poverty, Psychological Resources and Subjective Well-Being. *Social Indicators Research* 73: 375–408.

Levesque, Chantal S., Geoffrey C. Williams, Diane Elliot, Michael A. Pickering, Bradley Bodehamer, and Phillip J. Finley. 2007. Validating the Theoretical Structure of the Treatment Self-regulation Questionnaire (TSRQ) across Three Different Health Behaviors. *Health Education Research* 22 (5): 691–702.

Levin, Jeffrey S., and Linda M. Chatters. 1998. Research on Religion and Mental Health: An Overview on Empirical Findings and Theoretical Issues. In *Handbook of Religion and Mental Health*, 33–50, ed. Harold G. Konenig. San Diego, CA: Academic.

Levontin, Liat, and Anat Bardi. 2019. Using Personal Values to Understand the Motivational Basis of Amity Goal Orientation. *Frontiers in Psychology* 9: 2736.

Lewin-Epstein, Noah, Amit Kaplan, and Asaf Levanon. 2003. Distributive Justice and Attitudes toward the Welfare State. *Social Justice Research* 16 (1):1–27.

Lewinsohn, Peter M., Julie E. Redner, and John R. Selley. 1991. The Relationship between Life Satisfaction and Psychosocial Variables: New Perspectives. In *Subjective Well-Being: An Interdisciplinary Perspective*, 141–169, ed. Fritz Strack, Michael Argyle, and Norbert Schwarz. Oxford: Pergamon Press.

Lewis, Peter. 2007. *Growing apart, Oil, Politics, and Economic Change in Indonesia and Nigeria*. Ann Arbor, MI: University of Michigan Press.

Li, Babai, and Andrew G. Walder. 2001. Career-advancement as Party Patronage: Sponsored Mobility into the Chinese Administrative Elite, 1949–1996. *Americal Journal of Sociology* 106 (5): 1371–1408.

Li, Jingpeng, and Dingguo Song. 1992. *Political Consciousness and Political Behavior of Contemporary China's Youth*. Beijing, China: China's People Public Order University.

Li, Si.-ming. 2010. Mortgage Loan as a Means of Home Finance in Urban China: A Comparative Study of Guangzhou and Shanghai. *Housing Studies* 25 (6): 857–876.

Li, Yu.-sheng, and Ying-chih Chung. 2008. Neighborhood Effects on an Individual's Health Using Neighborhood Measurements Developed by Factor Analysis and Cluster Analysis. *Journal of Urban Health* 86 (1): 5–18.

Liao, Pei-Shan., Fu. Yang-Chih, and Chin-Chun. Yi. 2005. Perceived Quality of Life in Taiwan and Hong Kong: An Intra-culture Comparison. *Journal of Happiness Studies* 6: 43–67.

Lichter, Daniel T., and Rukamalie Jayakody. 2002. Welfare Reform: How Do We Measure Success? *Annual Review of Sociology* 28: 117–141.

Lichter, Daniel T., Christie D. Batson, and J. Brian Brown. 2004. Welfare Reform and Marriage Promotion: The Marital Expectations and Desires of Single and Cohabiting Mothers. *Social Service Review* 78: 2–25.

Lichter, David T., Diane K. McLaughlin, and David C. Ribar. 2002. Economic Restructuring and the Retreat from Marriage. *Social Science Research* 31: 230–256.

Lien, Pei-te. 1994. Ethnicity and Political Participation: A Comparison Between Asian and Mexican Americans. *Political Behavior* 16 (2): 237–264.

Lijphart, Arend. 1997. Unequal Participation: Democracy's Unresolved Dilemma. *American Political Science Review* 91 (1): 1–14.

Like, Taya Z. 2011. Urban Inequality and Racial Differences in Risk for Violent Victimization. *Crime & Delinquency* 57 (3): 432–457.

Lilleker, Darren G., and Thierry Vedel. 2013. The Internet in Campaigns and Elections. In *The Oxford Handbook of Internet Studies*, 401–420, ed. William H. Dutton. Oxford, UK: Oxford University Press.

Lilly, J. Robert, Francis T. Cullen, and Richard A. Ball. 2011. *Criminological Theory: Context and Consequences*. Los Angeles, CA: SAGE.

Lim, Chaeyoon, and Robert D. Putnam. 2010. Religion, Social Networks, and Life Satisfaction. *American Sociological Review* 75 (6): 914–933.

Lin, Chun-Hung A., Suchandra Lahiri, and Ching-Po. Hsu. 2015. Population Aging and Regional Income Inequality in Taiwan: A Spatial Dimension. *Social Indicators Research* 122 (3): 757–777.

Lin, Ka., Xu. Yun, Tianhai Huang, and Jiahua Zhang. 2013. Social Exclusion and Its Cause in East Asian Societies: Evidence from SQSQ Survey Data. *Social Indicators Research* 112 (3): 641–660.

Lin, Y.-J., C.-S. Chen, T.-C. Liu, and H.-C. Lin. 2008b. Taiwan's National Health Insurance System and the Application of Preventive Care: The Case of Pal Smear Testing. *Public Health* 122: 857–861.

Linares, Leticia, Paula Jauregui, David Herrero-Fernández, and Ana Estévez. 2016. Mediationg Role of Mindfulness as a Trait Between Attachment Styles and Depressive Symptoms. *Journal of Psychology* 150 (7): 881–896.

Lincoln, Karen D., Linda M. Chatters, and Robert Joseph Taylor. 2003. Psychological Distress Among Black and White Americans: Different Effects of Social Support, Negative Integration and Personal Control. *Journal of Health & Social Behavior* 44 (3): 390–407.

Lindenberg, Siegwart. 2001. Social Rationality versus Rational Egoism. In *Handbook of Sociological Theory*, 635–668, ed. Jonathan H. Turner. New York: Kluwer.

Lindh, Arvid. 2015. Public Opinion against Markets? Attitudes towards Market Distribution of Social Services: A Comparison of 17 Countries. *Social Policy & Administration* 49 (7): 887–910.

Lineres, L. Oriann. 2004. Social Connection to Neighbors, Multiple Victimization, and Current Health among Women Residing in High Crime Neighborhoods. *Journal of Family Violence* 19 (6): 355–366.

Linssen, Rik, Luuk van Kempen, and Gerbet Kraaykamp. 2011. Subjective Well-being in Rural India: The Curse of Conspicuous Consumption. *Social Indicators Research* 101: 57–72.

Lipford, Jody W., and Bruce Yandle. 2009. The Determinants of Purposeful Voluntarism. *Journal of Socio-Economics* 38 (1): 72–79.

Lippa, Richard A. 2005. *Gender, Nature, and Nurture*, 2nd ed. Mahwah, NJ: Lawrence Erlbaum.

Liska, Allen E., Fred E. Markowitz, Rachel Bridges Whaley, and Paul Bellair. 1999. Modeling the Relationship Between the Criminal Justice and Marital Health Systems. *American Journal of Sociology* 104 (6): 1744–1775.

Lister, Michael. 2007. Institutions, Inequality and Social Norms: Explaining Variations in Participation. *British Journal of Politics & International Relations* 9: 20–35.

Litman, Jordan A., Oliver C. Robinson, and James D. Demetre. 2017. Intrapersonal Curiosity: Inquisitiveness about the Inner Self. *Self & Identity* 16 (2): 231–250.

Litor, Lilach. 2019. Constitutionalism and Anti-privatisation Strikes: Introducing an Eclectic Model. *Israel Law Review* 52 (3): 327–366.

Littlejohn, Stephen W., Karen A. Foss, and John G. Oetzel. 2017. Theories of Human Communication. Long Grove, IL: Waveland.

Littman, Rebecca, and Elizabeth Levy Paluck. 2015. The Cycle of Violence: Understanding Individual Participation in Collective Violence. *Political Psychology* 36 (S1): 79–99.

Litwak, Eugene, and Henry J. Meyer. 1966. A Balance Theory of Coordination between Bureaucratic Organizations and Community Primary Groups. *Administrative Science Quarterly* 11: 31–58.

Livingstone, Sonia, Nick Couldry, and Tim Markham. 2007. Youthful Steps Towards Civic Participation: Does the Internet Help? In *Young Citizens in the Digital Age: Political Engagement, Young People and New Media*, 21–34, ed. Brian D. Loader. London: Routledge.

Lizardo, Omar. 2006. How Cultural Tastes Shape Personal Networks. *American Sociological Review* 71 (5): 778–807.

Lo, Alex Y.H.., and C.Y. Jim. 2012. Citizen Attitude and Expectation Towards Greenspace Provision in Compact. *Land Use Policy* 29: 577–586.

Lo, Sonny Shiu-Hing. 2021. *The Dynamics of Peaceful and Violent Protests in Hong Kong: The Anti-extradition Movement*, Singapore: Palgrave.

Loader, Brian D. 2007. Young Citizens in the Digital Age: Different or Displaced? In *Young Citizens in the Digital Age: Political Engagement, Young People and New Media*, 1–17, ed. Brian D. Loader. London: Routledge.

Lockerbie, Brad. 1999. The Partisan Component to the Incumbency Advantage: 1956–1996. *Political Research Quarterly* 52 (3): 631–646.

Lockwood, Penelope. 2006. Someone Like Me Can Be Successful: Do College Students Need Same-Gender Role Models? *Psychology of Women Quarterly* 30: 36–46.

Lodewijkx, Hein F. M., Gaby L. E. Kersten, and Martijn van Zomeren. 2008. Dual Pathways to Engage in 'Silent Marches' against Violence: Moral Outrage, Moral Cleansing and Modes of Identification. *Journal of Community & Applied Social Psychology* 18 (3): 153–167.

Lofors, Jonas, and Kristina Sundquist. 2007. Law-linking Social Capital as a Predictor of Mental Disorders: A Cohort Study of 4.5 Million Swedes. *Social Science & Medicine* 64: 21–34.

Logan, Jill M., and Rebecca J. Cobb. 2013. Trajectories of Relationship Satisfaction: Independent Contributions of Capitalization and Support Perceptions. *Personal Relationships* 20 (2): 277–293.

Logan, John R., Yanjie Bian, and Fuqin Bian. 1999. Housing Inequality in Urban China in the 1990s. *International Journal of Urban and Regional Research* 23: 7–25.

Lokot, Tetyana. 2020. Data Subjects Vs. People's Data: Competing Discourses of Privacy and Power in Modern Russia. *Media & Communication* 8 (2): 314–22 (\104-382).

London, Rebecca A. 2003. Which TANF Applicants Are Diverted and What Are Their Outcomes? *Social Service Review* 77 (3): 373–398.

Loo, Jeff Hai-chi. 2020. The Myth of Hong Kong Nationalism. *Asian Education & Development Studies* 9 (4): 535–545.

Lopez, Paola Hasbún, Borja Martinović, Magdalena Bobowik, Xenia Chryssochoou, Aleksandra Cichocka, Andreea Ernst-Vintila, Renata Franc, Éva. Fülöp, Djouaria Ghilani, Arshiya Kochar, Pia Lamberty, Giovanna Leone, Laurent Licata, and Iris Žeželj. 2019. Support for Collective Action against Refugees: The Role of National, European, and Global Identifications, and Autochthony Beliefs. *European Journal of Social Psychology* 49 (7): 1439–1455.

Lopez-Escobar, Esteban, Juan Pablo Llamas, and Maxwell McCombs. 1998. Agenda Setting and Community Consensus: First and Second Level Effects. *International Journal of Public Opinion Research* 10 (4): 335–348.

Lorenz, Lois. 1998. Selecting and Implementing Support Groups for Bereaved Adults. *Cancer Practice* 6 (3): 161–166.

Lou, Shi-Jer., C. Ru-Chu Shih, Ray Diez, and Kuo-Hung. Tseng. 2011. The Impact of Problem-Based Learning Strategies on STEM Knowledge Integration and Attitudes: An Exploratory Study Among Female Taiwanese Senior High School Students. *International Journal of Technology and Design Education* 21 (2): 195–215.

Louis, Vincent V., and Shanyang Zhao. 2002. Effects of Family Structure, Family SES, and Adulthood Experience on Life Satisfaction. *Journal of Family Issues* 23 (8): 986–1005.

Lowndes, Vivien, and Mark Roberts. 2013. *Why Institutions Matter: The New Institutionalism in Political Science*. Houndmills, UK: Palgrave.

Lu, Hong, Lening Zhang, and Terance D. Mieche. 2002. Interdependency, Communitarianism and Reintegrative Shaming in China. *Social Science Journal* 39: 189–201.

Lu, Luo, and Shu-fang Kao. 2002. Traditional and Modern Characteristics across the Generations: Similarities and Discrepancies. *Journal of Social Psychology* 142 (1): 45–59.

Lu, Yuhwa Eva, Doman Lum, and Sheying Chen. 2001. Cultural Competency and Achieving Styles in Clinical Social Work: A Conceptual and Empirical Exploration. *Journal of Ethnic & Cultural Diversity in Social Work* 9 (3/4): 1–630.

Lubbers, Mareel, Marcel Coenders, and Peer Scheepers. 2006. Objections to Asylum Seeker Centres: Individual and Contextual Determinants of Resistance to Small and Large Centres in the Netherlands. *European Sociological Review* 32 (3): 243–257.

Lubell, Mark. 2002. Environmental Activism as Collective Action. *Environment & Behavior* 34 (4): 431–454.

Lubell, Mark. 2003. Collaborative Institutions, Belief-Systems, and Perceived Policy Effectiveness. *Political Research Quarterly* 56 (3): 309–323.

Ludwig, Jens, and Philip J. Cook. 2001. The Benefits of Reducing Gun Violence: Evidence from Contingent-Valuation Survey Data. *Journal of Risk & Uncertainty* 22 (3): 207–226.

Luhmann, Maike, Richard E. Lucas, Michael Eid, and Ed Diener. 2013. The Prospective Effect of Life Satisfaction on Life Events. *Social Psychological & Personality Science* 4 (1): 39–45.

Lui, Hon-Kwong. 2011. The Widening Income Dispersion in Hong Kong: 1986–2006. *Journal of Income Distribution* 20 (2): 6–22.

Lum, Yat-sang, and Elizabeth Lightfoot. 2003. The Effect of Health on Retirement Saving Among Older Workers. *Social Work Research* 27 (1): 31–44.

Luna, Jessie K. 2019. The Ease of Hard Work: Embodied Neoliberalism Among Rocky Mountain Fun Runners. *Qualitative Sociology* 42 (2): 251–271.

Lundasen, Susanne Wallman, and Dag Wollebaek. 2013. Diversity and Community Trust in Swedish Local Communities. *Journal of Elections, Public Opinion & Parties* 23 (3): 299–321.

Luo, Lu., Robin Gilmour, and Shu-fang Kao. 2001. Cultural Values and Happiness: An East-West Dialogue. *Journal of Social Psychology* 14 (4): 477–493.

Lusardi, Annamaria, and Jason Beeler. 2007. Saving Between Cohorts: The Role of Planning. In *Redefining Retirement: How Will Boomers Fare?* 271–295, ed. Brigitte Madnan, Olivia S. Mitchell and Beth J. Soldo. Oxford, UK: Oxford University Press.

Luschen, G?nther, William Cockerham, and Gerhard Kunz. 1996. "The Sociocultural Context of Sport and Health Problems of Causal Relations and Structural Interdependence. *Sociology of Sport Journal* 13: 197–213.

Luthar, Timothy C. 2009. *Hegel's Critique of Modernity: Reconciling Individual Freedom and the Community*. Lanham, MD: Lexington.

Lydon-Staley, David M., Perry Zurn, and Danielle S. Bassett. 2019. Within-Person Variability in Curiosity During Daily Life and Associations with Well-Being. *Journal of Personality* 88 (4): 625–641.

Lynch, Julia, and Mikko Myrskyla. 2009. Always the Third Rail? Pension Income and Policy Preferences in European Democracies. *Comparative Political Studies* 42 (8): 1068–1097.

Lyubomirsky, Sonja, Chris Tkach, and M. Robin DiMatteo. 2006. What Are the Differences between Happiness and Self-esteem? *Social Indicators Research* 78: 363–404.

Ma, Josef, Todd Vachon, and Simon Cheng. 2019. National Income, Political Freedom, and Investments in R&D and Education: A Comparative Analysis of the Second Digital Divide among 15-Year-Old Students. *Social Indicators Research* 144 (1): 133–166.

Ma, Joyce L.C.., Timothy K.Y.. Wong, Yuk King Lau, and Shuk Han Pun. 2009. Perceived Family Functioning and Family Resources of Hong Kong Families: Implications for Social Work Practice. *Journal of Family Social Work* 12: 244–263.

MacDonald, Douglas A. 2000. Spirituality: Description, Measurement, and Relation to the Five-Factor Model of Personality. *Journal of Personality* 68 (1): 153–197.

MacDonald, Douglas A., and Harris L. Friedman. 2002. Assessment of Humanistic, Transpersonal, and Spiritual Constructs: States of the Science. *Journal of Humanistic Psychology* 42 (4): 102–125.

MacGregor, Casimir, Alan Petersen, and Christine Parker. 2021. Promoting a Healthier, Younger You: The Media Marketing of Anti-Ageing Superfoods. *Journal of Consumer Culture* 21 (2): 164–179.

Macias, Thomas. 2015. Risks, Trust, and Sacrifice: Social Structural Motivators for Environmental Change. *Social Science Quarterly* 96 (5): 1264–1276.

MacLeod, Andrew K. 2015. Well-Being: Objectivism, Subjectivism or Sobjectivism? *Journal of Happiness Studies* 16 (4): 1073–1089.

Madero-Hernandez, Ardys, and Bonnie S. Fisher. 2013. Routine Activity Theory. In *The Oxford Handbook of Criminological Theory*, 513–534, ed. Francis T. Cullen and Pamela Wilcox. New York: Oxford University Press.

Madlock, Paul E., and David Westerman. 2011. Hurtful Cyber-Teasing and Violence: Who's Laughing out Loud? *Journal of Interpersonal Violence* 26 (17): 3542–3560.

Madrid, Hector P., and Malcolm G. Patterson. 2016. Creativity at Work as a Joint Function Between Openness to Experience, Need for Cognition and Organizational Fairness. *Learning & Individual Differences* 51: 409–416.

Magaletta, Philip R., and J.M. Oliver. 1999. The Hope Construct, Will, and Ways: Their Relations with Self-efficacy, Optimism, and General Well-being. *Journal of Clinical Psychology* 55 (5): 539–551.

Magalhaes, Pedro C. 2014. Government Effectiveness and Support for Democracy. *European Journal of Political Research* 53 (1): 77–97.

Magdol, Lynn, and Diane R. Bessel. 2003. Social Capital, Social Currency, and Portable Assets: The Impacts of Residential Mobility on Exchanges of Social Support. *Personal Relationships* 10: 149–169.

Magee, Marc Porter. 2008. Civic Participation and Social Capital: A Social Network Analysis in Two American Counties. In *Social Capital: An International Research Program*, 308–327, ed. Nan Lin and Bonnie H. Erickson. Oxford, UK: Oxford University Press.

Mahoney, Dennis J. 2004. *Politics and Progress: The Emergence of American Political Science*. Lanham, MD: Lexington.

Mainemelis, Charalampos, et al. 2002. Learning Style and Adaptive Flexibility: Testing Experiential Learning Theory. *Management Learning* 33 (1): 5–33.

Mak, S., and Jason Mueller. 2000. Job Insecurity, Coping Resources and Personality Dispositions in Occupational Strain. *Work & Stress* 14 (4): 312–328.

Makhanova, Anastasia, and Melissa A. Shepherd. 2020. Behavioral Immune System Linked to Responses to the Threat of Covid-19. *Personality & Individual Differences* 167: 110221.

Malahy, Lori W., Michelle A. Rubinlicht, and Cheryl R. Kaiser. 2009. Justifying Inequality: A Cross-Temporal Investigation of U.S. Income Disparities and Just-World Beliefs from 1973 and 2006. *Social Justice Research* 22: 369–383.

Maldonado, Luis, Francisco Olivos, Juan Carlos Castillo, Jorge Atria, and Ariel Azar. 2019. Risk Exposure, Humanitarianism and Willingness to Pay for Universal Healthcare: A Cross-National Analysis of 28 Countries. *Social Justice Research* 32 (3): 349–383.

Malesevic, Sinisa. 2010. *The Sociology of War and Violence*. Cambridge, UK: Cambridge University Press.

Malinowski, Peter. 2014. Flourishing Through Meditation and Mindfulness. In *The Oxford Handbook of Happiness*, 384–396, ed. Susan A. David, Ilona Boniwell and Amanda Conley Ayers. Oxford, UK: Oxford University Press.

Malka, Ariel, and Christopher J. Soto. 2011. The Conflicting Influences of Religiosity on Attitude Toward Torture. *Personality & Social Psychology Bulletin* 37 (8): 1091–1103.

Mallard, Alison G.C.., Charles E. Lance, and Alex C. Michalos. 1997. Cultures as a Moderator of Overall Life Satisfaction: Life Facet Satisfaction Relationship. *Social Indicators Research* 40: 259–284.

Mallard, Graham. 2020. *Bounded Rationality*. Newcastle, UK: Agenda.

Maltseva, Kateryna. 2016. Prosocial Morality in Individual and Collective Cognition. *Journal of Cognition & Culture* 16 (1–2): 1–36.

Man, Derek C., and Simon S.K.. Lam. 2003. The Effects of Job Complexity and Autonomy on Cohesiveness in Collectivistic and Individualistic Work Groups: A Cross-Cultural Analysis. *Journal of Organizational Behavior* 24 (8): 979–994.

Mannarini, Terri, Michele Roccato, and Silvia Russo. 2015. The False Consensus Effect: A Trigger of Radicalization in Locally Unwanted Land Uses Conflicts? *Journal of Environmental Psychology* 42: 76–81.

Mannarini, Terri, Michele Roccato, Angela Fedi, and Alberto Rovere. 2009. Six Factors Fostering Protest: Predicting Participation in Locally Unwanted Land Uses Movements. *Political Psychology* 30 (6): 895–920.

Manstead, Antony S. R. 2011. The Benefits of a Critical Stance: A Reflection on Past Papers on the Theories of Reasoned Action and Planned Behaviour. *British Journal of Social Psychology* 50 (3): 366–373.

Mantena, Karuna. 2012. Another Realism: The Politics of Gandhian Nonviolence. *American Political Science Review* 106 (2): 455–470.

Manturuk, Kim, Mark Lindblad, and Roberto Quercia. 2010. Friends and Neighbors: Homeownership and Social Capital among Low- to Moderate-Income Families. *Journal of Urban Affairs* 32 (4): 471–488.

Mapelli, Vittorio. 1993. Health Needs, Demand for Health Services and Expenditure across Social Groups in Italy: An Empirical Investigation. *Social Science & Medicine* 36 (8): 999–1009.

Marcum, Christopher Steven. 2013. Age Differences in Daily Social Activities. *Research on Aging* 35 (5): 612–640.

Marcus, George E., and Michael MacKuen. 2001. "Emotions and Politics: The Dynamic Functions of Emotionality. In *Citizens and Politics: Perspectives from Political Psychology*, 41–67, ed. James H. Kuklinski. Cambridge, UK: Cambridge University Press.

Marcus, George E., W. Riussell Neuman, and Michael MacKuen. 2000. *Affective Intelligence and Political Judgment*. Chicago, IL: University of Chicago Press.

Marien, Sofie, and Marc Hooghe. 2011. Does Political Trust Matter? An Empirical Investigation into The Relation Between Political Trust and Support for Law Compliance. *European Journal of Political Research* 50 (2): 267–291.

Marien, Sofie. 2011. The Effect of Electoral Outcomes on Political Trust: A Multi-level Analysis of 23 Countries. *Electoral Studies* 30: 712–726.

Marier, Patrik, and Jean F. Mayer. 2007. Welfare Retrenchment as Social Justice: Pension Reform in Mexico. *Journal of Social Policy* 36 (4): 585–604.

Marion, Melanie. 2006. Democracy, Community, Trust: The Impact of Elections in Rural China. *Comparative Political Studies* 39 (3): 301–325.

Markauskaite, Lina. 2007. Exploring the Structure of Trainee Teachers' ICT Literacy: The Main Components of, and Relationships Between, General Cognitive and Technical Capabilities. *Educational Technology Research & Development* 55 (6): 547–572.

Markowitz, Fred E. 2001. Modeling Processes in Recovery from Mental Illness: Relationships between Symptoms, Life Satisfaction, and Self-concept. *Journal of Health & Social Behavior* 42 (1): 64–79.

Markowski, Radoslow. 2006. Political Accountability and Institutional Design in New Democracies. *International Journal of Sociology* 36 (2): 45–75.

Marks, Loren. 2004. Sacred Practices in Highly Religious Families: Christian, Jewish, Mormon, and Muslim Perspectives. *Family Process* 43 (2): 217–231.

Marks, Nadine F. 1996. Flying Solo at Midlife: Gender Marital Status and Psychological Well-Being. *Journal of Marriage and the Family* 58: 917–932.

Marks, Nic, and Hetan Shah. 2005. A Well-Being Manifesto for a Flourishing Society. In *The Science of Well-Being*, 503–531, ed. Felica A. Huppert, Nick Baylis and Barry Keverne. Oxford, UK: Oxford University Press.

Marschall, Melissa J., and Dietlind Stolle. 2004. Race and the City: Neighborhood Context and Development of Generalized Trust. *Political Behavior* 26 (2): 125–153.

Marsh, Robert M. 2005. Tolerance of Civil Liberties in a New Democracy. *Comparative Sociology* 4 (3–4): 313–338.

Martin, John E., and Jennifer Booth. 1999. Behavioral Approaches to Enhance Spirituality. In *Integrating Spirituality into Treatment: Resources for Practitioners*, 161–175, ed. William R. Miller. Washington, DC: American Psychological Association.

Martin, John Levi. 2011. *The Explanation of Social Action*. New York, NY: Oxford University Press.

Martin, Mike, and Gerben J. Westerhof. 2003. Do You Need to Have Them or Should You Believe You Have Them? Resources, Their Approval, and Well-being in Adulthood. *Journal of Adult Development* 10 (2): 99–112.

Martin, Virginia. 2000. The Effect of Neighborhood Racial Heterogeneity and Income Inequality on the Level of Home Ownership. *Research in Community Sociology* 10: 345–362.

Martinelli, Alberto. 2005. *Global Modernization: Rethinking the Project of Modernity*. London: SAGE.

Martinelli, Kathleen A., and Steven H. Chaffee. 1995. Measuring New-Voter Learning Via Three Channels of Political Information. *Journalism & Mass Communication Quarterly* 72: 18–32.

Marx, Paul. 2014. Labour Market Risks and Political Preferences: The Case of Temporary Employment. *European Journal of Political Research* 53 (1): 136–159.

Maslow, Abraham H. 1999. *Toward a Psychology of Being*, 3rd ed. New York: Wiley.

Mason, Andrew. 2012. *Living Together as Equals: The Demands of Citizenship*. Oxford, UK: Oxford University Press.

Mata, Fernando, and Ravi Pendakur. 2014. Social Capital, Diversity and Giving or Receiving Help Among Neighbours. *Social Indicators Research* 118 (1): 329–347.

Matheson, George, and Michael Wearing. 1999. Within and without: Labor Force Status and Political Views in Four Welfare States. In *The End of the Welfare State? Responses to State Retrenchment*, 135–160, ed. Stefan Svallfors and Peter Taylor-Gooby. London: Routledge.

Mattes, Robert, and Jennifer Christie. 1997. Personal versus Collective Quality of Life and Soth Africa's Evaluation of Democratic Government. *Social Indicators Research* 41: 205–228.

Mattes, Robert, and Roger Southall. 2004. Popular Attitudes toward the South African Electoral System. *Democratization* 11 (1): 51–76.

Matthewman, Steve. 2011. *Technology and Social Theory*. Houndmills, Palgrave.

Matthews, Gerald, Amanda K. Emo, Gregory Funke, Moshe Zeidner, Richard D. Roberts, Paul T. Costa, and Ralf Schulze. 2006. Emotional Intelligence, Personality, and Task-Induced Stress. *Journal of Experimental Psychology: Applied* 12 (2): 96–107.

Matthews, Gerald. 1997. An Introduction to the Cognitive Science of Personality and Emotion. In *Cognitive Science Perspectives on Personality and Emotion*, 3–30, ed. Gerald Matthews. Amsterdam, Netherlands: Elsevier.

Mau, Steffen. 2005. Democratic Demand for a Social Europe? Preferences of the European Citizenry. *International Journal of Social Welfare* 14: 76–85.

Maurer, Markus. 2011. Education and Social Integration: Comprehensive Schooling in Europe. *European Educational Research Journal* 10 (1): 160–167.

Mauro, Max. 2020. Media Discourse, Sport and the Nation: Narratives and Counter-Narratives in the Digital Age. *Media, Culture, & Society* 42 (6): 932–951.

Maxton-Lee, Bernice. 2020. Activating Responsible Citizens: Depoliticized Environmentalism in Hegemonic Neoliberalism. *Democratization* 27 (3): 443–460.

Mayer, Adam. 2017. Social Capital, Economic Hardship, and Health: A Test of the Buffering Hypothesis in Transition and Nontransition Countries. *Sociological Spectrum* 37 (2): 111–126.

McAulay, Brian, et al. 2006. Testing a Push-Pull Theory of Work Commitment among Organizational Professionals. *Social Science Journal* 43: 571–596.

McCabe, Brian J. 2014. Are Homeowners Better Citizens? Homeownership and Community Participation in the United States. *Social Forces* 91 (3): 929–954.

McCall, Leslie, and Lane Kenworthy. 2009. Americans' Social Policy Preferences in the Era of Rising Inequality. *Perspectives on Politics* 7 (3): 459–484.

McCammon, Holly J., and Minyoung Moon. 2015. Social Movement Coalitions. In *The Oxford Handbook of Social Movements*, 326–339, ed. Donatella Della Porta and Mario Diani. Oxford, UK: Oxford University Press.

McClurg, Scott D. 2006. The Electoral Resources of Political Talk: Examining Disagreement and Expertise Effects in Social Networks on Political Participation. *American Journal of Political Science* 50 (3): 737–754.

McCright, Aaron M., and Riley E. Dunlop. 2008. The Nature and Social Bases of Progressive Social Movement Ideology: Examining Public Opinion toward Social Movements. *Sociological Quarterly* 49: 825–848.

McCright, Aaron M., and Terry Nichols Clark. 2006. The Political Opportunity Structure of the Environmental Movement in U.S. Communities. *Research in Urban Policy* 10: 199–240.

McCullough, Michael E., and David B. Larson. 1999. Prayer. In *Integrating Spirituality into Treatment: Resources for Practitioners*, 85–110, ed. William R. Miller. Washington, DC: American Psychological Association.

McDonald, Kevin. 2013. *Our Violent World: Terrorism in Society*. Houndmills, UK: Palgrave.

McDowell, M.E., S. Occhipinti, M. Ferguson, J. Dunn, and S.K. Chambers. 2010. Predictors of Change in Unmet Supportive Care Needs in Cancer. *Psycho-Oncology* 19: 508–516.

McDowell, Michael and Nathan Robert Brown. 2009. *World Religions: At Your Fingertips*. New York, NY: Alpha.

McGrail, Stephen. 2011. Environmentalism in Transition? Emerging Perspectives, Issues and Futures Practices in Contemporary Environmentalism. *Journal of Futures Studies* 15 (3): 117–144.

McGraw, Kathleen M., Milton Lodge, and Jeffrey M. Jones. 2002. The Pandering Politician of Suspicious Minds. *Journal of Politics* 14 (2): 362–383.

McGregor, Shannon C. 2018. Personalization, Social Media, and Voting: Effects of Candidate Self-personalization on Vote Intention. *New Media & Society* 20 (3): 1139–1160.

McIlroy, John. 2014. Marxism and the Trade Unions: The Bureaucracy Versus the Rank and File. *Critique: Journal of Socialist Theory* 42 (4): 497–526.

McKenzie, Jordan. 2016. Happiness vs Contentment? A Case for a Sociology of the Good Life. *Journal for the Theory of Social Behaviour* 46 (3): 252–267.

McLaren, Lauren M. 2003. Anti-immigrant Prejudice in Europe: Contact, Threat Perception, and Preferences for the Exclusion of Migrants. *Social Forces* 81 (3): 909–930.

McLean, Scott. 2015. Individual Autonomy or Social Engagement? Adult Learners in Neoliberal Times. *Adult Education Quarterly* 65 (3): 196–214.

McMahon, Sarah, N. Andrew Peterson, Samantha C. Winter, Jane E. Palmer, Judy L. Postmus, and Ruth Anne Koenick. 2015. Predicting Bystander Behavior to Prevent Sexual Assault on College Campuses: The Role of Self-efficacy and Intent. *American Journal of Community Psychology* 56 (1–2): 46–56.

McMullin, Julie Ann, and John Cairney. 2004. Self-esteem and the Intersection of Age, Class, and Gender. *Journal of Aging Studies* 18 (1): 75–90.

McNally, Richard J. 1990. Psychological Approaches to Panic Disorder: A Review. *Psychological Bulletin* 108 (3): 403–419.

McNeeley, Susan, and Yue Yuan. 2017. A Multilevel Examination of the Code of the Street?s Relationship with Fear of Crime. *Crime & Delinquency* 63 (9): 1146–1167.

McPhail, Clark, and Charles W. Tucker. 2003. Collective Behavior. In *Handbook of Symbolic Interactionism*, 721–741, ed. Larry T. Reynolds and Nancy J. Herman-Kinney. Lanham, MD: Rowman.

McPherson, Miller, Lynn Smith-Lovin, and Matthew E. Brashears. 2006. Social Isolation in America: Changes in Core Discussion Networks over Two Decades. *American Sociological Review* 71 (3): 353–375.

McVeigh, Rory, and Christian Smith. 1999. Who Protests in America: An Analysis of Three Political Alternatives: Inaction, Institutionalized Politics, or Protest. *Sociological Forum* 14 (4): 685–702.

McVeigh, Rory. and David Sikkink. 2001. God, Politics, and Protest: Religious Beliefs and the Legitimation of Contentious Tactics. *Social Forces* 79 (4): 1425–1458 (\117-351).

Mechanic, David, and Sharon Meyer. 2000. Concepts of Trust among Patients with Serious Illness. *Social Science & Medicine* 51: 657–668.

Medvedovski, Dmitri, and Kirk Allison. 2017. Paternal Religious Affiliation and Practice in Lithuania: Spiritual Goods or Secular Utilities? *International Journal of Social Economics* 44 (12): 1758–1777.

Meerkerke, Gert-Jan, Regina J.J.M. van den Eijnden, and Henk F.L. Garrestsen. 2006. Predicting Compulsive Internet Use: It's All about Sex? *CyberPsychology & Behavior* 9 (1): 95–103.

Megone, Christopher. 1990. The Quality of Life: Starting from Aristotle. In *Quality of Life: Perspectives and Policies*, 28–54, ed. Sally Baldwin, Christine Godfrey, and Carol Propper. London: Routledge.

Meier, Kenneth J. 1994. *The Politics of Sin: Drugs, Alcohol, and Public Policy*. Armonk, NJ: Sharpe.

Meis, Mareike. 2017. When Is a Conflict a Crisis? On the Aesthetics of the Syrian Civil War in a Social Media Context. *Media, War & Conflict* 10 (1): 69–86.

Meisenberg, Gerhard, and Amandy Williams. 2008. Are Acquiescent and Extreme Response Styles Related to Low Intelligence and Education? *Personality & Individual Differences* 44: 1539–1550.

Meiser, B., P. Buton, V. Schnieden, M. Gattas, C. Gaff, K. Uarrop, A. Banker, M.A. Young, and K. Tucker. 2000. Psychological Adjustment of Women at Increased Risk of Developing Hereditary Breast Cancer. *Psychology, Health, & Medicine* 5 (4): 377–388.

Melton, Heather C. 2000. Stalking: A Review of the Literature and Direction for the Future. *Criminal Justice Review* 25 (2): 246–262.

Melzer, Silvia Maja. 2011. Does Migration Make You Happy? The Influence of Migration on Subjective Well-being. *Journal of Social Research & Policy* 2 (2): 73–92.

Menahem, Gila. 2001. Urban Civic Worlds: A Conceptual and Empirical Exploration. *Local Government Studies* 27 (1): 37–60.

Mendelsohn, Matthew, and Richard Nadeau. 1996. The magnification and Minimization of Social Cleavages by the Broadcast and Narrowcast News Media. *International Journal of Public Opinion Research* 8 (4): 374–389.

Meng, Chenli, and Eugene Abrokwah. 2021. Training and Support Relationship Influences on Volunteers' Public Advocacy Behaviours: Their Mediation by Psychological Empowerment. *Journal of Psychology in Africa* 31 (4): 430–433.

Meng, Tianguang, and He Chen. 2014. A Multilevel Analysis of Social Capital and Self-Rated Health: Evidence From China. *Health & Place* 27: 38–44.

Merrilees, Bill, Dale, and Carmel Herrington. 2009. Antecedents of Residents' City Brand Attitudes. *Journal of Business Research* 62: 362–367.

Mesch, Gustavo S. 1996. The Effect of Environmental Concerns and Governmental Incentives on Organized Action in Local Areas. *Urban Affairs Review* 31 (3): 346–366.

Mesch, Gustavo S. 2009. Social Bonds and Internet Pornographic Exposure among Adolescents. *Journal of Adolescence* 32: 601–618.

Mesch, Gustavo S., and Orit Manor. 1998. Social Ties, Environmental Perception, and Local Attachment. *Environment & Behavior* 30 (4): 504–519.

Mesch, Gustavo S., and Stephen Coleman. 2007. New Media and New Voters: Young People, the International the 2005 UK Election Campaign. In *Young Citizens in the Digital Age: Political Engagement, Young People and New Media*, 35–47, ed. Brian D. Loader. London: Routledge.

Mesirow, Jack. 2003. Transformative Learning as Discourse. *Journal of Transformative Education* 1 (1): 58–63.

Messner, Steven F. 1986. Modernization, Structural Characteristics, and Societal Rates of Crimes: An Application of Blau's Macrosociological Theory. *Sociological Quarterly* 27 (1): 27–41.

Messner, Steven F., Helmut Thome, and Richard Rosenfeld. 2008. Institutions, Anomie, and Violent Crime: Clarifying and Elaborating Institutional-anomie Theory. *International Journal of Conlfict & Violence* 2 (2): 163–181.

Messner, Steven F., Richard Rosenfeld, and Susanna Karstedt. 2013. Social Instituions and Crime. In *The Oxford Handbook of Criminological Theory*, 405–423, ed. Francis T. Cullen and Pamela Wilcox. New York: Oxford University Press.

Metzl, Einat S., and Malissa A. Morrell. 2008. The Role of Creativity in Models of Resilience: Theoretical Exploration and Practical Applications. *Journal of Creativity in Mental Health* 3 (3): 303–318.

Meulemann, Heiner. 2010. Self-concern, Self-transcendence, and Well-Being. *European Sociological Review* 26 (4): 385–399.

Meyer, David S. 2004. Protest and Political Opportunities. *Annual Review of Sociology* 30: 125–145.

Meyer, Katherine, Yousef Ali, and Sheri Locklear. 1998. Political Participation of Men and Women in Postwar Kuwait. *Research in Political Sociology* 8: 57–80.

Michael, Mike. 2017. *Actor-network Theory: Trials, Trails, and Translations*. London, UK: SAGE.

Michalos, Alex C., Bruno D. Zumbo, and Anita Hubley. 2000. Health and the Quality of Life. *Social Indicators Research* 51: 245–286.

Michalos, Alex C., Harvey V. Thommasen, Rua Read, Nancy Anderson, and Bruno D. Zumbo. 2005. Determinants of Health and the Quality of Life in the Bella Coola Valley. *Social Indicators Research* 72: 1–50.

Michalski, Joseph H. 2005. Explaining Intimate Partner Violence: The Sociological Limitation of Victimization Studies. *Sociological Forum* 20 (4): 623–640.

Migliaccio, Todd A. 2002. Abused Husbands: A Narrative Analysis. *Journal of Family Issues* 23 (1): 26–52.

Mikulincer, Mario, and Phillip R. Shaver. 2014. Adult Attachment and Happiness: Individual Differences in the Experience and Consequences of Positive Emotions. In *The Oxford Handbook of Happiness*, 834–846, ed. Susan A. David, Ilona Boniwell and Amanda Conley Ayers. Oxford, UK: Oxford University Press.

Milbraith, Lester W. 1982. A Conceptualization and Research Strategy for the Study of Ecological Aspects of the Quality of Life. *Social Indicators Research* 10: 133–157.

Milbrath, Lester W. 1986. Environmental Beliefs and Values. In *Political Psychology: Contemporary Problems and Issues*, 97–138, ed. Margaret G. Hermann. San Francisco, CA: Jossey-Bass.

Milgram, Roberta M., and Eunsook Hong. 1994. Creative Thinking and Creative Performance in Adolescents as Predictors of Creative Attainments in Adults: A Follow-up Study after 18 Years.In *Beyond Terman: Contemporary Longitudinal Studies of Giftedness and Talent*, 212–228, ed. Rena F. Subotnik, and Karen D. Arnold. Norwood, NJ: Ablex.

Miller, Alan S. 1995. A Rational Choice Model of Religious Behavior in Japan. *Journal for the Scientific Study of Religion* 34 (2): 234–244.

Miller, Melissa K. 2010. Membership Has Its Privileges. *Political Research Quarterly* 63 (2): 356–372.

Miller, Paul, and Charles Mulvey. 1991. Australian Evidence on the Exit/Voice Model of hte Labor Market. *Industrial & Labor Relations Review* 45 (1): 44–57.

Miller, Seumas. 2001. *Social Action: A Teleological Account*. Cambridge, UK: Cambridge University Press.

Miller, William L. 1991. *Media and Voters: The Audience Context and Influence of Press and Television at the 1987 General Election*. Oxford: Clarendon.

Miller, William R., and Carol E. Thoresen. 2003. Spirituality, Religion, and Health: An Emerging Research Field. *American Psychologist* 58 (1): 24–35.

Miller-Stevens, Katrina, Jennifer A. Taylor, John C. Morris, and Stephen E. Lanivich. 2018. Assessing Value Differences between Leaders of Two Social Venture Types: Benefit Corporations and Nonprofit Organizations. *VOLUNTAS: International Journal of Voluntary and Nonprofit Organizations* 29 (5): 938–950.

Milligan, Christine, and Nicholas R. Fyfe. 2005. Preserving Space for Volunteers: Exploring the Links Between Voluntary Welfare Organizations, Volunteering and Citizenship. *Urban Studies* 42 (3): 417–433.

Milner, Henry. 2002. *Civic Literacy: How Informed Citizens Make Democracy Work*. Hanover, NH: University Press of New England.

Mincer, Jacob. 1993. *Studies in Labor Supply*. Aldershot, UK: Elgar.

Miner-Rubino, Kathi, David G. Winter, and Abigail J. Stewart. 2004. Gender, Social Class, and the Subjective Experience of Aging: Self-perceived Personality Change from Early Adulthood to Late Midlife. *Personality & Social Psychology Bulletin* 30 (12): 1599–1610.

Minkov, Michael. 2011. *Cultural Differences in a Globally World*. Bingley, UK: Emerald.

Minogue, Kenneth. 2010. *The Servile Mind: How Democracy Erodes the Moral Life*. New York: Encounter.

Mirowsky, John, and Catherine E. Ross. 1998. Education, Personal Control, Lifestyle and Health: A Human Capital Hypothesis. *Research on Aging* 20 (4): 415–449.

Mirowsky, John, and Catherine E. Ross. 2001. Age and Effect of Economic Hardship on Depression. *Journal of Health & Social Behavior* 42: 132–150.

Mishler, William, and Richard Rose. 1997. Trust, Distrust and Skepticism: Popular Evaluation of Civil and Political Institutions in Post-communist Societies. *Journal of Politics* 59 (2): 418–451.

Mishna, Faye. 2012. *Bullying: A Guide to Research, Intervention, and Prevention*. New York< NY: Oxford University Press.

Mitchell, Katharyne. 2017. Factivism: A New Configuration of Humanitarian Reason. *Geopolitics* 22 (1): 110–128.

Mitoma, Glenn, and Kerry Bystrom. 2013. Humanitarianism and Responsibility. *Journal of Human Rights* 12 (1): 1–20.

Mitrut, Andreea, and Francois-Charles. Wolff. 2011. Do Private and Public Transfers Received Affect Life Satisfaction: Evidence from Romania. *Journal of Economic Psychology* 32: 969–979.

Miyata, Kakuto, and Tetsuro Kubayashi. 2008. Causal Relationship Between Internet Use and Social Capital in Japan. *Asian Journal of Social Psychology* 11: 42–52.

Mizen, Phil. 2015. The Madness That Is The World: Young Activists' Emotional Reasoning and Their Participation in a Local Occupy Movement. *Sociological Review* 63 (S2): 167–182.

Mizrahi, Shlomo. 2016. Economic Conditions, Government Effectiveness and Public Attitudes towards the Welfare State. *Journal of Poverty & Social Justice* 24 (2): 157–170.

Moeller, Scott J., Jennifer Crocker, and Brad J. Bushman. 2009. Creating Hostility and Conflict: Effects of Entitlement and Self-image Goals. *Journal of Experimental Social Psychology* 45 (2): 448–452.
Moen, Phyllis, Erin L. Kelly, and Jack Lam. 2013. Healthy Work Revisited: Do Changes in Time Strain Predict Well-Being? *Journal of Occupational Health Psychology* 18 (2): 157–172.
Moen, Phyllis, Mary Ann Erickson, and Donna Dempster-McClain. 1997. their Mother's Daughters: The Intergenerational Transmission of Gender Attitudes in a World of Changing Roles. *Journal of Marriage & the Family* 59 (2): 281–293.
Mogg, Karin, and Brendan P. Bradley. 1998. A Cognitive-Motivational Analysis of Anxiety. *Behavior Research & Therapy* 36: 809–848.
Moiseeva, V.V., and M.E. Pozniakova. 2009. Can Religion Counteract the Spread of Narcotics Abuse among Young People. *Russian Education & Society* 51 (3): 25–43.
Molana, Hanieh H., and Richard E. Adams. 2019. Evaluating Sense of Community in the Residential Environment from the Perspectives of Symbolic Interactionism and Architectural Design. *Journal of Community Psychology* 47 (7): 1591–1602.
Moller, Jorgen, and Svend-Erik. Skaaning. 2013. *Democracy and Democratization in Comparative Perspective: Conceptions, Conjunctures, Causes, and Consequences*. Abingdon, UK: Routledge.
Moller, Jorgen, and Svend-Erik. Skaaning. 2014. Respect for Civil Liberties During the Third Wave of Democratization: Presenting a New Dataset. *Social Indicators Research* 117 (3): 1069–1087.
Moller, Stephanie, and Huiping Li. 2009. Segregation in Organizations: Parties, Unions, Policies and Occupational Sex Segregation in the United States. *Social Forces* 87 (3): 1529–1560.
Moller, Stephanie, David Bradley, Everlyne Huber, Francois Nielsen, and John D. Stephens. 2003. Determinants of Relative Poverty in Advanced Capitalist Democracies. *American Sociological Review* 68 (1): 22–51.
Moller, Valerie. 2005. Resilient or Resigned? Criminal Victimisation and Quality of Life in South Africa. *Social Indicators Research* 72: 263–317.
Molz, Ashleigh R., Chelsea L. Black, Benjamin G. Shapero, Rachel E. Bender, Lauren B. Alloy, and Lyn Y. Abramson. 2013. Aggression and Impulsivity as Predictors of Stress Generation in Bipolar Spectrum Disorders. *Journal of Affective Disorders* 146 (2): 272–280.
Mommaas, Hans. 2004. Cultural Clusters and the Post-industrial City: Towards the Remapping of Urban Cultural Policy. *Urban Studies* 41 (3): 507–532.
Mondak, Jeffery J., and Jon Hurwitz. 2012. Examining the Terror Exception: Terrorism and Commitments to Civil Liberties. *Public Opinion Quarterly* 76 (2): 193–213.
Monfortia, Jessica Lavariega, and Adam J. McGlynn. 2015. The Awakening of the Sleeping Giant? An Examination of the Role of Ethnicity in the 2006 Immigrant Rights Protests. *Social Science Journal* 52 (4): 550–560.
Montet, Christian, and Daniel Serra. 2003. *Game Theory and Economics*. Houndmills, UK: Palgrave.
Montgomery, Diane, Pamela A. Hodges, and Judith S. Kuafman. 2004. An Exploratory Study of the Relationship Between Mood States and Creativity Self-perceptions. *Creativity Research Journal* 16 (2&3): 341–344.
Mooijman, Marlon, Joe Hoover, Ying Lin, Heng Ji, and Morteza Dehghani. 2018. Moralization in Social Networks and the Emergence of Violence during Protests. *Nature Human Behaviour* 2 (6): 389–396.
Mookerjee, Rajer, and Krista Beron. 2004. Gender, Religion, and Happiness. *Journal of Socio-Economics* 34: 674–685.
Moore, Dahlia, and Salem Aweiss. 2003. Outcome Expectations in Prolonged Conflicts: Perceptions of Sense of Control and Relative Deprivation. *Sociological Inquiry* 73 (2): 190–211.
Moore, Margaret. 2001. *The Ethics of Nationalism*. Oxford, UK: Oxford University Press.
Moore, Simon, and Jonathan P. Shepherd. 2006. The Cost of Fear: Shadow Pricing the Intangible Costs of Crime. *Applied Economics* 38 (3): 293–300.
Moran, Erin K., Neera Mehta, and Ann M. Kring. 2012. Emotional Responding in Depression: Distinctions in the Time Course of Emotion. *Cognition & Emotion* 26 (7): 1153–1175.

Morenoff, Jeffrey D., Ana V. Diez Roux, Ben B. Hansen, and Theresa L. Osypuk. 2008. Residential Environments and Obesity: What Can We Learn about Policy Interventions from Observational Studies? In *Making American Healthier: Social and Economic Policy as Health Policy*, 309–343, ed. Robert F. Schoeni, James S. House, George A. Kaplan, and Harold Pollack. New York: Russell Sage.

Morgan, G. Scott., and Wing Yi Chan. 2016. Different Paths to Protest: Predictors of Collective Action in the Occupy Movement: Collective Action and Occupy. *Journal of Applied Social Psychology* 46 (10): 565–582.

Morgan, Jessica, and Oliver Robinson. 2013. Intrinsic Aspirations and Personal Meaning across Adulthood: Conceptual Interrelations and Age/Sex Differences. *Developmental Psychology* 49 (5): 999–1010.

Morgan, Susan E., Jenny K. Miller, and Lily A. Abrasaratnam. 2003. Similarities and Differences Between African Americans and European Americans' Attitudes, Knowledge, and Willingness to Communicate about Organ Donation. *Journal of Applied Social Psychology* 33 (4): 693–715.

Morin, Aysel. 2016. Framing Terror. *Journalism & Mass Communication Quarterly* 93 (4): 986–1005.

Morody, Mioslawa, and Anna Giza-Poleszczuk. 2018. *Transformation of Social Bonds: The Outline of the Theory of Social Change*. Berlin, Germany: Lang.

Morris, Stephen D., and Joseph L. Klesner. 2010. Corruption and Trust: Theoretical Considerations and Evidence from Mexico. *Comparative Political Studies* 43 (10): 1258–1285.

Morrison, Elizabeth Wolfe, and Corey C. Phelps. 1999. Taking Charge at Work: Extrarole Efforts to Institute Workplace Change. *Academy of Management Journal* 42 (4): 403–419.

Morrow, Raymond D., with David D. Brown. 1994. *Critical Theory and Methodology*. Thousand Oaks, CA: SAGE.

Morselli, Davide, and Stefano Passini. 2018. Exclusive and Inclusive Protest in Europe: Investigating Values, Support for Democracy, and Life Conditions. *Journal of Community & Applied Social Psychology* 28 (3): 123–141.

Mortimer, Jeylan T., and Heather McLaughlin. 2014. Theoretical and Substantive Approaches to Socialization and Inequality in Social Psychology. In *Handbook of the Social Psychology of Inequality*, 243–272, ed. Jane D. McLeod, Edward J. Lawler, and Michael Schwalbe. Dordrecht, Netherland: Springer.

Mortimer, Jeylan T., and Jan Lorence. 1989. Satisfaction and Involvement: Disentangling a Deceptively Simple Relationship. *Social Psychology Quarterly* 52 (4): 249–265.

Morton, Thomas A., and Julie M. Duck. 2001. Communication and Health Beliefs: Mass and Interpersonal Influences on Perceptions of Risk to Self and Others. *Communication Research* 28 (5): 602–626.

Mosca, Lorenzo, and Donatella della Porta. 2009. Unconventional Politics Online: Internet and the Global Justice Movement. In *Democracy in Social Movements*, 194–216, ed. Donatella della Porta. Houndmills, UK: Palgrave.

Moschis, George P., and Fon Sim Ong. 2011. Religiosity and Consumer Behavior of Older Adults: A Study of Subcultural Influences in Malaysia. *Journal of Consumer Behavior* 10: 8–17.

Moscoso-Sanchez, David, Álvaro. Rodríguez-Díaz, and Jesús Fernández-Gavira. 2015. Elitist Rhetoric and the Sports Gap. Examining the Discourse and Reality of Sport in Spain. *European Journal for Sport & Society* 12 (1): 31–51.

Moskolenko, Sophia, and Clark McCauley. 2009. Measuring Political Mobilization: The Distinction between Activism and Radicalism. *Terrorism & Political Violence* 21: 239–260.

Moss, Dana M., and David A. Snow. 2016. Theorizing Social Movements. In *Handbook of Contemporary Sociological Theory*, 547–569, ed. Seth Abrutyn. Cham, Switzerland: Springer.

Mouzelis, Nicos. 1999. Modernity: A Non-European Conceptualization. *British Journal of Sociology* 50 (1): 141–159.

Moy, Jane W. 2006. Are Employers Assessing the right Traits in Hiring: Evidence from Hong Kong Companies. *International Journal of Human Resource Management* 17 (4): 734–754.

Moy, Patricia, and Michael Pfau. 2000. *With Malice toward All? The Media and Public Confidence in Democratic Institutions*. Westport, CT: Praeger.

Muennig, Peter, Alison K. Cohen, Aileen Palmer, and Wenyi Zhu. 2013. The Relationship between Five Different Measures of Structural Social Capital, Medical Examination Outcomes, and Mortality. *Social Science & Medicine* 85: 18–26.

Muffels, Ruud, and Didier Fouarge. 2004. The Role of European Welfare States in Explaining Resources Deprivation. *Social Indicators Research* 68: 299–330.

Muhlau, Peter. 2014. Middle Class Squeeze? Social Class and Perceived Financial Hardship in Ireland, 2002–2012. *Economic and Social Review* 45 (4): 485–509.

Mukherjee, Rabin. 2000. *Democracy: A Failure, Shefocracy: The Solution for Human Welfare*. Lanham, MD: University Press of America.

Mulatu, Mesfin Samuel, and Carmi Schooler. 2002. Causal Connections Between Socio-economic Status and Health: Reciprocal Effects and Mediating Mechanisms. *Journal of Health & Social Behavior* 43 (1): 22–41.

Mulder, Clara H., and Michael Wagner. 1998. First-time Home-Ownership in the Family Life Course: A West German-Dutch Comparison. *Urban Studies* 35 (4): 687–713.

Mummendey, Amelie, Thomas Kessler, Andreas Klink, and Rosemarie Mielke. 1999. Strategies to Cope with Negative Social Identity: Predictions by Social Identity Theory and Relative Deprivation Theory. *Journal of Personality & Social Psychology* 76 (2): 229–245.

Munch, Richard. 1987. *Theory of Action: Towards a New Synthesis Going beyond Parsons*. London: Routledge & Kegan Paul.

Munch, Richard. 1988. *Understanding Modernity: Toward a New Perspective Going beyond Durkheim and Weber*. London: Routledge.

Munck, Ronaldo. 2005. *Globalization and Social Exclusion: A Transformationalist Perspective*. Bloomfield, CT: Kumarian.

Munck, Ronaldo. 2018. Development and Social Change: A Genealogy for an Era of Complexity. In *Handbook on Development and Social Change*, 1–18, ed. G. Honor Fagan and Ronaldo Munck. Northampton, MA: Elgar.

Munk, Martin D. 2003. Institutionalized Legitimate Informational Capital on the Welfare State: Has Policy Failed? In *The International Assessment of New Research and Theory*, ed. Carlos Alberto Torres and Ari Antikainen. Lanham, MD: Rowman.

Muntaner, Carles, and John Lynch. 2002. Income Inequality, Social Cohesion, and Class Relations: Critique of Wilkinson's Neo-Durkheimian Research Program. In *The Political Economy of Social Inequalities: Consequences for Health and Quality of Life*, 325–346, ed. Vicente Navarro. Amityville, NY: Baywood.

Muris, Peter, Cor Meesters, and Silvia van den Berg. 2003. Internalizing and Externalizing Problems as Correlates of Self-Reported Attachment Style and Perceived Parental Rearing in Normal Adolescents. *Journal of Child & Family Studies* 12 (2): 171–183.

Murphy, Kristina. 2009. Public Satisfaction with Police: The Importance of Procedural Justice and Police Performance in Police–Citizen Encounters. *Australian & New Zealand Journal of Criminology* 42 (2): 159–178.

Murphy, Patricia L. 2000. The Commodified Self in Consumer Culture: A Cross-cultural Perspective. *Journal of Social Psychology* 140 (5): 636–647.

Murray, Sandra L., Dale W. Griffin, Jaye L. Derrick, Brianna Harris, Maya Aloni, and Sadie Leder. 2011. Tempting Fate or Inviting Happiness? Unrealistic Idealization Prevents the Decline of Marital Satisfaction. *Psychological Science* 22 (5): 619–626.

Murrell, Stanley A., and Fran H. Norris. 1991. Differential Social Support and Life Changes as Contributors to the Social Class-Distress Relationship in Older Adults. *Psychology and Aging* 6 (2): 223–231.

Musick, Marc A. 2000. Race and Formal Volunteering: The Differential Effects of Class and Religion. *Social Forces* 78 (4): 1539–1570.

Musick, Marc A., and John Wilson. 2008. *Volunteers: A Social Profile*. Bloomington, IN: Indiana University Press.

Mutz, Diana C. 1998. *Impersonal Influence: How Perceptions of Mass Collectives Affect Political Attitudes*. Cambridge, UK: Cambridge University Press.

Myer, Landon, Dan J. Stein, Anna Grimsrud, Soraya Seedat, and David R. Williams. 2008. Social Determinants of Psychological Distress in a Nationally Representative Sample of South African Adults. *Social Science & Medicine* 60: 1828–1840.

Myers, David G. 2008. Religion and Human Flourishing. In *The Science of Subjective Well-Being*, 323–343, ed. Michael Eid and Randy J. Larsen. New York: Guilford.

Myers, David G. 2014. Religious Engagement and Well-Being. In *The Oxford Handbook of Happiness*, 88–100, ed. Susan A. David, Ilona Boniwell and Amanda Conley Ayers. Oxford, UK: Oxford University Press.

Myers, Jane E., and Thomas J. Sweeney. 2008. Wellness Counseling: The Evidence Base for Practice. *Journal of Counseling & Development* 86 (4): 482–493.

Nabi, Robin L., and Jennifer R. Horner. 2001. Victims with Voices: How Abused Women Conceptualize the Problem of Spousal Abuse and Implications for Intervention and Prevention. *Journal of Family Violence* 16 (3): 237–253.

Nabi, Robin L., and Abby Prestin. 2017. The Tie that Binds: Reflection Emotion's Role in the Relationship between Media Use and Subjective Well-Being. In *The Routledge Handbook of Media Use and Well-Being: International Perspectives on Theory and Research on Positive Media Effects*, 51–64, ed. Leonard Reinecke and Mary Beth Oliver. New York, NY: Routledge.

Nabi, Robin L., and John L. Sullivan. 2001. Does Television Viewing Relate to Engagement in Protective Action Against Crime? A Cultivation Analysis from a Theory of Reasoned Action Perspective. *Communication Research* 28 (6): 802–825.

Nackers, Kimberly. 2015. Framing the Responsibility to Protect: The 2009 Sri Lankan Civil War. *Global Responsibility to Protect* 7 (1): 81–108.

Nagayoshi, Kikuko, and Yoshimichi Sato. 2014. Who Supports Redistributive Policies in Contemporary Japan? An Integrative Approach To Self-interest And Trust Models. *International Sociology* 29 (4): 302–323.

Nahum-Shani, Inbal, Melanie M. Henderson, Sandy Lim, and Amiram D. Vinokur. 2014. Supervisor Support Does Supervisor Support Buffer or Exacerbate the Adverse Effects of Supervisor Undermining? *Journal of Applied Psychology* 99 (3): 484–503.

Nai, Jared, Jayanth Narayanan, Ivan Hernandez, and Krishna Savani. 2018. People in More Racially Diverse Neighborhoods Are More Prosocial. *Journal of Personality & Social Psychology* 114 (4): 497–515.

Namini, Sussan, Claudia Appel, Ralph Jurgensen, and Sebastian Murken. 2010. How is Well-Being Related to Membership in New Religious Movements? An Application of Person-Environment Fit Theory. *Applied Psychology: An International Review* 59 (2): 181–201.

Napier, Jaime L., and John T. Jost. 2008. Why Are Conservatives Happier Than Liberals? *Psychological Science* 19 (6): 565–572.

Narayan, Despa, and Michael F. Cassidy. 2001. A Dimensional Approach to Measuring Social Capital: Development and Validation of a Social Capital Inventory. *Current Sociology* 49 (2): 59–102.

Neal, JoAnne, Robert J. Edelman, and Martin Glachan. 2002. Behavioral Inhibition and Symptoms of Anxiety and Depression: Is There a Specific Relationship with Social Phobia? *British Journal of Clinical Psychology* 41: 361–374.

Neckerman, Kathryn M., and Florencia Toche. 2007. Inequality: Causes and Consequences. *Annual Review of Sociology* 33: 335–357.

Nederveen Pieterse, Jan. 2010. *Development Theory: Deconstructions/Reconstructions*. London: SAGE.

Neilson, Lisa A. 2010. Boycott or Buycott? Understanding Political Consumerism. *Journal of Consumer Behavior* 9 (3): 214–227.

Nelson, Julie A. 2015. Fearing Fear: Gender and Economic Discourse. *Mind & Society* 14 (1): 129–139.

Nepal, Mani, Alok K. Bohara, and Kishore Gawande. 2011. More Inequality, More Killings: The Maoist Insurgency in Nepal. *American Journal of Political Science* 55 (4): 886–906.

Nes, Lise Soblerg, and Suzanne C. Segerstrom. 2006. Dispositional Optimism and Coping: A Meta-Analytic Review. *Personality & Social Psychology Review* 10 (3): 235–251.

Neto, Felix, and Jose Barros. 2003. Predictors of Loneliness Among Students and Nuns in Angola and Portugal. *Journal of Psychology* 137 (4): 351–362.

Neumayer, Eric, and Thomas Plumper. 2009. International Terrorism and the Clash of Civilizations. *British Journal of Political Science* 39: 711–734.

Nevarez, Leonard. 2011. *Pursuing Quality of Life: From the Affluent Society to the Consumer Society*. New York: Routledge.

Newey, Glen. 2001. *After Politics: The Rejection of Politics in Contemporary Liberal Philosophy*. Houndmills, UK: Palgrave.

Ney, Steven, and Nadia Molenaars. 1999. Cultural Theory as a Theory of Democracy. *Innovation* 12 (4): 489–509.

Ng, Aik Kwang, David Y.F.. Ho, Shyh-hin Wong, and Ian Smith. 2003. In Search of the Good Life: A Cultural Odyssey in the East and West. *Genetic, Social, and General Psychology Monographs* 129 (4): 317–363.

Ng, Eddie Chi Wai, and Adrian T. Fisher. 2016. Protestant Spirituality and Well-Being of People in Hong Kong: The Mediating Role of Sense of Community. *Applied Research in Quality of Life* 11 (4): 1253–1267.

Ng, Kok-Yee., Soon Ang, and Kim-Yin. Chan. 2008. Personality and Leader Effectiveness: A Moderated Mediation Model of Leadership Self-Efficacy, Job Demands, and Job Autonomy. *Journal of Applied Psychology* 93 (4): 733–743.

Nickerson, Carol, Norbert Schwarz, and Ed Diener. 2007. Financial Aspirations, Financial Success, and Overall Life Satisfaction: Who? And How? *Journal of Happiness Studies* 8: 467–515.

Nickerson, David W. 2007. Quality Is Job One: Professional and Volunteer Voter Mobilization Calls. *American Journal of Political Science* 51 (2): 269–282.

Nie, Norman, and D. Sunshine Hillygus. 2001. Education and Democratic Citizenship. In *Making Good Citizens: Education and Civil Society*, 30–57, ed. Diane Ravitch, and Joseph P. Viteritti. New Haven, CT: Yale University Press.

Nie, Norman, Sidney Verba, and John R. Petrocik. 1979. *The Changing American Voter*. Cambridge, MA: Harvard University Press.

Nielsen, Ingrid, and Russell Smyth. 2008. Who Wants Safer Cities? Perceptions of Public Safety and Attitudes to Migrants among China's Urban Population. *International Review of Law & Economics* 28: 46–55.

Nielsen, Sara, Kerstine Kaya, Nicole Lønfeldt, Kate B. Wolitzky-Taylor, Ida Hageman, Signe Vangkilde, Sarah Ingrid, and Franksdatter Daniel. 2017. Adult Attachment Style and Anxiety: The Mediating Role of Emotion Regulation. *Journal of Affective Disorders* 218: 253–259.

Niemi, Richard G., John Bremer, and Michael Heel. 1999. Determinants of State Economic Perceptions. *Political Behavior* 21 (2): 175–193.

Niemiec, Christopher P., and Richard M. Ryan. 2014. What Makes for a Life Well Lived? Autonomy and Its Relation to Full Functioning and Organismic Wellness. In *The Oxford Handbook of Happiness*, 214–226, ed. Susan A. David, Ilona Boniwell and Amanda Conley Ayers. Oxford, UK: Oxford University Press.

Nilson, Linda Burzotta. 1981. Reconsidering Ideological Lines: Beliefs about Poverty in America. *Sociological Quarterly* 22: 531–548.

Nimmo, Dan, and Robert L. Savage. 1976. *Candidates and Their Images: Concepts, Methods, and Findings*. Santo Monica, CA: Goodyear.

Niu, Weihua, and James C. Kaufman. 2013. Creativity of Chinese and American Cultures: A Synthetic Analysis. *Journal of Creative Behavior* 47 (1): 77–87.

Njoh, Ambe J. 2009. Ideology and Public Health Elements of Human Settlement Policies in Sub-Saharan Africa. *Cities* 26 (1): 9–18.

Noack, Peter, Christine Krettek, and Sabine Walper. 2001. Peer Relations of Adolescents from Nuclear and Separated Families. *Journal of Adolescence* 24: 535–548.

Noe, Kelly, and Dana A. Forgione. 2014. Economic Incentives in the Hospice Care Setting: A Comparison of for-Profit and Nonprofit Providers. *Journal of Public Budgeting, Accounting & Financial Management* 26 (2): 233–270.

Noguera, Carles Simo, Teresa Castro Martin, and Asuncion Soro Bonmati. 2005. The Spanish Case: The Effects of the Globalization Process on the Transition to Adulthood. In *Globalization, Uncertainty and Youth in Society*, 375–402, ed. Hans-Peter Blossfeld, Erik Klijzing, Melinda Mills and Karin Kurz. London: Routledge.

Nolan, Brian. 2009. Income Inequality and Public Policy. *Economic & Social Review* 40 (4): 489–510.

Norcross, John C. 2006. Integrating Self-help into Psychotherapy: 16 Practical Suggestions. *Professional Psychology* 37 (6): 683–693.

Nordin, Andreas. 2011. Making the Lisbon Strategy Happen: A New Phase of Lifelong Learning Discourse in European Policy? *European Educational Research Journal* 10 (1): 11–20.

Norris, Pippa, and Ronald Inglehart. 2009. *Cosmopolitan Communications: Cultural Diversity in a Globalized World*. Cambridge, UK: Cambridge University Press.

Norris, Pippa. 1991. Gender Differences in Political Participation in Britain: Traditional, Radical, and Revisionist Models. *Government and Opposition* 26 (1): 44–55.

Norris, Pippa. 1999a. Institutional Explanations for Political Support. In *Critical Citizens: Global Support for Democratic Government*, 217–235, ed. Pippa Norris. Oxford, UK: Oxford University Press.

Norris, Pippa. 1999b. The Growth of Critical Citizens and Its Consequences. In *Critical Citizens: Global Support for Democratic Government*, 257–272, ed. Pippa Norris. Oxford, UK: Oxford University Press.

Norris, Pippa. 2001a. *Digital Divide: Civic Engagement, Information, Poverty, and the Intrernet Worldwide*. Cambridge, UK: Cambridge Univesity Press.

Norris, Pippa. 2001b. *Digital Divide: Civic Engagement, Information, Poverty, and the Internet Worldwide*. Cambridge, UK: Cambridge University Press.

Norris, Pippa. 2002. *Democratic Phoenix: Reinventing Political Activism*. Cambridge, UK: Cambridge University Press.

Norris, Pippa. 2011. *Democratic Deficit: Critical Citizens Revisited*. New York: Cambridge University Press.

Novak, Deanna L., and Mara Mather. 2007. Aging and Variety Seeking. *Psychology & Aging* 22 (4): 728–737.

Ntoumanis, Nikos, Vassilis Barkoukis, and Cecilie Thogersen-Ntoumani. 2009. Developmental Trajectories of Motivation in Physical Education: Course, Demographic Differences, and Antecedents. *Journal of Educational Psychology* 101 (3): 717–728.

Nugent, Gwen, Bradley Barker, Neal Grandgenett, and Viacheslav I. Adamchuk. 2010. Impact of Robotics and Geospatial Technology Interventions on Youth STEM Learning and Attitudes. *Journal of Research on Technology in Education* 42 (4): 391–408.

Nunkoo, Robin, and Stephen L.J.. Smith. 2013. Political Economy of Tourism: Trust in Government Actors, Political Support, and Their Determinants. *Tourism Management* 36: 120–132.

Nunkoo, Robin. 2015. Tourism Development and Trust in Local Government. *Tourism Management* 46: 623–634.

Nussio, Enzo. 2019. Can Crime Foster Social Participation as Conflict Can? *Social Science Quarterly* 100 (3): 653–665.

Nyenhuis, Robert. 2020. The Political Struggle for the People: Populist Discourse in the 2019 South African Elections. *Commonwealth & Comparative Politics* 58 (4): 409–432.

O'Boyle, Garrett. 2002. Theories of Justification and Political Violence: Examples from Four Groups. *Terrorism & Political Violence* 14 (23): 23–46.

O'Byrne, Darren J. and Alexander Hensby. 2011. *Theorizing Global Studies*. Houndmills, UK: Palgrave.

O'Connor, Robert E., Richard J. Bord, Brent Yarnel, and Nancy Wiefele. 2002. Who Wants to Reduce Greenhouse Gas Environments? *Social Science Quarterly* 83 (1): 1–17.

O'Connor, Seini, and Ronald Fischer. 2012. Predicting Societal Corruption across Time. *Journal of Cross-Cultural Psychology* 43 (4): 644–659.

O'Dwyer, Shaun. 2003. Democracy and Confucian Values. *Philosophy East & West* 53 (1): 39–63.

O'Mahony, Patrick. 2013. *The Contemporary Theory of the Public Sphere*. Bern, Switzerland: Lang.

O'Neill, John, Alan Holland, and Andrew Light. 2008. *Environmental Values*. Abingdon, UK: Routledge.

O'Neill, Shane. 2000. The Politics of Inclusive Agreements towards a Critical Discourse Theory of Democracy. *Political Studies* 48: 503–521.

Obben, James, and Monique Waayer. 2011. New Zealand's Old-Age Pension Scheme and Household Saving. *International Journal of Social Economics* 38 (9): 767–788.

O'Brien, Robert M. 1990. Estimating the Reliability of Aggregate-level Variables Based on Individual-level Characteristics. *Sociological Methods & Research* 18 (4): 473–504.

Obschonk, Martin, Michael Stuetzer, David B. Audretsch, Peter J. Rentfrow, Jeff Potter, and Samuel D. Gosling. 2016. Macropsychological Factors Predict Regional Economic Resilience During a Major Economic Crisis. *Social Psychological & Personality Science* 7 (2): 95–104.

Obucina, Ognjen. 2013. The Patterns of Satisfaction Among Immigrants. *Social Indicators Research* 113: 1105–1127.

O'Cass, Aron, and Anthony Pecotich. 2005. Political Opinion Leadership and Electoral Behavior. *Journal of Nonprofit & Public Sector Marketing* 14 (1/2): 285–307.

Oesterle, Sabrina, Monica Kirkpatrick Johnson, and Jeylan T. Mortimer. 2004. Volunteerism during the Transition to Adulthood: A Life Course Perspective. *Social Forces* 82 (3): 1123–1149.

Oettingen, Gabriele, and Malin Patricia Chromick. 2018. How Hope Influences Goal-directed Behavior. In *The Oxford Handbook of Hope*, 69–79, ed. Matthew W. Gallagher and Shane J. Lopez. New York, NY: Oxford University Press.

Oettingen, Garbiele, and Julie Y.A. Cachia. 2016. Problems with Positive Thinking and How to Overcome Them. In *Handbook of Self-regulation: Research, Theory, and Application*, 547–570, ed. Kathleen D. Vohs, and Roy F. Baumeister. New York, NY: Guilford.

Ohmer, Mary L. 2007. Citizen Participation in Neighborhood Organizations and Its Relationship to Volunteers' Self- and Collective Efficacy and Sense of Community. *Social Work Research* 31 (2): 109–120.

Oishi, Shigehiro, and Minkyung Koo. 2008. Two New Questions about Happiness: Is Happiness Good? And Is Happier Beter. In *The Science of Subjective Well-Being*, 290–306, ed. Michael Eid and Randy J. Larsen. New York: Guilford.

Oishi, Shigehiro, Edward F. Diener, Richard E. Lucas, and Eunkook M. Suh. 1999. Cross-Cultural Variations in Predictors of Life Satisfaction: Perspectives from Needs and Values. *Personality and Social Psychology Bulletin* 25 (8): 980–990.

Oishi, Shigehiro, Robert S. Wyer, Jr., and Stanley J. Colombe. 2000. Cultural Variation in the Use of Current Life Satisfaction to Predict the Future. *Journal of Personality & Social Psychology* 78 (3): 434–445.

Oishi, Shigehiro, Selin Kesebir, and Ed Diener. 2011. Income Inequality and Happiness. *Psychological Science* 22 (9): 1095–1100.

Oishi, Shigehiro. 2000. Goals as Cornerstones of Subjective Well-being: Linking Individuals and Cultures. In *Culture and Subjective Well-Being*, 87–112, ed. Ed Diener and Eunkook M. Suh. Cambridge, MA: MIT.

Oksanen, Atte, James Hawdon, Emma Holkeri, Matti Nosi, Pekka Rosonen, and M. Nicole Warehime. 2014. Exposure to Online Hate Among Young Social Media Users. *Sociological Studies of Children & Youth* 18: 267–273.

Okulicz-Kozaryn, Adam. 2012. Income and Well-Being Across Provinces. *Social Indicators Research* 106: 371–392.

Okun, Morris A., Alicia Barr, and A. Regula Herzog. 1998. Motivation to Volunteer by Older Adults: A Test of Competing Measurement Models. *Psychology & Aging* 13 (4): 608–621.

Olcese, Cristiana, Clare Saunders, and Nikos Tzavidis. 2014. In the Streets with a Degree: How Political Generations, Educational Attainment and Student Status Affect Engagement in Protest Politics. *International Sociology* 29 (6): 525–545.

Oliver, J. Eric., and Tali Mendelberg. 2000. Reconsidering the Environment at Determinants of White Racial Attitudes. *American Journal of Political Science* 44 (3): 574–589.

Oliver, J. Eric. 2003. Mental Life and the Metropolis in Suburban America: The Psychological Correlates of Metropolitan Place Characteristics. *Urban Affairs Review* 39 (2): 228–253.

Oliver, Pamela E., and Gerald Marwell. 2002. Recent Developments in Critical Mass Theory. In *New Directions in Contemporary Sociological Theory*, 172–193, ed. Joseph Berger and Morris Zelditch, Jr. Lanham, MD: Rowman & Littlefield.

Olivera, Javier. 2015. Changes in Inequality and Generalized Trust in Europe. *Social Indicators Research* 124 (1): 21–41.

Olson, Amanda, Stephanie Reiland, Susan Davies, and Amy Reitmaier Koehler. 2016. Learning about the Experience of Living With Chronic Conditions: A Framework Analysis of Nursing Students' Reflections on Their Conversations with Older Adults. *Gerontology & Geriatrics Education* 17: 1–21.

Olssen, Mark, John Codd, and Anne-Marie O'Neill. 2004. *Education Policy: Globalization, Citizenship and Democracy*. London, UK: SAGE.

Olsson, Christian, and Sinia Maleevi. 2018. War. In *The SAGE Handbook of Political Sociology*, 715–733, ed. William Outhwaite and Stephen Turner. London, UK: SAGE.

Olthof, Tjeert, and Frits A. Grossens. 2007. Bullying and the Need to Belong: Early Adolescents Bullying-related Behavior and the Acceptance They Desire and Receive from Particular Classmates. *Social Development* 17 (1): 24–46.

Omoto, Allen M., Mark Snyder, and Justin D. Hackett. 2010. Personality and Motivation Antecedents of Activism and Civic Engagement. *Journal of Personality* 78 (6): 1703–1734.

Oneal, John R., Bruce Russett, and Michael L. Berbaum. 2003. Causes of Peace: Democracy, Independence, and International Organizations, 1885–1992. *International Studies Quarterly* 47: 371–393.

Onu, Diana, Thomas Kessler, Daniela Andonovska-Trajkovska, Immo Fritsche, Georgia R. Midson, and Joanne R. Smith. 2016. Inspired by the Outgroup: A Social Identity Analysis of Intergroup Admiration. *Group Processes & Intergroup Relations* 19 (6): 713–731.

Onursal, Recep, and Daniel Kirkpatrick. 2021. Is Extremism the 'New' Terrorism? The Convergence of Extremism and Terrorism in British Parliamentary Discourse. *Terrorism & Political Violence* 33 (5): 1094–1116.

Opp, Karl-Dieter., and Bernhard Kittel. 2009. The Dynamics of Political Protest: Feedback Effects and Interdependence in the Explanation of Protest Participation. *European Sociological Review* 26 (1): 97–109.

Opp, Karl-Dieter. 1989. *The Rationality of Political Protest: A Comparative Analysis of Rational Choice Theory*. Boulder, CO: Westview.

Opp, Karl-Dieter. 2002. When Do Norms Emerge by Human Design and When by the Unintended Consequences of Human Action? *Rationality & Society* 14 (2): 131–158.

Oppedal, Brit, Espen Roysamb, and David Lackland Sam. 2004. The Effect of Acculturation and Social Support Change in Mental Health among Young Immigrants. *International Journal of Behavioral Development* 28 (6): 481–494.

O'Rand, Angela M. 1996. The Cumulative Stratification of the Life Course. In *Handbook of Aging and the Social Sciences*, 188–207, ed. Robert H. Binstock and Linda K. George. San Diego, CA: Academic.

Orend, Brian. 2006. *The Morality of War*. Peterborough, Canada: Broadview.

Orr, Allan. 2012. Terrorism: A Philosophical Discourse. *Journal of Applied Security Research* 7 (1): 93–106.

Oshio, Takashi, and Miki Kobayashi. 2010. Income Inequality, Perceived Happiness, and Self-rated Health: Evidence from Nationwide Surveys in Japan. *Social Science & Medicine* 70: 1358–1366.

Oshio, Takashi, Kayo Nozaki, and Miki Kobayoshi. 2011. Relative Income and Happiness in Asia: Evidence from Nationwide Surveys in China, Japan, and Korea. *Social Indicators Research* 104: 351–367.

Ostberg, Viveca. 2003. Children in Classrooms: Peer Status, Status Distribution and Mental Well-Being. *Social Science & Medicine* 56: 17–29.

Ostrom, Elinor, and T.K. Ahn. 2009. The Meaning of Social Capital and Its Link to Collective Action. In *Handbook of Social Capital: The Troika of Sociology, Political Science and Economics*, 17–35, ed. Gert Tinggaard Svendsen and Gunnar Linad Haase Svendsen. Cheltenham, UK: Elgar.

Ousey, Graham C., and Matthew R. Lee. 2013. Community Inequality and Crime. In *The Oxford Handbook of Criminological Theory*, 352–388, ed. Francis T. Cullen and Pamela Wilcox. New York: Oxford University Press.

Outlaw, Lucius T., Jr. 1999. On Race and Philosophy. In *Racism and Philosophy*, 50–75, ed. Susan E. Babbitt and Sue Campbell. Ithaca, NY: Cornell University Press.

Owen, Stephen. 2017. Monitoring Social Media and Protest Movements: Ensuring Political Order through Surveillance and Surveillance Discourse. *Social Identities* 23 (6): 688–700.

Owens, Patricia. 2010. The Ethics of War: Critical Alternatives. In *Ethics and World Politics*, 309–323, ed. Duncan Bell. Oxford, UK: Oxford University Press.

Oyserman, Daphna, Heather M. Coon, and Markus Kemmelmeier. 2002. Rethinking Individualism and Collectivism: Evaluation of Theoretical Assumptions and Meta-analyses. *Psychological Bulletin* 128 (1): 3–72.

Ozbay, Ozben. 2008. Does Social Capital Deter Youth from Cheating, Alcohol Use and Violence in Turkey? Bringing Torpil in. *Journal of Criminal Justice* 36: 403–415.

Packe, Alexander C., and Benjamin Radcliff. 2008. Welfare Policy and Subjective Well-being across Nations: An Individual-level Assessment. *Social Indicators Research* 89: 179–191.

Page, Kyle S., and Sue C. Jacobs. 2011. Surviving the Shift: Rural Police Stress and Counseling Services. *Psychological Services* 8 (1): 12–22.

Pai, Manacy, and Joongbaeck Kim. 2017. Neighborhood Physical Disorder and Psychological Distress: Does the Risk Increase With Age? *International Journal of Aging & Human Development* 84 (4): 378–402.

Pal, Sarmistha. 2000. Economic Reform and Household Welfare in Rural China: Evidence from Household Survey Data. *Journal of International Development* 12: 187–206

Paletz, Susannah B.F., and Kaiping Peng. 2009. Problem Finding and Contradiction: Examining the Relationship between Naive Dialectical Thinking, Ethnicity, and Creativity. *Creativity Research Journal* 21 (2–3): 139–151.

Palker-Corell, Ann, and David K. Marcus. 2004. Partner Abuse, Learned Helplessness, and Trauma Symptoms. *Journal of Social & Clinical Psychology* 23 (4): 445–462.

Pallante, Virginia, Roscoe Stanyon, and Elisabetta Palagi. 2018. Calming an Aggressor through Spontaneous Post-Conflict Triadic Contacts: Appeasement in Macaca Tonkeana. *Aggressive Behaviour* 44 (4): 406–415.

Pallas, Aaron M. 2002. Educational Participation Across the Life Course: Do the Rich Get Richer? *Advances in Life Course Research* 7: 327–354.

Palmer, Neal A., Douglas D. Perkins, and Xu. Qingwen. 2011. Social Capital and Community Participation among Migrant Workers in China. *Journal of Community Psychology* 39 (1): 89–105.

Palmer, Tom G. 2010. Classical Liberalism, Poverty, and Morality. In *Poverty and Morality: Religious and Secular Perspectives*, 83–114, ed. William A. Galston and Peter H. Hoffenberg. Cambridge, UK: Cambridge University Press.

Panagopoulos, Costas. 2010. Affect, Social Pressure, and Prosocial Motivation: Field Experimental Evidence of the Mobilizing Effects of Pride, Shame and Publicizing Voting Behavior. *Political Behavior* 32: 369–386.

Papadakis, Elim. 2000. Environmental Values and Political Action. *Journal of Sociology* 36 (1): 81–97.

Papadopoulos, Konstantinos, Anthony J. Montgomery, and Elena Chronopoulou. 2013. The Impact of Visual Impairments in Self-esteem and Locus of Control. *Research in Developmental Disabilities* 34: 4565–4570.

Papastephanou, Marianna. 2015. The Lifeblood of Science and Its Politics: Interrogating Epistemic Curiosity as an Educational Aim. *Education Sciences* 6 (4): 1.

Pappas, Takis S. 2019. *Populism and Liberal Democracy: A Comparative and Theoretical Analysis.* Oxford, UK: Oxford University Press.

Pardos-Prado, Sergi. 2011. Framing Attitudes Towards Immigrants in Europe: When Competition Does Not Matter. *Journal of Ethnic & Migration Studies* 37 (7): 999–1015.

Parducci, Allen. 1995. *Happiness, Pleasure, and Judgment: The Contextual Theory and Its Applications.* Mahwah, NJ: Lawrence Erlbaum.

Parent, Mike C., Tyler C. Bradstreet, Makenzie Wood, Eddy Ameen, and Jennifer L. Callahan. 2016. The Worst Experience of My Life: The Internship Crisis and Its Impact on Students. *Journal of Clinical Psychology* 72 (7): 714–742.

Pargament, Kenneth I., and Annette Mahoney. 2009. Spirituality: The Search for the Sacred. In *Oxford Handbook of Positive Psychology*, 611–619, ed. C. R. Synder and Shane J. Lopez. New York, NY: Oxford University Press.

Park, Chang Sup, and Barbara K. Kaye. 2017. The Tweet Goes On: Interconnection of Twitter Opinion Leadership, Network Size, and Civic Engagement. *Computers in Human Behavior* 69: 174–180.

Park, Crystal L. 2010. Making Sense of the Meaning Literature: An Integrative Review of Meaning Making and Its Effects on Adjustment to Stressful Life Events. *Psychological Bulletin* 136 (2): 257–301.

Park, Rhokeun, and Deborah Searcy. 2012. Job Autonomy as a Predictor of Mental Well-Being: The Moderating Role of Quality-Competitive Environment. *Journal of Business & Psychology* 27 (3): 305–316.

Parker, Mitchell S. 1985. Identity and the Development of Religious Thinking. *New Directions for Child Development* 30: 43–60.

Parker, Sharon K., Carolyn M. Axtell, and Nick Turner. 2001. Designing a Safer Workplace: Importance of Job Autonomy Communication Quality, and Supportive Supervisors. *Journal of Occupational Health Psychology* 6 (3): 211–228.

Parkes, Alison, Ade Kearns, and Rowland Atkinson. 2002. What Makes People Dissatisfied with Their Neighbourhoods? *Urban Studies* 39 (13): 2413–2438.

Parks, Acacia C., Stephen M. Schueller, and Arber Tasimi. 2014. Increasing Happiness in the General Population: Empirically Supported Self-help? In *The Oxford Handbook of Happiness*, 962–977, ed. Susan A. David, Ilona Boniwell and Amanda Conley Ayers. Oxford, UK: Oxford University Press.

Parrado, Emilio A. 2005. Globalization and the Transition to Adulthood in Mexico. In *Globalization, Uncertainty and Youth in Society*, 327–348, ed. Hans-Peter Blossfeld, Erik Klijzing, Melinda Mills and Karin Kurz. London: Routledge.

Parson, Sean. 2015. Parks, Permits, and Riot Police: San Francisco Food Not Bombs and Autonomous Occupations of Space. *New Political Science* 37 (3): 346–362.

Parsons, Talcott. 1968. *The Structure of Social Action.* New York: Free.

Pasek, Josh, Lauren Feldman, Daniel Romer, and Kathleen Hall Jamieson. 2008. Schools as Incubators of Democratic Participation: Building Long-Term Political Efficacy with Civic Education. *Applied Developmental Science* 12 (1): 26–37.

Passini, Stefano, and Davide Morselli. 2011. In the Name of Democracy: Disobedience and Value-Oriented Citizenship. *Journal of Community & Applied Social Psychology* 21 (3): 255–267.

Passini, Stefano. 2019. Promoting or Opposing Social Change: Political Orientations, Moral Convictions and Protest Intentions. *Europe's Journal of Psychology* 15 (4): 671–88.

Passy, Florence, and Marco Giugni. 2000. Life-spheres, Networks, and Sustained Participation in Social Movement: A Phenomenological Approach to Political Commitment. *Sociologial Forum* 15 (1): 117–144.

Patall, Erika A., Harris Cooper, and Jorgianne Civey Robinson. 2008. The Effects of Choice of Intrinsic Motivation and Related Outcomes: A Meta-analysis of Research Findings. *Psychological Bulletin* 134 (2): 270–300.

Patch, Kartikeya C. 2012. Eastern Traditions, Consciousness, and Spirituality. In *The Oxford Handbook of Psychology and Spirituality*, 343–357, ed. Lisa J. Miller. New York, NY: Oxford University Press.

Patel, Meghna, Jeshmin Bhaju, Martie Thompson, and Nadine Kaslow. 2012. Life Stress as Mediator of the Childhood Maltreatment - Intimate Partner Violence Link in Low-Income, African American Women. *Journal of Family Violence* 27 (1): 1–10.

Paterson, Lindsay. 2008. Political Attitudes, Social Participation and Social Mobility: A Longitudinal Analysis. *British Journal of Sociology* 59 (3): 413–434.

Pattie, Charles, Patrick Seyd, and Paul Whiteley. 2004. *Citizenship in Britain: Values, Participation and Democracy*. Cambridge, UK: Cambridge University Press.

Pauwels, Lieven, and Maarten De Waele. 2014. Youth Involvement in Politically Motivated Violence: Why Do Social Integration, Perceived Legitimacy, and Perceived Discrimination Matter. *International Journal of Conflict & Violence* 8 (1): 134–153.

Pavot, William, Ed Diener, and Eunkook Suh. 1998. Temporal Satisfaction with Life Scale. *Journal of Personality Assessment* 70 (2): 340–354.

Paxton, Pamela, and Stephen Knack. 2012. Individual and Country-Level Factors Affecting Support For Foreign Aid. *International Political Science Review* 33 (2): 171–192.

Paxton, Pamela. 1999. Is Social Capital Declining in the United States? A Multiple Indicator Assessment. *American Journal of Sociology* 105 (1): 88–127.

Pearlman, Wendy. 2013. Emotions and the Microfoundations of the Arab Uprisings. *Perspectives on Politics* 11 (2): 387–409.

Pearson-Merkowitz, Shanna, and Joshua J. Dyck. 2017. Crime and Partisanship: How Party Id Muddles Reality, Perception, and Policy Attitudes on Crime and Guns. *Social Science Quarterly* 98 (2): 443–454.

Pebley, Anne, R., and Narayan Sastry. 2004. Neighborhoods, Poverty and Children's Well-Being. In *Social Inequality*, 119–145, ed. Kathryn M. Neckerman. New York: Russell Sage.

Pedahzur, Ami, and Daphna Canetti-Nisim. 2004. Support for Right-wing Extremist Ideology: Socio-economic Indicators and Socio-psychological Mechanisms of Social Identification. *Comparative Sociology* 3 (1): 1–36.

Peet, Richard, and Elaine Hatwick. 2009. *Theories of Development: Contentions, Arguments, Alternatives*. New York: Guilford.

Peffer, R.G. 1990. *Marxism, Morality, and Social Justice*. Princeton, NJ: Princeton University Press.

Pehrson, Samuel, Roberto Gonzalez, and Rupert Brown. 2011. Indigenous Rights in Chile: National Identity and Majority Group Support for Multicultural Policies. *Political Psychology* 32 (4): 667–690.

Pei, Zhijun, and Yingchun Pan. 2018. Political Efficacy, Social Network and Involvement in Public Deliberation in Rural China. *Social Indicators Research* 139 (2): 453–471 (184-189).

Peifer, J.L. 2010. The Economics and Sociology of Religious Giving: Instrumental Rationality or Communal Bonding? *Social Forces* 88 (4): 1569–1594.

Peiro, Amado. 2006. Happiness, Satisfaction and Socio-Economic Conditions: Some International Evidence. *Journal of Socio-Economics* 35: 348–365.

Pelters, Britta, and Barbro Wijma. 2016. Neither a Sinner nor a Saint: Health as a Present-Day Religion in the Age of Healthism. *Social Theory & Health* 14 (1): 129–148

Peltonen, Kirsi, Samir Quota, Eyad Elsarraj, and Raija-Leena. Punamaki. 2010. Military Trauma and Social Development: The Moderating and Mediating Roles of Peer and Sibling Relations in Mental Health. *International Journal of Behavioral Development* 34: 554–563.

Pena, Pablo A. 2020. Relative Age and Investment in Human Capital. *Economics of Education Review* 78: 102039.

Pena-Lopez, José Atilano., and José Manuel. Sanchez-Santos. 2016. Individual Social Capital: Accessibility and Mobilization of Resources Embedded in Social Networks. *Social Networks* 49: 1–11.

Peng, Yisheng, Wenqin Zhang, Xu. Xiaohong, Russell Matthews, and Steve Jex. 2019. When Do Work Stressors Lead to Innovative Performance? An Examination of the Moderating Effects of Learning Goal Orientation and Job Autonomy. *International Journal of Stress Management* 26 (3): 250–260.

Peng, Zongchao, Ben Ma, and Taoxiong Liu. 2017. *Chinese Cooperative-Harmonious Democracy*. Abington, UK: Routledge.

Peritore, N. Patrick, and Galve-Peritore Ana Karina. 2000. Ecopolitics in the Global South: A Q Method Study of Elites in Seven Nations. In *Social Discourse and Environmental Policy: An Application of Q Methodology*, 196–217, ed. Helen Addams. Cheltenham, UK: Edward Elgar.

Perks, Thomas, and Michael Haan. 2011. Youth Religious Involvement and Adult Community Participation: Do Levels of Youth Religious Involvement Matter? *Nonprofit and Voluntary Sector Quarterly* 40 (1): 107–129.

Perlin, Jonah. 2011. Religion as a Conversation Starter: What Liberal Religious Political Advocates Add to the Debate About Religion's Place in Legal and Political Discourse. *Georgetown Law Journal* 100 (1): 331–365.

Perotin, Virginie. 2001. The Voluntary Sector: Job Creation and Social Policy: Illusions and Opportunities. *International Labour Review* 140 (3): 327–362.

Perren, Kim, Sara Arber, and Kate Davidson. 2004. Neighboring in Later Life: The Influence of Socio-economic Resources, Gender and Household Comparison on Neighbourly Relationship. *Sociology* 38 (5): 965–984.

Persell, Caroline Hodges. 1997. The Interdependence of Social Justice and Civil Society. *Sociological Forum* 12 (3): 149–171.

Peruzzi, Agnese. 2014. Understanding Social Exclusion from a Longitudinal Perspective: A Capability-Based Approach. *Journal of Human Development & Capabilities* 15 (4): 335–354.

Peter, Fabienne. 2009. *Democratic Legitimacy*. New York: Routledge.

Peter, Jochen, and Patti M. Valkenburg. 2007. Who Looks for Casual Dates on the Internet? A Test of the Compensation and the Recreation Hypotheses. *New Media & Society* 9 (3): 455–474.

Petersen, Alan R. 1996. Risk and the Regulated Self: The Discourse of Health Promotion as Politics of Uncertainty. *Australian & New Zealand Journal of Sociology* 32 (1): 44–57.

Peterson, Bill E., and Eva C. Klohnen. 1995. Realization of Generativity in Two Samples of Women at Midlife. *Psychology & Aging* 10 (1): 20–29.

Peterson, Carol B., James E. Mitchell, Sara Engbloom, Sean Nugent, Melissa Pederson Mussell, Scott J. Crow, and Paul Thuras. 2001. Self-help versus Therapist-led Group Cognitive-behavioral Treatment of Binge Eating Disorder at Follow-up. *International Journal of Eating Disorder* 30: 363–374.

Peterson, Christopher, and Martin E.P.. Seligman. 2004. *Character Strengths and Virtues: A Handbook and Classification*. Washington, DC: American Psychological Association.

Peterson, Christopher, Nansook Park, and Patrick J. Sweeney. 2008. Group Well-Being: Morale from a Positive Psychology Perspective. *Applied Psychology* 57: 19–36.

Petrocik, John R. 1991. An Algorithm for Estimating Turnout as a Guide to Predicting Elections. *Public Opinion Quarterly* 55: 643–647.

Petrou, Michalis, and George Kandylis. 2016. Violence and Extreme Right Activism: The Neo-Nazi golden Dawn in a Greek Rural Community. *Journal of Intercultural Studies* 37 (6): 589–604.

Pettigrew, Thomas F. 2002. Relative Deprivation as a Key Social Psychological Concept. In *Relative Deprivation: Specification, Development, and Integration*, 351–373, ed. Iain Walker and Heather J. Smith. Cambridge, UK: Cambridge University Press.

Pettit, Philip. 2012. *On the People's Terms: A Republican Theory and Model of Democracy*. Cambridge, UK: Cambridge University Press.

Pevnick, Ryan. 2015. Should Civil Liberties Have Strict Priority? *Law & Philosophy* 34 (5): 519–549.

Pfaff, Steven, and Hyojoung Kim. 2003. Exit-Voice Dynamics in Collective Action: An Analysis of Emigration and Protest in the East German Revolution. *American Journal of Sociology* 109 (2): 401–444.

Pfattheicher, Stefan, Mattis Geiger, Johanna Hartung, Selina Weiss, and Simon Schindler. 2017. Old Wine in New Bottles? The Case of Self-compassion and Neuroticism. *European Journal of Personality* 31 (2): 160–169.

Pfau-Effingere, Birgit. 2012. Women's Employment in the Institutional and Cultural Context. *International Journal of Sociology & Social Policy* 32 (9/10): 530–543.

Pfeifer, Hanna. 2019. The Normative Power of Secularism. Tunisian Ennahda's Discourse on Religion, Politics, and the State (2011–2016). *Politics & Religion* 12 (3): 478–500.

Pfeiffer, Jens P., and Martin Pinquart. 2012. Goal Engagement and Goal Attainment in Adolescents with and without Visual Impairment. *Journal of Adolescence* 35: 909–916.

Phalet, Karen, Gulseli Baysu, and Maykel Verkuyten. 2010. Political Mobilization of Dutch Muslims: Religious Identity, Salience, Goal Framing and Normative Constraints. *Journal of Social Issues* 66 (4): 759–779.

Pham-Kanter, Genevieve. 2009. Social Comparisons and Health: Can Having Richer Friends and Neighbors Make Your Sick? *Social Science & Medicine* 69: 335–344.

Phan, Mai B., Nadine Blumer, and Erin I. Demaiter. 2009. Helping Hands: Neighborhood Diversity, Deprivation, and Reciprocity of Support in Non-kin Networks. *Journal of Social & Personal Relationships* 26 (6–7): 899–918.

Phillips, David. 2006. *Quality of Life: Concept, Policy and Practice*. London: Routledge.

Pichler, Florian. 2009. Down-to-Earth Cosmopolitanism: Subjective and Objective Measurements of Cosmopolitanism in Survey Research. *Current Sociology* 57 (5): 704–732.

Piliavin, Jane Allyn, and Peter L. Callero. 1991. *Giving Blood: The Development of an Altruistic Identity*. Baltimore, MY: Johns Hopkins University Press.

Piliavin, Jane Allyn. 2008. Long-term Benefits of Habitual Helping: Doing Well by Doing Good. In *Cooperation: The Political Psychology of Effective Human Interaction*, 241–258, ed. Brandon A. Sullivan, Mark Snyder and John L. Sullivan. Malden, MA: Blackwell.

Pilisuk, Marc, JoAnn McAllister, and Jack Rothman. 1996. Coming Together for Action: The Challenge of Contemporary Grassroots Community Organizing. *Journal of Social Issues* 52 (1): 15–37.

Pilling, David. 2014. *Ending Adversity: Japan and the Art of Survival*. London, UK: Lane.

Piquero, Alex R., and Matthew Hickman. 2002. The Rational Choice Implications of Control Balance Theory. In *Rational Choice and Criminal Behavior: Recent Research and Future Challenges*, 85–107, ed. Alex R. Piquero and Stephen G. Tibbetts. New York: Routledge.

Pistrang, Nancy, Chris Barker, and Keith Humphreys. 2008. Mutual Help Groups for Mental Health Problems: A Review of Effectiveness Studies. *American Journal of Community Psychology* 42: 110–124.

Piven, Frances Fox, and Richard A. Cloward. 2005. Rule Making, Rule Breaking, and Power. In *The Handbook of Political Sociology: States, Civil Societies, and Globalization*, 33–53, ed. Thomas Janoski, Robert Alford, Alexander Hicks, and Mildred A. Schwartz. Cambridge, UK: Cambridge University Press.

Plagnol, Anke C. 2011. Financial Satisfaction over the Life Course: The Influence of Assets and Liabilities. *Journal of Economic Psychology* 32: 45–64.

Plagnol, Anke, and Richard A. Easterlin. 2008. Aspirations, Attainments, and Satisfaction: Life Cycle Differences between American Women and Men. *Journal of Happiness Studies* 9: 601–619.

Pleasants, Nigel. 2018. Ordinary Men: Genocide, Determinism, Agency, and Moral Culpability. *Philosophy of the Social Sciences* 48 (1): 3–32.

Pleasants, Nigel. 2019. Free Will, Determinism and the Problem of Structure and Agency in the Social Sciences. *Philosophy of the Social Sciences* 49 (1): 3–30.

Plucker, Jonathan A., and Robert Q. Dana. 1998. Alcohol, Tobacco, and Marijuana Use: Relationships to Undergraduate Students' Creative Achievement. *Journal of College Student Development* 39 (5): 472–483.

Plutzer, Eric, Adith Maney, and Robert E. O'Connor. 1998. Ideology and Elite's Perceptions of the Safety of New Technologies. *American Journal of Political Science* 42: 190–209.

Plutzer, Eric. 1987. Determinants of Leftist Radical Belief in the United States: A Test of Competing Theories. *Social Forces* 65: 1002–1019.

Pollio, Howard R., Tracy B. Henley, and Craig J. Thompson. 1997. *The Phenomeonology of Everyday Life*. Cambridge, UK: Cambridge University Press.

Polson, Edward C. 2017. Religious Environments and the Distribution of Anti-poverty Nonprofit Organizations. *Nonprofit & Voluntary Sector Quarterly* 46 (1): 156–174.

Ponti, Lucia, and Franca Tani. 2019. Attachment Bonds as Risk Factors of Intimate Partner Violence. *Journal of Child & Family Studies* 28 (5): 1425–1432.

Pontusson, Jonas, and David Rueda. 2010. The Politics of Inequality: Voter Mobilization and Left Parties in Advances Industrial States. *Comparative Political Studies* 43 (6): 675–705.

Poortinga, Wouter, Lorraine Whitmarsh, and Christine Suffolk. 2014. The Introduction of a Single-Use Carrier Bag Charge in Wales: Attitude Change and Behavioural Spillover Effects. *Journal of Environmental Psychology* 36: 240–247.

Popovic, Nash. 2014. Sjould Education Have Happiness Lessons? In *The Oxford Handbook of Happiness*, 551–562, ed. Susan A. David, Ilona Boniwell and Amanda Conley Ayers. Oxford, UK: Oxford University Press.

Portes, Alejandro, and Erik Vickstrom. 2011. Diversity, Social Capital, and Cohesion. *Annual Review of Sociology* 37: 467–479.

Portes, Alejandro, and Ruben G. Rumbaut. 2001. *Legacies: The Story of the Immigrant Second Generation*. Berkeley, CA: University of California Press.

Posel, Dorrit Ruth, and Daniela Maria Casale. 2011. Relative Standing and Subjective Well-Being in South Africa: The Role Perceptions, Expectations and Income Mobility. *Social Indicators Research* 104: 195–223.

Pospech, Pavel. 2020. The Spectre of the Queue: Resignifying the Past in the Post-Communist Czech Republic. *American Journal of Cultural Sociology* 8 (2): 191–213.

Posthumus, Hanneke, Gideon Bolt, and Ronald van Kempen. 2013. Why Do Displaced Residents Move to Socioeconomically Disadvantaged Neighborhoods? *Housing Studies* 28 (2): 272–293.

Poveda, Alexander Cotte. 2011. Economic Development, Inequality, and Poverty: An Analysis of Urban Violence in Columbia. *Oxford Development Studies* 39 (4): 453–468.

Powdthavee, Nattavadh. 2009. How Important Is Rank to Individual Perception of Economic Standing? A Within-community Analysis. *Journal of Economic Inequality* 7: 225–248.

Prabhu, Veena, Charlotte Sutton, and William Sauser. 2008. Creativity and Certain Personality Traits: Understanding the Mediating Effect of Intrinsic Motivation. *Creativity Research Journal* 20 (1): 53–66.

Pradel-Miquel, Marc. 2017. Crisis, (Re-)Informalization Processes and Protest: The Case of Barcelona. *Current Sociology* 65 (2): 209–221.

Pratt, Michael W., Rhett Diessner, Adelle Pratt, Bruce Hunsberger, and S. Mark Pancer. 1996. Moral and Social Reasoning and Perceptive Testing in Later Life: A Longitudinal Study. *Psychology & Aging* 11 (1): 66–73.

Pratt, Travis C., Kristy Holtfreter, and Michael D. Reisig. 2010. Routine Online Activity and Internet Fraud Targeting: Extending the Generality of Routine Activity Theory. *Journal of Research in Crime & Delinquency* 47 (3): 267–296.

Prenda, Kimberly M., and Margie E. Lachman. 2001. Planning for the Future: A Life Management Strategy for Increasing Control and Life Satisfaction in Adulthood. *Psychology & Aging* 16 (2): 206–216.

Prezza, Miretta, Matilde Amici, Tiziana Roberti, and Gloria Tedeschi. 2001. Sense of Community Referred to the Whole Town: Its Relations with Neighboring, Homelessness, Life Satisfaction and Area of Residence. *Journal of Community Psychology* 29 (1): 29–52.

Price, Vincent, Clarissa David, Brian Goldthorpe, Marci Mccoy Roth, and Joseph N. Cappella. 2006. Locating the Issue Public: The Multi-dimensional Nature of Engagement with Health Care Reform. *Public Behavior* 28 (1): 33–63.

Prins, R.G., M.A. Beenackers, M.C. Boog, F.J. Van Lenthe, J. Brug, and A. Oenema. 2014. Neighbourhood Social Capital as a Moderator Between Individual Cognitions and Sports Behaviour among Dutch Adolescents. *Social Science & Medicine* 105: 9–15.

Prior, Marcus. 2019. *Hooked: How Politics Captures People's interest*. Cambridge: Cambridge, UK.

Probst, Tahira. 2000. Wedded to the Job: Moderating Effects of Job Involvement on the Consequences of Job Insecurity. *Journal of Occupational Health Psychology* 5 (1): 63–73.

Prouteau, Liopel, and Francois-Charles. Wolff. 2008. On the Relational Motive for Volunteer Work. *Journal of Economic Psychology* 29: 314–335.

Puccio, Gerard J., Reginald J. Talbot, and Andrew J. Joniak. 2000. Examining Creative Performance in the Workplace through a Person-Environment Fit Model. *Journal of Creative Behavior* 34 (4): 227–247.

Pujol, Joan. 1999. Deconstructing and Reconstructing: Producing a Reading on Human Reproductive Technologies. In *Applied Discourse Analysis: Social and Psychological Interventions*, 87–109, ed. Carla Willig. Buckingham, UK: Open University Press.

Pulkkinen, Lea, Anna-Liisa. Lyyra, and Katja Kokko. 2009. Life Success of Males on Nonoffender, Adolescence-limited, Persistent, and Adult-onset Antisocial Pathways: Follow-up from Age 8 to 42. *Aggressive Behavior* 35: 117–135.

Pulkkinen, Lea. 2018. Longitudinal Study of Personality and Social Development: Insights about Aggression after Five Decades. In *The Cambridge Handbook of Violent Behavior and Aggression*, 31–51, ed. Alexander T. Vazsonyi, David J. Flannery and Matt DeLisi. Cambridge, UK: Cambridge University Press.

Putnam, Robert D. 2007. E Pluribus Unum: Diversity and Community in the Twenty-first Century. *Scandinavian Political Studies* 30 (2): 137–174.

Qian, Meihua, Jonathan A. Plucker, and Jiliang Shen. 2010. A Model of Chinese Adolescents' Creative Personality. *Creativity Research Journal* 22 (1): 62–67.

Qouta, Samir, Raija-Leona. Punamaki, Edith Montgoery, and Eyad El Sarray. 2007. Predictors of Psychological Distress and Positive Resources among Palestinian Adolescents: Trauma, Child, and Mothering Characteristics. *Child Abuse & Neglect* 31: 699–717.

Quah, Stella R. 2003. *Home and Kin: Families in Asia*. Singapore: Eastern Universities.

Quaranta, Mario. 2016. Protesting in Hard Times: Evidence from a Comparative Analysis of Europe, 2000–2014. *Current Sociology* 64 (5): 736–756.

Queralt, Magaly, and Ann Dryden Witte. 1999. Estimating the Unmet Need for Services: A Middling Approach. *Social Science Review* 73 (4): 524–559.

Quinn, Dennis P., and John T. Woolley. 2001. Democracy and National Economic Performance: The Preference for Stability. *American Journal of Political Science* 45 (3): 634–657.

Quinn, Jane. 1995. Positive Effects of Participation in Youth Organizations. In *Psychosocial Disturbances in Young People: Challenges for Prevention*, 274–304, ed. Michael Rutter. Cambridge, UK: Cambridge University Press.

Raab, Jurgen. 2019. *Erving Goffman: From the Perspective of the New Sociology of Knowledge*. Abington, UK: Routledge.

Rabbani, Martha Jalali. 2011. *The Development and Antidevelopment Debate: Critical Reflections on the Philosophical Foundations*. Farnham, UK: Ashgate.

Radcliff, Benjamin. 2001. Politics, Market, and Life Satisfaction: The Political Economy of Human Happiness. *American Political Science Review* 85 (4): 938–952.

Radcliff, Benjamin. 2008. The Politics of Human Happiness. In *Cooperation: The Political Psychology of Effective Human Interaction*, 305–321, ed. Brandon A. Sullivan, Mark Snyder and John L. Sullivan. Malden, MA: Blackwell.

Rader, Nicole E., Jeralynn S. Cossman, and Jeremy R. Porter. 2012. Fear of Crime and Vulnerability: Using a National Sample of Americans to Examine Two Competing Paradigms. *Journal of Criminal Justice* 40 (2): 134–141.

Rahe, William M., and Michael A. Stegman. 1994. The Impact of Home Ownership on the Social and Political Involvement of Low-income People. *Urban Affairs Review* 30 (1): 152–172.

Raijman, Rebeca, Moshe Semyonov, and Peter Schmidt. 2003. Do Foreigners Deserve Rights? Determinants of Public Views towards Foreigners in Germany and Israel. *European Sociological Review* 19 (4): 379–392.

Ram, Rati. 2009. Government Spending and Happiness of the Population: Additional Evidence from Large Cross-country Samples. *Public Choice* 138: 483–490.

Ram, Rati. 2010. Social Capital and Happiness: Additional Cross-country Evidence. *Journal of Happiness Studies* 11: 409–418.

Ramarajan, Lakshmi, Ida E. Berger, and Itay Greenspan. 2017. Multiple Identity Configurations: The Benefits of Focused Enhancement for Prosocial Behavior. *Organization Science* 28 (3): 495–513.

Ramone, Jenni. 2011. *Postcolonial Theories*. Houndmills, UK: Palgrave.

Rampichini, Carla, and Silvana Schifini D'Andrea. 1998. A Hierarchical Ordinal Probit Model for the Analysis of Life Satisfaction in Italy. *Social Indicators Research* 44 (1): 41–69.

Rashad, Ahmed Shoukry, Mesbah Fathy Sharaf, and El Hussien Mansour. 2019. Does Income Inequality Increase Violence against Women? An Instrumental Variable Approach. *European Journal of Development Research* 31 (4): 779–808.

Rasmussen, Douglas, and Douglas J. Den Uyl. 2005. *Norms of Liberty: A Perfectionist Basis for Non-perfectionist Politics*. University Park, PA: Pennsylvania State University Press.

Rasmussen, Stig Hebbelstrup Rye, and AsbjØRn Sonne NØRgaard. 2018. When and Why Does Education Matter? Motivation and Resource Effects in Political Efficacy. *European Journal of Political Research* 57 (1): 24–46.

Ratcliffe, Matthew. 2008. *Feelings of Being: Phenomenology*. Psychiatry and the Sense of Reality: Oxford, UL Oxford University Press.

Ravanera, Zenaida R., Fernando Rajalton, and Pierre Turcotta. 2003. Youth Integration and Social Capital: An Analysis of the Canadian Social Surveys in Time Use. *Youth & Society* 35 (2): 158–182.

Reardon, Sean F., and Kendra Bischoff. 2011. Income Inequality and Income Segregation. *American Journal of Sociology* 116 (4): 1092–1153.

Reber, Rolf. 2016. *Critical Feeling: How to Use Feelings Strategically*. Cambridge, UK: Cambridge University Press.

Redmond, Gerry, and Jennifer Skattebol. 2019. Material Deprivation and Capability Deprivation in the Midst of Affluence: The Case of Young People in Australia. *Children & Youth Services Review* 97: 36–48.

Reed, Paul B., and L. Kevin Selbee. 2003. Do People Who Volunteer Have a Distinctive Ethos? A Canadian Study.In *The Values of Volunteering: Cross-Cultural Perspectives*, 91–109, ed. Paul Dekker and Loek Halman. New York: Kluwer.

Reese, Bianka M., May S. Chen, Manali Nekkanti, and Marta I. Mulawa. 2021. Prevalence and Risk Factors of Women's Past-Year Physical Ipv Perpetration and Victimization in Tanzania. *Journal of Interpersonal Violence* 36 (3–4): 1141–1167.

Reese, Gerhard, Amir Rosenmarnn, and James E. Cameron. 2019. *The Psychology of Globalization: Identity, Ideology, and Action*. London, UK: Academic.

Reeskens, Tim, and Leen Vandecasteele. 2017. Hard Times and European Youth. The Effect of Economic Insecurity on Human Values, Social Attitudes and Well-Being. *International Journal of Psychology* 52 (1): 19–27.

Reeskens, Tim, and Wim van Oorschot. 2013. Equity, Equality, or Need? A Study of Popular Preferences for Welfare Redistribution: Principles across 24 European Countries. *Journal of European Public Policy* 20 (8): 1174–1195.

Reeve, Johnmarshall, Edward L. Deci, and Richard M. Ryan. 2004. Self-determination Theory: A Dialectical Framework for Understanding Sociocultural Influences on Student Motivation. In *Big Theories Revisited*, 31–60, ed. Dennis M. McInerney, and Shawn Van Etten. Greenwich, CT: Information Age.

Remmer, Karen L. 2012. The Rise of Leftist-populist Governance in Latin America: The Roots of Electoral change. *Comparative Political Studies* 45 (8): 947–972.

Renger, Daniela, and Gerhard Reese. 2017. From Equality-Based Respect to Environmental Activism: Antecedents and Consequences of Global Identity. *Political Psychology* 38 (5): 867–879.

Renger, Daniela, Silke Eschert, Mimke L. Teichgräber, and Sophus Renger. 2020. Internalized Equality and Protest against Injustice: The Role of Disadvantaged Group Members' Self-Respect in Collective Action Tendencies. *European Journal of Social Psychology* 50 (3): 547–560.

Rentziou, Aikaterini, Christina Milioti, Konstantina Gkritza, and Matthew G. Karlaftis. 2011. Urban Road Pricing: Modeling Public Acceptance. *Journal of Urban Planning & Development* 137 (1): 56–64.

Requena, Miguel, and Mikolaj Stanek. 2014. Religiosity and Politics in Spain and Poland: A Period Effect Analysis. *Sociological Compass* 61 (3): 348–367.

Rettig, Kathryn D., Ronit D. Leichtentritt, and Laura M. Stanton. 1999. Understanding Noncustodial Fathers' Family and Life Satisfaction from Resource Theory Perspective. *Journal of Family Issues* 20 (4): 507–538.

Reznek, Lawrie. 2010. *Delusions and the Madness of the Masses*. Lanham, MD: Rowman.

Rhoades, Linda, and Robert Eisenberger. 2002. Perceived Organizational Support: A Review of the Literature. *Journal of Applied Psychology* 87 (4): 698–714.

Rhodes, Jeremy. 2011. Choosing Sides: An Exploration of Role Conflict among Evangelical Democrats. *Sociology of Religion* 72 (1): 28–49.

Rhomberg, Chris. 2010. A Signal Juncture: The Detroit Newspaper Strike and Post-accord Labor Relations in the United States. *American Journal of Sociology* 115 (6): 1853–1894.

Riad, Jasmin K., and Fran H. Norris. 1992. The Influence of Relocation on the Environmental, Social, and Psychological Stress Experienced by disaster Victims. *Environment & Behavior* 28 (2): 163–182.

Ribeiro, Raquel Barbosa, and Isabel Soares. 2017. Insights and Directions for Sociological Approaches to Saving: The Case of a Financial Education Programme for Children in Portugal. *Journal of Consumer Culture* 17 (3): 845–863.

Rice, Julie Steinkopf. 2013. Homo Economicus and Consumer Activist Subjectivity: Anti-Capitalist Activism through Alternative Trade. *New Political Economy* 18 (6): 845–861.

Richards, Lindsay. 2016. For Whom Money Matters Less: Social Connectedness as a Resilience Resource in the UK. *Social Indicators Research* 125 (2): 509–535.

Richards, P. Scott. 2012. Honoring Religious Diversity and Universal Spirituality in psychotherapy. In *The Oxford Handbook of Psychology and Spirituality*, 237–254, ed. Lisa J. Miller. New York, NY: Oxford University Press.

Richards, Ruth. 2001. A New Aesthetic for Environmental Awareness: Chaos Theory, the Beauty of Nature, and Our Broader Humanistic Identity. *Journal of Humanistic Psychology* 41: 59–95.

Richey, Sean. 2007. Manufacturing Trust: Community Currencies and the Creation of Social Capital. *Political Behavior* 29: 69–88.

Richey, Sean. 2009. Hierarchy in Political Discussion. *Political Communication* 26 (2): 137–152.

Richmond, David A. 2003. Embeddedness in Voluntary Associations and the Timing of Geographic Moves. *Sociological Forum* 18 (2): 295–322.

Riddle, Karyn. 2010. Always on My Mind: Exploring How Frequent, Recent, and Vivid Television Portrayals Are Used in the Formation of Social Reality Judgments. *Media Psychology* 13 (2): 155–179.

Riemer, Hila, Minkyung Koo SharonShavitt, and Hazel Rose Markus. 2014. Preferences Don't Have to Be Personal: Expanding Attitude Theorizing with a Cross-Cultural Perspective. *Psychological Review* 121 (4): 619–648.

Rigby, C. Scott, and Richard M. Ryan. 2017. Time well-spent? Motivation for Entertainmenbt Media and Its Eudaimonic Aspects through the Lens of Self-determination Theory. In *The Routledge Handbook of Media Use and Well-being: International Perspectives on Theory and Research on Positive Media Effects,* 34–48, ed. Leonard Reinecke and Mary Beth Oliver. New York, NY: Routledge.

Rijken, Mieke, and Peter P. Groenewegen. 2008. Money Does Not Bring Well-being, But It Does Help? The Relationship between Financial Resources and Life Satisfaction of the Chronically Ill Meidated by Social Deprivation and Loneliness. *Journal of Community & Applied Social Psychology* 18: 3–33.

Riley, Matilda White, and John W. Riley, Jr. 1999. Sociological Research on Age: Legacy and Challenge. *Ageing & Society* 19: 123–132.

Rindermann, H., and A.C. Neubauer. 2004. Processing Speed, Intelligence, Creativity, and School Performance: Testing and Causal Hypotheses Using Structural Equation Models. *Intelligence* 32: 573–589.

Rindermann, Heiner. 2008. Relevance of Education and Intelligence for the Political Development of Nations: Democracy, Rule of Law and Political Liberty. *Intelligence* 36 (4): 306–322.

Ringen, Stein. 2007. *What Democracy Is for: On Freedom and Moral Goernment*. Princeton, NJ: Princeton University Press.

Rip, Blanka, Robert J. Vallerand, and Mare-Andre K. Lafreniere. 2012. Passion for a Cause, Passion for a Creed: On Ideological Passion, Identity Threat, and Extremism. *Journal of Personality* 80 (3): 573–602.

Ritchie, Liesel Ashley. 2012. Individual Stress, Collective Trauma, and Social Capital in the Wake of the Exxon Valdez Oil Spill: Individual Stress, Collective Trauma, and Social Capital. *Sociological Inquiry* 82 (2): 187–211.

Ritzer, George, and Douglas Goodman. 2001. Postmodern Social Theory. In *Handbook of Sociological Theory*, 151–169, ed. Jonathan H. Turner. New York: Kluwer.

Ritzer, George. 1997. *Postmodern Social Theory*. New York: McGraw-Hill.

Rivera, Jason D. 2018. Reliance on Faith-Based Organizations for Tangible Assistance in Times of Disaster: Exploring the Influence of Bonding Social Capital. *Sociological Spectrum* 38 (1): 39–50.

Rivera, Lauren. 2008. Managing Spoiled National Identity: War, Tourism, and Memory in Croatia. *American Sociological Review* 73: 613–634.

Roazen, Paul. 2003. Freud and His Followers. In *The Cambridge History of Twentieth-century Political Thought*, 392–411, ed. Terence Ball and Richard Bellamy. Cambridge, UK: Cambridge University Press.

Robert, Peter, and Erzsebet Bukodi. 2005. The Effects of the Globalization Process in the Transition to Adulthood in Hungary. In *Globalization, Uncertainty and Youth in Society*, 177–213, ed. Hans-Peter Blossfeld, Erik Klijzing, Melinda Mills and Karin Kurz. London: Routledge.

Roberts, Alasdair. 2012. Why the Occupy Movement Failed. *Public Administration Review* 72: 754–762.

Roberts, Donald F., Lisa Henriksen, and Ulla G. Foehr. 2009. Adolescence, Adolescents, and Media. In *Handbook of Adolescent Psychology, Vol.2: Contextual Influences and Adolescent Development*, 314–344, ed. Richard M. Lerner and Laurence Steinberg. Hoboken, NJ: Wiley.

Roberts, Ken. 2004. Leisure Inequalities, Class Divisions and Social Exclusion in Present-day Britain. *Cultural Trends* 13 (2): 57–71.

Robichau, Robbie W., and Billie Sandberg. 2022. Creating Meaningfulness in Public Service Work: A Qualitative Comparative Analysis of Public and Nonprofit Managers' Experience of Work. *American Review of Public Administration* 52 (2): 122–138.

Robila, Mihaela. 2006. Economic Pressure and Social Exclusion in Europe. *Social Science Journal* 43: 85–97.

Robinaugh, Donald J., Christine Mauro, Eric Bui, Lauren Stone, Riva Shah, Yuanjia Wang, Natalia A. Skritskaya, Charles F. Reynolds, Sidney Zisook, Mary-Frances. O'Connor, Katherine Shear, and Naomi M. Simon. 2016. Yearning and Its Measurement in Complicated Grief. *Journal of Loss & Trauma* 21 (5): 410–420.

Robinson, John P., and Steven P. Martin. 2009. Social Attitude Differences between Internet Users and Non-Users: Evidence from the General Social Survey. *Information, Communication & Society* 12 (4): 508–524.

Rochelle, Tina L. 2015. Diversity and Trust in Hong Kong: An Examination of Tin Shui Wai, Hong Kong's City of Sadness. *Social Indicators Research* 120: 437–454.

Rocke, Christina, and Margie E. Lachman. 2008. Perceived Trajectories of Life Satisfaction across Past, Present, and Future: Profiles and Correlates of Subjective Change in Young, Middle-aged, and Older Adults. *Psychology & Aging* 23 (4): 833–847.

Roderick, Ian. 2016. *Critical Discourse Studies and Technology: A Multimodal Approach to Analyzing Technoculture*. London, UK: Bloomsbury.

Roepstorff, Kristina. 2020. A Call for Critical Reflection on the Localisation Agenda in Humanitarian Action. *Third World Quarterly* 41 (2): 284–301.

Rojek, Chris. 1995. *Decentring Leisure: Rethinking Leisure Theory*. London: Sage.

Rojek, Chris. 2005. Leisure and Tourism. In *The SAGE Handbook of Sociology*, 302–313, ed. Craig Calhoun, Chris Rojek, and Bryan Turner. London, UK: SAGE.

Rojo, Luisa Martin. 2014. Occupy: The Spatial Dynamics of Discourse in Global Protest Movements. *Journal of Language & Politics* 13 (4): 583–598.

Roscigno, Vincent J. 1999. The Black-White Adolescent Gap, Family-school Link, and the Importance of Place. *Sociological Inquiry* 69 (2): 159–186.

Roscigno, Vincent J., and Randy Hodson. 2004. The Organizational and Social Foundations of Worker Resistance. *American Sociological Review* 69 (1): 14–39.

Rose, Lawrence E., and Per Arnt Pettersen. 2000. The Legitimacy of Local Government: What Makes a Difference? Evidence from Norway. *Research on Urban Policy* 8: 25–65.

Rosen, Jeffrey B., and Jay Schulkin. 1998. From Normal Fear to Pathological Anxiety. *Psychological Review* 105 (2): 325–350.

Rosenau, Pauline Marie. 1992. *Postmodernism and the Social Sciences: Insights, Inroads, and Intrusions*. Princeton, NJ: Princeton University Press.

Rosenfeld, Jake. 2010. Economic Determinants of Voting in an Era of Union Decline. *Social Science Quarterly* 91 (2): 379–395.

Rosenfeld, Lawrence B., and Jack M. Richman. 1997. Developing Effective Social Support: Team Building and the Social Support Process. *Journal of Applied Sport Psychology* 9: 133–153.

Ross, Catherine E. 1995. Reconceptualizing Marital Status as a Continuum of Social Attachment. *Journal of Marriage & the Family* 57: 129–140.

Ross, Catherine E., and John Mirowsky. 1989. Explaining the Social Patterns of Depression: Control and Problem Solving–or Support and Talking? *Journal of Health & Social Behavior* 30 (2): 206–219.

Ross, Catherine E., and John Mirowsky. 1995. Does Employment Affect Health? *Journal of Health & Social Behavior* 36 (3): 230–243.

Ross, Catherine E., and John Mirowsky. 1996. Economic and Interpersonal Work Rewards: Subjective Utilities of Men's and Women's Compensation. *Social Forces* 75 (1): 223–246.

Ross, Catherine E., and John Mirowsky. 2009. Neighborhood Disorder, Subjective Alienation, and Distress. *Journal of Health & Social Behavior* 50: 49–64.

Ross, Catherine E., John R. Reynolds, and Karlyn J. Geis. 2000. The Contingent Meaning of Neighborhood Stability for Residents' Psychological Well-being. *American Sociological Review* 65: 581–597.

Rossen, Isabel L., Patrick D. Dunlop, and Carmen M. Lawrence. 2015. The Desire to Maintain the Social Order and the Right to Economic Freedom: Two Distinct Moral Pathways to Climate Change Scepticism. *Journal of Environmental Psychology* 42: 42–47.

Rossi, Alice S. 2001. Contemporary Dialogue on Civil Society and Social Responsibility. In *Caring and Doing for Others: Social Responsibility in the Domain of Family, Work, and Community*, 3–74, ed. Alice S. Rossi. Chicago, IL: University of Chicago Press.

Rossi, Alice S. 2004a. The Menopausal Transition and Aging Processes. In *How Healthy Are We: A National Study of Well-being at Midlife*, 153–201, ed. Orville Gilbert Brim, Carol D. Ryff and Ronald C. Kessler. Chicago, IL: University of Chicago Press.

Rothstein, Bo., and Eric M. Uslaner. 2005. All for All: Equality, Corruption, and Social Trust. *World Politics* 58 (1): 41–72.

Rothstein, Bo. 2005. *Social Traps and the Problem of Trust*. Cambridge, UK: Cambridge University Press.

Rowan, John. 2001. *Ordinary Ecstasy: The Dialectics of Humanistic Psychology*. Hove, UK: Brunner-Routledge.

Rowatt, Wade C., Jordan LaBouff, Megan Johnson, Paul Froese, and Jo-Ann. Tsang. 2009. Associations among Religiousness, Social Attitudes, and Prejudice in a National Random Sample of American Adults. *Psychology of Religion & Spirituality* 1 (1): 14–24.

Roy, Kakoli, and Anoshua Chaudhuri. 2008. Influence of Socioeconomic Status, Wealth and Financial Empowerment on Gender Differences in Health and Healthcare Utilization in Later Life: Evidence from India. *Social Science & Medicine* 66: 1951–1962.

Roy, Sanjit Kumar. 2009. Internet Uses and Gratifications: A Survey in the Indian Context. *Computers in Human Behavior* 25: 878–886.

Rozer, Jesper, and Gerbert Kraaykamp. 2013. Income Inequality and Subjective Well-being: A Cross-national Study on the Conditional Effects of Individual and National Characteristics. *Social Indicators Research* 113: 1009–1023.

Rubenstein, Dorothy J. 2000. Stimulating Children's Creativity and Curiosity: Does Content and Medium Matter? *Journal of Creative Behavior* 34 (1): 1–17.

Rubinstein, David. 1993. Capitalism, Social Mobility, and Distributive Justice. *Social Theory & Practice* 19 (2): 183–204.

Rucht, Dieter. 2007. The Spread of Protest Politics. In *The Oxford Handbook of Political Behavior*, 708–723, ed. Russell J. Dalton and Hans-Dieter Klingemann. New York: Oxford University Press.

Rudel, Thomas K., J. Timmons Roberts, and JoAnn Carmin. 2011. Political Economy of the Environment. *Annual Review of Sociology* 37: 221–238.

Rudig, Wolfgang, and Georgios Karyotis. 2014. Who Protests in Greece? Mass Opposition to Austerity. *British Journal of Political Science* 44 (3): 487–513.

Rudowicz, Elisabeth, and Anna Hui. 1997. The Creative Personality: Hong Kong Perspective. *Journal of Social Behavior & Personality* 12 (1): 139–157.

Rudra, Nita, and Stephan Haggard. 2005. Globalization, Democracy, and Effective Welfare Spending in the Developing World. *Comparative Political Studies* 38 (9): 1015–1049.

Ruggiero, Vincenzo. 2017. The Radicalization of Democracy: Conflict, Social Movements and Terrorism. *Critical Criminology* 25 (4): 593–607.

Ruiter, Robert A.C., Bas Verplanken, Gerjo Kok, and Marieke Q. Werri. 2003. The Role of Coping Appraisal in Reactions to Fear Appeals: Do We Need Threat Information? *Journal of Health Psychology* 8 (4): 465–474.

Runco, Mark A. 2010. Divergent Thinking, Creativity, and Ideation. In *The Cambridge Handbook of Creativity*, 413–446, ed. James C. Kaufman and Robert J. Sternberg. New York: Cambridge University Press.

Runco, Mark A. 2014. *Creativity: Theories and Themes: Research, Development, and Practice*. San Diego, CA: Academic.

Rundman, Laurie A., and Peter Glick. 2008. *The Social Psychology of Gender: How Power and Intimacy Shape Gender Relations*. New York, NY: Guilford.

Rupasingha, Anil, Stephan J. Coetz, and David Freshwater. 2006. The Production of Social Capital in U.S. Counties. *Journal of Socio-Economics* 35: 83–101.

Ruppanner, Leah. 2010. Conflict and Housework: Does Country Context Matter? *European Sociological Review* 26 (5): 557–570.

Russo, Silvia, and Michele Roccato. 2010. How Long Does Victimization Foster Fear of Crime? A Longitudinal Study. *Journal of Community Psychology* 38 (8): 960–974.

Ruta, Simona, and Costin Cernescu. 2008. Influence of Social Changes on the Evolution of Hiv Infection in Romania. *International Journal of Environmental Studies* 65 (4): 501–513.

Ryan, Holly Eva. 2015. Affect's Effects: Considering Art-Activism and the 2001 Crisis in Argentina. *Social Movement Studies* 14 (1): 42–57.

Ryan, Richard M., and Edward L. Deci. 2006. Self-Regulation and the Problem of Human Autonomy: Does Psychology Need Choice, Self-determination, and Will? *Journal of Personality* 74 (6): 1557–1586.

Ryan, Richard M., and Edward L. Deci. 2017. *Self-determination Theory: Basic Psychological Needs in Motivation, Development, and Wellness*. New York, NY: Guilford.

Ryan, Richard M., Veronika Huta, and Edward L. Deci. 2008. Living Well: A Self-determination Theory Perspective on Eudaimonia. *Journal of Happiness Studies* 9: 139–170.

Ryckman, Kirssa Cline. 2019. A Turn to Violence: The Escalation of Nonviolent Movements. *Journal of Conflict Resolution* 64 (2–3): 318–343.

Rydgren, Jens. 2007. The Sociology of the Radical Right. *Annual Review of Sociology* 33: 241–262.

Ryff, Carol D. 1989. Happiness Is Everything, or Is It? Explorations on the Meaning of Psychological Well-Being. *Journal of Personality and Social Psychology* 57 (6): 1069–1081.

Ryff, Carol D. 2013. Psychological Well-being Revisited: Advances in the Science and Practice of Eudaimonia. *Psychotherapy & Psychosomatics* 83: 10–28.

Ryff, Carol D., and Burton Singer. 1998. The Contours of Positive Human Health. *Psychological Inquiry* 9 (1): 1–28.

Ryff, Carol D., L. Carey, M. Keyes, and Diane L. Hughes. 2003. Status Inequalities, Perceived Discrimination and Eudaimonic Well-being: Do the Challenge of Minority Life Hone Purpose and Growth? *Journal of Health & Social Behavior* 44 (3): 275–291.

Ryff, Carol D., Corey L.M. Keyes, and Diane L. Hughes. 2004. Psychological Well-being in MIDUS: Profiles of Ethnic/racial Diversity and Life-course Uniformity. In *How Healthy Are We: A National Study of Well-being at Midlife*, 398–422, ed. Orville Gilbert Brim, Carol D. Ryff and Ronald C. Kessler. Chicago, IL: University of Chicago Press.

Sa'di, Ahmad H. 2015. Social Protest under Authoritarianism: A Critique of Regime Type and Instrumental Rationality-Based Explanations. *Sociology* 49 (3): 455–470.

Saab, Rim, Nicole Tausch, Russell Spears, and Wing-Yee. Cheung. 2015. Acting in Solidarity: Testing an Extended Dual Pathway Model of Collective Action by Bystander Group Members. *British Journal of Social Psychology* 54 (3): 539–560.

Sabelli, Hector C., and Linnen Carlson-Sabelli. 1991. Process Theory as a Framework for Comprehensive Psychodynamic Formulations. *Genetic, Social & General Psychology Monographs* 117 (1): 7–27.

Sabucedo, José-Manuel., Marcos Dono, Mónica. Alzate, and Gloria Seoane. 2018. The Importance of Protesters' Morals: Moral Obligation as a Key Variable to Understand Collective Action. *Frontiers in Psychology* 9: 418.

Sachs, John. 2003. Validation of the Satisfaction with Life Scale in a Sample of Hong Kong University Students. *Psychologia* 46: 225–234.

Sacks, Audrey, and Margaret Levi. 2010. Measuring Government Effectiveness and Its Consequences for Social Welfare in Sub-Saharan. *Social Forces* 88 (5): 2325–2351.

Sadurski, Wojciech. 1999. *Freedom of Speech and Its Limits*. Dordrecht, Netherlands: Kluwer.

Safford, John L. 2002. *Democracy Is Dangerous: Resisting the Typranny of the Majority*. Lanham, MD: University Press of America.

Sahar, Gail. 2008. Patriotism, Attributions for the 9/11 Attacks and Support for War: Then and Now. *Basic & Applied Social Psychology* 30: 189–197.

Sahi, Shalini Kalra. 2017. Psychological Biases of Individual Investors and Financial Satisfaction. *Journal of Consumer Behaviour* 16 (6): 511–535.

Salagame, Kiran Kumar K. 2014. Well-Being from the Hindu/Sanatana Dharma Perspective. In *The Oxford Handbook of Happiness*, 371–396, ed. Susan A. David, Ilona Boniwell and Amanda Conley Ayers. Oxford, UK: Oxford University Press.

Salamon, Lester M., and S. Wojciech Sokolowski. 2016. Beyond Nonprofits: Re-conceptualizing the Third Sector. *VOLUNTAS: International Journal of Voluntary and Nonprofit Organizations* 27 (4): 1515–1545.

Salamon, Lester M., and S. Wojciech Sokolowski. 2003. Institutional Roots of Volunteering: Toward a Macro-structural Theory of Individual Voluntary Action. In *The Values of Volunteering: Cross-Cultural Perspectives*, 71–90, ed. Paul Dekker and Loek Halman. New York: Kluwer.

Salehi, Esmail. 2012. The Impacts of Environmental Factors in Crime Occurrence and Safety of Tehran's Citizens. *Crime, Law, & Social Change* 58 (4): 457–467.

Salinas-Jimenez, Madel Mar, Joaquin Artes, and Javier Salinas-Jimerrez. 2011. Education as a Positional Good: A Life Satisfaction Approach. *Social Indicators Research* 103: 409–426.

Salotti, Simone. 2010. Global Imbalances and Household Savings: The Role of Wealth. *Social Science Journal* 47: 21–44.

Salzer, Mark S., Julian Rappaport, and Lisa Segre. 1999. Professional Appraisal of Professionally Led and Self-help Groups. *American Journal of Orthopsychiatry* 69: 536–540.

Sampson, Edward E. 1999. The Romantic and the Postmodern. *Journal of Humanistic Psychology* 39 (3): 47–55.

Sampson, Robert J. 1991. Linking the Micro- and Macrolevel Dimensions of Community Social Organization. *Social Forces* 70 (1): 43–64.

Sampson, Robert J., and Stephen W. Raudenbush. 2004. Social Disorder: Neighborhood Stigma and the Social Construction of Broken Windows. *Social Psychology Quarterly* 67 (4): 319–342.

Sampson, Robert J., Doug McAdam, Heather MacIndoe, and Simon Weffer Elizondo. 2005. Civil Society Reconsidered: The Durable Nature and Community Structure of Collective Civic Action. *American Journal of Sociology* 111 (3): 673–714.

Sanchez, Maria Luisa Martinez. 2007. *The Effect of Social Capital in Women's Participation in the Labor Force in Mexico: A Neighborhood in Monterry*. Doctoral Dissertation, University of Texas at Arlington.

Sandeerson, Cynthia, and Marsha M. Linehan. 1999. Acceptance and Forgiveness. In *Integrating Spirituality into Treatment: Resources for Practitioners*, 199–216, ed. William R. Miller. Washington, DC: American Psychological Association.

Sanders, Jimy M. 1990. Public Transfers: Safety Net or Inducement into Poverty? *Social Forces* 68 (3): 813–834.

Sangster, Roberta L., and Robert W. Reynolds. 1996. A Test of Inglehart's Socialization Hypothesis for the Acquisition of Materialist/postmaterialist Values: The Influence of Childhood Poverty on Adult Values. *Political Psychology* 17 (2): 253–269.

Santoro, Wayne A., and Lisa Broidy. 2014. Gendered Rioting: A General Strain Theoretical Approach. *Social Forces* 93 (1): 329–354.

Sanyal, Paromita. 2006. Capacity Building Through Partnership: Intermediary Nongovernmental Organizations as Local and Global Actors. *Nonprofit & Voluntary Sector Quarterly* 35 (1): 66–82.

Saraglou, Vassilis. 2004. Being Religious Implies Being Different in Humour: Evidence from Self- and Peer-rations. *Mental Health, Religion & Culture* 7 (3): 255–267.

Sarasa, Sebastian. 2008. Do Welfare Benefits Affect Women's Choices of Adult Care Giving? *European Sociological Review* 24 (1): 37–51.

Sargent-Cox, Kerry A., Peter Butterworth, and Kaarin J. Anstey. 2015. Role of Physical Activity in the Relationship between Mastery and Functional Health. *Gerontologist* 55 (1): 120–131.

Saris, Willem E. 2001. The Strength of the Causal Relationship between Living Conditions and Satisfaction. *Sociological Methods & Research* 30 (1): 11–34.

Sarkheyli, Elnaz, Ayyoob Sharifi, Mojtaba Rafieian, Mohammad reza Bemanian, and Akito Murayama. 2012. An Investigation of the Reasons for Non-compliance with FAR Regulations in Tehran. *Cities* 29: 223–233.

Sarkisian, Natalia. 2006. Doing Family Ambivalence: Nuclear and Extended Families in Single Mothers' Lives. *Journal of Marriage & Family* 68: 804–811.

Saroglou, Vassilis, and Lydwine Anciaux. 2004. Liking Sick Humor: Coping Styles and Religion as Predictors. *Humor: International Journal of Humor Research* 17 (3): 257–277.

Sarracino, Francesco. 2010. Social Capital and Subjective Well-being Trends: Comparing 11 Western European Countries. *Journal of Socio-Economics* 39: 482–517.

Saucier, Gerard, and Katarzyna Skrzypinska. 2006. Spiritual but Not Religious? Evidence for Two Independent Dispositions. *Journal of Personality* 74 (5): 1257–1292.

Saunders, Peter, and Melissa Wong. 2012. Examining Australian Attitudes to Inequality and Redistribution. *Journal of Australian Political Economy* 71: 51–75.

Saunders, Peter, Hung Wong, and Wo Ping Wong. 2014. Deprivation and Poverty in Hong Kong. *Social Policy & Administration* 48 (5): 556–575.

Savage, Stephen P. 1981. *The Theories of Talcott Parsons: The Social Relations of Action*. London: Macmillan Press.

Savolainen, Jukka. 2009. Work, Family and Criminal Desistance, Adult Social Bonds in a Nordic Welfare State. *British Journal of Criminology* 49: 285–304.

Saward, Michael. 1998. *The Terms of Democracy*. Cambridge, UK: Polity.

Saxton, Gregory D., and Michelle A. Benson. 2006. Structure, Politics, and Action: An Integrated Model of Nationalist Protest and Rebellion. *Nationalism & Ethnic Politics* 12 (2): 137–175.

Scabini, Eugenia, and Vittorio Cigoli. 1997. Young Adult Families: An Evlutionary Slowdown or a Breakdown in the Generational Transition? *Journal of Family Issues* 18 (6): 608–626.

Scaff, Lawrence A. 2000. Weber on the Cultural Situation of the Modern Age. In *The Cambridge Companion to Weber*, 99–116, ed. Stephen Turner. Cambridge, UK: Cambridge University Press.

Scaff, Lawrence. 2014. *Weber and the Weberians*. Houndmills, UK: Palgrave. (HM585.S3234)

Scafuto, Francesca, and Francesco La Barbera. 2016. Protest Against Waste Contamination in the Land of Fires: Psychological Antecedents for Activists and Non-activists. *Journal of Community & Applied Social Psychology* 26 (6): 481–495.

Scambler, Graham. 2002. *Health and Social Change: A Critical Theory*. Buckingham, UK: Open University Press.

Schaie, K. Warner. 2013. *Developmental Influences on Adult Intelligence: The Seattle Longitudinal Study*. New York: Oxford University Press.

Scharrer, Erica. 2008. Media Exposure and Sensitivity to Violence in News Reports: Evidence of Desensitization? *Journalism & Mass Communication Quarterly* 85 (2): 291–310.

Schatzman, Christina. 2005. Political Challenge in Latin America: Rebellion and Collective Protest in an Era of Democratization. *Journal of Peace Research* 42 (3): 291–310.

Schecter, David L. 2009. Legislating Morality Outside of the Legislature: Direct Democracy, Voter Participation and Morality Politics. *Social Science Journal* 46 (1): 89–110.

Schellenberg, Kathryn. 1996. Taking It or Leaving It: Instability and Turnover in a High-Tech Firm. *Work & Occupations* 23 (2): 190–213.

Scherger, Simone. 2009. Cultural Practices, Age and the Life Course. *Cultural Trends* 18 (1): 23–45.

Schiebel, Julien, Omrani Hichem, and Gerber Philippe. 2015. Border Effects on the Travel Mode Choice of Resident and Crossborder Workers in Luxembourg. *European Journal of Transport & Infrastructure Research* 15 (4): 570–596.

Schieman, Scott, and Atsushi Narisada. 2014. In Control or Fatalistically Ruled? The Sense of Mastery among Working Canadians. *Canadian Review of Sociology* 51 (4): 343–374.

Schieman, Scott, and Paul Glavin. 2017. Ironic Flexibility: When Normative Role Blurring Undermines the Benefits of Schedule Control. *Sociological Quarterly* 58 (1): 51–71.

Schieman, Scott, Karen van Gundy, and John Taylor. 2001. Status, Role, and Resource Explanations for Age Patterns in Psychological Distress. *Journal of Health & Social Behavior* 42: 80–96.

Schieman, Scott. 2001. Age, Education, and the Sense of Contrl: A Test of the Cumulative Advantage Hypothesis. *Research on Aging* 23 (2): 153–178.

Schieman, Scott. 2002. Socioeconomic Status, Job Conditions, and Well-Being: Self-concept Explanations for Gender-contingent Effects. *Sociological Quarterly* 43 (4): 627–646.

Schieman, Scott. 2013. Job-Related Resources and the Pressures of Working Life. *Social Science Research* 42 (2): 271–282.

Schiff, Miriam, and David Bargal. 2000. Helping Characteristics of Self-help and Support Groups: Their Contribution to Participants' Subjective Well-being. *Small Group Research* 31 (3): 275–304.

Schindler, Ines, Christopher P. Fagundes, and Kyle W. Murdock. 2010. Predictors of Romantic Relationship Formation: Attachment Style, Prior Relationships, and Dating Goals. *Personal Relationships* 17 (1): 97–105.

Schinkel, Willem. 2004. The Will to Violence. *Theoretical Criminology* 8 (1): 5–31 (\85-198).

Schlozman, Kay Lehma, Nancy Burns, and Sidney Verba. 1994. Gender and the Pathways to Participation: The Role of Resources. *Journal of Politics* 56 (4): 963–990.

Schmidt, Laura I., Monika Sieverding, Fabian Scheiter, and Julia Obergfell. 2015. Predicting and Explaining Students' Stress with the Demand-Control Model: Does Neuroticism Also Matter? *Educational Psychology* 35 (4): 449–465.

Schmidt, Steffen. 2010. A Challenge-response Model in Research on Social Change. In *Social Change and Human Development: Concept and Results*, 31–49, ed. Rainer K. Silbereisen. Los Angeles, CA: SAGE.

Schneck, Stefan. 2014. Why the Self-employed Are Happier: Evidence from 25 European Countries. *Journal of Business Research* 67: 1043–1048.

Schneider, Silke L. 2007. Anti-immigrant Attitudes in Europe: Outgroup Size and Perceived Ethnic Threat. *European Sociological Review* 24 (1): 53–67.

Schnittker, Jason, and Jere R. Behrman. 2012. Learning to Do Well or Learning to Do Good? Estimating the Effects of Schooling on Civic Engagement, Social Cohesion, and Labour Market Outcomes in the Presence of Endowments. *Social Science Research* 41: 306–320.

Schofer, Evan, and Francisco J. Cranados. 2006. Environmentalism, Globalization and National Economies, 1980–2000. *Social Forces* 85 (2): 965–991.

Schofer, Evan, and Marion Fourcade-Gourinchas. 2001. The Structural Contexts of Civic Engagement: Voluntary Association Membership in Comparative Perspective. *American Sociological Review* 66: 806–828.

Schofer, Evan. 2004. Cross-national Differences in the Expansion of Science, 1970–1990. *Social Forces* 83 (1): 215–248.

Scholte, Jan Aart. 1993. *International Relations of Social Change*. Buckingham, UK: Open University Press.

Scholz, John T., and Mark Lubell. 1998. Trust and Taxpaying: Testing the Heuristic Approach to Collective Action. *American Journal of Political Science* 42 (2): 398–417.

Scholz, John T., and Neil Pinney. 1995. Duty, Fear and Tax Compliance: The Heuristic Bases of Critizenship Behavior. *American Journal of Political Science* 39 (2): 490–512.

Schoon, Ingrid. 2006. *Risk and Resilience: Adaptations in Changing Times*. Cambridge, UK: Cambridge University Press.

Schram, Danford. 2015. *The Return of Ordinary Capitalism: Neoliberalism, Precarity, Occupy*. New York: Oxford University Press.

Schrijvers, Lieke L., and Jelle Wiering. 2018. Religious/Secular Discourses and Practices of Good Sex. *Culture & Religion* 19 (2): 139–159.

Schroeder, Ralph, and Richard Swedberg. 2002. Weberian Perspectives on Science, Technology and the Economy. *British Journal of Sociology* 53 (3): 383–401.

Schroeder, Ralph. 2013. *An Age of Limits: Social Theory for the 21st Century*. Houndmills, UK: Palgrave.

Schuessler, K.F., and G.A. Fisher. 1985. Quality of Life Research and Sociology. *Annual Review of Sociology* 11: 129–149.

Schulz, Wolfgang. 1995. Multiple-Discrepancies Theory Versus Resource Theory. *Social Indicators Research* 34: 153–169.

Schunk, Dale H., and Ellen L. Usher. 2019. Social Cognitive Theory and Motivation. In *The Oxford Handbook of Human Motivation*, 11–26, ed. Richard M. Ryan. New York, NY: Oxford University Press.

Schur, Chaudia L., Marc L. Berk, and Jill M. Yegiap. 2004. Public Perceptions of Cost Containment Strategies: Mix or Signals for Managed Care. *Health Affairs* W4: 516–525.

Schutte, Sebastian. 2015. Geography, Outcome, and Casualties. *Journal of Conflict Resolution* 59 (6): 1101–1128.

Schwadel, Philip. 2012. Social Class and Finding a Congregation: How Attendees Are Introduced to Their Congregations. *Review of Religious Research* 54: 543–554.

Schwartz, David, Andrea Hopmeyer-Gorman, Robin L. Toblin, and Tania Abau-ezzeddine. 2003. Mutual Antipathies in the Peer Group as a Moderating Factor in the Association between Community Violence Exposure and Psychosocial Maladjustment. *New Directions for Child & Adolescent Development* 102: 39–72.

Schwartz, Gary E. 2012. Consciousness, Spirituality, and Postmaterialist Science: An Empirical and Experiential Approach. In *The Oxford Handbook of Psychology and Spirituality*, 584–597, ed. Lisa J. Miller. New York, NY: Oxford University Press.

Schwartz, Seth J., Erin Phelps, Jacqueline V. Lerner, Shi Huang, C. Hendricks Brown, Selva Lewin-Bizan, Yibing Li, and Richard M. Lerner. 2010. Promotion as Prevention: Positive Youth Development as Protective against tobacco, Alcohol, Illicit Drug, and Sex Initiation. *Applied Developmental Science* 1494: 197–211.

Schwartz, Shalom H., and Gila Melech. 2000. National Differences in Mirco and Macro Worry: Social, Economic, and Cultural Explanations. In *Culture and Subjective Well-Being*, 219–256, ed. Ed Diener and Eunkook M. Suh. Cambridge, MA: MIT.

Schwarz, Norbert, and Fritz Strack. 1999. Reports of Subjective Well-being: Judgmental Processes and Their Methodological Implications. In *Well-Being: The Foundations of Hedonic Psychology*, 61–84, ed. Daniel Kahneman, Ed Diener and Norbert Schwarz. New York: Russell Sage.

Schwinn, Thomas. 1998. False Connections: Systems and Action Theories in Neofunctionalism and in Jurgen Habermas. *Sociological Theory* 16 (1): 75–95.

Schwirian, Kent P., Timothy J. Curry, and Rachael A. Woldoff. 2001. Community Conflict over Arena and Stadium Funding: Competitive Framing, Social Action, and the Socio-Spatial Perspective. *Sociological Focus* 34 (1): 1–20.

Schyns, Peggy. 2001. Income and Satisfaction in Russia. *Journal of Happiness Studies* 2: 173–204.

Scourfield, Jonathan, and Ian Welsh. 2003. Risk, Reflexivity and Social Control in Child Protection: New Times or Same Old Story? *Critical Social Theory* 23 (3): 398–420.

Scruggs, Lyle. 2003. *Sustaining Abundance: Environmental Performance on Industrial Democracies*. Cambridge, UK: Cambridge University Press.

Scruton, Roger. 2014. *How to Be a Conservative*. London, UK: Bloomsbury.

Seaton, Cherisse L., and Sherry L. Beaumont. 2008. Individual Differences in Identity Styles Predict Proactive Forms of Positive Adjustment. *Identity* 8 (3): 249–268.

Seccombe, Karen. 1996. Health Insurance Coverage among the Working Poor. *Research in the Sociology of Health Care* 13A: 199–227.

Sedziafa, Alice Pearl, and Eric Y. Tenkorang. 2016. Kin Group Affiliation and Marital Violence against Women in Ghana. *Violence & Victims* 31 (3): 486–509.

Seidl, David, and Hannah Mormann. 2014. Niklas Luhmann as Organization Theorist. In *The Oxford Handbook of Sociology, Social theory, and Organization Studies: Contemporary Currents*, 125–157, ed. Paul Alder, Paul Du Gay, Glenn Morgan and Mike Reed. Oxford, UK: Oxford University Press.

Seidlitz, Larry, Alexis D. Abernethy, Paul R. Duberstein, James S. Evinger, Theresa H. Chang, and Barbara L. Lewis. 2002. Development of the Spiritual Transcendence Index. *Journal of the Scientific Study of Religion* 41 (3): 439–453.

Seippel, Ornulf. 1999. Political Environmentalism: Class Interests, Modern Values or Postmodern Feelings? *Innovation: European Journal of Social Sciences* 12 (2): 129–153.

Seligman, Martin E.P.. 2002. *Authentic Happiness: Using the New Positive Psychology to Realize Your Potential for Lasting Fulfillment*. New York: Free.

Selim, Sibel. 2008. Life Satisfaction and Happiness in Turkey. *Social Indicators Research* 88: 531–562.

Sell, Jane, Zeng-yin Chen, Pam Hunter-Holmes, and Anna C. Johnnsson. 2002. A Cross-Cultural Comparison of Public Good and Resource Good Settings. *Social Psychology Quarterly* 65 (3): 285–297.

Selvanathan, Hema Preya, and Brian Lickel. 2019. Empowerment and Threat in Response to Mass Protest Shape Public Support for a Social Movement and Social Change: A Panel Study in the Context of the Bersih Movement in Malaysia. *European Journal of Social Psychology* 49 (2): 230–243.

Selznick, Philip. 2002. *The Communitarian Persuasion*. Washington, DC: Woodrow Wilson.

Selznick, Philip. 2008. *A Humanistic Science: Values and Ideals in Social Inquiry*. Stanford, CA: Stanford University Press.

Semetko, Holli A., and Klaus Schoenbach. 1994. *Germany's Unity Election: Voters and the Media*. Cresskill, NJ: Hampton.

Semple, Randye J. and Sean P. Hott. 2012. Translation of Eastern Meditation Disciplines into Western Psychotherapy. In *The Oxford Handbook of Psychology and Spirituality*, 326–342, ed. Lisa J. Miller. New York, NY: Oxford University Press.

Semyonov, Moshe, Rebecca Raijman, and Anat Yom-Tov. 2002. Labor Market Competition, Perceived Threat, and Endorsement of Economic Discrimination Against Foreign Workers in Israel. *Social Problems* 49 (3): 416–431.

Senjo, Scott R. 2011. Dangerous Fatigue Conditions: A Study of Police Work and Law Enforcement Administration. *Police Practice & Research* 12 (3): 235–252.

Seoighe, Rachel. 2016. Discourses of Victimization in Sri Lanka's Civil War. *Social & Legal Studies* 25 (3): 355–380.

Settersten, Richard A., Jr., and Tanetta E. Andersson. 2002. Moving and Still: Neighborhoods, Human Development, and the Life Course. *Advances in Life Course Research* 7: 186–227.

Settle, Jaime E. 2018. *Frenemies: How Social Media Polarizes America*. Cambridge, UK: Cambridge University Press.

Shah, Dhavan V., and Dietram A. Scheufele. 2006. Explicating Opinion Leadership: Nonpolitical Dispositions, Information Consumption, and Civic Participation. *Political Communication* 23 (1): 1–22.

Shan, Hongxia. 2017. Lifelong Education and Lifelong Learning with Chinese Characteristics: A Critical Policy Discourse Analysis. *Asia Pacific Education Review* 18 (2): 189–201.

Shapira, Nathan A., toby D. Goldsmith, Paul E. Kerk, Jr., Uday M. Khosla, and Susan L. McElroy. 2000. Psychiatric Features of Individuals with Problematic Internet Use. *Journal of Affective Disorders* 57: 267–272.

Sharp, Elaine B., and Mark R. Josyla. 2008. Culture, Segregation, and Tolerance in Urban America. *Social Science Quarterly* 89 (3): 573–591.

Shaw, William H. 1999. *Contemporary Ethics: Taking Account of Utilitarianism*. Malden, MA: Blackwell.

Shek, Daniel T.L. 2010. The Spirituality of the Chinese People: A Critical Review. In *The Oxford Handbook of Chinese Psychology*, 343–366, ed. Michael Harris Bond. Oxford, UK: Oxford University Press.

Sheldon, Kennon M., and Tim Kasser. 2001. Getting Older, Getting Better? Personal Strivings and Psychological Maturity across the Life Span. *Developmental Psychology* 37 (4): 491–501.

Shen, Junyi, and Tatsuyoshi Saijo. 2008. Reexamining the Relations between Socio-demographic Characteristics and Individual Environmental Concern: Evidence from Shanghai Data. *Journal of Environmental Psychology* 28: 42–50.

Sherkat, Darren E., and Christopher G. Ellison. 2007. Structuring the Religion-Environment Connection: Identifying Religious Influences on Environmental Concern and Activism. *Journal of the Scientific Study of Religion* 46 (1): 71–85.

Shi, Leiyu. 1993. Health Promotion, Medical Care Use, and Costs in a Sample of Worksite Employees. *Evaluation Review* 17 (5): 475–487.

Shi, Tianjian. 2000. Cultural Values and Democracy in the People's Republic of China. *China Quarterly* 540–559.

Shields, David Light, and Brenda Light Bredemeier. 2008. Sport and the Development of Character. In *Handbook of Moral and Character Education*, 500–519, ed. Larry P. Nucci and Darcia Narvaez. New York, NY: Routledge.

Shimai, Satoshi, Keiko Otake, Nansook Park, Christopher Peterson, and Martin E.P.. Seligman. 2006. Convergence of Character Strengths in American Young Adults. *Journal of Happiness Studies* 7: 311–322.
Shin, Doh Chull. 2012. *Confucianism and Democratization in East Asia*. New York: Cambridge University Press.
Shin, Kwang-Yeong. 2013. Economic Crisis, Neoliberal Reforms, and the Rise of Precarious Work in South Korea. *American Behavioral Scientist* 57 (3): 335–353.
Shindler, Ines, Ursula M. Staudinger, and John R. Nesselroade. 2006. Development and Structural Dynamics of Personal Life Investment in Old Age. *Psychology & Aging* 21 (4): 737–753.
Shippee, Nathan D. 2012. Victimization, Fear of Crime, and Perceived Risk: Testing a Vulnerability Model of Personal Control. *Sociological Perspectives* 55 (1): 117–140.
Shmueli, Amir. 1999. Survival vs. Quality of Life: A Study of the Israeli Public Priorities in Medical Care. *Social Science & Medicine* 49: 297–302.
Shockley, Ellie, and Amir Shawn Fairdosi. 2015. Power to the People? Psychological Mechanisms of Disengagement from Direct Democracy. *Social Psychology & Personality Science* 6 (5): 529–586.
Shor, Eran, and Yuval Yonay. 2010. Sport, National Identity, and Media Discourse over Foreign Athletes in Israel. *Nationalism & Ethnic Politics* 16 (3–4): 483–503.
Shorey, Hal S., Steve Bisgaier, and Scott R. Thien. 2018. Attachment Process and the Social Developmental Bases of Hope. In *The Oxford Handbook of Hope*, 313–325, ed. Matthew W. Gallagher and Shane J. Lopez. New York, NY: Oxford University Press.
Shorthose, Jim, and Neil Maycroft. 2017. *Where in Creativity? A Multi-disciplinary Approach*. Abington, UK: Routledge.
Shriver, Thomas E., Amy Chasteen Miller, and Sherry Cable. 2003. Women's Work: Women's Involvement in the Gulf War Illness Movement. *Sociological Quarterly* 44 (4): 639–658.
Shuman, Carolyn R., Glenn P. Fournet, Paul F. Zelhart, and Billy C. Roland. 1992. Attitudes of Registered Nurses toward Euthanasia. *Death Studies* 16 (1): 1–15.
Siahpush, Mohammad, Ron Borland, Janet Taylor, Gopal K. Singh, Zahid Ansari, and Adrian Serraglio. 2006. The Association of Smoking with Perception of Income Inequality, Relation Material Well-being, and Social Capital. *Social Science & Medicine* 63: 2801–2812.
Sidanius, Jim, and Felicia Pratto. 2012. Social Dominance Theory. In *Handbook of Theories of Social Psychology*, vol. 2, 418–438, ed. Paul A.M. Van Lange, Arie W. Kruglanski and E. Tory Higgins. London, CA: SAGE.
Sidanius, Jim. 1988. Political Sophistication and Political Deviance: A Structure Equation Examination of Context Theory. *Journal of Personality & Social Psychology* 55 (1): 37–51.
Signorielli, Nancy. 1998. Health Images in Television. In *Health Communication Research: A Guide to Developments and Directions*, 163–179, ed. Lorraine D. Jackson and Bernard K. Duffy. Westport, CT: Greenwood.
Silbereisen, Rainer K., Martin Pinquart, and Martin J. Tomasik. 2010. Demands of Social Change and Psychosocial Adjustment: Results from the Jena Study. In *Social Change and Human Development: Concept and Results*, 125–147, ed. Rainer K. Silbereisen. Los Angeles, CA: SAGE.
Silver, Daniel. 2011. The Moodiness of Action. *Sociological Theory* 29 (3): 199–222.
Silverman, E. Reed., and Raj Decker Miller. 2011. Male Perpetration of Teen Dating Violence: Associations with Neighborhood Violence Involvement, Gender Attitudes, and Perceived Peer and Neighborhood Norms. *Journal of Urban Health* 88 (2): 226–239.
Silverstein, Merril, and Sarah Ruiz. 2006. Breaking the Chain: How Grandparents Moderate the Transmission of Maternal Depression to Their Grandchildren. *Family Relations* 55: 601–612.
Silvia, Paul J., and Nathan A. Kimbrel. 2010. A Dimensional Analysis of Creativity and Mental Illness: Do Anxiety and Depression Symptoms Predict Creative Cognition, Creative Accomplishments, and Creative Self-Concepts? *Psychology of Aesthetics, Creativity, & the Arts* 4 (1): 2–10.
Silvia, Paul J., Benjamin Wigert, Roni Reiter-Palmon, and James C. Kaufman. 2012. Assessing Creativity with Self-Report Scales: A Review and Empirical Evaluation. *Psychology of Aesthetics, Creativity, & the Arts* 6 (1): 19–34.

Simon, Robin W., and Kathryn Lively. 2010. Sex, Anger and Depression. *Social Forces* 88 (4): 1543–1568.

Simon-Bemd, Stefan Sturmer, and Kerstin Steffens. 2000. Helping Individuals or Group Members? The Role of Individuals and Collective Identification in AIDS Volunteerism. *Personality & Social Psychology Bulletin* 26 (4): 497–506.

Simonton, Deah Keith. 2003. Scientific Creativity as Constrained Stochastic Behavior: The Integration of Product, Person, and Process Perspectives. *Psychological Bulletin* 129 (4): 475–494.

Simpkins, Sandra D., Jennifer A. Fredricks, Pamela E. Davis-Kean, and Jacquelynne S. Eccles. 2006. Healthy Mind, Healthy Habits: The Influence of Activity Involvement and Middle Childhood. In *Developmental Contexts in Middle Childhood: Bridges to Adolescence and Adulthood*, 283–302, ed. Aletha C. Huston, and Marika N. Ripke. Cambridge, UK: Cambridge University Press.

Simpson, Patricia A., and Michelle Kaminski. 2005. Rising Income Inequality in a Time of Plenty: The Influence of Micro-Justice Standards and Group Membership on Macro-Justice Perceptions. *Employee Responsibilities & Rights Journal* 17 (1): 47–61.

Sing, Ming, and K.M. Lee. 1999. The Support of Hong Kong Chinese for Democratic Reform. *East Asia* 17 (2): 47–80.

Sing, Ming. 2004. *Hong Kong's Tortuous, Democratization: A Comparative Analysis*. London: RoutledgeCurzon.

Sing, Ming. 2020. Explaining Public Participation in Anti-Authoritarian Protests in Hong Kong. *Communist & Post-Communist Studies* 53 (4): 2–21.

Singer, Alexa J., Cecilia Chouhy, Peter S. Lehmann, Jessica N. Walzak, Marc Gertz, and Sophia Biglin. 2019. Victimization, Fear of Crime, and Trust in Criminal Justice Institutions: A Cross-National Analysis. *Crime & Delinquency* 65 (6): 822–844.

Singer, Eleanor, Amy D. Corning, and Toni Antonucci. 1999. Attitudes toward Genetic Testing and Fetal Diagnosis, 1990–1996. *Journal of Health & Social Behavior* 40: 429–455.

Singh, Mala. 2011. The Place of Social Justice in Higher Education and Social Change Discourses. *Compare* 41 (4): 481–494.

Sinn, Jeffrey S., and Matthew W. Hayes. 2017. Replacing the Moral Foundations: An Evolutionary-Coalitional Theory of Liberal-Conservative Differences. *Political Psychology* 38 (6): 1043–1064.

Sirgy, M. Joseph., David Efraty, Phillip Siepel, and Doag-jin Lee. 2001. A New Measure of Quality of Work Life (QWL) Based on Need Satisfaction and Spillover Theories. *Social Indicators Research* 55: 241–302.

Sirgy, M. Joseph., Dong-jie Lee, Chad Miller, and James E. Littlefield. 2004. The Impact of Globalization on a Country's Quality of Life: Toward an Integrated Model. *Social Indicators Research* 68: 251–298.

Sirgy, M. Joseph. 2001. *Handbook of Quality-of-Life Research: An Ethical Marketing Perspective*. Dordrecht, Netherlands: Kluwer Academic.

Sirgy, M. Joseph. 2012. *The Psychology of Quality of Life: Hedonic Well-Being, Life Satisfaction, and Eudaimonia*. Dordrecht, Netherlands: Springer.

Siu, Kin Wai Michael, and Jia Xin Xiao. 2015. Quality of Life and Recycling Behaviour in High-Rise Buildings: A Case in Hong Kong. *Applied Research in Quality of Life* 11 (4): 1137–1154.

Sjoberg, Lennart. 2003. Distal Factors in Risk Perception. *Journal of Risk Research* 6 (3): 187–211.

Skerkart, Darren E., and Christopher G. Ellison. 1999. Recent Developments and Current Controversies in the Sociology of Religion. *Annual Review of Sociology* 25: 363–394.

Skerkat, Darren E. 1998. Counterculture or Continuity? Competing Influence on Baby Boomers' Religious Orientation and Participation. *Social Force* 76 (3): 1087–1104.

Skitka, Linda J. and G. Scott Morgan. 2014. The Social and Political Implications of Moral Conviction. *Political Psychology* 35 (SUPPL.1): 95–110.

Skyttner, Lars. 2005. *General Systems Theory: Problems, Perspecgives, Practices*. Singapore: World Scientific.

Slater, Don. 2005. The Sociology of Consumption and Lifestyle. In *The SAGE Handbook of Sociology*, 174–187, ed. Craig Calhoun, Chris Rojek, and Bryan Turner. London, UK: SAGE.

Slavina, Anna, and Robert Brym. 2020. Demonstrating in the Internet Age: A Test of Castells' Theory. *Social Movement Studies* 19 (2): 201–221.

Smart, Alan. 2001. Unruly Places: Urban Governance and the Persistence of Illegality in Hong Kong¡¯s Urban Squatter Areas. *American Anthropologist* 103 (1): 30–44.

Smidt, Hannah. 2020. Mitigating Election Violence Locally: UN Peacekeepers' Election-Education Campaigns in Côte D'Ivoire. *Journal of Peace Research* 57 (1): 199–216.

Smit, Brandon W., Liam C. Ryan, and Courtney A. Nelson. 2016. Does Autonomy Increase or Decrease Negative Emotional Displays from Service Workers? *Journal of Personnel Psychology* 15 (3): 134–138.

Smith, Brian N., and Mark F. Stasson. 2000. A Comparison of Health Behavior Constructs: Social Psychological Predictors of AIDS-preventive Behavioral Intentions. *Journal of Applied Social Psychology* 30 (3): 443–462.

Smith, David A. 2004. Global Cities in East Asia: Empirical and Conceptual Analysis. *International Social Science Journal* 181: 399–412.

Smith, Elizabeth, Fiona Ross, Sheila Donovan, Jill Manthorpe, Sally Brearley, John Sitzia, and Peter Beresford. 2006. Service User Involvement in Nursing, Midwifery and Health Visiting Research: A Review of Evidence and Practice. *International Journal of Nursing Studies* 45 (2): 298–315.

Smith, Michael D., Richard S. Kranich, and Lori M. Hunter. 2001. Growth, Decline, Stability, and Disruption: A Longitudinal Analysis of Sociaal Well-being in Four Western Rural Communities. *Rural Sociology* 66 (3): 425–450.

Smith, Philip D. 2002. *The Virtue of Civility in the Practice of Politics*. Lanham, MD: University Press of America.

Smith, Steven R. 2011. *Equality and Diersity: Value Incommensurability and the Politics of Recognition*. Bristol, UK: Polity.

Smith, Suzanne R., and Raeann R. Hamon. 2012. *Exploring Family Theories*. New York: Oxford University Press.

Smith, Tom W. 2005. Generation Gaps in Attitudes and Values from the 1970s to the 1990s. In *On the Frontier of Adulthood: Theory, Research, and Public Policy*, 177–221, ed. Richard A. Settersten Jr., Frank F. Furstenberg Jr., and Ruben G. Rumbaut. Chicago, IL: University of Chicago Press.

Smyth, Lisa, and Martina McKnight. 2013. Maternal Situations: Sectarianism and Civility in a Divided City. *Sociological Review* 61 (2): 304–322.

Sneed, Joel R., Susan Krauss Whitbourne, and Michelle E. Culang. 2006. Trust, Identity, and Ego Integrity: Modeling Erikson's Core Stages over 34 Years. *Journal of Adult Development* 13: 148–157.

Snow, David A., and Peter B. Owens. 2014. Social Movements and Social Inequality: Toward a More Balanced Assessment of the Relationship. In *Handbook of the Social Psychology of Inequality*, 657–681, ed. Jane D. McLeod, Edward J. Lawler, and Michael Schwalbe. Dordrecht, Netherlands: Springer.

Snyder, C.R. 2000. Hypothesis: There is Hope. In *Handbook of Hope: Theory, Measures, Applications*, 3–21, ed. C.R. Snyder. San Diego, CA: Academic.

Sobieraj, Sarah, and Deborah White. 2004. Taxing Political Life: Reevaluating the Relationship Between Voluntary Association Membership, Political Engagement, and the State. *Sociological Quarterly* 45 (4): 739–764.

Soderberg, Inga-Lill., and Misse Wester. 2012. Lay Actions in the Face of Crisis—Swedish Citizens' Actions in Response to the Global Financial Crisis of 2008. *Journal of Socio-Economics* 41 (6): 796–805.

Soenens, Bart, and Maarten Vansteenkiste. 2005. Antecedents and Outcomes of Self-determination in 3 Life Domains: The Role of Parents' and Teachers' Autonomy Support. *Journal of Youth & Adolescence* 34 (6): 589–604.

Sokolowski, S. Wojciech. 1996. Show Me the Way to the Next Worthy Seed: Towards a Microstructural Theory of Volunteering and Giving. *VOLUNTAS: International Journal of Voluntary and Nonprofit Organizations* 7 (3): 259–278.

Soler-i-Marti, Roger. 2015. Youth Political Involvement Update: Measuring The Role of Cause-Oriented Political Interest in Young People's Activism. *Journal of Youth Studies* 18 (3): 396–416.

Soliman, Abdrabo, Tarek Bellaj, and Maher Khelifa. 2016. An Integrative Psychological Model for Radicalism: Evidence from Structural Equation Modeling. *Personality & Individual Differences* 95: 127–133.

Solomon, Lewis D. 2006. *From Athens to America: Virtues and the Formulation of Public Policy.* Lanham, MD: Lexington.

Solomon, Sheldon, Jeff Greenberg, and Tom Pyszczynski. 1991. A Terror Management Theory of Social Behavior: The Psychological Functions of Self-esteem and Cultural Worldviews. *Advances in Experimental Social Psychology* 24: 93–159.

Solt, Frederick. 2015. Economic Inequality and Nonviolent Protest. *Social Science Quarterly* 96 (5): 1314–1327.

Solt, Frederick. 2016. The Standardized World Income Inequality Database. *Social Science Quarterly* 97 (5): 1267–1281.

Somma, Nicolás M., Matías Bargsted, and Felipe Sánchez. 2020. Protest Issues and Political Inequality in Latin America. *American Behavioral Scientist.* 64 (9): 1299–1323.

Son, Joonmo, and John Wilson. 2012. Using Normative Theory to Explain the Effect of Religion and Education on Volunteering. *Sociological Perspectives* 55 (3): 473–499.

Sonderlund, Anders L., Thomas A. Morton, and Michelle K. Ryan. 2017. Multiple Group Membership and Well-Being: Is There Always Strength in Numbers? *Frontiers in Psychology* 8: 1038.

Sonderskov, Kim Mannemar. 2011. Does Generalized Social Trust Led to Associational Membership? Unravelling a Bowl of Well-tossed Spaghetti. *European Sociological Review* 27 (4): 419–434.

Soons, Judith P.M.., Aart C. Liefbroer, and Matthijs Kalmijn. 2009. The Long-Term Consequences of Relationship Formation for Subjective Well-Being. *Journal of Marriage & Family* 71: 1254–1270.

Soper, Kate. 2007. Re-Thinking the Good Life: The Citizenship Dimension of Consumer Disaffection with Consumerism. *Journal of Consumer Culture* 7 (2): 205–229.

Sorell, Tom. 2013. *Emergencies and Politics: A Sober Hobbesian Approach.* Cambridge, UK: Cambridge University Press.

Sorens, Jason. 2011. Mineral Production, Territory, and Ethnic Rebellion: The Role of Rebel Constituencies. *Journal of Peace Research* 48 (5): 571–585.

Sorensen, Mads P., and Allan Christiansen. 2013. *Ulrich Beck: An Introduction to the Theory of Second Modernity and the Risk Society.* Abington, UK: Routledge.

Sorial, Sarah. 2012. *Sedition and the Advocacy of Violence: Free Speech and Counter-Terrorism.* Abingdon, UK: Routledge.

Sotirovic, Mira. 2000. Effects of Media Use on Audience Framing and Support for Welfare. *Mass Communication & Society* 3 (2&3): 269–296.

Sotirovic, Mira. 2001. Media Use and Perceptions of Welfare. *Journal of Communication* 51: 750–774.

South, Scott J., and Kyle D. Crowder. 2000. The Declining Significance of Neighborhood? Marital Transitions in Community Context. *Social Forces* 78 (3): 1067–1099.

Spicker, Paul. 2013. *Reclaiming Individualism: Perspectives on Public Policy.* Bristol, UK: Policy.

Spitzberg, Brian H. 2013. Intimate Partner Violence. In *The SAGE Handbook of Conflict Communication,* 187–210, ed. John G. Oetzel and Stelle Ting-Toomey. Thousand Oaks, CA: SAGE. Bufacchi, Vittorio. 2007. *Violence and Social Justice.* Houndmills, UK: Palgrave.

Spohn, Ryan E., and Howard B. Kaplan. 2000. Adolescent Substance Use and Adult Health Status: A Critical Analysis of a Problematic Relationship. *Advances in Medical Sociology* 7: 45–65.

Stafford, Ian. 2000. Children with Movement Difficulties, Primary Education and the Development of Performance Indicators. *British Journal of Special Education* 27 (2): 81–86.

Stafford, M., S. Cummins, S. Macintyre, A. Ellaway, and M. Marmot. 2005. Gender Differences in the Associations between Health and Neighborhood Environment. *Social Science & Medicine* 60: 1681–1692.

Stalker, Glenn John. 2008. Measuring Diversity in Daily Social Contact: The Contribution of Social Context, Work and Leisure on the Opportunity for Engagement. *Social Indicators Research* 86 (2): 275–295.

Stanley, Ian H., Yeates Conwell, Connie Bowen, and Kimberly A. Van Orden. 2014. Pet Ownership May Attenuate Loneliness among Older Adult Primary Care Patients Who Live Alone. *Aging & Mental Health* 18 (3): 394–399.

Stanley, John K., David A. Heasher, Janet R. Stanley, and Dianne Vella-Brodrick. 2011. Mobility, Social Exclusion, and Well-being: Exploring the Links. *Transportation Research Part A* 45: 789–801.

Stansfeld, S.A., and M.G. Marmot. 1992. Social Class and Minor Psychiatric Disorder in British Civil Servants: A Validated Screening Survey Using the General Health Questionnaire. *Psychological Medicine* 22: 739–749.

Stanton, Glenn T., and Bill Maier. 2004. *Marriage on Trial*. Downers Grove, IL: InterVarsity.

Staples, Susan L., Randolph R. Cornelius, and Margaret S. Gibbs. 1999. Noise Disturbance from a Developing Airport: Perceived Risk or General Annoyance? *Environment & Behavior* 31 (5): 692–710.

Starrin, Bengt, Cecilia Aslund, and Kent W. Nilsson. 2009. Financial Stress, Shaming Experiences and Psychosocial Ill-health: Studies into the Finances-shame Model. *Social Indicators Research* 91: 283–298.

Starrs, Claire J., John R. Z. Abela, David C. Zuroff, Rhonda Amsel, Josephine H. Shih, Shuqiao Yao, Xiong Zhao Zhu, and Wei Hong. 2017. Predictors of Stress Generation in Adolescents in Mainland China. *Journal of Abnormal Child Psychology* 45 (6): 1207–1219.

Staub, Ervin, and Johanna Vollhardt. 2008. Altruism Born of Suffering: The Roots of Caring and Helping after Victimization and Other Trauma. *American Journal of Orthopsychiatry* 78 (3): 267–780.

Staudinger, Ursula M., William Fleeson, and Paul B. Baltes. 1999. Predictors of Subjective Physical Health and Global Well-being: Similarities and Differences between the United States and Germany. *Journal of Personality & Social Psychology* 76 (2): 305–329.

Stavrova, Olga, and Daniel Ehlebracht. 2018. Education as an Antidote to Cynicism. *Social Psychological & Personality Science* 9 (1): 59–69.

Stavrova, Olga, and Pascal Siegers. 2014. Religious Prosociality and Morality Across Cultures. *Personality & Social Psychology Bulletin* 40 (3): 315–333.

Stavrova, Olga. 2014. *Fitting in and Getting Happy: How Conformity to Societal Norms Affect Subjective Well-Being*. Frankfurt, Germany: Campus.

Steel, Brent S. 1999. Public Perceptions and Preferences Concerning Pacific Salmon Recovery: An Oregon Voluntary and Grassroots Perspective. *Social Science Journal* 36: 497–513.

Steel, Liz, Warren Kidd, and Anne Brown. 2012. *The Family*. Houndmills, UK: Palgrave.

Steele, Jeanne Rogge. 1999. Teenage Sexuality and Media Practice: Factoring in the Influences of Family, Friends and School. *Journal of Sex Research* 36 (4): 331–341.

Steger, Michael F., Shigehiro Oishi, and Todd B. Kashdan. 2009. Meaning in Life Across the Life Span: Levels and Correlates of Meaning in Life from Emerging Adulthood to Older Adulthood. *Journal of Positive Psychology* 4 (1): 43–52.

Stehr, Nico. 2008. *Moral Markets: How Knowledge and Affluence Change Consumers and Products*. Boulder, CO: Paradigm.

Steinberg, Dominique Moyse. 2004. *The Mutual-aid Approach to Working with Groups Helping People Help One Another*, 2nd ed. New York: Haworth.

Steinberg, Marc W. 2003. Capitalist Development, the Labor Process, and the Law. *American Journal of Sociology* 109 (2): 445–495.

Steiner, Jurg. 2012. *The Foundations of Deliberative Democracy: Empirical Research and Normative Implications*. New York: Cambridge University Press.

Steinhardt, H. Christoph., and Jan Delhey. 2020. Socio-Economic Modernization and the Crisis of Trust in China: A Multi-level Analysis of General and Particular Trust. *Social Indicators Research* 152: 923–949.

Stenberg, Sten-ake. 2000. Inheritance of Welfare Recipiency: An Intergenerational Study of Social Assistance Recipiency in Postwar Sweden. *Journal of Marriage & the Family* 62: 229–239.

Stephan, Ekkehard. 1989. A Net of Psychological Utility Theories. In *Psychological Theories from a Structuralist Point of View*, 63–102. Berlin, Germany: Springer.

Stephan, Walter G., and Cookie White Stephan. 2000. An Integrated Threat Theory of Prejudice.In *Reducing Prejudice and Discrimination*, 23–45, ed. Stuart Oskamp. Mahwah, NJ: Lawrence Erlbaum.

Sternberg, Robert J. 2001. What is the Common Thread Of Creativity? Its Dialectical Relation To Intelligence And Wisdom. *American Psychologist* 56 (4): 360–362.

Stets, Jan E. 1995. Job Autonomy and Contro. over One's Spouse: A Compensatory Process. *Journal of Health & Social Behavior* 36 (3): 244.

Stets, Jan E., and Ryan Trettevik. 2014. Emotions in Identity Theory. In *Handbook of the Sociology of Emotions*, vol II, 33–75, ed. Jan E. Stets and Jonathan H. Turner. Dordrecht, Netherlands: Springer.

Stevens, Fred C.J.., Charles D. Kaplan, Rudolf W.H.M.. Ponds, and Jellemer Jolles. 2001. The Importance of Active Lifestyles for Memory Performance and Memory Self-knowledge. *Basic & Applied Social Psychology* 23 (2): 137–145.

Stevenson, Fiona A., Miranda Leontowitsch, and Catherine Duggan. 2008. Over-the-Counter Medicines: Professional Expertise and Consumer Discourses. *Sociology of Health & Illness* 30 (6): 913–928 (\d12-4.14, 102–288).

Stevenson, Nick. 2011. *Education and Cultural Citizenship*. Los Angeles, CA: SAGE.

Stewart, Charles J., Craig Allen Smith, and Robert E. Denton, Jr. 2012. *Persuasion and Social Movements*. Long Grove, IL: Waveland.

Stier, Haya, and Noah Lewin-Epstein. 2003. Time-to-work: A Comparative Analysis of Preferences for Working Hours. *Work & Occupations* 30 (1): 302–326.

Stiglbauer, Barbara, and Carrie Kovacs. 2018. The More, the Better? Curvilinear Effects of Job Autonomy on Well-Being from Vitamin Model and PE-Fit Theory Perspectives. *Journal of Occupational Health Psychology* 23 (4): 520–536.

Stogner, John, Chris L. Gibson, and J. Mitchell Miller. 2014. Examining the Reciprocal Nature of the Health-Violence Relationship: Results from a Nationally Representative Sample. *Justice Quarterly* 31 (3): 473–499.

Stokman, Frans N., Jelle Van Der Knoop, and Reinier C.H. Van Oosten. 2013. Modeling Collective Decision-Making.In *The Handbook of Rational Choice Social Research*, 51–182, ed. Rafael Wittek, Tom A. H. Snijders, and Victor Nee. Stanford, CA: Stanford University Press.

Stolle, Dietlind. 2001. Clubs and Congregations: The Benefits of Joining an Association. In *Trust in Society*, 202–244, ed. Karen S. Cook. New York: Russell Sage Foundation.

Stolzenberg, Ross M. 2001. It's about Time and Gender: Spousal Employment and Health. *American Journal of Sociology* 107 (1): 61–100.

Stone, Walter J., and Matthew K. Buttice. 2010. Voters in Context: The Politics of Citizen Behavior. In *The Oxford Handbook of American Elections and Political Behavior*, 555–576, ed. Jan E., Leighley. Oxford, UK: Oxford University Press.

Stone, William F. 1993. Psychodynamic, Cognitive Functioning, or Group Orientation: Research and Theory in the 1980s. In *Strength and Weakness: The Authoritarian Personality Today*, 159–181, ed. William F. Stone, Gerda Lederer and Richard Christie. New York: Springer-Verlag.

Stott, Clifford, John Drury, and Steve Reicher. 2017. On the Role of a Social Identity Analysis in Articulating Structure and Collective Action: The 2011 Riots in Tottenham and Hackney. *British Journal of Criminology* 57 (4): 964–981.

Stoyan, Alissandra T., Sara Niedzwiecki, Jana Morgan, Jonathan Hartlyn, and Rosario Espinal. 2016. Trust in Government Institutions: The Effects of Performance and Participation in the Dominican Republic and Haiti. *International Political Science Review* 37 (1): 18–35.

Straughn, Jeremy Brooke, and Angie L. Andriot. 2011. Education, Civic Patriotism and Democratic Citizenship: Unpacking the Education Effect on Political Involvement. *Sociological Forum* 26 (3): 556–580.

Stretesky, Paul B., and Michael J. Lynch. 2009. A Cross-National Study of the Association between Per Capita Carbon Dioxide Emissions and Exports to the United States. *Social Science Research* 38 (1): 239–250.

Stride, Helen, and Malcolm Higgs. 2014. An Investigation into the Relationship between Values and Commitment: A Study of Staff in the U.K. Charity Sector. *Nonprofit & Voluntary Sector Quarterly* 43 (3): 455–479.

Stromblad, Per, and Gunnar Myrberg. 2013. Urban Inequality and Political Recruitment. *Urban Studies* 50 (5): 1049–1065.

Sturmer, Stefan, and Bernd Simon. 2009. Pathways to Collective Protest: Calculation, Identification, or Emotion? A Critical Analysis of the Role of Group-Based Anger in Social Movement Participation. *Journal of Social Issues* 65 (4): 681–705.

Stutzer, Alois. 2004. The Role of Income Aspirations in Individual Happiness. *Journal of Economic Behavior & Organization* 54: 89–109.

Su, Li Ping, Richard B. Miller, Jerevie M. Canlas, Tsui-Shan. Li, Ying-Ling. Hsiao, and Brian J. Willoughby. 2015. A Cross-Cultural Study of Perceived Marital Problems in Taiwan and the United States. *Contemporary Family Therapy* 37 (2): 165–175.

Su, Lujun, Binli Tang, and Jeroen Nawijn. 2021. How Tourism Activity Shapes Travel Experience Sharing: Tourist Well-Being and Social Context. *Annals of Tourism Research* 91: 103316.

Su, Wei, Sylvie Mrug, and Michael Windle. 2010. Social Cognitive and Emotional Mediators Link Violence Exposure and Parental Nurturance to Adolescent Aggression. *Journal of Clinical Child & Adolescent Psychology* 39 (6): 814–824.

Su, Yang, and Shizheng Feng. 2013. Adapt or Voice: Class, Guanxi, and Protest Propensity in China. *Journal of Asian Studies* 72 (1): 45–67.

Subramanian, S.V., and Ichiro Kawachi. 2006. Whose Health is Affected by Income Inequality? A Multilevel Intervention Analysis of Contemporaneous and Legal Effects of State Income Inequality on Individual Self-rated Health in the United States. *Health & Place* 12: 141–156.

Suchweh, Patrick. 2012. The Moral Economy of Inequality: Popular Views on Income Differentiation, Poverty and Wealth. *Socio-Economic Review* 10: 419–445.

Suh, Chan S., Ion Bogdan Vasi, and Paul Y. Chang. 2017. How Social Media Matter: Repression and the Diffusion of the Occupy Wall Street Movement. *Social Science Research* 65: 282–293.

Suh, Chan S., Paul Y. Chang, and Yisook Lim. 2012. Spill-Up and Spill-Over of Trust: An Extended Test of Cultural and Institutional Theories of Trust in South Korea. *Sociological Forum* 27 (2): 504–526.

Suh, Eunkook M. 2002. Culture, Identity Consistency, and Subjective Well-being. *Journal of Personality & Social Psychology* 83 (6): 1378–1391.

Suh, Eunkook M., and Jayoung Koo. 2008. Comparing Subjective Well-being across Cultures and Nations: The What and Why Questions. In *The Science of Subjective Well-Being*, 414–427, ed. Michael Eid and Randy J. Larsen. New York: Guilford.

Suldo, S.M. 2004. The Role of Life Satisfaction in The Relationship Between Authoritative Parenting Dimensions and Adolescent Problem Behavior. *Social Indicators Research* 66 (1–2): 165–195.

Suler, John R. 2016. *Psychology of the Digitial Age: Human Become Electric*. New York, NY: Cambridge University Press.

Sullivan, Alice. 2001. Cultural Capital and Education Attainment. *Sociology* 35 (4): 893–912.

Sullivan, Daniel, Sheridan A. Stewart, and Joseph Diefendorf. 2015. Simmel's Time-Space Theory: Implications for Experience of Modernization and Place. *Journal of Environmental Psychology* 41: 45–57.

Summers-Effler, Erika. 2002. The Micro Potential for Social Change: Emotion, Consciousness, and Social Movement Formation. *Sociological Theory* 20 (1): 41–60.

Sun, Gong, Steven D'Alessandro, and Lester Johnson. 2014. Traditional Culture, Political Ideologies, Materialism and Luxury Consumption in China. *International Journal of Consumer Studies* 38 (6): 578–585.
Sun, Ivan Y., Jessica C.M.. Li, and Wu. Yuning. 2011. Chinese and American College Students' Preferences for Police Response to Domestic Violence. *Policing & Society* 21 (2): 214–232.
Sun, Ivan Y., Hu. Rong, Daniel F. K. Wong, Xuesong He, and Jessica C. M. Li. 2013. One Country, Three Populations: Trust in Police among Migrants, Villagers, and Urbanites in China. *Social Science Research* 42: 1737–1749.
Sun, Jiming, and Xun Wang. 2010. Value Differences between Generations in China: A Study in Shanghai. *Journal of Youth Studies* 13 (1): 65–81.
Sun, Moon-Gi. 2011. State Intervention, Economic Growth and Income Inequality in South Korea. *Korea Observer* 42 (3): 413–429.
Sun, Shaojing, Alan M. Rubin, and Paul M. Haridakis. 2008. The Role of Motivation and Media Involvement in Explaining Internet Dependency. *Journal of Broadcasting & Electronic Media* 52 (3): 408–431.
Sun, Wenkai, and Xianghong Wang. 2012. Do Government Actions Affect Trust? Cross-city Evidence in China. *Social Science Journal* 49: 447–457.
Sundararajan, Louise, and Maharaj K. Raina. 2016. Mind and Creativity: Insights From Rasa Theory With Special Focus On Sahrdaya (the Appreciative Critic). *Theory & Psychology* 26 (6): 788–809.
Sundquist, Kristina, and Min Yang. 2007. Linking Social Capital and Self-rated Health: A Multilevel Analysis of 11,775 Men and Women in Sweden. *Health & Place* 13: 324–334.
Sung, Pei-Fen., and Meng-Li. Yang. 2009. National Identity and Its Relationship with Teachers' Historical Knowledge and Pedagogy: The Case of Taiwan. *Asia Pacific Journal of Education* 29 (2): 179–194.
Sussman, Steve, and Susan L. Ames. 2001. *The Social Psychology of Drug abuse*. Buckingham, UK: Open University Press.
Sutherland, Claire. 2005. Nation-Building Through Discourse Theory. *Nations & Nationalism* 11 (2): 185–202.
Suzuki, Tadashi, and Joel Best. 2003. The Emergence of Trendsetters for Fashions and Fads: Kogaru in 1990s Japan. *Sociological Quarterly* 44 (1): 61–79.
Svebak, Sven, Rod A. Martin, and Jostein Holmen. 2004. The Prevalence of Sense of Humor in a Large, Unselected County Population in Norway: Relations with Age, Sex, and some Health Indicators. *Humor: International Journal of Humor Research* 17 (1/2): 121–134.
Svensson, Lennart G. 2006. New Professionalism, Trust and Competence. *Current Sociology* 54 (4): 579–593.
Swader, Christopher S., and Irina D. Vorobeva. 2015. Receiving Gifts for Sex in Moscow, Kyiv, and Minsk: A Compensated Dating Survey. *Sexuality & Culture* 19 (2): 321–348.
Swank, Eric, and Breanne Fahs. 2016. Gay Rights Activism: Collection Action Frames, Networks, and Protesting among Gays, Lesbians, and Bisexuals. *Journal of Civil Society* 12 (4): 430–447.
Swanson, Jeffrey W., Arthur O. Linskey, Ruben Quintero-Salinas, Andres J. Pumariega, and Charles E. Holzer, III. 1992. A Binational School Survey of Depressive Symptoms, Drug Use, and Suicidal Ideation. *Journal of the American Academy of Child & Adolescent Psychiatry* 31 (4): 669–678.
Swaroop, Sapna, and Jeffrey D. Morenoff. 2006. Building Community: The Neighborhood Context of Social Organization. *Social Forces* 84 (3): 1665–1695.
Swart, Lu-Anne., Sarah Day, Rajen Govender, and Mohamed Seedat. 2020. Participation in (Non)Violent Protests and Associated Psychosocial Factors: Sociodemographic Status, Civic Engagement, and Perceptions of Government's Performance. *South African Journal of Psychology* 50 (4): 480–492.
Swartz, David L. 2013. *Symbolic Power, Politics, and Intellectuals: The Political Sociology of Pierre Bourdieu*. Chicago, IL: University of Chicago Press.
Szondi, Gyorgy. 2010. From Image Management to Relationship Building: A Public Relations Approach to Nation Building. *Place Branding & Public Diplomacy* 6 (4): 333–343.

Tacher, Elisa Levy, and Christine Anderson Readdick. 2006. The Relation between Aggression and Creativity among Second Graders. *Creativity Research Journal* 18 (3): 261–267.

Tadjoeddin, Mohammad Zulfan. 2013. Educated but Poor: Explaining Localized Ethnic Violence During Indonesia's Democratic Transition. *International Area Studies Review* 16 (1): 24–49.

Tak, Sangdong. 2017. Cooperative Membership and Community Engagement: Findings from a Latin American Survey. *Sociological Forum* 32 (3): 566–586.

Takahashi, Lois M., and Sharon Lord Gaber. 1998. Controversial Facility Siting in the Urban Environment: Resident and Planner Perceptions in the United States. *Environment & Behavior* 30 (2): 184–215.

Talisse, Robert B. 2009. *Democracy and Moral Conflict*. Cambridge, UK: Cambridge University Press.

Tam, Kim-Pong. 2013. Dispositional Empathy with Nature. *Journal of Environmental Psychology* 35: 92–104.

Tam, May, and Chung Yan Ip. 2017. Experience and Coping of Employment Risks in Hong Kong. *International Journal of Sociology & Social Policy* 37 (3–4): 166–185.

Tamres, Lisa K., Denise Janicki, and Vicki S. Helgeson. 2002. Sex Differences in Coping Behavior: A Meta-analytic Review and an Examination of Relative Coping. *Personality & Social Psychology Review* 6 (1): 2–30.

Tan, Sor-hoon. 2003. *Confucian Democracy: A Deweyan Reconstruction*. Albany, NY: State University of New York.

Tang, Min. 2011. The Political Behavior of the Chinese Middle Class. *Journal of Chinese Political Sciences* 16: 373–387.

Tang, Wenfang. 2001. Religion and Society in China and Taiwan. In *Chinese Political Culture, 1989–2000*, 298–319, ed. Shiping Hua. Armonk, NY: Sharpe.

Tanggaard, Lene. 2009. Resisting an Isolated Learning Discourse. *International Journal of Lifelong Education* 28 (6): 693–703.

Taniguchi, Hiromi, and Leonard Thomas. 2011. The Influences of Religious Attitudes on Volunteering. *Voluntas: International Journal of Voluntary & Nonprofit Organizations* 22 (2): 335–355.

Taniguchi, Hiromi. 2013. The Influence of Generalized Trust on Volunteering in Japan. *Nonprofit & Voluntary Sector Quarterly* 42 (1): 127–147.

Tankebe, Justice. 2009. Public Cooperation With the Police in Ghana: Does Procedural Fairness Matter? *Criminology* 47 (4): 1265–1293.

Tanner-Smith, Emily E., Sandra J. Wilson, and Mark W. Kipsey. 2013. Risk Factors and Crime. In *The Oxford Handbook of Criminological Theory*, 89–111, ed. Francis T. Cullen and Pamela Wilcox. New York: Oxford University Press.

Taormina, Robert J., and Jennifer H. Gao. 2010. A Research Model for Guanxi Behavior: Antecedents, Measures, and Outcomes of Chinese Social Networking. *Social Science Research* 39: 1195–1212.

Taplin, Ross H., Rosemary Kerr, and Alistair M. Brown. 2013. Who Pays for Blended Learning? A Cost-Benefit Analysis. *Internet & Higher Education* 18: 61–68.

Tapper, James, and Koji Kobayashi. 2018. It's a Harsh Fact of Life with the Rma: Neo-Liberalism and the Realities of Community Sports Facility Development by the Private Sector in New Zealand. *Leisure Studies* 37 (3): 282–294.

Targgort Murphy, R. 2014. *Japan and the Shackles of the Past*. Oxford, UK: Oxford University Press.

Tavares, Susana M., Daan van Knippenberg, and Rolf van Dick. 2016. Organizational Identification and Currencies of Exchange: Integrating Social Identity and Social Exchange Perspectives. *Journal of Applied Social Psychology* 46: 34–45.

Taylor, Dorceta A. 2000. The Rise of the Environmental Justice Paradigm: Injustice Framing and the Social Construction of Environmental Discourses. *American Behavior Scientist* 43 (4): 568–580.

Taylor, Graham, Andrew Mathers, and Martin Upchurch. 2011. Beyond Political Economism: New Identities for Unions in Western Europe? *Capital & Class* 36 (1): 17–34.

Taylor, Issac. 2018. *The Ethics of Counterterrorism*. New York, NY: Routledge.

Taylor, Jeanette, Matt McGue, William G. Iacono, and David T. Lykken. 2000. A Behavioral Genetic Analysis of the Relationship between the Socialization Scale and Self-reported Delinquency. *Journal of Personality* 68 (1): 29–50.

Taylor, Ralph B., Brian R. Wyant, and Brian Lockwood. 2015. Variable Links within Perceived Police Legitimacy? Fairness and Effectiveness across Races and Places. *Social Science Research* 49: 234–248.

Taylor, Verta, Katrina Kimport, Nella Van Dyke, and Ellen Ann Andersen. 2009. Culture and Mobilization: Tactical Repertoires, Same-sex Weddings, and the Impact on Gay Activism. *American Sociological Review* 74: 865–890.

Taylor-Gooby, Peter, Charlotte Hastie, and Catherine Bromley. 2003. Querulous Citizens: Welfare Knowledge and the Limits to Welfare Reform. *Social Policy & Administration* 37 (1): 1–20.

Taylor-Gooby, Peter. 2001. Risk Contingency and the Third Way: Evidence from the BHPS and Qualitative Studies. *Social Policy & Administration* 35 (2): 195–211.

Tedin, Kent L., Richard E. Matland, and Gregory R. Weiher. 2001. Age, Race, Self-interest, and Financing Public Schools through Referenda. *Journal of Politics* 63 (1): 270–294.

TenHouten, Warren D. 2007. *A General Theory of Emotions and Social Life*. Abingdon, UK: Routledge.

TenHouten, Warren D. 2017. *Alienation and Affect*. Abingdon, UK: Routledge.

Tenorio, Kimberly A., and Celia C. Lo. 2011. Social Location, Social Integration, and the Co-Occurrence of Substance Abuse and Psychological Distress. *American Journal of Drug & Alcohol Abuse* 37 (4): 218–223.

Teodoro, Antonio. 2003. Educational Policies and New Ways of Governance on a Transitionalization Period. In *The International Assessment of New Research and Theory*, 183–210, ed. Carlos Alberto Torres and Ari Antikainen. Lanham, MD: Rowman.

Teorell, Jan. 2003. Linking Social Capital to Political Participation: Voluntary Associations and Networks of Recruitment in Sweden. *Scandinavian Political Studies* 26 (1): 49–66.

Tester, Keith. 2004. *The Social Thought of Zygmunt Bauman*. Houndmills, UK: Palgrave.

Teymoori, Ali, Jolanda Jetten, Brock Bastian, Amarina Ariyanto, Frederique Autin, Nadia Ayub, Constantina Badea, Tomasz Besta, Fabrizio Butera, Rui Costa-Lopes, Lijuan Cui, Carole Fantini, Gillian Finchilescu, Lowell Gaertner, Mario Gollwitzer, Angel Gomez, Roberto Gonzalez, Ying Yi Hong, Dorthe Hoj Jensen, and Minoru Karasawa. 2016. Revisiting the Measurement of Anomie. *PLoS ONE* 11 (7): 1–27.

Thapa, Shreena, Shelley L. Brown, and Tracey A. Skilling. 2021. The Relationship between Self-Esteem, Gender, Criminal Attitudes, and Recidivism in a Youth Justice Sample. *Criminal Justice & Behavior* 48 (4): 539–555.

Tharp, Roland G. 2012. *Delta Theory and Psychosocial Systems: The Practice of Influence and Change*. New York, NY: Cambridge University Press.

Thiede, Michael, and Stefan Traub. 1997. Mutual Influences of Health and Poverty: Evidence from German Panel Data. *Social Science & Medicine* 45 (6): 867–877.

Thin, Neil. 2012. *Social Happiness: Theory into Policy and Practice*. Bristol, UK: Polity.

Thoits, Peggy A., and Lyndi N. Hewitt. 2001. Volunteer Work and Well-being. *Journal of Health & Social Behavior* 42: 115–131.

Thomas, Diez, Paul C. Stern, and Gregory A. Guagnano. 1998. Social Structural and Social Psychological Bases of Environmental Concern. *Environment & Behavior* 30 (4): 450–471.

Thomas, Emma F., and Winnifred R. Louis. 2013. Doing Democracy: The Social Psychological Mobilization and Consequences of Collective Action. *Social Issues & Policy Review* 7 (1): 173–200.

Thompson, Brian L., and James Daniel Lee. 2004. Who Cares if Police Become Violent? Explaning Approval of Police Use of Force Using a National Sample. *Sociological Inquiry* 74 (3): 381–410.

Thompson, Cynthia A., Laura L. Beauvais, and Karen S. Lyness. 1999. When Work-family Benefits and Not Enough: The Influence of Work-family Culture on Benefit Utilization, Organization Attachment, and Work-family Conflict. *Journal of Vocational Behavior* 54: 392–415.

Thompson, Martie P., Linda E. Saltzman, and Holly Johnson. 2003. A Comparison of Risk Factors for Intimate Partner Violence-Related Injury across Two National Surveys on Violence against Women. *Violence against Women* 9 (4): 438–457.

Thomson, A.J.P. 2005. *Deconstruction and Democracy: Derrida's Politics of Friendship*. London: Continuum.

Thornton, Arland, William G. Axinn, and Yu. Xie. 2007. *Marriage and Cohabitation*. Chicago, IL: University of Chicago Press.

Thorson, James A. 1998. Religion and Anxiety: Which Anxiety? Which Religion? In *Handbook of Religion and Mental Health*, 147–160, ed. Harold G. Konenig. San Diego, CA: Academic.

Thyen, Kressen, and Johannes Gerschewski. 2018. Legitimacy and Protest under Authoritarianism: Explaining Student Mobilization in Egypt and Morocco during the Arab Uprisings. *Democratization* 25 (1): 38–57.

Tiliouine, Habib, Robert A. Cummins, and Melanie Davern. 2006. Measuring Wellbeing in Developing Countries: The Case of Algeria. *Social Indicators Research* 75: 1–30.

Tilley, James. 2002. Is Youth a Better Predictor of Sociopolitical Values than Is Nationality? *Annals of the American Academy of Political & Social Science* 580: 226–256.

Tilly, Charles. 2009. Power and Democracy. In *The SAGE Handbook of Power*. 70–88, ed. Stewart R. Clegg and Mark Haugaard. London, UK: SAGE.

Tink, Lisa N., Danielle Peers, Candace I. J. Nykiforuk, and Bethan C. Kingsley. 2020. Moving Beyond Ideology: Contemporary Recreation and the Neoliberal Discourses of New Public Health. *Leisure Studies* 39 (6): 767–781.

Todd, Mary K., and Ellis L. Gesten. 1999. Predictors of Child Abuse Potential in At-risk Adolescents. *Journal of Family Violence* 14 (4): 417–436.

Toews, David. 2018. *Social and Politica. Life in the Era of Digital Media: Higher Diversities*. Abington, UK: Routledge.

Tokunaga, Robert S. 2016. An Examination of Functional Difficulties from Internet Use: Media Habit and Displacement Theory Explanations. *Human Communication Research* 42 (3): 339–370.

Tolsma, Jochem, Tom van der Meer, and Maurice Gesthuizen. 2009. The Impact of Neighborhood and Municipality Characteristics on Social Cohesion in the Netherlands. *Acta Politica* 44 (3): 286–313.

Tom, Shelley R., David Schwartz, Lei Chang, Jo Ann M. Farver, and Yiyuan Xu. 2010. Correlates of Victimization in Hong Kong Children's Peer Groups. *Journal of Applied Developmental Psychology* 31: 27–37.

Tomer, John F. 2002. Human Well-Being: A New Approach Based on Overall and Ordinary Functionings. *Review of Social Economy* 60 (1): 23–45.

Tomhave, Alan. 2012. Civility as a Condition of Citizenship. In *Civility in Politics and Education*, 154–188, ed. Deborah S. Mower and Wade L. Robison. New York: Routledge.

Tomich, Patricia L., and Vicki S. Helgeson. 2002. Five Years Later: A Cross-Sectional Comparison of Breast Cancer Survivors with Healthy Women. *Psycho-Oncology* 11: 154–169.

Tonglet, Michele, Paul S. Phillips, and Margaret Bates. 2004. Determining the Drivers for Households Pro-environmental Behavior: Waste Minimisation Compared to Recycling. *Resources, Conservation & Recycling* 42: 27–48.

Torche, Florencia. 2011. Is a College Degree Still the Great Equalizer? Intergenerational Mobility across Levels of Schooling in the United States. *American Journal of Sociology* 117 (3): 763–807.

Torfing, Jacob. 1999. *New Theories of Discourse: Laclau, Mouffe and Zizek*. Oxford, UK: Blackwell.

Tov, William, and Ed Diener. 2008. The Well-Being of Nations: Linking together Trust, Cooperation, and Democracy. In *Cooperation: The Political Psychology of Effective Human Interaction*, 323–342, ed. Brandon A. Sullivan, Mark Snyder and John L. Sullivan. Malden, MA: Blackwell.

Townley, Barbara. 2014. Bourdieu and Organizational Theory: A Ghostly Apparition? In *The Oxford Handbook of Sociology, Social theory, and Organization Studies: Contemporary Currents*, 39–63, ed. Paul Alder, Paul Du Gay, Glenn Morgan and Mike Reed. Oxford, UK: Oxford University Press.

Tracy, Jessica A., Joey T. Cheng, Richard W. Robins, and Kali H. Trzesniewski. 2009. Authentic and Hubristic Pride: The Affective Core of Self-esteem and Narcissism. *Self & Identity* 8: 196–213.

Tracy, Karen, and Jessica M. F. Hughes. 2014. Democracy-Appealing Partisanship: A Situated Ideal of Citizenship. *Journal of Applied Communication Research* 42 (3): 307–324.

Trainor, Brian T. 2008. Politics as the Quest for Unity. *Philosophy & Social Criticism* 34 (8): 905–924.

Tranter, Bruce, and Mark Western. 2009. The Influence of Green Parties on Postmaterialist Values. *British Journal of Sociology* 60 (1): 145–167.

Traunmuller, Richard. 2011. Moral Communities? Religion as a Source of Social Trust in a Multilevel Analysis of 97 German Regions. *European Sociological Review* 27 (3): 346–363.

Travers, Eva F. 1982. Ideology and Political Participation among High School Students: Changes from 1970 to 1979. *Youth & Society* 13 (3): 327–352.

Treharne, Gareth J., Antonia C. Lyons, and Rachel E. Tupling. 2001. The Effects of Optimism, Pessimism, Social Support, and Mood on the Lagged Relationship between Daily Stress and Symptoms. *Current Research on Social Psychology* 7 (5): 1–13.

Treiman, Thomas, and Justine Gartner. 2006. Are Residents Willing to Pay for Their Community Forests? Results of a Contingent Valuation Survey in Missouri, USA. *Urban Studies* 43 (9): 1537–1547.

Treno, Andrew J., and Harold D. Holder. 1997. Community Mobilization, Organizing, and Media Advocacy. *Evaluation Review* 21 (2): 166–190.

Triandis, Harry C. 1995. *Individualism and Collectivism.* Boulder, CO: Westview.

Triandis, Harry C. 2000. Cultural Syndromes and Subjective well-being. In *Culture and Subjective Well-Being*, 13–36, ed. Ed Diener and Eunkook M. Suh. Cambridge, MA: MIT.

Triandis, Harry C., and Eunkook M. Suh. 2002. Cultural Influences on Personality. *Annual Review Psychology* 53: 133–160.

Triandis, Harry C., and Michele J. Gelfand. 2012. A Theory of Individualism and Collectivism. In *Handbook of Theories of Social Psychology*, vol. 2, 498–520, ed. Paul A.M. Van Lange, Arie W. Kruglanski and E. Tory Higgins. London, CA: SAGE.

Truelove, Heather Barnes, P. Wesley Schultz, and Ashley Jade Gillis. 2019. Using Social Psychology to Protect the Environment. In *The SAGE Handbook of Applied Social Psychology*, 491–514, ed. Kieran C. O'Doherty and Darrin Hodgetts. London, UK: SAGE.

Trumbo, Craig W., Katherine A. McComas, and John C. Besley. 2008. Individual-and-Community-Level Effects on Risk Perception in Cancer Cluster Investigations. *Risk Analysis* 28 (1): 161–178.

Tsai, Chia-hung. 2019. Unfolding the Pattern of Contentious Participation in Taiwan. *Electoral Studies* 58: 94–102.

Tsai, Ming-chang. 2006. Does Globalization Affect Human Well-Being. Paper presented in *16th ISA World Congress of Sociology*, July 23–29, 2006, Durban, South Africa.

Tsai, Ming-Tien., and Chun-Chen. Huang. 2007. The Relationship among Ethical Climate Types, Facets of Job Satisfaction, and the Three Components of Organizational Commitment: A Study of Nurses in Taiwan. *Journal of Business Ethics* 80 (3): 565–581.

Tseloni, Andromachi, Karin Wittebrood, Graham Farrell, and Ken Pease. 2004. Burglary, Victimization in England and Wales, the United States and the Netherlands. *British Journal of Criminology* 44: 66–91.

Tsfati, Yario, Riva Turkachinsky, and Yorom Peri. 2009. Exposure to News, Political Comedy, and Entertainment Talk Shows: Concern about Security and Political Mistrust. *International Journal of Public Opinion Research* 21 (4): 399–423.

Tsiotsou, Rodoula H. 2015. The Role of Social and Parasocial Relationships on Social Networking Sites Loyalty. *Computers in Human Behavior* 48: 401–414.

Tuason, Ma., and G. Teresa. 2008. Those Who Were Born Poor: A Qualitative Study of Philippine Poverty. *Journal of Counseling Psychology* 55 (2): 158–171.

Tukachinsky, Riva, and Keren Eyal. 2018. The Psychology of Marathon Television Viewing: Antecedents and Viewer Involvement. *Mass Communication & Society* 21 (3): 275–295.

Tulin, Marina, Bram Lancee, and Beate Volker. 2018. Personality and Social Capital. *Social Psychology Quarterly* 81 (4): 295–318.

Tung, An-chi, and Wen Shan Yang. 2006. Fertility Decision and Women Labor Market Status: A Case Study in Taiwan. *Demography Studies* 39: 39–55.

Turiel, Elliot. 2014. Morality: Epistemology, Development, and Social Opposition. In *Handbook of Moral Development*, 3–22, ed. Melanie Killen and Judith G. Smetana. New York: Psychology.

Turner, Bryan S. 2009. Talcott Parsons's Sociology of Religion and the Expressive Revolution. *Journal of Classical Sociology* 5 (3): 303–318.

Turner, Bryan. 2005a. The Sociology of the Family. In *The SAGE Handbook of Sociology*, 135–153, ed. Craig Calhoun, Chris Rojek, and Bryan Turner. London, UK: SAGE.

Turner, John C., and Katherine J. Reynolds. 2012. Self-categorization Theory. In *Handbook of Theories of Social Psychology*, vol. 2, 399–417, ed. Paul A.M. Van Lange, Arie W. Kruglanski and E. Tory Higgins. London, CA: SAGE.

Turner, Jonathan H. 1984. *Social Stratification: A Theoretical Analysis*. New York: Columbia University Press.

Turner, Jonathan H. 2003. *Human Institutions: A Theory of Societal Evolution*. Lanham, MD: Rowman & Littlefield.

Turner, Jonathan H. 2010. *Theoretical Principles of Sociology, Volume 2: Microdynamics*. New York: Springer.

Turner, Jonathan H. 2013. *Contemporary Sociological Theory*. Thousand Oaks, CA: SAGE.

Turner, Jonathan H., and Jan E. Stets. 2005. *The Sociology of Emotions*. Cambridge, UK: Cambridge University Press.

Turnipseed, Patricia H., and David L. Turnipseed. 2013. Testing the Proposed Linkage between Organizational Citizenship Behaviours and in Innovative Organizational Climate. *Creativity & Innovation Management* 22 (2): 209–216.

Twenge, Jean M., and W. Keith Campbell. 2003. Isn't It Fun to Get the Respect That We're Going to Deserve? Narcissism, Social Rejection, and aggression. *Personality & Social Psychology Bulletin* 29 (2): 261–272.

Tybur, Joshua M., Willem E. Frankenhuis, and Thomas V. Pollet. 2014. Behavioral Immune System Methods: Surveying the Present to Shape the Future. *Evolutionary Behavioral Sciences* 8 (4): 274–283.

Tyler, Tom R. 1998. Trust and Democratic Governance. In *Trust and Governance*, 269–294, ed. Valerie Braithwaite and Margaret Levi. New York; Russell Sage.

Tyler, Tom R. 2012. Justice Theory. In *Handbook of Theories of Social Psychology*, vol. 2, 344–361, ed. Paul A.M. Van Lange, Arie W. Kruglanski and E. Tory Higgins. London, CA: SAGE.

Tyler, Tom R., Robert J. Boerkmann, Heather J. Smith, and Yuen J. Huo. 1997. *Social Justice in a Diverse Society*. Boulder, CO: Westview.

Tyron, Warren W. 1997. Introduction to the Bidirectional Associative Memory Model: Implications for Psychopathology, Treatment, and Research. In *Cognitive Science Perspectives on Personality and Emotion*, 65–122, ed. Gerald Matthews. Amsterdam, Netherlands: Elsevier.

Uchino, Bert N., Julianne Holt-Lunstad, Darcy Uno, and Jeffrey B. Flinders. 2001. Heterogeneity in the Social Networks of Yung and Older Adults: Prediction of Mental Health and Cardiovascular Reactivity during Acute Stress. *Journal of Behavioral Medicine* 24 (4): 361–382.

Uddin, Emaj. 2011. Cross-Cultural Social Stress among Muslim, Hindu, Santal and Oraon Communities in Rasulpur of Bangladesh. *International Journal of Sociology & Social Policy* 31 (5–6): 335–360.

Ulbig, Stacy G. 2002. Policies, Procedures, and People: Sources of Support for Government? *Social Science Quarterly* 83 (3): 789–809.

Ullrich, Simone, David P. Farrington, and Jeremy W. Cold. 2007. Dimensions of DSM-IV Personality Disorders and Life-success. *Journal of Personality Disorders* 21 (6): 657–663.

Umberson, Debra, Kristi Williams, Daniel A. Powers, Meichu D. Chen, and Anna M. Campbell. 2005. As Good as It Gets? A Life Course Perspective on Marital Quality. *Social Forces* 84 (1): 493–511.

Umeh, Kanayo, and Reema Patel. 2004. Theory of Planned Behaviour and Ecstasy Use: Analysis of Moderator-interactions. *British Journal of Health Psychology* 9: 25–38.

Umeh, Kanayo. 2004. Cognitive Appraisals, Maladaptive Coping, and Past Behavior in Protective Motivation. *Psychology & Health* 19 (6): 719–735.

Ungar, Sheldon. 2001. Moral Panic versus the Risk Society: The Implications of the Changing Sites of Social Anxiety. *British Journal of Sociology* 52 (2): 271–291.

Uppal, Charu. 2021. Mobilizing Citizens at Their Level: A Case Study of Public Engagement. *Journalism Practice* 15 (5): 601–619.

Urbatsch, R. 2014. *Families' Values: How Parents, Siblings, and Children Affect Political Attitudes.* New York: Oxford University Press.

Uslaner, Eric M. 2002. *The Moral Foundations of Trust.* Cambridge, UK: Cambridge University Press.

Uslaner, Eric M. 2008. *Corruption, Inequality, and the Rule of Law: The Bulging Pocket Makes the Easy Life.* Cambridge, UK: Cambridge University Press.

Uslaner, Eric M., and Mitchell Brown. 2005. Inequality, Trust, and Civic Engagement. *American Politics Research* 33 (6): 868–894.

Valentino, Nicholas A., and David O. Sears. 1998. Event-driven Political Communication and the Preadult Socialization of Partisanship. *Political Behavior* 20 (2): 127–154.

Valera, Sergi, and Joan Guardia. 2014. Perceived Insecurity and Fear of Crime in a City with Low-Crime Rates. *Journal of Environmental Psychology* 38: 195–205.

Valiente, Celia. 2018. Gender and Political Sociology. In *The SAGE Handbook of Political Sociology*, 143–154, ed. William Outhwaite and Stephen Turner. London, UK: SAGE.

van Bruggen, Alinda C. 2000. Social Participation and Subjective Well-being of Long-term Unemployed: Why is Paid Work So Hard to Substitute for? In *Advances in Quality of Life Theory and Research*, 111–128, ed. Ed Diener and Don R. Rahtz. Dordrecht, Netherlands: Kluwer Academic.

van de Vliert, Evert S., Kluwer Esther, and Richard Lynn. 2000. Citizens of Warmer Countries are More Competitive and Poorer: Culture or Chance? *Journal of Economic Psychology* 21: 143–165.

Van de Vyver, Julie and Dominic Abrams. 2018. The Arts as a Catalyst for Human Prosociality and Cooperation. *Social Psychological & Personality Science* 9 (6): 664–674.

van de Werfhorst, Herman G., and Gerbert Kraaykamp. 2001. Four Field-related Educational Resources and Their Impact on Labor, Consumption, and Sociopolitical Orientation. *Sociology of Education* 74: 296–317.

van den Bos, Kees, Jitse van Ameijde, and Hein van Gorp. 2001. On the Psychology of Religion: The Role of Personal Uncertainty in Religious Worldview Defense. *Basic & Applied Social Psychology* 28 (4): 333–341.

Van den Broeck, Evert, Karolien Poels, and Michel Walrave. 2015. Older and Wiser? Facebook Use, Privacy Concern, and Privacy Protection in the Life Stages of Emerging, Young, and Middle Adulthood. *Social Media + Society* 1(2):2056305115616l4.

van der Bracht, Koen, Hélène. Flaam, Koen Vlassenroot, and Bart Van de Putte. 2017. Conflict and Insecurity: A Sociological Perspective on Perceptions of Insecurity in Conflict-Affected Democratic Republic of Congo. *Current Sociology* 65 (3): 336–355.

Van der Meer, T.W.G., and J. van Ingen. 2009. Schools of Democracy: Disentangling the Relationship between Civic Participation and Political Action in 17 European Countries. *European Journal of Political Research* 48: 281–308.

van der Toorn, Jojanneke, Miholy Berkics, and John T. Jost. 2010. System Justification, Satisfaction, and Perceptions of Fairness and Typicality at Work: A Cross-System Comparison Involving the U.S. and Hungary. *Social Justice Research* 23 (2): 189–210.

Van Dyke, Nella and Marc Dixon. 2013. Activist Human Capital: Skills Acquisition and the Development of Commitment to Social Movement Activism. *Mobilization* 18 (2): 197–212.

van Eijck, Koen, and Wim Knulst. 2005. No More Need for Snobbism: Highbrow Cultural Participation in a Taste Democracy. *European Sociological Review* 21 (5): 513–528.

Van Eijck, Koen. 2001. Social Differentiation in Musical Taste Patterns. *Social Forces* 79 (3): 1163–1185.

Van Haaften, E., Zhenrong Yu Heleen, and Fons J.R.. Van de Vijver. 2004. Human Resilience in a Degrading Environment: A Case Study in China. *Asian Journal of Social Psychology* 7: 205–219.
van Hemert, Dianne A., Fons J.R.. van de Viver, Ype H. Poortinger, and James Georgas. 2002. Structural and Functional Equivalence of the Eysenck Personality Questionnaire within and between-countries. *Personality & Individual Differences* 33: 1229–1249.
van Ingen, Erik, and René Bekkers. 2015. Generalized Trust through Civic Engagement? Evidence from Five National Panel Studies. *Political Psychology* 36 (3): 277–294.
Van Knippenberg, Barbara, Daan Van Knippenberg, and David De Cremer. 2007. Why People Resort to Coercion: The Role of Utility and Legitimacy. *European Journal of Social Psychology* 37: 276–287.
Van Leeuwen, Wouter, and Matthijs Baas. 2017. Creativity Under Attack: How People's Role in Competitive Conflict Shapes Their Creative Idea Generation. *Creativity Research Journal* 29 (4): 354–369.
Van Ness, Justin, and Erika Summers-Effler. 2016. Reimaging Collective Behavior. In *Handbook of Contemporary Sociological Theory*, 527–546, ed. Seth Abrutyn. Cham, Switzerland: Springer.
van Oorschot, Wim, and Wil Arts. 2005. The Social Capital of European Welfare States: The Crowding out Hypothesis Revisited. *Journal of European Social Policy* 15 (1): 5–26.
van Praag, B.M.S., P. Frijters, and A. Ferrer-i-Carbonell. 2003. The Anatomy of Subjective Well-being. *Journal of Economic Behavior & Organization* 51: 29–49.
van Praag, Bernard M.S., and Paul Frijters. 1999. The Measurement of Welfare and Well-being: The Layden Approach. In *Well-being: The Foundations of Hedonic Psychology*, 413–433, ed. Daniel Kahneman, Ed Diener and Norbert Schwarz. New York: Russell Sage.
van Praag, Bernard, and Ada Ferrer-I-Carbonell. 2004. *Happiness Quantified: A Satisfaction Calculus Approach*. Oxford, UK: Oxford University Press.
van Prooijen, J.W., M. Gallucci, and G. Toeset. 2008. Procedural Justice in Punishment Systems: Inconsistent Punishment Procedures Have Detrimental Effects on Cooperation. *British Journal of Social Psychology* 47 (2): 311–324.
van Riper, Carena J., Jee In Yoon, Gerard T. Kyle, Kenneth E. Wallen, Adam C. Landon, and Christopher Raymond. 2019. The Antecedents of Place Attachment in the Context of an Australian National Park. *Journal of Environmental Psychology* 61: 1–9.
van Tienen, Marike, Peer Scheepers, Jan Reitsma, and Hans Schulderman. 2011. The Role of Religiosity for Formal and Informal Volunteering in the Netherlands. *VOLUNTAS: International Journal of Voluntary and Nonprofit Organizations* 22: 365–389.
van Troost, Dunya, Bert Klandermans, and Jacquelien van Stekelenburg. 2018. Friends in High Places. Anger and Frustration among Protesters When Their Political Allies Fail Them. *Humanity & Society* 42 (4): 455–479.
Vugt, Van, Keith Dowding Mark, Peter John, and Eric van Dijk. 2003. The Exit of Residential Mobility or the Voice of Political Action: Strategies for Problem Solving in Residential Communities. *Journal of Applied Social Psychology* 33 (2): 321–338.
van Wilsem, Johan. 2007. Cross-national Research on Violent Victimization. In *The Cambridge Handbook of Violent Behavior and Aggression*, 486–500, ed. Daniel J. Flannery, Alexander T. Vazsonyi and Irwin D. Waldman. Cambridge, UK: Cambridge University Press.
Van Zomeren, Martijn. 2009. Metaphors of Protest: A Classification of Motivations for Collective Action. *Journal of Social Issues* 65 (4): 661–679.
Vanderstraeten, Raf. 2003. Explorations in the Systems-theoretical Study of Education. In *The International Assessment of New Research and Theory*, 42–57, ed. Carlos Alberto Torres and Ari Antikainen. Lanham, MD: Rowman.
Vansteenkiste, Maarten, Timmermans Willy Tinneke, Bart Soenens Lens, and Aya Van den Broeck. 2008. Does Extrinsic Goal Faming Enhance Extrinsic Goal-oriented Individuals' Learning and Performance? An Experimental Test of the Match Perspective versus Self-determination Theory. *Journal of Education Psychology* 100 (2): 387–397.
Varady, David P., and Jeffrey A. Raffel. 1995. *Allocating Homebuyers Through Schools and Housing Programs*. Albany, NY: State University of New York Press.

Varga, Mihai. 2008. How Political Opportunities Strengthen the Far Right: Understanding the Rise in Far-right Militancy in Russia. *European Asia Studies* 60 (4): 561–579.

Vargas-Lagos, Veronica. 1991. How Should Resources Be Reallocated between Physicians and Nurses in Africa and Latin America? *Social Science & Medicine* 33 (6): 723–727.

Varner, Gary. 2008. Utilitarianism and the Evolution of Ecological Ethics. *Science & Engineering Ethics* 14: 551–573.

Vartanian, Thomas P. 1999. Adolescent Neighborhood Effects on Labor Market and Economic Outcomes. *Social Service Review* 73 (2): 142–167.

Vartanian, Thomas P., and Justine M. McNamara. 2004. The Welfare Myth: Disentagling the Long-term Effects of Poverty and Welfare Receipt for Young Single Mothers. *Journal of Sociology & Social Welfare* 31 (4): 105–140.

Veenhoven, Ruut. 1984. *Conditions of Happiness*. Dordrecht, Holland: D. Reidel.

Veenhoven, Ruut. 2000. Freedom and Happiness: A Comparative Study in Forty-four Nations in the Early 1990s. In *Culture and Subjective Well-being*, 257–288, ed. Ed Diener and Eunkook M. Suh. Cambridge, MA: MIT.

Veenhoven, Ruut. 2005. Return of Inequality in Modern Society? Test by Dispersion of Life-satisfaction across Time and Nations. *Journal of Happiness Studies* 6: 457–487.

Veenhoven, Ruut. 2008. Sociological Theories of Subjective Well-being. In *The Science of Subjective Well-being*, 44–61, ed. Michael Eid and Randy J. Larsen. New York: Guilford.

Veenhoven, Ruut. 2014. Notions of the Good Life. In *The Oxford Handbook of Happiness*, v, ed. Susan A. David, Ilona Boniwell and Amanda Conley Ayers. Oxford, UK: Oxford University Press.

Veenstra, Gerry, Isaac Luginnah, Sarah Wakefield, Stephen Birth, John Eyles, and Susan Elliott. 2005. Why You Know, Where You Live: Social Capital, Neighbourhood and Health. *Social Science & Medicine* 60: 2799–2818.

Venkatesh, Alladi. 1999. Postmodernism Perspectives for Macromarketing: An Inquiry into the Global Information and Sign Economy. *Journal of Macromarketing* 19 (2): 153–169.

Vera-Toscano, Esperanza, Victoria Ateca-Amestoy, and Rafael Serrano-Del-Rosal. 2006. Building Financial Satisfaction. *Social Indicators Research* 77: 211–243.

Verba, Sidney, Kay Lehman Schlozman, and Henry E. Brady. 1995. *Voice and Equality: Civic Voluntarism in American Politics*. Cambridge, MA: Harvard.

Verkuyten, Maykel, and Borja Martinovic. 2015. Majority Member¡¯s Recognition and Protest against Discrimination of Immigrants: The Role of Power Threat, Deprovincialization and Common National Identity. *Social Justice Research* 28 (3): 257–273.

Vernby, Kare, and Henning Finseraas. 2010. Xenophobia and Left Voting. *Politics & Society* 38 (4): 490–516.

Verschuur, Margot J., Marija Maric, and Philip Spinhoven. 2010. Differences in Changes in Health–Related Anxiety Between Western and Non–Western Participants in a Trauma?Focused Study. *Journal of Traumatic Stress* 23 (2): 300–303.

Vesalon, Lucian, and Remus Cretan. 2015. We Are Not the Wild West: Anti-Fracking Protests in Romania. *Environmental Politics* 24 (2): 288–307.

Vestergaard, Anne. 2013. Humanitarian Appeal and the Paradox of Power. *Critical Discourse Studies* 10 (4): 444–467.

Vestergren, Sara, John Drury, and Eva Hammar Chiriac. 2017. The Biographical Consequences of Protest and Activism: A Systematic Review and a New Typology. *Social Movement Studies* 16 (2): 203–221.

Veugelers, John W.P.. 2000. Right-wing Extremism in Contemporary France: A Silent Counterrevolution? *Sociological Quarterly* 41 (1): 19–40.

Viewiebe, Roland, and Bernd Wegener. 2000. Social Inequality and the Perceived Income Justice Gap. *Social Justice Research* 13 (2): 123–149.

Villarreal, Andres, and Braulio F. A. Silva. 2006. Social Cohesion, Criminal Victimization and Perceived Risk Crime in Brazilian Neighborhoods. *Social Forces* 84 (3): 1725–1753.

Vincens, Natalia, Maria Emmelin, and Martin Stafström. 2018. Social Capital, Income Inequality and the Social Gradient in Self-Rated Health in Latin America: A Fixed Effects Analysis. *Social Science & Medicine* 196: 115–122.
Viola, Thiago Wendt, Giovanni Abrahio Salum, Bruno Kluwe-Schiavon, Breno Sanvicente-Vieira, Mateus Luz Levandowski, and Rodrigo Grassi-Oliveir. 2016. The Influence of Geographical and Economic Factors in Estimates of Childhood Abuse and Neglect Using the Childhood Trauma Questionnaire: A Worldwide Meta-Regression Analysis. *Child Abuse & Neglect* 51: 1–11.
Visher, Glenn S. 1997. *Human Values: From the Greeks to Modern Times*. Commack, NY: Nova.
Visser, Miranda, Melinda Mills, Liesbet Heyse, Rafael Wittek, and Vincenzo Bollettino. 2016. Work?Life Balance among Humanitarian Aid Workers. *Nonprofit & Voluntary Sector Quarterly* 45 (6): 1191–1213.
Vitak, Jessica. 2017. A Digital Path to Happiness? Applying Communication Privacy Management Theory to Mediated Interactions. In *The Routledge Handbook of Media Use and Well-being: International Perspectives on Theory and Research on Positive Media Effects*, 274–287, ed. Leonard Reinecke and Mary Beth Oliver. New York, NY: Routledge.
Vitoroulis, Irene, and Katholiki Georgiades. 2017. Bullying among Immigrant and Non-Immigrant Early Adolescents: School- and Student-Level Effects. *Journal of Adolescence* 61: 141–151.
Volker, Beate, and Henk Flap. 2007. Sixteen Million Neighbors: A Multilevel Study of the Role of Neighbors in the Personal Networks of the Dutch. *Urban Affairs Review* 43 (2): 256–284.
Volker, Beate, Henk Flap, and Siegwart Lindenberg. 2007. When Are Neighborhoods Communities? Community in Dutch Neighborhoods. *European Sociological Review* 23 (1): 99–114.
Von Krogh, Georg, and Martin W. Wallin. 2011. The Firm, Human Capital and Knowledge Creation. In *The Oxford Handbook of Human Capital*, 261–286, ed. Alan Burton-Jones and J.C. Spender. Oxford, UK: Oxford University Press.
von Stuckrad, Kocku. 2013. Secular Religion: A Discourse-Historical Approach to Religion in Contemporary Western Europe. *Journal of Contemporary Religion* 28 (1): 1–14.
Vuori, Miika Vuori. 2015. Revisiting Local Responses to Mass Violence. *Journal of Risk Research* 19 (4): 515–532.
Wacquant, Loic. 2008. *Urban Outcasts: A Comparative Sociology of Advanced Marginality*. Cambridge, UK: Polity.
Wadsworth, Tim. 2014. Sex and the Pursuit of Happiness: How Other People¡¯s Sex Lives and Related to Our Sense of Well-being. *Social Indicators Research* 116: 115–135.
Wager, Nadia M. 2012. Respondents' Experiences of Completing a Retrospective Web-Based, Sexual Trauma Survey: Does a History of Sexual Victimization Equate with Risk for Harm? *Violence & Victims* 27 (6): 991–1004.
Wagner, Jenny, and Frieder R. Lang. 2011. Principles of Interpersonal Competence and Motivational Distinguishing Reciprocity and Affect in Social Contexts of Leanring. In *The Oxford Handbook of Reciprocal Adult Development Learning*, 155–170, ed. Carol Hoare, New York: Oxford University Press.
Wahlstrom, Mattias. 2011. Taking Control or Losing Control? Activist Narratives of Provocation and Collective Violence. *Social Movement Studies* 10 (4): 367–385.
Waiton, Stuart. 2008. *The Politics of Antisocial Behaviour: Amoral Panics*. New York: Routledge.
Walder, Andrew G. 2002. Markets and Income Inequality in Rural China: Political Advantage in an Expanding Economy. *American Sociological Review* 67 (2): 231–253.
Walder, Andrew G., and Xiasbin He. 2014. Public Housing with Private Assets: Wealth Creation in Urban China. *Social Science Research* 46: 85–99.
Walen, Heather R., and Margie E. Lachman. 2016. Social Support and Strain from Partner, Family, and Friends: Costs and Benefits for Men and Women in Adulthood. *Journal of Social & Personal Relationships* 17 (1): 5–30.
Walker, Alan. 2005. Towards an International Political Economy of Ageing. *Ageing & Society* 25: 815–839.
Walker, Gordon J., Jinyang Deng, and Rodney B. Bleser. 2001. Ethnicity, Acculturation, Self-construal, and Motivations of Outdoor Recreation. *Leisure Sciences* 23: 263–283.

Walker, Robert, Mark Tomlinson, and Glenn Williams. 2010. The Problem with Poverty: Definition, Measurement and Interpretation. In *The SAGE Handbook of Measurement*, 353–376, ed. Geoffrey Walford, Eric Tucker, and Madhu Viswanathan. London, UK: SAGE.

Walkerdine, Valerie, and Peter Bansel. 2010. Neoliberalism, Work and Subjectivity: Towards a More Complex Account. In *The SAGE Handbook of Identities*, 492–507, ed. Margaret Wetherell and Chandra Talpade Mohanty. London, UK: SAGE,

Wallace, Claire, and Florian Pichler. 2009. More Participation, Happier Society? A Comparative Study of Civil Society and the Quality of Life. *Social Indicators Research* 93: 255–274.

Wallace, Patricia. 2016. *The Psychology of the Internet*. New York: Cambridge.

Walter-Ginzburg, Adrian, Dov Shmotkin, Tzvia Blumstein, and Aviva Shorek. 2005. A Gender-based Dynamic Multidimensional Longitudinal Analysis of Resilience and Mortality in the Old-old in Israel: The Cross-sectional and Longitudinal Aging Study (CALAS). *Social Science & Medicine* 60: 1705–1715.

Walters, Glenn D. 2020. Perceived Peer Delinquency, Proactive Criminal Thinking, Neighborhood Disorder, and Serious Offending: Moderated Mediation and Theoretical Integration. *Journal of Crime & Justice* 43 (4): 467–485.

Walters, William. 2012. *Governmentality: Critical Encounters*. Abington, UK: Routledge.

Walton-Moss, Benita J., Jennifer Manganello, Victoria Frye, and Jacquelyn C. Campbell. 2005. Risk Factors for Intimate Partner Violence and Associated Injury among Urban Women. *Journal of Community Health* 30 (5): 377–389.

Wan, Po-san. 1992. Subjective Quality of Life. In *Indicators of Social Development: Hong Kong 1990*, 173–201, ed. Siu-kai Lau, Ming-kwan Lee, Po-san Wan, and Siu-lun Wong. Hong Kong: Hong Kong Institute of Asia-Pacific Studies.

Wang, Chin-Sheng., and Wen-Bin. Chiou. 2006. Psychological Motives and Online Game Addiction: A Test of Flow Theory and Humanistic Needs Theory for Taiwanese Adolescents. *CyberPsychology & Behavior* 9 (3): 317–324.

Wang, Dan J., and Sarah A. Soule. 2016. Tactical Innovation in Social Movements: The Effects of Peripheral and Multi-Issue Protest. *American Sociological Review*. 81 (3): 517–548.

Wang, Hui, Juer Tong, Su. Fubing, Guoxue Wei, and Ran Tao. 2011. To Reallocate or Not: Reconsidering the Dilemma in China¡¯s Agricultural Land Tenure Policy. *Land Use Policy* 28: 805–814.

Wang, Kate Yeong-Tsyr., Chack-kie Wong, and Kwong-leung Tang. 2013. Citizens' Attitudes towards Economic Insecurity and Government after the 2007 Financial Tsunami: A Hong Kong and Taiwan Comparison. *International Journal of Social Welfare* 22: 152–163.

Wang, Lili, and Elizabeth Graddy. 2008. Social Capital, Volunteering, and Charitable Giving. *VOLUNTAS: International Journal of Voluntary and Nonprofit Organizations* 19: 23–42.

Wang, Ning. 2012. *The Rise of the Consumer in Modern China*. Reading, UK: Paths International.

Wang, Peigang, and Tyler J. VanderWeele. 2011. Empirical Research on Factors Related to the Subjective Well-being of Chinese Urban Residents. *Social Indicators Research* 101: 447–459.

Wang, Xiao. 2013. Negotiating Safer Sex: A Detailed Analysis of Attitude Functions, Anticipated Emotions, Relationship Status and Gender. *Psychology & Health* 28 (7): 800–817.

Wang, Yanlai, Nicholas Rees, and Bernadette Andreosso-O'Callaghan. 2004. Economic Change and Political Development in China: Findings from a Public Opinion Survey. *Journal of Contemporary China* 13 (39): 203-222.

Wang, Ying, Shaojing Sun, and Yiping Song. 2010. Motivation for Luxury Consumption: Evidence from a Metropolitan City in China. *Research in Consumer Behavior* 12: 161–181.

Wansink, Brian, and Robert van Itterum. 2012. Fast Food Restaurant Lighting and Music Can Reduce Calorie Intake and Increase Satisfaction. *Psychology Reports* 111 (1): 228–232.

Warren, Mark E. 2011. Democracy. In *The Oxford Handbook of the History of Political Philosophy*, 517–529, ed. George Klosko. Oxford, UK: Oxford University Press.

Waterman, Alan S. 2008. Reconsidering Happiness: A Eudaimonist's Perspective. *Journal of Positive Psychology* 3 (4): 234–252.

Waterman, Alan S. 2013. The Humanistic Psychology-Positive Psychology Divide: Contrasts in Philosophical Foundations. *American Psychologist* 68 (3): 124–133.

Waterman, Alan S., Seth J. Schwartz, Edie Goldbacher, Hope Green, Christine Miller, and Susheel Philip. 2003. Predicting the Subjective Experience of Intrinsic Motivation: The Role of Self-determination, the Balance of Challenges and Skills and Self-realization Values. *Personality & Social Psychology Bulletin* 29 (11): 1447–1458.

Watkins, Philip C. 2016. *Positive Psychology*. New York, NY: Springer.

Watt, Margo C., and Sherry H. Stewart. 2003. Dyscontrol Experiences Questionnaire: Development, Reliability and Validity. *Journal of Psychopathology & Behavioral Assessment* 25 (3): 155–165.

Watts, Duncan J. 2014. Common Sense and Sociological Explanations. *American Journal of Sociology* 120 (2): 313–351.

Waugh, Christian. 2014. The Regulatory Power of Positive Emotions in Stress; A Temporal-functional Approach. In *The Resilience Handbook: Approaches to Stress and Trauma*, 73–85, ed. Martha Kent, Mary C. Davis and John W. Reich. New York: NY: Routledge.

Weakliem, David L., and Casey Borch. 2006. Alienation in the United States: Uniform or Group-specific Change? *Sociological Forum* 21 (3): 415–438.

Webber, Martin P., and Peter J. Huxley. 2007. Measuring Access to Social Capital: The Validity and Reliability of the Resource Generator-UK and Its Association with Common Mental Disorder. *Social Science & Medicine* 65: 481–492.

Weber, Peter C. 2021. Cross-Partisanship and the Vulnerability Democracy: How Civility and Nonpartisanship Undermined Civil Society in Interwar Germany. *Journal of Civil Society* 17 (2): 179–198.

Webley, Paul, and Ellen K. Nyhus. 2006. Parents' Influence on Children's Future Orientation and Saving. *Journal of Economic Psychology* 27: 140–164.

Webster, Jeffrey Dean, Ernst T. Bohlmeijer, and Gerben J. Westerhof. 2014. Time to Flourish: The Relationship of Temporal Perspective to Well-Being and Wisdom across Adulthood. *Aging & Mental Health* 18 (8): 1046–1056.

Weeber, Stan C., and Daniel G. Rodenheaver. 2003. Militias at the Millennium: A Test of Smelser's Theory of Collective Behavior. *Sociological Quarterly* 44 (2): 181–204.

Wei, Ran. 2007. Effects of Playing Violent Videogames on Chinese Adolescents' Pro-violence Attitudes, Attitudes toward Others, and Aggressive Behavior. *CyberPsychology & Behavior* 10 (3): 371–379.

Wei, Wei. 2017. Good Gay Buddies for Lifetime: Homosexually Themed Discourse and the Construction of Heteromasculinity among Chinese Urban Youth. *Journal of Homosexuality* 64 (12): 1667–1683.

Weimann, Gabriel, and Hans-Bernd. Brosius. 1994. Is There a Two-Step Flow of Agenda-Setting? *International Journal of Public Opinion* 6 (4): 323–341.

Weinberg, Michael, Sharon Gil, Avi Besser, and Jasmin Bass. 2021. Personality Traits and Trauma Exposure: The Relationship between Personality Traits, Ptsd Symptoms, Stress, and Negative Affect Following Exposure to Traumatic Cues. *Personality & Individual Differences* 177: 110802.

Weinschenk, Aaron C. and Christopher T. Dawes. 2022. Civic Education in High School and Voter Turnout in Adulthood. *British Journal of Political Science*.

Weinstein, Netta, and Richard M. Ryan. 2010. When Helping Helps: Autonomous Motivation for Prosocial Behavior and Its Influence on Well-being for the Helper and Recipient. *Journal of Personality & Social Psychology* 98 (2): 222–244.

Weisberg, Herbert F. 2005. The Structure and Effects of Moral Predispositions in Contemporary American Politics. *Journal of Politics* 67 (3): 646–668.

Wellman, Barry. 1990. The Place of Kinfolk in Personal Community Network. *Marriage & Family Review* 15 (1/2): 195–228.

Wells, Thomas, Gary D. Sandfur, and Dennis P. Hogan. 2003. What Happens after the High School Years among Young Persons with Disabilities? *Social Forces* 82 (2): 803–832.

Welsch, Heinz. 2002. Preferences over Prosperity and Pollution: Environmental Valuation Based on Happiness Surveys. *Kyklos* 55 (4): 473–494.

Welzel, Christian, and Ronald Inglehart. 2010. Agency, Values, and Well-being: A Human Development Model. *Social Indicators Research* 97: 43–63.

Welzel, Christian. 2013. *Freedom Rising: Human Empowerment and the Quest for Emanicpaiton.* New York: Cambridge University Press.

Wen, Ming, Jessie Fan, Lei Jin, and Guixin Wang. 2010. Neighborhood Effects on Health among Migrants and Natives in Shanghai, China. *Health & Place* 16 (3): 452–460.

Wenz, Peter S. 2009. *Beyond Red and Blue: How Twelve Political Philosophies Shape American Debates.* Cambridge, MA: MIT Press.

Wenzel, Michael. 2000. Justice and Identity: The Significance of Inclusion for Perceptions of Entitlement and the Justice Motive. *Personality & Social Psychology Bulletin* 26 (2): 157–176.

Werbner, Pnina. 2010. Religious Identity. In *The SAGE Handbook of Identities*, 233–257, 45–62, ed. Margaret Wetherell and Chandra Talpade Mohanty. London, UK: SAGE,

Wernet, Christine A., Cheryl Elman, and Brian F. Pendleton. 2005. The Postmodern Individual: Structural Determinants of Attitudes. *Comparative Sociology* 4 (3–4): 339–364.

Western, Mark. 1999. Who Thinks What about Capitalism? Class Consciousness and Attitudes to Economic Institutions. *Journal of Sociology* 35 (3): 351–370.

Wetterbeng, Anna. 2007. Crisis, Connection, and Class: How Social Ties Affect Household Welfare. *World Development* 35 (4): 585–606.

Wheatley, Daniel, and Sarah L. Buglass. 2019. Social Network Engagement and Subjective Well-Being: A Life-Course Perspective. *British Journal of Sociology* 70 (5): 1971–1995.

Whelan, Christopher T., and Bertrand Maitre. 2010. Identifying Economically Vulnerable Groups as the Economic Crisis Emerged. *Economic & Social Review* 41 (4): 501–525.

Whelan, Christopher T., and Bertrand Maitre. 2013. Material Deprivation, Economic Stress, and Reference Groups in Europe: An Analysis of EU-SILC 2009. *European Sociological Review* 29 (6): 1162–1174.

Whelan, Christopher T., Helen Russell, and Bertrand Maitre. 2016. Economic Stress and the Great Recession in Ireland: Polarization, Individualization or Middle Class Squeeze? *Social Indicators Research* 126 (2): 503–526.

Whigham, Stuart. 2019. Nationalism, Party Political Discourse and Scottish Independence: Comparing Discursive Visions of Scotland's Constitutional Status. *Nations & Nationalism* 25 (4): 1212–1237.

White, Diana L., Alexis J. Walker, and Leslie N. Richards. 2008. Intergenerational Family Support Following Infant Death. *International Journal of Aging & Human Development* 67 (3): 187–208.

White, James M., David M. Klein, and Todd F. Martin. 2015. *Family Theories: An Introduction.* Thousand Oaks, CA: SAGE.

White, Mathew A. 2014. Positive Education at Geelong Grammar School. In *The Oxford Handbook of Happiness*, 657–668, ed. Susan A. David, Ilona Boniwell and Amanda Conley Ayers. Oxford, UK: Oxford University Press.

White, Melanie. 2006. An Ambivalent Civility. *Canadian Journal of Sociology* 31 (4): 445–460.

Whitham, Monica M. 2012. Community Connections: Social Capital and Community Success. *Sociological Forum* 27 (2): 441–457.

Whiting, Sophie A. 2012. The Discourse of Defence: Dissident Irish Republican Newspapers and the Propaganda War. *Terrorism & Political Violence* 24 (3): 483–503.

Whitton, Joy. 2018. *Fostering Imagination in Higher Education: Disciplinary and Professional Practices.* Abingdon, UK: Routledge.

Whynes, David K., and Tracey H. Sach. 2007. WTP and WTA: Do People Think Differently? *Social Science & Medicine* 65: 947–957.

Whyte, Martin King, and Maocan Gao. 2009. How Angry Are Chinese Citizens about Current Inequalities? Evidence from a National Survey. *Social Transformations in Chinese Societies* 5: 17–54.

Wiepking, Pamala, and Ineke Maas. 2009. Resources That Make You Generous: Effects of Social and Human Resources on Charitable Giving. *Social Forces* 87 (4): 1973–1995.

Wiest, Amber L., David L. Andrews, and Michael D. Giardina. 2015. Training the Body for Healthism: Reifying Vitality in and through the Clinical Gaze of the Neoliberal Fitness Club. *Review of Education/Pedagogy/Cultural Studies* 37 (1): 21–40.

Wiklund, Hans. 2005. A Habermasian Analysis of the Deliberative Democratic Potential of ICT-enabled Services in Swedish Municipalities. *New Media & Society* 7 (5): 701–723.

Wilder, Jesse Bryant. 2007. *Art History for Dummies*. Hobokin, NJ: Wiley.

Wilking, Jennifer R., and Guang Zhang. 2013. Accepting the Bargain? An Experimental Study of Political Rights, Economic Development and Support for Government in Rural China. *Journal of Chinese Political Science: Official Journal of the Association of Chinese Political Studies* 18 (3): 241–257.

Wilkinson, Richard G., and Kate E. Pickett. 2017. The Enemy between Us: The Psychological and Social Costs of Inequality. *European Journal of Social Psychology* 47 (1): 11–24.

Wilkinson, Steven I. 2009. Riots. *Annual Review of Political Science* 12: 329–343.

Williams, Kipling D., Christopher K. T. Cheung, and Wilma Choi. 2000. Cyberostracism: Effects of Being Ignored over the Internet. *Journal of Personality & Social Psychology* 79 (5): 748–762.

Williamson, John B., and Ulrike Bochmer. 1997. Female Life Expectancy, Gender Stratification, Health Status, and Level of Economic Development: A Cross-national Study of Less Developed Countries. *Social Science & Health* 45 (2): 305–317.

Williamson, K.M. 2002. Civility Proxies and Social Tolerance in American Marketplaces. *Sociological Inquiry* 72 (3): 486–499.

Willmann, Elke, Kimberly Feldt, and Manfred Amelang. 1997. Prototypical Behavior Patterns of Social Intelligence: An Intercultural Comparison between Chinese and German Subjects. *International Journal of Psychology* 32 (5): 329–346.

Wilson, Franklin D., and Roger B. Hammer. 2001. Ethnic Residential Segregation and Its Consequences. In *Urban Inequality: Evidence from Four Cities*, 272–303, ed. Alice O'Connor, Chris Tilly and Lawrence D. Bobo. New York: Russell Sage.

Wilson, George. 2001. Support for Redistributive Policies among the African American Middle Class: Race and Class Effects. *Research in Social Stratification & Mobility* 18: 97–115.

Wilson, John, and Marc A. Musick. 1997. Work and Volunteering: The Long Arm of the Job. *Social Forces* 76 (1): 251–272.

Wilson, Melvin N., Deanna Y. Cooke, and Edith G. Arrington. 1997. African-American Adolescents and Academic Achievement: Family and Peer Influences. In *Social and Emotional Adjustment and Family Relations in Ethnic Minority Families*, 145–155, ed. Ronald D. Taylor and Margaret C. Wang. Mahwah, NJ: Lawrence Erlbaum.

Wilson, Shaun, Gabrielle Meagher, and Kersti Hermes. 2012. The Social Division of Welfare Knowledge: Policy Stratification and Perceptions of Welfare Reform in Australia. *Policy & Politics* 40 (3): 323–346.

Wink, Paul, and Michele Dillon. 2003. Religiousness, Spirituality and Psychological Functioning in Late Adulthood: Findings from a Longitudinal Study. *Psychology & Aging* 18 (4): 916–924.

Winkelmann, Liliana, and Rainer Winkelmann. 2010. Does Inequality Harm the Middle Class? *Kyklos* 63 (2): 301–316.

Winterdyk, John, and Nikki Thompson. 2008. Student and Non-Student Perceptions and Awareness of Identity Theft. *Canadian Journal of Criminology & Criminal Justice* 50 (2): 153–186.

Wittebrood, Karin, and Paul Nieuwbeerta. 2000. Criminal Victimization during One's Life Course: The Effects of Previous Victimization and Patterns of Routine Activities. *Journal of Research in Crime & Delinquency* 37 (1): 91–122.

Wituk, Scott, Matthew D. Shepherd, Susan Slavich, Mary L. Warren, and Greg Meissen. 2000. A Topography of Self-help Groups: An Empirical analysis. *Social Work* 45 (2): 157–165.

Wnuk-Lipinski. 2007. Civil Society and Democratization. In *The Oxford Handbook of Political Behavior*, 675–692, ed. Russell J. Dalton and Hans-Dieter Klingemann. New York: Oxford University Press.

Wo, James C. 2018. Understanding the Density of Nonprofit Organizations across Los Angeles Neighborhoods: Does Concentrated Disadvantage and Violent Crime Matter? *Social Science Research* 71: 56–71.

Wodtke, Geoffrey T. 2012. The Impact of Education on Intergroup Attitudes. *Social Psychology Quarterly* 75 (1): 80–106.

Wojcieszak, Magdalena E., and Diana C. Mutz. 2009. Online Groups and Political Discourse: Do Online Discussion Spaces Facilitate Exposure to Political Disagreement? *Journal of Communication* 59: 40–56.

Woldoff, Rachael A., and Seth Ovadia. 2009. Not Getting Their Money's Worth: African-American Disadvantages in Converting Income, Wealth, and Education into Residential Quality. *Urban Affairs Review* 45 (1): 66–91.

Wolfe, Scott E., Justin Nix, Robert Kaminski, and Jeff Rojek. 2016. Is the Effect of Procedural Justice on Police Legitimacy Invariant? Testing the Generality of Procedural Justice and Competing Antecedents of Legitimacy. *Journal of Quantitative Criminology* 32 (2): 253–282.

Wolff, Richard D., and Stephen A. Resnick. 2012. *Contending Economic Theories: Neoclassical, Keynesian, and Marxian*. Cambridge, MA: MIT.

Wollschleger, Jason. 2012. Interaction Ritual Chains and Religious Participation. *Sociological Forum* 27 (4): 896–912.

Wong, Chack-kie, and Angela Wai-yan Shik. 2011. Renewed Conception of Harmonious Society, Governance, and Citizenship: Evidence for the Study of Chinese Perceptions in Hong Kong. *Asian Social Work & Policy Review* 5: 1–19.

Wong, Chack-kie, Ka.-ying Wong, and Bong-ho Mok. 2005a. Emotions, Self-interest and Support for Social Welfare in Chinese Society with Reference to a Dutch Study on Welfare Legitimacy. *International Journal of Social Welfare* 15 (4): 302–313.

Wong, Kevin Tze-wai, Victor Zheng, and Po.-san Wan. 2016. The Impact of Cross-border Integration with Mainland China on Hong Kong's Local Politics: The Individual Visit Scheme as a Double-edged Sword for Political Trust in Hong Kong. *China Quarterly* 228: 1081–1104.

Wong, Tai-Chee., Mun-Ching. Yeow, and Xuan Zhu. 2005b. Building a Global City: Negotiating the Massive Influx of Floating Population in Shanghai. *Journal of Housing & the Built Environment* 20: 21–50.

Wong, Timothy Ka-ying, and Po.-san Wan. 2011. Perceptions and Determinants of Environmental Concern: The Case of Hong Kong and Its Implications for Sustainable Development. *Sustainable Development* 19: 235–249.

Wong, Timothy Ka-ying, Po.-san Wan, and Kenneth Wing-kin Law. 2010. The Public's Changing Perception of the Condition of Social Welfare in Hong Kong: Lessons from Social Development. *Social Policy & Administration* 44 (5): 620–640.

Wong, Yu Cheung, Chi Kwong Law, and John Wat Chu. 2010. Digital Divide and Social Inclusion: Policy Challenge for Social Development in Hong Kong and South Korea. *Journal of Asian Public Policy* 3 (1): 37–52.

Wood, Donald N. 2003. *The Unraveling of the West: The Rise of Postmodernism and the Decline of Democracy*. Westport, CT: Praeger.

Wood, Helen. 2010. From Media and Identity to Mediated Identity. In *The SAGE Handbook of Identities*, 258–276, ed. Margaret Wetherell and Chandra Talpade Mohanty. London, UK: SAGE.

Wood, Joanne V., and Karen VanderZee. 1997. Social Comparison among Cancer Patients: Under What Conditions Are Comparisons Upward and Downward? In *Health, Coping, and Well-being: Perspectives from Social Comparison Theory*, 299–328, ed. Bram P. Buunk and Fredercik X. Gibbons. Mahwah, NJ: Lawrence Erlbaum.

Woodrum, Eric. 1992. Pornography and Moral Attitudes. *Sociological Spectrum* 12: 329–347.

Woodrum, Eric. 1997. Religious Effect on Environmentalism. *Sociological Spectrum* 17: 221–234.

Woolcock, Michael. 1998. Social Capital and Economic Development: Toward a Theoretical Synthesis and Policy Framework. *Theory & Society* 27: 151–208.

Wright, Emily M., Gillian M. Pinchevsky, Michael L. Benson, and Dana L. Radatz. 2015. Intimate Partner Violence and Subsequent Depression: Examining the Roles of Neighborhood Supportive Mechanisms. *American Journal of Community Psychology* 56 (3): 342–356.

Wright, Stephen C. 2010. Collective Action and Social Change. In *The SAGE Handbook of Prejudice, Stereotyping and Discrimination*, 577–595, ed. John F. Dovidio, Miles Hewstone, Peter Glick and Victoria M. Esses. London, UK: SAGE.

Wu, Homer C., Abby Liu, and Chih-Hung. Wang. 2010. Taiwanese University Students' Perceived Freedom and Participation in Leisure. *Annals of Leisure Research* 13 (4): 679–700.

Wu, Zheng, and Lindy MacNeill. 2003. Education, Work, and Childbearing after Age 30. *Journal of Comparative Family Studies* 191–212.

Wulff, Stephen, Mary Bernstein, and Verta Taylor. 2015. New Theoretical Directions from the Study of Gender and Sexually Movements: Collective Identity, Multi-institutional Politics, and Emotions. In *Oxford Handbook of Social Movements*, 108–130, ed. Donatella della Porta and Mario Diani. Oxford, UK: Oxford University Press.

Wuthnow, Joel. 2006. The Integration of Cooptation and Coercion: China's Taiwan Strategy since 2001. *East Asia* 23 (3): 22–45.

Wuthnow, Robert J. 2011. Taking Talk Seriously: Religious Discourse as Social Practice. *Journal for the Scientific Study of Religion* 50 (1): 1–21.

Wuthnow, Robert. 1992. How Religious Groups Promote Forgiving: A National Study. *Journal for the Scientific Study of Religion* 125–139.

Wuthnow, Robert. 2002. The United States: Bridging the Privileged and the Marginalized? In *Democracies in Flux: The Evolution of Social Capital in Contemporary Society*, 59–102, ed. Robert Putnam. New York: Oxford University Press.

Wuthnow, Robert. 2004. *Saving America? Faith-Based Services and the Future of Civil Society*. Princeton, NJ: Princeton University Press.

Xanthopoulou, Despoina, Arnold B. Bakker, Evangelia Demerouti, and Wilmar B. Schaufeli. 2009. Reciprocal Relationships between Job Resources, Personal Resources, and Work Engagement. *Journal of Vocational Behavior* 74: 235–244.

Xiao, Hong. 2000. Structure of Child-rearing Values in Urban China. *Sociological Perspectives* 43 (3): 457–471.

Xu, Qingwen, Douglas D. Perkins, and Julan Chun-Chung. Chow. 2010. Sense of Community, Neighboring, and Social Capital as Prediction of Local Political Participation in China. *American Journal of Community Psychology* 45: 259–271.

Xu, Xiaohe, and Shu-chuan Lai. 2002. Resources, Gender Ideologies, and Marital Power: The Case of Taiwan. *Journal of Family Issues* 23 (2): 209–245.

Yack, Bernard. 2012. *Nationalism and the Moral Psychology of Community*. Chicago, IL: University of University Press.

Yagci, Alper H. 2017. The Great Recession, Inequality and Occupy Protests around the World. *Government & Opposition* 52 (4): 640–670.

Yahne, Carolina E., and William R. Miller. 1999. Evoking Hope. In *Integrating Spirituality into Treatment: Resources for Practitioners*, 217–233, ed. William R. Miller. Washington, DC: American Psychological Association.

Yair, Gad. 2003. Decisive Movements and Key Experiences: Expanding Paradigmatic Boundaries in the Study of School Effects. In *The International Assessment of New Research and Theory*, 124–142, ed. Carlos Alberto Torres and Ari Antikainen. Lanham, MD: Rowman.

Yamaoka, Kazue. 2008. Social Capital and Health and Well-being in East Asia: A Population-based Study. *Social Science & Medicine* 66: 885–899.

Yan, Gang. 1995. *Inner Saint and Outer Ruler: Confucian Life Philosophy*. Chengdu, China: Sichuan People.

Yanagisawa, Anton. 2011. Poverty: Social Control over Our Labor Force. *International Journal of Social Economics* 38 (4): 316–329.

Yanez, Betina, Donald Edmondson, Annette L. Stanton, Crystal L. Park, Lorna Kwan, and Patricia A. Granz. 2009. Facets of Spirituality as Predictors of Adjustment to Cancer: Relative Contributors of Having Facts and Findings Meaning. *Journal of Consulting & Clinical Psychology* 77 (4): 730–741.

Yang, Ming-Ching., Jen-Son. Cheng, and Yu. Shu-Wen. 2012. Leisure Lifestyle and Health-Related Quality of Life of Taiwanese Adults. *Social Behavior & Personality* 40 (2): 301–317.

Yang, Philip, and Nadine Barrett. 2006. Understanding Public Attitudes towards Social Security. *International Journal of Social Welfare* 15: 95–109.

Yang, Qing, and Wenfang Tang. 2010. Exploring the Sources of Institutional Trust in China: Culture, Mobilization, or Performance? *Asian Politics & Policy* 2 (3): 415–436.

Yang, Wen-Shan., and Pei-Chin. Yen. 2012. A Comparative Study of Marital Dissolution in East Asian Societies: Gender Attitudes and Social Expectations towards Marriage in Taiwan, Korea and Japan. *Asian Journal of Social Science* 39: 751–755.

Yankow, Jeffrey J. 2006. Why Do Cities Pay More? An Empirical Examination of Some Competing Theories of the Urban Wage Premium. *Journal of Urban Economics* 60: 139–161.

Yates, Adam, Ye. Luo, Catherine Mobley, and Erin Shealy. 2015. Changes in Public and Private Environmentally Responsible Behaviors by Gender: Findings from the 1994 and 2010 General Social Survey. *Sociological Inquiry* 85 (4): 503–531.

Yee, Nick. 2006. Motivations for Play in Online Games. *CyberPsychology & Behavior* 9 (6): 772–775.

Yeganeh, Hamid. 2017. Cultural Modernization and Work-Related Values and Attitudes. *International Journal of Development Issues* 16 (2): 130–146.

Yeh, Kuang-Hui., and Yung-Jui. Yang. 2006. Construct Validation of Individuating and Relating Autonomy Orientations in Culturally Chinese Adolescents. *Asian Journal of Social Psychology* 9 (2): 148–160.

Yetim, Nalan, and Ünsal. Yetim. 2014. Sense of Community and Individual Well-Being: A Research on Fulfillment of Needs and Social Capital in the Turkish Community. *Social Indicators Research* 115 (1): 93–115.

Yeung, Irs, S.H. Kong, and Janet Lee. 2000. Attitudes towards Organ Donation in Hong Kong. *Social Service & Medicine* 50: 1643–1654.

Yeung, W. Jean., Miriam R. Linver, and Jeanne Brooks-Gunn. 2002. How Money Matters for Young Children's Development: Parental Investment and Family Processes. *Child Development* 73 (6): 1861–1879.

Yienprugsawan, V., S. Seubsman, S. Kohamman, L.L.-Y. Lim, A.C. Sleigh, and the Thai Cohort Study Team. 2010. Personal Wellbeing Index in a National Cohort of 87134 Thai Adults. *Social Indicators Research* 98: 201–215.

Yip, Ngai Ming, Ray Forrest, and Adrienne La Grange. 2007. Cohort, Trajectories in Hong Kong's Housing System: 1981–2001. *Housing Studies* 22 (1): 121–136.

Yngfalk, Carl. 2016. Bio-Politicizing Consumption: Neo-Liberal Consumerism and Disembodiment in the Food Marketplace. *Consumption, Markets & Culture* 19 (3): 275–295.

Yogeeswaran, Kumar, and Nilanjana Dasgupta. 2014. Conceptions of National Identity In A Globalised World: Antecedents And Consequences. *European Review of Social Psychology* 25 (1): 189–227.

Yoo, Ji Hye, and Eui Jun Jeong. 2017. Psychosocial Effects of SNS Use: A Longitudinal Study Focused on the Moderation Effect of Social Capital. *Computers in Human Behavior* 69: 108–119.

Yoon, Jeongkoo. 2001. The Role of Structure and Motivation for Workplace Empowerment: The Case of Korean Employees. *Social Psychology Quarterly* 64 (2): 195–206.

Yoos, George E. 2007. *Reframing Rhetoric: A Liberal Politics without Dogma*. New York: Palgrave.

York, Richard, Eugene A. Rosa, and Thomas Dietz. 2003. Footprints on the Earth: The Environmental Consequences of Modernity. *American Sociological Review* 68 (2): 279–300.

Young, Anne F., Annette J. Dobson, and Julie E. Byles. 2001. Determinants of General Practitioner Use among Women in Australia. *Social Science & Medicine* 53: 1641–1651.

Young, Janette, Hazel Maxwell, and Nicole Peel. 2021. Leisure Meets Health: Important Intersections and Alternative Discourses. *Annals of Leisure Research* 24 (3): 275–282.

Young, Michael, and Peter Willmont. 1957. *Family and Kinship*. London: Routledge & Kegan Paul.

Young, Stephanie L., and D'Arcy J. Reynolds. 2017. You Can Be an Agent of Change: The Rhetoric of New Age Self-Help in Enlightened. *Western Journal of Communication* 81 (1): 1–20.

Youngs, Richard. 2019. *Civic Activism Unleashed: New Hope or False Dawn for Democracy*. New York, NY: Oxford University Press.

Younts, C. Wesley., and Charles W. Mueller. 2001. Justice Processes: Specifying the Mediating Role of Perceptions of Distributive Justice. *American Sociological Review* 66 (1): 125–145.

Yu, Wei-hsin, and Chi-Tsun. Chiu. 2016. Growing Pains: Changes in Psychological Well-Being in Urban China. *Social Indicators Research* 129 (3): 1349–1382.

Yuan, Guiyan, Qingxiang Han. 2003. *On the Man's Holistic Development. Nanning*, China: Guanxi People.

Yuchtman-Yaar, Ephraim, and Tamar Hermann. 1998. The Latitude of Acceptance. *Journal of Conflict Resolution* 42 (6): 721–743.

Yuchtman-Yaar, Ephraim, and Yasmin Alkalay. 2007. Religious Zones, Economic Development and Modern Value Orientations: Individual versus Contextual Effects. *Social Science Research* 36: 789–807.

Yuchtman-Yaar, Ephraime. 2002. Value Priorities in Israeli Society: An Examination of Inglehart's Theory of Modernization and Cultural Variation. *Comparative Sociology* 1 (3–4): 347–367.

Yukl, Gary. 2011. Contingency Theories of Effective Leadership. In *The SAGE Handbook of Leadership*, 286–298, ed. Alan Bryman, David Collinson, Keith Grint, Brad Jackson and Mary Uhl-Bien. London: SAGE.

Yzerbyt, Vincent Y. 2010. Motivational Process. In *The SAGE Handbook of Prejudice, Stereotyping and Discrimination*, 146–162, ed. John F. Dovidio, Miles Hewstone, Peter Glick and Victoria M. Esses. London, UK: SAGE.

Zaff, Jonathan F., Kristin A. Moore, Angela Romano Papillo, and Stephanie Williams, Jr. 2003. Implications of Extracurricular Activity Participation during Adolescence on Positive Outcomes. *Journal of Adolescent Research* 18 (6): 599-630.

Zafirovski, Milan. 2010. The Merton Theorem Revisited and Restated: Conservatism and Fascism as Functional Analogues. *American Sociologist* 41: 142–173.

Zagorski, Krzysztof. 2011. Income and Happiness in Time of Post-communist Modernization. *Social Indicators Research* 104: 331–349.

Zalewski, Maureen, Stephanie F. Thompson, and Liliana J. Lengua. 2017. Parenting as a Moderator of the Effects of Maternal Depressive Symptoms on Preadolescent Adjustment. *Journal of Clinical Child & Adolescent Psychology* 46 (4): 563–572.

Zanin, Luca. 2017. Education and Life Satisfaction in Relation to the Probability of Social Trust: A Conceptual Framework and Empirical Analysis. *Social Indicators Research* 132 (2): 925–947.

Zarychta, Alan. 2015. Community Trust and Household Health: A Spatially-Based Approach with Evidence from Rural Honduras. *Social Science & Medicine* 146: 85–94.

Zatepilina-Monacell, Olga. 2012. High Stakes: U.S. Nonprofit Organizations and the U.S. Standing Abroad. *Public Relations Review* 38 (3): 471–476.

Zavala, Egbert, and Xavier Guadalupe-Diaz. 2019. Testing Target Congruence Theory on Emotional Abuse Victimization Experienced by Heterosexual and LGBQ College Students. *Journal of Aggression, Maltreatment & Trauma* 28 (9): 1069–1090.

Zeidner, Moshe, and Gerald Matthews. 2011. *Anxiety 101*. New York: Springer.

Zelditch, Morris, Jr. 2001. Theories of Legitimacy. In *The Psychology of Legitimacy: Emerging Perspectives on Ideology, Justice, and Intergroup Relations*, 33–53, ed. John T. Jost and Brenda Major. Cambridge, UK: Cambridge University Press.

Zhang, Jie, and Junsen Zhang. 2004. How Does Social Security Affect Economic Growth? Evidence from Cross-country Data. *Journal of Population Economics* 17: 473–500.

Zhang, Lening, Steven F. Messner, and Jianhong Liu. 2007a. A Multilevel Analysis of the Risk of Household Burglary in the City of Tianjin, China. *British Journal of Criminology* 47: 918–937.

Zhang, Li-fang, and Robert J. Sternberg. 2012. Cultured and Intellectual Styles. In *Handbook of Intellectual Styles: Preferences in Cognition, Learning, and Thinking*, 131–152. New York: Springer.

Zhang, Tony Huiquan. 2022. Political Freedom, Education, and Value Liberalization and Deliberalization: A Cross-National Analysis of the World Values Survey, 1981–2014. *Social Science Journal*.

Zhang, Wei-Bin. 1999. *Confucianism and Modernization: Industrialization and Democratization of the Confucian Regions*. New York: St. Martin.

Zhang, Yaoqi, Anwar Hussain, Jinyang Deng, and Neil Letson. 2007b. Public Attitudes toward Urban Trees and Supporting Urban Tree Programs. *Environment & Behavior* 39 (6): 797–814.

Zhang, Yingqiang, and Tor Eriksson. 2010. Inequality of Opportunity and Income Inequality in Nine Chinese Provinces, 1989–2006. *China Economic Review* 21 (4): 607–616.

Zhao, Ruohui, and Liqun Cao. 2010. Social Change and Anomie: A Cross-national Study. *Social Forces* 80 (3): 1209–1230.

Zhong, Lena Y. 2010. Bystander Intervention and Fear of Crime: Evidence from Two Chinese Communities. *International Journal of Offender Therapy & Comparative Criminology* 54 (2): 250–263.

Zhou, Xueguang, and Olga Suhomlinova. 2001. Redistribution under State Socialism: A USSR and PRC Comparison. *Research in Social Stratification & Mobility* 18: 163–204.

Zhou, Yunqing. 2000. *Chinese National Affairs Social Development in Twenty-first Century*. Zhengzhou, China: Henan People.

Zhu, Jian-hua. 1996. I Don't Know in Public Opinion Surveys in China: Individual and Contextual Causes of Item Nonresponses. *Journal of Contemporary China* 5 (12): 223–244.

Zhu, Jonathan J.H.., and Zhou He. 2002. Perceived Characteristics, Perceived Needs, and Perceived Popularity: Adoption and Use of the Internet in China. *Communication Research* 29 (4): 460–495.

Zhu, Jonathan Jian-hua, and Huixin Ke. 2001. Political Culture as Social Construction of Reality: A Case Study of Hong Kong's Image in Mainland China. In *Chinese Political Culture, 1989–2000*, 188–215, ed. Shiping Hua. Armonk, NY: Sharpe.

Zhu, Yazong. 1995. *Critical History of Chinese Science and Technology*. Chengsha, China: National Defense, Science, and Technology University.

Zhuang, Meixi. 2020. Rules Consciousness or Rights Consciousness? A Structural Equation Model of the Relationship between Sociopolitical Values and the Protest Potential among Chinese Citizens. *Chinese Journal of Political Science* 25 (3): 457–476.

Ziersch, Anna M., Fran E. Baum, Colin MacDougall, and Christine Putland. 2005. Neighborhood Life and Social Capital: The Implications for Health. *Social Science & Medicine* 60: 71–86.

Zimran, Adiel. 2020. The Theological Value of Autonomy. *International Journal of Constitutional Law* 18 (3): 687–713.

Zitek, Emily M., and Alexander H. Jordan. 2019. Psychological Entitlement Predicts Failure to Follow Instructions. *Social Psychological & Personality Science* 10 (2): 172–180.

Zittoun, Tania, and Alex Gillespie. 2016. *Imagination in Human and Cultural Development*. Hove, UK: Routledge.

Zmerli, Sonja, and Juan Carlos Castillo. 2015. Income Inequality, Distributive Fairness and Political Trust in Latin America. *Social Science Research* 52: 179–192.

Zotti, Roberto, Nino Speziale, and Cristian Barra. 2016. On the Causal Effect of Religiosity on Life Satisfaction Using a Propensity Score Matching Technique. *International Journal of Social Economics* 43 (10): 1031–1048.

Zsido, Andras N., Nikolett Arato, Andras Lang, Beatrix Labadi, Diana Stecina, and Szabolcs A. Bandi. 2021. The Role of Maladaptive Cognitive Emotion Regulation Strategies and Social Anxiety in Problematic Smartphone and Social Media Use. *Personality & Individual Differences* 173: 110647.

Zumbrunnen, John, and Amy Gangl. 2008. Conflict, Fusion, or Coexistence? The Complexity of Contemporary American Conservatism. *Political Behavior* 30 (2): 199–221.

Zurbriggen, Eileen L. 2013. Objectification, Self-Objectification, and Societal Change. *Journal of Social and Political Psychology* 1 (1): 188–215.

Zurcher, Jessica D. 2017. Exploring Descriptive Norms of Parent-Child Communication about Pornography among Parents of Middle-Schoolers in the US. *Journal of Children & Media* 11 (4): 381–398.

Zweifel, Peter, and Friedrich Breyer. 1997. *Health Economics*. New York: Oxford University Press.

The manufacturer's authorised representative in the EU is Springer
Nature Customer Service Centre GmbH, Europaplatz 3, 69115 Heidelberg,
Germany. If you have any concerns regarding our products, please
contact ProductSafety@springernature.com

Printed and bound by CPI Group (UK) Ltd, Croydon, CR0 4YY
30/09/2026
02225237-0016